AF360692

Current Insights on Lipid-Based Nanosystems 2023

Current Insights on Lipid-Based Nanosystems 2023

Editors

Ana Catarina Silva

João Nuno Moreira

José Manuel Sousa Lobo

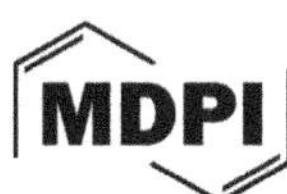

Basel • Beijing • Wuhan • Barcelona • Belgrade • Novi Sad • Cluj • Manchester

Editors

Ana Catarina Silva
Faculty of Health Sciences
University Fernando Pessoa
Porto
Portugal

João Nuno Moreira
Faculty of Pharmacy
University of Coimbra
Coimbra
Portugal

José Manuel Sousa Lobo
Laboratory of Pharmaceutical
Technology
University of Porto
Porto
Portugal

Editorial Office
MDPI
St. Alban-Anlage 66
4052 Basel, Switzerland

This is a reprint of articles from the Special Issue published online in the open access journal *Pharmaceuticals* (ISSN 1424-8247) (available at: www.mdpi.com/journal/pharmaceuticals/special_issues/NLC4Y2M84S).

For citation purposes, cite each article independently as indicated on the article page online and as indicated below:

Lastname, A.A.; Lastname, B.B. Article Title. *Journal Name* **Year**, *Volume Number*, Page Range.

ISBN 978-3-0365-9806-2 (Hbk)
ISBN 978-3-0365-9805-5 (PDF)
doi.org/10.3390/books978-3-0365-9805-5

Contents

About the Editors

Ana Catarina Silva

Associate Professor of Pharmaceutical Technology and Pharmaceutical Biotechnology, Faculty of Health Sciences, University Fernando Pessoa, Porto, Portugal.

Senior Researcher at UCIBIO, REQUIMTE, Faculty of Pharmacy, University of Porto, Portugal. Researcher at FP-I3ID, FP-BHS, University Fernando Pessoa, Porto, Portugal. European PhD in Pharmaceutical Sciences with specialization in Pharmaceutical Technology from University of Porto. Graduation in Pharmaceutical Sciences from University Fernando Pessoa.

Author of several works in the areas of Pharmaceutical Technology and Pharmaceutical Biotechnology (h-index of 25). Included in the World's Top 2% Scientists List in 2021, 2022, and 2023 by Stanford University, USA.

Current research interests are focused on the development of lipid-based nanosystems to improve drug delivery. In particular, nose-to-brain delivery and cutaneous delivery; the quality-by-design (QbD) approach to optimize formulations of lipid-based nanosystems; and the development of Biopharmaceuticals and Advanced Therapy Medicinal Products (ATMPs).

João Nuno Moreira

Associate Professor, with Habilitation and Tenure, and Researcher. Scientific activity is focused on the design of lipid-based nanosystems for anticancer drug and nucleic acid-targeted delivery, addressing the impact on the tumor microenvironment at the cellular and molecular levels, both in vitro and in animal models of cancer. With this, novel antitumor targeted strategies are expected to be generated against tumors associated with clear, unmet medical needs.

José Manuel Sousa Lobo

Emeritus Professor at University of Porto. Full Professor (in the area of Pharmaceutical Technology) since 1997. Teacher at the Faculty of Pharmacy (University of Porto) since 1974. Lectures on Galenic Pharmacy.

Research interests are focused on pharmaceutical technology, industrial pharmacy, biopharmaceutics and pharmacokinetics.

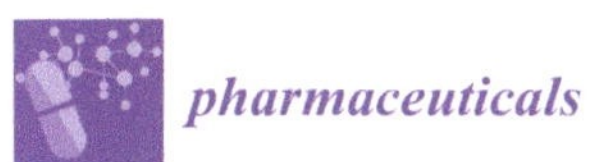 *pharmaceuticals*

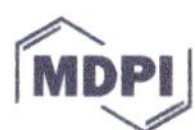

Editorial

Current Insights on Lipid-Based Nanosystems 2023

Ana Catarina Silva [1,2,3,*] , João Nuno Moreira [4,5] and José Manuel Sousa Lobo [1,2]

1. UCIBIO (Research Unit on Applied Molecular Biosciences), REQUIMTE (Rede de Química e Tecnologia), MEDTECH (Medicines and Healthcare Products), Laboratory of Pharmaceutical Technology, Department of Drug Sciences, Faculty of Pharmacy, University of Porto, 4050-313 Porto, Portugal; slobo@ff.up.pt
2. Associate Laboratory i4HB-Institute for Health and Bioeconomy, Faculty of Pharmacy, University of Porto, 4050-313 Porto, Portugal
3. FP-BHS (Biomedical and Health Sciences Research Unit), FP-I3ID (Instituto de Investigação, Inovação e Desenvolvimento), Faculty of Health Sciences, University Fernando Pessoa, 4249-004 Porto, Portugal
4. CNC—Center for Neurosciences and Cell Biology, Center for Innovative Biomedicine and Biotechnology (CIBB), Faculty of Medicine (Polo 1), University of Coimbra, Rua Larga, 3004-504 Coimbra, Portugal; jmoreira@ff.uc.pt
5. Faculty of Pharmacy, Univ Coimbra—University of Coimbra, CIBB, Pólo das Ciências da Saúde, Azinhaga de Santa Comba, 3000-548 Coimbra, Portugal
* Correspondence: anacatsil@gmail.com

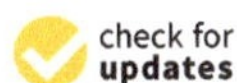

Citation: Silva, A.C.; Moreira, J.N.; Sousa Lobo, J.M. Current Insights on Lipid-Based Nanosystems 2023. *Pharmaceuticals* **2023**, *16*, 1700. https://doi.org/10.3390/ph16121700

Received: 20 November 2023
Accepted: 24 November 2023
Published: 8 December 2023

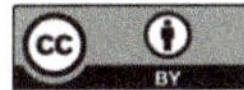

Among the different types of nanosystems that have been investigated for therapeutic use, lipid-based ones are the most explored, as they have advantages over non-lipid nanosystems, especially for improving the transport and efficacy of drugs through different routes of administration, such as ocular, cutaneous, intranasal, and intravenous [1–18].

The concept of lipid-based nanosystems is broad and includes solid lipid nanoparticles (SLN), nanostructured lipid carriers (NLC), cationic lipid nanoparticles, liposomes, exosomes, nanoemulsions, microemulsions, and self-nanoemulsifying systems. Studies have shown that these nanosystems are promising for improving the efficacy of lipophilic drugs or nucleic acids in different therapeutic applications, especially those that respond to unmet medical needs [2,4,19–26].

In the second edition of the Special Issue on lipid-based nanosystems, we notice that research in this field remains very active, as we published 16 works, including 10 research articles and 6 review articles, which were the following:

1. Aljuffali, I.A.; Anwer, M.K.; Ahmed, M.M.; Alalaiwe, A.; Aldawsari, M.F.; Fatima, F.; Jamil, S. Development of Gefitinib-Loaded Solid Lipid Nanoparticles for the Treatment of Breast Cancer: Physicochemical Evaluation, Stability, and Anticancer Activity in Breast Cancer (MCF-7) Cells. *Pharmaceuticals* **2023**, *16*, 1549. https://doi.org/10.3390/ph16111549.
2. Ocaña-Arakachi, K.; Martínez-Herculano, J.; Jurado, R.; Llaguno-Munive, M.; Garcia-Lopez, P. Pharmacokinetics and Anti-Tumor Efficacy of PEGylated Liposomes Co-Loaded with Cisplatin and Mifepristone. *Pharmaceuticals* **2023**, *16*, 1337. https://doi.org/10.3390/ph16101337.
3. Arif, S.T.; Khan, M.A.; Zaman, S.u.; Sarwar, H.S.; Raza, A.; Sarfraz, M.; Bin Jardan, Y.A.; Amin, M.U.; Sohail, M.F. Enhanced Antidepressant Activity of Nanostructured Lipid Carriers Containing Levosulpiride in Behavioral Despair Tests in Mice. *Pharmaceuticals* **2023**, *16*, 1220. https://doi.org/10.3390/ph16091220.
4. Tyagi, R.; Waheed, A.; Kumar, N.; Ahad, A.; Bin Jardan, Y.A.; Mujeeb, M.; Kumar, A.; Naved, T.; Madan, S. Formulation and Evaluation of Plumbagin-Loaded Niosomes for an Antidiabetic Study: Optimization and In Vitro Evaluation. *Pharmaceuticals* **2023**, *16*, 1169. https://doi.org/10.3390/ph16081169.
5. Ahalwat, S.; Bhatt, D.C.; Rohilla, S.; Jogpal, V.; Sharma, K.; Virmani, T.; Kumar, G.; Alhalmi, A.; Alqahtani, A.S.; Noman, O.M.; et al. Mannose-Functionalized Isoniazid-Loaded Nanostructured Lipid Carriers for Pulmonary Delivery: In Vitro

Prospects and In Vivo Therapeutic Efficacy Assessment. *Pharmaceuticals* **2023**, *16*, 1108. https://doi.org/10.3390/ph16081108.

6. Peczek, S.H.; Tartari, A.P.S.; Zittlau, I.C.; Diedrich, C.; Machado, C.S.; Mainardes, R.M. Enhancing Oral Bioavailability and Brain Biodistribution of Perillyl Alcohol Using Nanostructured Lipid Carriers. *Pharmaceuticals* **2023**, *16*, 1055. https://doi.org/10.3390/ph16081055.

7. Satyanarayana, S.D.; Abu Lila, A.S.; Moin, A.; Moglad, E.H.; Khafagy, E.-S.; Alotaibi, H.F.; Obaidullah, A.J.; Charyulu, R.N. Ocular Delivery of Bimatoprost-Loaded Solid Lipid Nanoparticles for Effective Management of Glaucoma. *Pharmaceuticals* **2023**, *16*, 1001. https://doi.org/10.3390/ph16071001.

8. Garrós, N.; Bustos-Salgados, P.; Domènech, Ò.; Rodríguez-Lagunas, M.J.; Beirampour, N.; Mohammadi-Meyabadi, R.; Mallandrich, M.; Calpena, A.C.; Colom, H. Baricitinib Lipid-Based Nanosystems as a Topical Alternative for Atopic Dermatitis Treatment. *Pharmaceuticals* **2023**, *16*, 894. https://doi.org/10.3390/ph16060894.

9. Tong, Y.; Shi, W.; Zhang, Q.; Wang, J. Preparation, Characterization, and In Vivo Evaluation of Gentiopicroside-Phospholipid Complex (GTP-PC) and Its Self-Nanoemulsion Drug Delivery System (GTP-PC-SNEDDS). *Pharmaceuticals* **2023**, *16*, 99. https://doi.org/10.3390/ph16010099.

10. Rincón, M.; Espinoza, L.C.; Silva-Abreu, M.; Sosa, L.; Pesantez-Narvaez, J.; Abrego, G.; Calpena, A.C.; Mallandrich, M. Quality by Design of Pranoprofen Loaded Nanostructured Lipid Carriers and Their Ex Vivo Evaluation in Different Mucosae and Ocular Tissues. *Pharmaceuticals* **2022**, *15*, 1185. https://doi.org/10.3390/ph15101185.

11. Paiva, D.d.F.; Matos, A.P.d.S.; Garófalo, D.d.A.; do Nascimento, T.; Monteiro, M.S.d.S.d.B.; Santos-Oliveira, R.; Ricci-Junior, E. Use of Nanocarriers Containing Antitrypanosomal Drugs for the Treatment of Chagas Disease. *Pharmaceuticals* **2023**, *16*, 1163. https://doi.org/10.3390/ph16081163.

12. Korzun, T.; Moses, A.S.; Diba, P.; Sattler, A.L.; Taratula, O.R.; Sahay, G.; Taratula, O.; Marks, D.L. From Bench to Bedside: Implications of Lipid Nanoparticle Carrier Reactogenicity for Advancing Nucleic Acid Therapeutics. *Pharmaceuticals* **2023**, *16*, 1088. https://doi.org/10.3390/ph16081088.

13. Subhan, M.A.; Filipczak, N.; Torchilin, V.P. Advances with Lipid-Based Nanosystems for siRNA Delivery to Breast Cancers. *Pharmaceuticals* **2023**, *16*, 970. https://doi.org/10.3390/ph16070970.

14. Gugleva, V.; Andonova, V. Recent Progress of Solid Lipid Nanoparticles and Nanostructured Lipid Carriers as Ocular Drug Delivery Platforms. *Pharmaceuticals* **2023**, *16*, 474. https://doi.org/10.3390/ph16030474.

15. Richards, T.; Patel, H.; Patel, K.; Schanne, F. Endogenous Lipid Carriers—Bench-to-Bedside Roadblocks in Production and Drug Loading of Exosomes. *Pharmaceuticals* **2023**, *16*, 421. https://doi.org/10.3390/ph16030421.

16. Torres, J.; Costa, I.; Peixoto, A.F.; Silva, R.; Sousa Lobo, J.M.; Silva, A.C. Intranasal Lipid Nanoparticles Containing Bioactive Compounds Obtained from Marine Sources to Manage Neurodegenerative Diseases. *Pharmaceuticals* **2023**, *16*, 311. https://doi.org/10.3390/ph16020311.

Among the articles published in this Special Issue on lipid-based nanosystems, the lipid nanoparticles, specifically NLC, are the most explored, which suggests the potential of these systems to reach clinic in the upcoming years. Regarding the most investigated diseases, these include cancer, brain diseases, ocular diseases, skin diseases, microbial infections, and metabolic diseases. Thereby, we hope that all these works will contribute to the advancement of these scientific fields.

We would like to thank all the authors of this Special Issue for contributing high-quality articles, as well as all the reviewers who critically evaluated these works. We also thank to the assistant editor Evelyn Du for her kind help in managing this Special Issue.

Author Contributions: Conceptualization, A.C.S.; writing—original draft preparation, A.C.S.; writing—review and editing, J.N.M. and J.M.S.L. All authors have read and agreed to the published version of the manuscript.

Funding: The Applied Molecular Biosciences Unit—UCIBIO, which is financed by national funds from Fundação para a Ciência e a Tecnologia—FCT (UIDP/04378/2020 and UIDB/04378/2020), supported this work.

Conflicts of Interest: The authors declare no conflict of interest.

References

1. Almeida, H.; Silva, A.C. Nanoparticles in Ocular Drug Delivery Systems. *Pharmaceutics* **2023**, *15*, 1675. [CrossRef] [PubMed]
2. Correia, A.C.; Monteiro, A.R.; Silva, R.; Moreira, J.N.; Sousa Lobo, J.M.; Silva, A.C. Lipid nanoparticles strategies to modify pharmacokinetics of central nervous system targeting drugs: Crossing or circumventing the blood–brain barrier (BBB) to manage neurological disorders. *Adv. Drug Deliv. Rev.* **2022**, *189*, 114485. [CrossRef] [PubMed]
3. Garcês, A.; Amaral, M.H.; Sousa Lobo, J.M.; Silva, A.C. Formulations based on solid lipid nanoparticles (SLN) and nanostructured lipid carriers (NLC) for cutaneous use: A review. *Eur. J. Pharm. Sci.* **2018**, *112*, 159–167. [CrossRef] [PubMed]
4. Kon, E.; Ad-El, N.; Hazan-Halevy, I.; Stotsky-Oterin, L.; Peer, D. Targeting cancer with mRNA–lipid nanoparticles: Key considerations and future prospects. *Nat. Rev. Clin. Oncol.* **2023**, *20*, 739–754. [CrossRef] [PubMed]
5. Gugleva, V.; Andonova, V. Recent Progress of Solid Lipid Nanoparticles and Nanostructured Lipid Carriers as Ocular Drug Delivery Platforms. *Pharmaceuticals* **2023**, *16*, 474. [CrossRef] [PubMed]
6. Han, H.; Li, S.; Xu, M.; Zhong, Y.; Fan, W.; Xu, J.; Zhou, T.; Ji, J.; Ye, J.; Yao, K. Polymer-and lipid-based nanocarriers for ocular drug delivery: Current status and future perspectives. *Adv. Drug Deliv. Rev.* **2023**, *7*, 114770. [CrossRef] [PubMed]
7. Wang, X.; Liu, S.; Sun, Y.; Yu, X.; Lee, S.M.; Cheng, Q.; Wei, T.; Gong, J.; Robinson, J.; Zhang, D. Preparation of selective organ-targeting (SORT) lipid nanoparticles (LNPs) using multiple technical methods for tissue-specific mRNA delivery. *Nat. Protoc.* **2023**, *18*, 265–291. [CrossRef]
8. Mohammed, H.A.; Khan, R.A.; Singh, V.; Yusuf, M.; Akhtar, N.; Sulaiman, G.M.; Albukhaty, S.; Abdellatif, A.A.; Khan, M.; Mohammed, S.A. Solid lipid nanoparticles for targeted natural and synthetic drugs delivery in high-incidence cancers, and other diseases: Roles of preparation methods, lipid composition, transitional stability, and release profiles in nanocarriers' development. *Nanotechnol. Rev.* **2023**, *12*, 20220517. [CrossRef]
9. Czajkowska-Kośnik, A.; Szekalska, M.; Winnicka, K. Nanostructured lipid carriers: A potential use for skin drug delivery systems. *Pharmacol. Rep.* **2019**, *71*, 156–166. [CrossRef]
10. Nguyen, T.-T.-L.; Maeng, H.-J. Pharmacokinetics and Pharmacodynamics of Intranasal Solid Lipid Nanoparticles and Nanostructured Lipid Carriers for Nose-to-Brain Delivery. *Pharmaceutics* **2022**, *14*, 572. [CrossRef]
11. Abla, K.K.; Mehanna, M.M. The battle of lipid-based nanocarriers against blood-brain barrier: A critical review. *J. Drug Target.* **2023**, *31*, 832–857. [CrossRef]
12. Ilić, T.; Đoković, J.B.; Nikolić, I.; Mitrović, J.R.; Pantelić, I.; Savić, S.D.; Savić, M.M. Parenteral Lipid-Based Nanoparticles for CNS Disorders: Integrating Various Facets of Preclinical Evaluation towards More Effective Clinical Translation. *Pharmaceutics* **2023**, *15*, 443. [CrossRef]
13. Jiang, Y.; Pan, X.; Yu, T.; Wang, H. Intranasal administration nanosystems for brain-targeted drug delivery. *Nano Res.* **2023**, *12*, 1–23. [CrossRef]
14. Almawash, S. Solid lipid nanoparticles, an effective carrier for classical antifungal drugs. *Saudi Pharm. J.* **2023**, *31*, 1167–1180. [CrossRef]
15. Xu, Y.; Fourniols, T.; Labrak, Y.; Préat, V.; Beloqui, A.; des Rieux, A. Surface modification of lipid-based nanoparticles. *ACS Nano* **2022**, *16*, 7168–7196. [CrossRef] [PubMed]
16. Akbari, J.; Saeedi, M.; Ahmadi, F.; Hashemi, S.M.H.; Babaei, A.; Yaddollahi, S.; Rostamkalaei, S.S.; Asare-Addo, K.; Nokhodchi, A. Solid lipid nanoparticles and nanostructured lipid carriers: A review of the methods of manufacture and routes of administration. *Pharm. Dev. Technol.* **2022**, *27*, 525–544. [CrossRef] [PubMed]
17. Das, B.; Nayak, A.K.; Mallick, S. Lipid-based nanocarriers for ocular drug delivery: An updated review. *J. Drug Deliv. Sci. Technol.* **2022**, *15*, 103780. [CrossRef]
18. Henostroza, M.A.B.; Tavares, G.D.; Yukuyama, M.N.; De Souza, A.; Barbosa, E.J.; Avino, V.C.; dos Santos Neto, E.; Lourenço, F.R.; Löbenberg, R.; Bou-Chacra, N.A. Antibiotic-loaded lipid-based nanocarrier: A promising strategy to overcome bacterial infection. *Int. J. Pharm.* **2022**, *621*, 121782. [CrossRef] [PubMed]
19. Silva, A.C.; Moreira, J.N.; Lobo, J.M.S. Editorial—Current Insights on Lipid-Based Nanosystems. *Pharmaceuticals* **2022**, *15*, 1267. [CrossRef] [PubMed]
20. Chapa González, C.; Martínez Saráoz, J.V.; Roacho Pérez, J.A.; Olivas Armendáriz, I. Lipid nanoparticles for gene therapy in ocular diseases. *DARU J. Pharm. Sci.* **2023**, *15*, 75–82. [CrossRef]
21. Zeng, L.; Gowda, B.J.; Ahmed, M.G.; Abourehab, M.A.; Chen, Z.-S.; Zhang, C.; Li, J.; Kesharwani, P. Advancements in nanoparticle-based treatment approaches for skin cancer therapy. *Mol. Cancer* **2023**, *22*, 10. [CrossRef] [PubMed]

22. Correia, A.; Moreira, J.; Sousa Lobo, J.; Silva, A. Design of experiment (DoE) as a quality by design (QbD) tool to optimize formulations of lipid nanoparticles for nose-to-brain drug delivery. *Expert Opin. Drug Deliv.* **2023**, *31*, 1–18. [CrossRef]
23. Zong, Y.; Lin, Y.; Wei, T.; Cheng, Q. Lipid Nanoparticle (LNP) Enables mRNA Delivery for Cancer Therapy. *Adv. Mater.* **2023**, e2303261. [CrossRef] [PubMed]
24. Akanda, M.; Mithu, M.S.H.; Douroumis, D. Solid lipid nanoparticles: An effective lipid-based technology for cancer treatment. *J. Drug Deliv. Sci. Technol.* **2023**, *3*, 104709. [CrossRef]
25. Jeong, M.; Lee, Y.; Park, J.; Jung, H.; Lee, H. Lipid nanoparticles (LNPs) for in vivo RNA delivery and their breakthrough technology for future applications. *Adv. Drug Deliv. Rev.* **2023**, *7*, 114990. [CrossRef]
26. Tenchov, R.; Sasso, J.M.; Zhou, Q.A. PEGylated Lipid Nanoparticle Formulations: Immunological Safety and Efficiency Perspective. *Bioconjug. Chem.* **2023**, *34*, 941–960. [CrossRef]

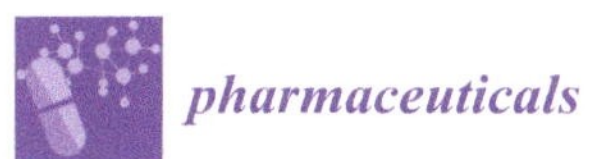 *pharmaceuticals*

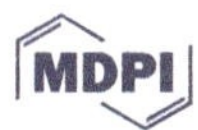

Article

Development of Gefitinib-Loaded Solid Lipid Nanoparticles for the Treatment of Breast Cancer: Physicochemical Evaluation, Stability, and Anticancer Activity in Breast Cancer (MCF-7) Cells

Ibrahim A. Aljuffali [1], Md. Khalid Anwer [2,*], Mohammed Muqtader Ahmed [2], Ahmed Alalaiwe [2], Mohammed F. Aldawsari [2], Farhat Fatima [2] and Shahid Jamil [3]

[1] Department of Pharmaceutics, College of Pharmacy, King Saud University, P.O. Box 2457, Riyadh 11451, Saudi Arabia; ialjuffali@ksu.edu.sa
[2] Department of Pharmaceutics, College of Pharmacy, Prince Sattam Bin Abdulaziz University, Al-kharj 11942, Saudi Arabia; mo.ahmed@psau.edu.sa (M.M.A.); a.alalaiwe@psau.edu.sa (A.A.); moh.aldawsari@psau.edu.sa (M.F.A.); f.soherwardi@psau.edu.sa (F.F.)
[3] Department of Pharmacy, College of Pharmacy, Knowledge University, Erbil 44001, Iraq; shahidjamil07@gmail.com
* Correspondence: m.anwer@psau.edu.sa

Abstract: In the current study, the toxic effects of gefitinib-loaded solid lipid nanoparticles (GFT-loaded SLNs) upon human breast cancer cell lines (MCF-7) were investigated. GFT-loaded SLNs were prepared through a single emulsification–evaporation technique using glyceryl tristearate (Dynasan™ 114) along with lipoid® 90H (lipid surfactant) and Kolliphore® 188 (water-soluble surfactant). Four formulae were developed by varying the weight of the lipoid™ 90H (100–250 mg), and the GFT-loaded SLN (F4) formulation was optimized in terms of particle size (472 ± 7.5 nm), PDI (0.249), ZP (-15.2 ± 2.3), and EE ($83.18 \pm 4.7\%$). The optimized formulation was further subjected for in vitro release, stability studies, and MTT assay against MCF-7 cell lines. GFT from SLNs exhibited sustained release of the drug for 48 h, and release kinetics followed the Korsmeyer–Peppas model, which indicates the mechanism of drug release by swelling and/or erosion from a lipid matrix. When pure GFT and GFT–SLNs were exposed to MCF-7 cells, the activities of p53 (3.4 and 3.7 times), caspase-3 (5.61 and 7.7 times), and caspase-9 (1.48 and 1.69 times) were enhanced, respectively, over those in control cells. The results suggest that GFT-loaded SLNs (F4) may represent a promising therapeutic alternative for breast cancer.

Keywords: gefitinib; lipid; surfactant; solid lipid nanoparticles; stability; breast cancer cell; MTT assay; anticancer

Citation: Aljuffali, I.A.; Anwer, M.K.; Ahmed, M.M.; Alalaiwe, A.; Aldawsari, M.F.; Fatima, F.; Jamil, S. Development of Gefitinib-Loaded Solid Lipid Nanoparticles for the Treatment of Breast Cancer: Physicochemical Evaluation, Stability, and Anticancer Activity in Breast Cancer (MCF-7) Cells. *Pharmaceuticals* **2023**, *16*, 1549. https://doi.org/10.3390/ph16111549

Academic Editors: Ana Catarina Silva, João Nuno Moreira and José Manuel Sousa Lobo

Received: 4 September 2023
Revised: 25 October 2023
Accepted: 30 October 2023
Published: 2 November 2023

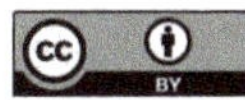

1. Introduction

Gefitinib (GFT) is a small molecule that belongs to the quinazoline family with molecular formula $C_{22}H_{24}ClFN_4O_3$, and the IUPAC name is 4-Quinazolinamine, N-(3-chloro-4-fluorophenyl)-7-methoxy-6-[3-(4-morpholinyl)propoxy]. The molecular weight of GFT is 446.9 g/mol, with a partition coefficient (logP) of about 3.5, which indicates that it has a moderate lipophilicity and can cross cell membranes [1,2]. It is a pale yellow powder, sensitive to light, and prone to degradation upon exposure to UV radiation. It is slightly soluble in water (0.1 mg/mL) but more soluble in organic solvents such as methanol, DMSO, ethanol, and acetone [3,4].

GFT was first developed by AstraZeneca and was approved by the U.S. Food and Drug Administration (FDA) in May 2003 [5]. GFT is used in the targeted therapy category due to its ability to block the epidermal growth factor receptor (EGFR), which is overexpressed in many types of cancer and promotes the growth and spread of cancer cells. As an EGFR tyrosine kinase inhibitor, GFT disrupts EGFR signaling and thus leads to the inhibition of cell proliferation, migration, and survival and the inducement of apoptosis in cancer cells. Reported side effects of GFT include skin rash, diarrhea, and liver toxicity [6–8]. In addition to its use in non-small-cell lung cancer, GFT has also been investigated for the treatment of other types of cancer, such as breast cancer, ovarian cancer, and head and neck cancer [9,10]. It has been suggested that GFT alone or in combination can be used in breast cancer treatment. MCF-7 is a type of breast cancer cell that expresses EGFR [11–14]. GFT was found to have a synergistic impact with the tamoxifen treatment, inhibiting the proliferation of endocrine-resistant MCF-7 breast cancer cells via lowering AKT and MAPK phosphorylation [15,16].

A study on the effects of GFT in combination with docetaxel, a commonly used chemotherapy drug, on MCF-7 cells found that the combination of GFT and docetaxel resulted in greater antiproliferative effects than either drug alone, suggesting that combining GFT with other chemotherapy drugs may enhance anticancer efficacy [13]. However, its use in these cancers is not yet well established and is still being studied in clinical trials.

To improve the bioavailability and therapeutic efficacy of GFT, researchers have been investigating various drug delivery systems. Nanoliposomes were developed for GFT to improve the solubility, stability, bioavailability, and efficacy of GFT in the treatment of lung cancer [15]. Using ionic gelation, Gupta et al. prepared polymeric nanoparticles to encapsulate drugs and improve their delivery and release at the target tumor cells more precisely [16]. In another study, PEGylated solid lipid nanoparticles were developed as a promising approach for lymphatic delivery of GFT [17]. Similarly, studies on GFT-loaded nanomicelles, self-assembled structures made of surfactants to target lung cancer stem cells, have the potential significantly to impact cancer therapy [18].

The development of stable GFT-loaded SLNs and further investigation of their potential application in the treatment of breast cancer are the goals of this study. Lipid Dynasan™ 114, lipid surfactant (lipoid 90H), and water-soluble surfactant (Kolliphore® 188) were used to create the GFT-loaded SLNs. The developed SLNs were tested against the MCF-7 breast cancer cell lines. GFT represents an established in vitro experimental model to study cytotoxicity effects, which is why the MCF-7 cell lines were chosen [19]. If the newly synthesized formulation demonstrates the desired cytotoxic action, the results of this study may eventually be used to treat breast cancer.

2. Results and Discussion

2.1. Particle Characterization and Drug Encapsulation

Among the four SLNs, GFT-loaded SLNs (F4) (Lipoid 90H, 250 mg) had better particle properties (Table 1). In general, the particle size varied, ranging from 378 to 472 nm. They have the benefit of allowing the drug entrapped within SLNs to pass through physiological drug barriers. Endocytosis allows for the passage of particles smaller than 500 nm through the epithelial cell membrane [20–22]. It is obvious that an increase in the concentration of lipid surfactant in the formulation results in an increase in particle size. It was found that the zeta potential increases with an increase in the Lipoid 90H amount in the formulation. As a result, a zeta potential of -15.2 mV was found to be more stable for GFT-loaded SLNs (F4) than for other formulations. At various lipid concentrations, the entrapment efficiency (EE) of GFT was also investigated in SLNs. It was found that the quantity of lipid surfactant affected the extent of GFT entrapment from 64.07 to 83.18%.

Table 1. Particle characterization of developed GFT-loaded SLNs.

GFT-Loaded SLNs	Particle Size (nm)	PDI	ZP (mV)	EE (%)
F1	378 ± 7.4	0.162 ± 0.002	−10.5 ± 1.3	64.07 ± 4.8
F2	405 ± 8.3	0.328 ± 0.014	−12.8 ± 1.2	66.67 ± 3.8
F3	465 ± 6.3	0.223 ± 0.011	−14.4 ± 0.8	71.69 ± 7.6
F4	472 ± 7.5	0.249 ± 0.004	−15.2 ± 2.3	83.18 ± 4.7

PDI, ZP, and EE stand for polydispersity index, zeta potential, and entrapment efficiency, respectively. "Particle size—significant difference ($p < 0.0001$) among all SLNs except F3 vs. F4 (non-significant); PDI—significant difference ($p < 0.0001$) among all SLNs; Zeta potential—non-significant among all SLNs except F1 vs. F4 (significant) ($p < 0.05$); EE%—significant difference ($p < 0.05$) between F1 vs. F4 and F2 vs. F4 and non-significant difference among F1 vs. F2, F1 vs. F3, F2 vs. F3, and F3 vs. F4. One-way ANOVA and Tukey's multiple comparison between formulations are used to test these findings".

2.2. Thermal Studies

A comparison of the thermal spectra of pure GFT and GFT-loaded SLNs (F2–F4) is shown in Figure 1. The DSC spectra of pure GFT showed a distinct endothermic peak at 199 °C, which was consistent with the literature [23–25]. GFT-loaded SLNs (F2) showed a reduced endothermic peak of GFT with minor shifting, while GFT-loaded SLN (F3) and SLN (F4) showed a complete disappearance of GFT peaks, demonstrating that there was no interaction or incompatibility between the drug and the excipients used, which is consistent with the diluting effect caused by the presence of lipids.

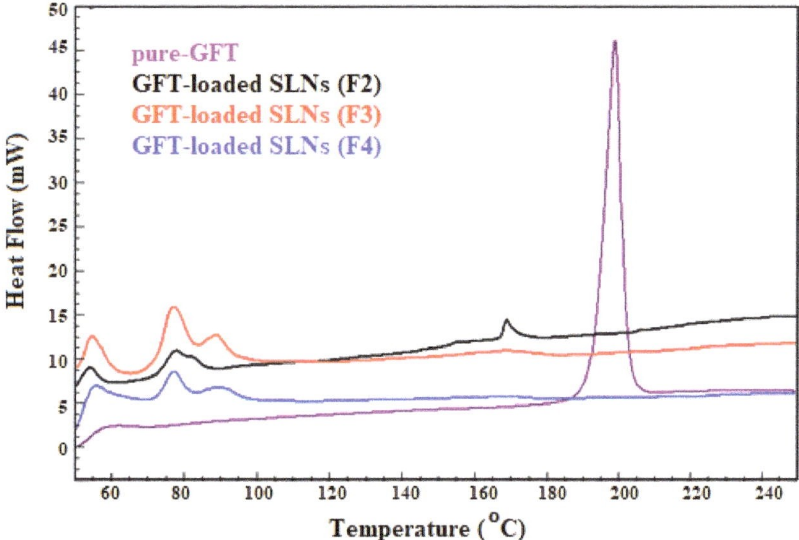

Figure 1. Characterization of pure GFT and GFT-loaded SLNs (F1-F4) using DSC spectra.

2.3. In Vitro Release Studies

SLNs are composed of dynasan lipids that can encapsulate GFT. These nanoscale particles were stabilized by a combination of poloxomer and lipoid stabilizers. Prepared GFT-loaded SLNs (F4) could serve as sustained drug carriers and also as drug stabilizers (Figure 2). The release interpretation of the pure drug at pH 7.4 demonstrates that initially, there was no release. Over time, however, GFT release increased gradually at 0.5 h (36.8%). The release continued to increase reaching 36.8%, 69.8%, and 83.2% at 1, 2, and 4 h, respectively. The drug release further progressed to 94.3% at 6 h and 99.4% at 8 h. The SLN formulation appears to have a sustained release rate compared to pure GFT. Further, it appears that the release reached a plateau or near-complete release at later time points. Since Dynasan™ 114 is a solid lipid with a high melting point, it can provide a sustained release effect by delaying the diffusion of the drug molecules from the Lipid Matrix. Lipid Dynasan™ 114 is a synthetic lipid used in SLNs [26]. Lipid surfactant (e.g., Lipoid 90H) could be instrumental in improving GFT drug release over a prolonged period by promoting its solubility in the lipid matrix and sustaining its release. The presence of Lipoid 90H at the particle surface helps prevent particle aggregation and also contributes to a controlled drug release profile by inhibiting burst release and promoting sustained release over time [27]. Water-soluble surfactants such as Kolliphore® 188 are used in combination with lipid surfactants to stabilize SLNs. Kolliphore® 188 is a block copolymer composed of hydrophilic poly(ethylene oxide) (PEO) and hydrophobic poly(propylene oxide) (PPO) segments. The PEO chains can adsorb onto the surface of SLNs, creating a stearic barrier similar to the lipid surfactants, avoiding agglomeration and keeping particles small in size, thereby improving the effective surface area for dissolution of the drug substance from the carriers [28]. The presence of Kolliphore® 188 can alter the release kinetics by regulating the diffusion of the drug through the surfactant layer. Additionally, the hydrophilic nature of Kolliphore® 188 can enhance the release of hydrophilic drugs by facilitating their dissolution and diffusion through the aqueous media [29,30]. Using a combination of lipid Dynasan™ 114, Lipoid 90 H, and Kolliphore® 188 in the preparation of GFT-loaded SLNs exerts a synergistic influence on the drug release profile.

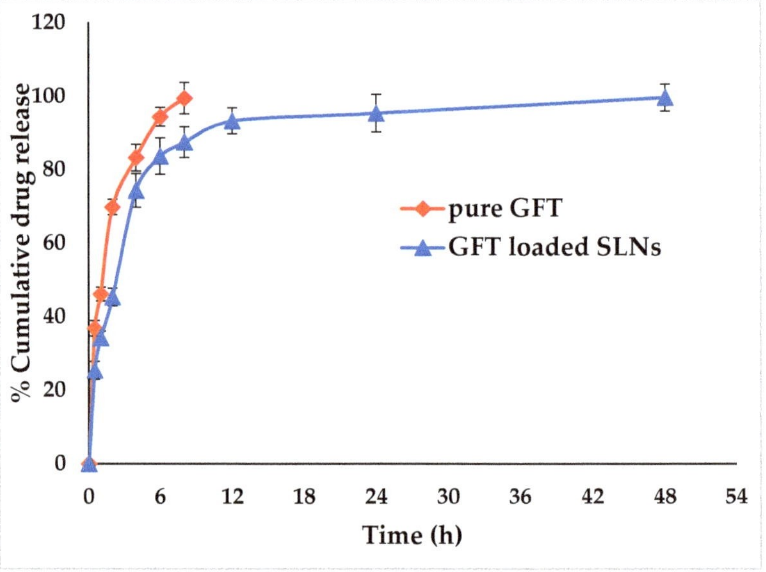

Figure 2. In vitro release of pure GFT and optimized GFT-loaded SLNs (F4).

The release kinetics data of GFT-loaded SLNs (F4) show the correlation coefficients (R^2 values) for different drug release kinetic models at pH 7.4. The zero-order model suggests that the drug is released at a constant rate over time at an R^2 value of 0.714, which suggests that the GFT released was independent of the drug concentration. The first-order model assumes an exponential decay in GFT release over time, with an R^2 value of 0.878, which indicates a better fit to the first-order model compared to the zero-order model. The Higuchi model describes drug release based on Fickian diffusion, where the release rate is proportional to the square root of time. The R^2 was found to be 0.715, indicating a moderate fit to the Higuchi model. Conversely, the R^2 of SLNs was found to be 0.909, indicating a reasonable fit to the Korsmeyer–Peppas model. The release exponent (n value) falls between 0.45 and 0.89; it indicates a combination of diffusion and other factors, such as swelling, erosion, or relaxation of the matrix. The n value observed by us was 0.309. The postulated mechanism of drug release may involve swelling and/or erosion of the lipid matrix because a higher R2 was seen in the Korsmeyer–Peppas model and along with an n value of less than 0.3 from optimized SLNs [31].

2.4. Morphology

The scanning electron microscopy (SEM) images of optimized GFT-loaded SLNs (F4) appeared smooth, spherical, and aggregated. The size observations of these particles conform with their DLS data. The lyophilizing aqueous SLN dispersions may encourage nanoparticle aggregation, particularly when freeze drying is performed without the application of a cryoprotectant (Figure 3).

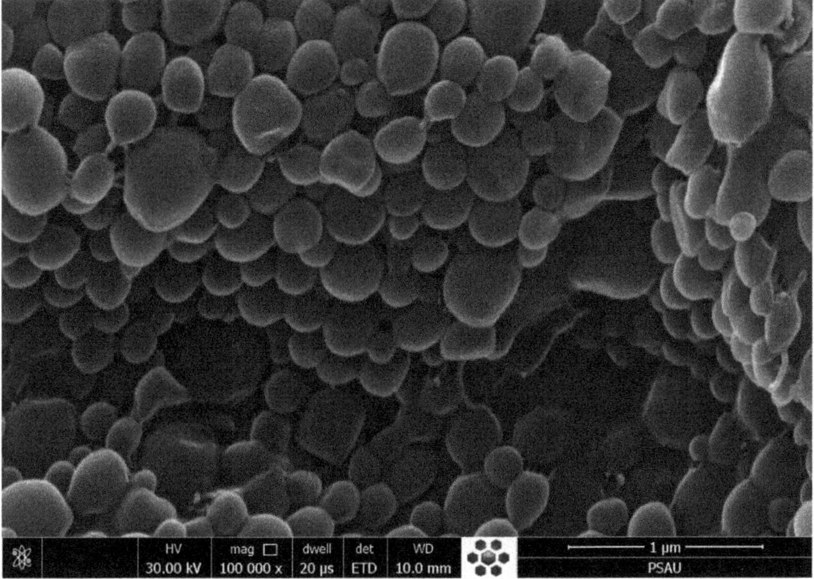

Figure 3. SEM characterization of optimized GFT-loaded SLNs (F4).

2.5. Stability Studies

The size, polydispersity index (PDI), zeta potential (ZP), and EE of the optimized GFT-loaded SLNs (F4) were studied at different time intervals (1, 2, and 3 months) after storage at 25 ± 1 °C and 37 ± 1 °C. The results are tabulated in Table 2. No significant changes were observed ($p < 0.05$) in the size, PDI, ZP, and EE at either storage temperature. The EE analysis revealed that the GFT was present at a 77.8% level after 3 months, even at 37 °C, indicating that the GFT-loaded SLNs (F4) were chemically stable and did not undergo any drug alteration or decomposition. According to the results of the drug content study, the probe sonication procedure used to prepare the SLNs could not have affected the drug's chemical stability. As a result, the developed GFT-loaded SLNs can be kept for up to three months at room temperature without significantly losing their drug content or other physical properties.

Table 2. Results of particle characterization of GFT-loaded SLNs (F4) after stability study.

Months	Conditions	Size (nm ± SD)	PDI (±SD)	ZP (mV) (±SD)	EE (% ± SD)
0	-	473 ± 7.5	0.249 ± 0.004	−15.7 ± 2.3	83.2 ± 4.7
1		474 ± 7.7	0.256 ± 0.009	−15.4 ± 2.0	82.3 ± 1.8
2	25 °C	481 ± 2.6	0.266 ± 0.009	−14.5 ± 1.1	80.3 ± 3.2
3		488 ± 2.7	0.273 ± 0.005	−13.9 ± 5.5	79.2 ± 1.9
1		490 ± 8.5	0.263 ± 0.036	−14.3 ± 0.6	79.3 ± 1.0
2	37 °C	496 ± 8.0	0.281 ± 0.006	−14.2 ± 0.5	78.9 ± 2.3
3		500 ± 10.0	0.278 ± 0.005	−14.0 ± 1.8	77.8 ± 1.8

2.6. MTT Assay on Breast Cancer Cell Lines

Figure 4 illustrates the cytotoxicity of pure GFT and GFT–SLNs towards MCF-7 cells. The IC50 of pure GFT and GFT–SLNs against MCF-7 were 4.0822 µM and 2.7814 µM, respectively. The GFT-loaded SLNs (F4) indicated a significant reduction in cell viability (100.93%, 85.98%, 82.00%, 76.16%, 60.19%, 49.73%, 25.642%, 13.817%, 5.565%, and 4.82% at 0.098, 0.195, 0.39, 0.78, 1.56, 3.125, 6.25, 12.50, 25, and 100 µM, respectively) in comparison to pure GFT (98.214%, 92.866%, 87.898%, 85.884%, 78.28%, 64.79%, 43.93%, 36.53%, 25.08%, and 19.84% at 0.098, 0.195, 0.39, 0.78, 1.56, 3.125, 6.25, 12.50, 25, and 100 µM, respectively), as depicted in Figure 4, against MCF-7 cells. In the MTT assay using MCF-7 cells, the cytotoxic effect of GFT-loaded SLNs was significantly ($p < 0.001$) increased in comparison to pure GFT and blank SLNs. The GFT-loaded SLNs improve GFT's anticancer activity in MCF-7 cells, which is thought to be due to the increased bioavailability and cellular uptake of drugs in the SLNs. As a result, the use of SLNs with GFT could be a replacement for the current method of treating human cancer with pure GFT.

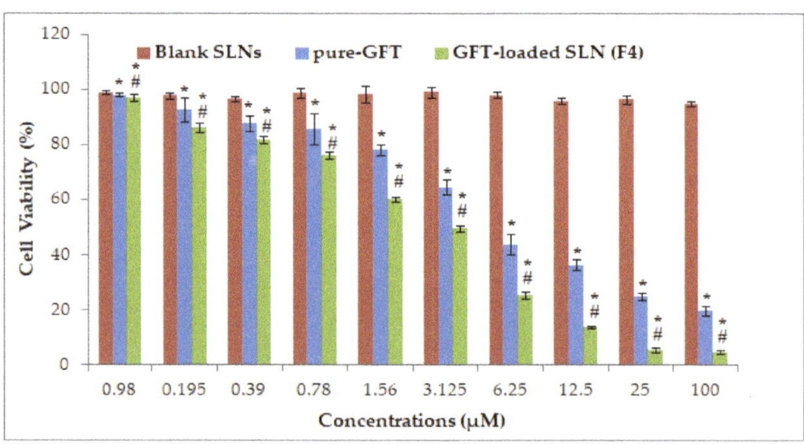

Figure 4. Cytotoxicity profile of blank SLNs, pure GFT, and optimized GFT-loaded SLNs (F4) at varying concentrations (0.98 to 100 µg/mL). "Data are expressed as mean ± SD (n = 3). Significant difference (* $p < 0.05$) was observed in blank SLNs vs. pure GFT; pure GFT vs. F4; and ($^{\#}$ $p < 0.001$) in blank SLNs vs. F4".

2.7. Morphological Changes in MCF-7 Cells Treated with GFT-Loaded SLNs

Figure 5 shows the morphological changes of MCF-7 cell lines after treatment with control, pure GFT, and GFT-loaded SLNs (F4). Compared to the control and pure GFT cells, cells treated with GFT-loaded SLNs showed the greatest amount of cell death after 24 h of incubation. Shrinkage and reduction in the number of adherent viable cells and increase in floating dead cells were observed in MCF-7 cells treated with pure GFT and GFT-loaded

SLNs (F4). This corresponds to the data from the MTT assay. The morphological changes are caused by damage to the cell organelles. Untreated MCF-7 cells typically exhibit an epithelial-like morphology; cells appear to be densely packed together. Individual MCF-7 cells often have a round or polygonal shape. When cultured at high density, MCF-7 cells tend to be tightly packed together, forming cohesive cellular clusters or islands. GFT-treated MCF-7 cells exhibit a reduced size compared to untreated cells. This shrinkage can result from various phenomena, such as cytoskeletal rearrangements or cellular dehydration. Treated cells display irregular or elongated shapes, differing from the typical round or polygonal morphology of untreated MCF-7 cells. Also treated cells exhibited a disruption in cell–cell junctions, leading to a loss of the well-defined cobblestone-like appearance. GFT-treated cells appear more scattered. GFT-loaded SLNs reduced the proliferation of MCF-7 cells, resulting in fewer cells compared to pure GFT-treated cells and untreated MCF-7 cells, as observed under a microscope. Cell-to-cell adhesion properties of MCF-7 cells were also found to be modified with F4 treatment. This may result in altered cell clustering, a loss of tight junctions, or changes in the formation of adherens junctions. GFT treatment with SLN F4 may induce programmed cell death, such as apoptosis, in MCF-7 cells.

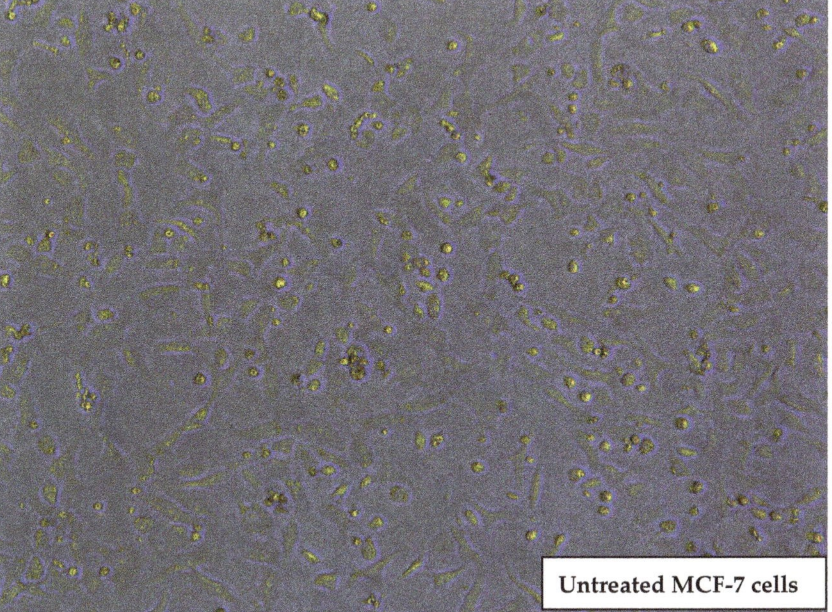

Figure 5. *Cont.*

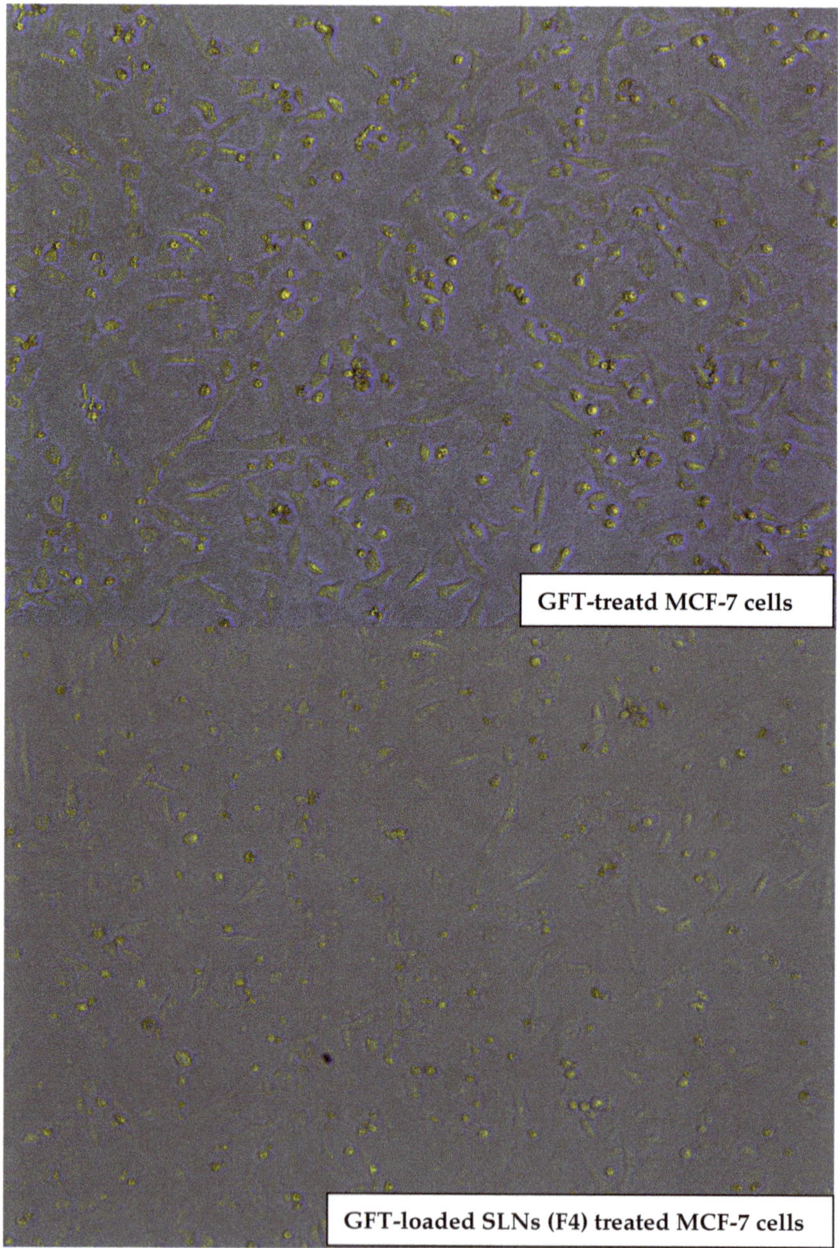

Figure 5. Morphological changes in MCF-7 treated cells. (magnification 200×).

2.8. ELISA Assay of P53, Caspase-3, and Caspase-9

Apoptosis, or programmed cell death, is mostly carried out through activated caspase-3 and the activation of p53 [32–34]. It selectively disassembles many intracellular components without harming or inflaming the neighboring normal cells. T chemotherapy-induced cell death and cancer cell apoptosis have been linked to p53, caspase-3, and caspase-9 activities. In this study, p53 expression in pure GFT and GFT–SLN groups was significantly increased compared to the untreated group ($p < 0.05$), indicating that GFT-loaded SLN (F4) > pure GFT has many characteristics. Strong apoptotic activity was exhibited when pure GFT and GFT–SLNs were exposed to MCF-7 cells; the activities of p53 (3.4 and 3.7 times), caspase-3 (5.61 and 7.7 times), and caspase-9 (1.48 and 1.69 times) were enhanced in those samples, respectively, compared to the control cells (Figure 6). The greater efficacy of GFT in SLNs raises a potential explanation for the triggering of apoptosis in cancer cells.

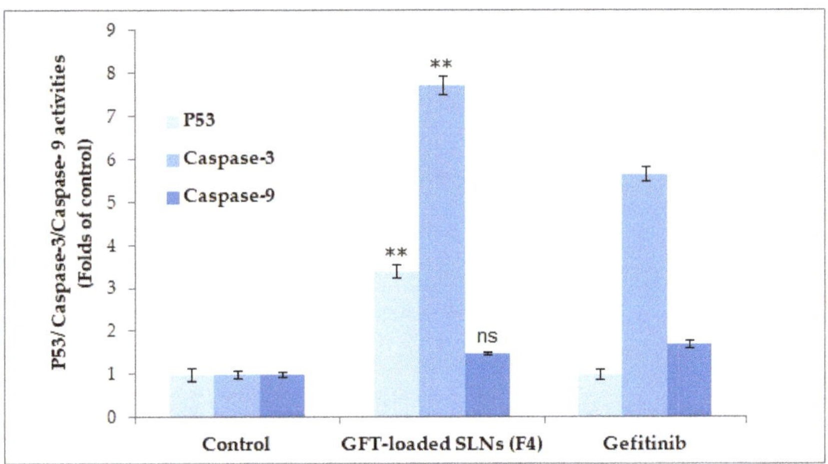

Figure 6. Effects of GFT-loaded SLNs on the level of p53, caspase-3, and caspase-9. Data were observed to show significant difference (** $p < 0.05$) in GFT-loaded SLNs (F4) vs. control and pure GFT (P53 and caspase-3) and non-significant difference ($p > 0.05$) between GFT-loaded SLNs (F4) and pure GFT (caspase-9).

3. Materials and Methods

3.1. Materials

The GFT was bought from "Mesochem Technology in Beijing, China". Glyceryl trimyristate (Dynasan 114), Kolliphore® 188, Lipoid 90H, and dichloromethane were bought from "Sigma Aldrich, St. Louis, MO, USA". All solvents/chemicals and purified water (MilliQ) used throughout the study were of analytical grade.

3.2. Preparation of GFT-Loaded SLNs

Four batches of GFT-loaded SLNs (F1-F4) were prepared by keeping a constant amount of pure drug (100 mg), lipid (Dynasan™ 114, 100 mg), and surfactant (Kolliphore 188, 0.5% w/v) and varying the amount of Lipoid 90H (as 100, 150, 200, and 250 mg) following the reported single emulsification technique [35–37]. Briefly, GFT (100 mg) was dissolved in a previously prepared solution of lipid Dynasan 114 and lipoid 90H in 5 mL of dichloromethane. On the other hand, the aqueous phase containing Kolliphore® 188 (20 mL, 0.5%, w/v) was prepared separately. By adding the aqueous phase with a syringe at a rate of 0.3 mL/min while using a probe sonicator "(model CL-18, Fisher Scientific; Hampton, NH, USA)" for 3 min at 65% W voltage efficiency and 5 sec ON/OFF cycles, the lipid phase was emulsified. On a magnetic stirrer, the organic solvent was evaporated for six hours. GFT-loaded SLNs were collected after high-speed (15,000 rpm) centrifugation "(HermleLabortechnik, Z216MK, Wehingen, Germany)", washed thrice with deionized water, and freeze dried. Collected drug-loaded SLNs were then lyophilized "(Millrock Technologies, Kingston, NY, USA)" and preserved for further studies. Table 3 lists the composition of four developed GFT-loaded SLNs (F1–F4). The percent entrapment efficiency (%EE) of developed formulations was measured indirectly by separating aqueous free drug in supernatant after high speed centrifugation (10,000 rpm). The amount of drug that was free was determined using

UV spectrophotometry at 331 nm [38], and EE% was calculated using the formula shown below [39]:

$$EE(\%) = \frac{\text{Total GFT} - \text{free GFT}}{\text{Total GFT}} \times 100$$

Table 3. Developed GFT-loaded SLN composition.

GFT-Loaded SLNs	GFT (mg)	Dynasan 114 (mg)	Lipoid 90H (mg)	Kolliphore® 188 (%*w/v*)
F1	100	100	100	0.5
F2	100	100	150	0.5
F3	100	100	200	0.5
F4	100	100	250	0.5

3.3. Particle Characterization and Drug Encapsulation

The mean particle size, PDI, and ZP of the GFT-loaded SLN preparation were evaluated through the dynamic scattering light (DLS) method using a Malvern zetasizer (ZEN-3600, Malvern Instruments Ltd., Worcestershire, UK). The mean particle size and PDI were determined using an appropriately diluted (200 times) fresh colloidal dispersion placed into a plastic disposable cuvette. The zeta potential of the nanoparticles was measured to determine their surface charge, which also denotes surface modifications. The procedure for ZP measurement was the same as that for mean particle size and PDI, except that a glass electrode cuvette was used.

3.4. Thermal Studies

Differential scanning calorimetry was used with the Korean-made Scinco-N650 instrument for the thermal characterization of pure GFT and GFT-loaded SLNs (F2–F4). In addition, 5 mg of the test samples was compressed in an aluminum pan and placed in a sample holder for comparison with the reference sample (an empty aluminum pan). With nitrogen gas flowing continuously at a rate of 15 mL/min, scanning was carried out in the temperature range of 50 to 250 °C.

3.5. In Vitro Release Studies

In vitro release assessments of pure GFT and optimized GFT-loaded SLNs (F4) have been completed in a phosphate buffer (pH 7.4). Accurately weighed amounts of pure GFT (10 mg) and GFT-loaded SLNs (equivalent to ten mg of natural GFT) were suspended in a dissolution medium (10 mL) and poured into a dialysis bag "(molecular weight reduce off at 12,000 Daltons)". After that, the dialysis bag was put into a beaker with 40 mL of the appropriate medium and kept on a biological shaker "(LBS-030S-Lab Tech, Jeju, Republic of Korea)" at 100 rpm and 37 °C. The sink condition was maintained by taking 1 mL of the sample at regular intervals and replacing it right away with the media. The collected samples were then appropriately diluted before being tested for drug content using UV spectroscopy at a maximum wavelength of 331 nm [38]. Furthermore, by incorporating the drug release findings into various mathematical kinetics models, the GFT drug release mechanism from the GFT-loaded SLNs (F4) at pH 7.4 could be estimated [40,41].

3.6. Morphology

The gold-sputter technique was used to characterize the morphology of optimized GFT-loaded SLNs (F4) using "SEM (Zeiss EVO LS10, Cambridge, UK)". Using the "Q-150R Sputter Unit" from "Quorum Technologies Ltd. (Laughton, East Sussex, UK)" for 60 s at 20 mA in an argon atmosphere, the freeze-dried SLNs were coated with gold. Imaging was conducted using an accelerating voltage of 30 kV and a magnification of 10–50 KX.

3.7. Stability Studies

The stability of optimized GFT-loaded SLNs (F4) was assessed in terms of size, PDI, ZP, and EE% by following previously published reports [42,43]. This was accomplished by simply packaging 10 mg of freeze-dried GFT-loaded SLNs (F4) in an amber glass vial and storing it at 25 °C and 37 °C for three months. The changes in the size, PDI, ZP, and drug content were recorded periodically (i.e., the seventh day, first month, third month, and sixth month). To assess these parameters, the previously stored GFT-loaded SLNs (F4) were re-suspended in PBS (pH 7.4).

3.8. MTT Cytotoxicity Studies

3.8.1. Cell Growth

The MCF-7 breast cancer cells were bought from the American Type Cutler Collection (ATCC) in Manassas, Virginia, in the United States. Cells were cultured in "Dulbecco's modified Eagle's medium (DMEM) (UFC Biotech, Riyadh, Saudi Arabia)" using tissue culture flasks with an area of 50 cm^2 in a humidified incubator at 37 °C, 5% CO_2. Supplementary media contained 10% fetal calf serum "(Alpha Chemika, Mumbai, India)", 1% penicillin mixture (100 units/mL), streptomycin (100 µg/mL), and 1% L-glutamic acid. The MTT detection kit was bought from "Sigma Aldrich (St. Louis, MO, USA)". In 96-well cell culture plates containing DMEM, cells were seeded.

3.8.2. MTT Assay on Breast Cancer Cell Lines

The anticancer potentials of GFT–SLNs and the pure drug were compared through the MTT assay using MCF-7 cells. Due to mitochondria-mediated apoptosis, the MTT test largely determines the viability of cells. In this test, 3-(4,5-dimethylthiazol-2-yl)-2,5-diphenyltetrazolium bromide, a water-soluble dye, is enzymatically converted to insoluble formazan, and the amount of formazan reveals the relative viability of the cell [44–47]. According to the experimental protocol, cell viability was determined using trypan blue dye before the experiment, and cell viability was found to be 95%. Cells were treated with the formulation when they were between passages 10 and 12. Briefly, 100 µL of medium was used to seed the cells in a 96-well microplate and kept overnight. The suspensions of blank SLNs, pure GFT, and GFT–SLNs (F4) were prepared using the medium as a diluent, while the GFT concentration ranged from 0.98 to 100 µg/mL [48]. The medium was taken out; the cells were exposed to the GFT formulations; and a control experiment (cells only receiving medium) was also performed. The drug-exposed cells were treated with 100 µL of MTT solution (5 mg/mL in PBS) after 48 h. Fresh medium devoid of medication was substituted for the media for the growing cells, and the cells were then incubated for an additional 4 h at 37 °C after being treated with 20 µL of MTT. The culture fluid was then discarded, and MTT crystals were then dissolved for 15 min at working temperature in a solution of DMSO, acetic acid, and sodium dodecyl sulfate (99.5 mL, 0.6 mL, and 10 g). Then, using a spectrophotometric microplate reader (Synergy HT, BioTek Instruments, Winooskim, VT, USA), the optical density (OD) of this solution was determined at 570 nm. Equation (1) was then used to calculate the cell viability (%). The data were plotted as a function of drug concentration (g/mL) versus cell viability (%), with the values normalized to those obtained for viable control cells (considered as 100%). The IC50 values were calculated using log(inhibitor) against the normalized response curve.

$$\% \text{ Cell viability} = \frac{\text{OD of sample} - \text{OD of blank}}{\text{OD of control} - \text{OD of blank}} \times 100 \tag{1}$$

3.8.3. Morphological Changes in MCF-7 Cells Treated with GFT-Loaded SLNs

For morphological studies through phase contrast microscopy, the MCF-7 cells were seeded in 6-well plates (1 × 10^5 per well) containing DMEM and were incubated at 37 °C in 5% CO_2 for 24 h. Thereafter, cells were treated with the GFT–SLN formulations containing 3.21 µg/mL of GFT and were incubated for 48 h. Then, cells were observed using phase contrast microscopes (Olympus CLX 41, Olympus Corporation, Tokyo, Japan) for changes in the cell structure/apoptosis, and the photographs were recorded.

3.8.4. ELISA Assay of P53, Caspase-3, and Caspase-9

Following the manufacturer's instructions and published studies [34,49], the activities of p53, caspase-3, and caspase-9 were assayed through ELISA. The MCF-7 cells were seeded in 96-well plates (5×10^4 cells/well), followed by treatment with pure GFT and GFT–SLNs. The pure GFT, GFT–SLNs, and untreated control cells were subsequently given time to acclimate in 96-well plates at room temperature. Then, 100 µL of the p53, caspase-3, and caspase-9 reagents were added to each of the corresponding wells of the plate that was pre-filled with 100 µL of culture media. After the treatment, the plates were covered, stirred at 500 rpm for 1–2 min, and then incubated at room temperature for 1 h. Finally, the OD was measured using a microplate reader at the wavelength of 405 nm.

4. Conclusions

In recent years, SLNs with different sizes and characteristics have been developed and extensively analyzed. SLNs are highly effective in enhancing the therapeutic effects and minimizing the side effects of anticancer drugs. Considering their advantages, characteristics, and high efficacy, it was suggested that GFT be formulated in SLNs and their efficacy evaluated. In this study, four batches of GFT-loaded SLNs were developed, and their particle size, PDI, ZP, and drug encapsulation were evaluated. MTT assay revealed that optimized GFT-loaded SLNs (F4) exert significant cytotoxicity on MCF-7 breast cancer cells. Overall, our results indicate that SLNs may use p53, caspase-3, and caspase-9 pathways to trigger apoptosis in MCF-7 cells. The study therefore concludes that GFT-loaded SLNs are promising chemotherapeutics for the treatment of breast cancer. However, further pre-clinical and clinical evaluations are needed on the findings of this study.

Author Contributions: Conceptualization, M.K.A. and I.A.A.; methodology, M.M.A. and F.F.; validation, S.J.; formal analysis, S.J.; investigation, I.A.A. and M.K.A.; resources, M.F.A.; writing—original draft preparation, M.K.A. and M.M.A.; writing—review and editing, M.K.A. and A.A.; supervision, A.A.; project administration, M.K.A.; funding acquisition, M.K.A. All authors have read and agreed to the published version of the manuscript.

Funding: This study was also supported via funding from Prince Sattam bin Abdulaziz University, project number (PSAU/2023/R/1444).

Institutional Review Board Statement: Not applicable.

Informed Consent Statement: Not applicable.

Data Availability Statement: The data presented in this study are available on request from the corresponding author.

Conflicts of Interest: The authors declare no conflict of interest.

References

1. Chavda, H.; Patel, C.; Anand, I. Biopharmaceutics classification system. *Syst. Rev. Pharm.* **2010**, *1*, 62–71. [CrossRef]
2. Elsayed, M. Controlled release alginate-chitosan microspheres of tolmetin sodium prepared by internal gelation technique and characterized by response surface modeling. *Braz. J. Pharm. Sci.* **2021**, *56*, e18414. [CrossRef]
3. Garizo, A.R.; Castro, F.; Martins, C.; Almeida, A.; Dias, T.P.; Fernardes, F.; Barrias, C.C.; Bernardes, N.; Fialho, A.M.; Sarmento, B. p28-functionalized PLGA nanoparticles loaded with gefitinib reduce tumor burden and metastases formation on lung cancer. *J. Control. Rel.* **2021**, *337*, 329–342. [CrossRef] [PubMed]
4. Amin, H.; Osman, S.K.; Mohammed, A.M.; Zayed, G. Gefitinib-loaded starch nanoparticles for battling lung cancer: Optimization by full factorial design and in vitro cytotoxicity evaluation. *Saudi Pharm. J.* **2023**, *31*, 29–54. [CrossRef]
5. National Cancer Institute. With FDA Approval, Gefitinib Returns to U.S. Market for Some Patients with Lung Cancer. August 2015. Available online: https://www.cancer.gov/news-events/cancer-currents-blog/2015/fda-gefitinib (accessed on 3 September 2023).
6. Armour, A.A.; Watkins, C.L. The challenge of targeting EGFR: Experience with gefitinib in nonsmall cell lung cancer. *Eur. Resp. Rev.* **2010**, *19*, 186–196. [CrossRef]

7. Gerber, D.E. EGFR Inhibition in the Treatment of Non-Small Cell Lung Cancer. *Drug Dev. Res.* **2008**, *69*, 359–372. [CrossRef] [PubMed]
8. Sordella, R.; Bell, D.W.; Haber, D.A.; Settleman, J. Gefitinib-sensitizing EGFR mutations in lung cancer activate anti-apoptotic pathways. *Science* **2004**, *305*, 1163–1167. [CrossRef] [PubMed]
9. Cohen, E.E.W.; Stenson, K.; Gustin, D.M.; Lamont, E.; Mauer, A.M.; Blair, E.; Stadler, W.M.; Dekker, A.; Mallon, W.; Vokes, E.E. A phase II study of 250-mg gefitinib (ZD1839) monotherapy in recurrent or metastatic squamous cell carcinoma of the head and neck (SCCHN). *Proc. Am. Soc. Clin. Oncol.* **2003**, *22*, 502. [CrossRef]
10. Blackledge, G.; Averbuch, S. Gefitinib ('Iressa', ZD1839) and new epidermal growth factor receptor inhibitors. *Br. J. Cancer* **2004**, *90*, 566–572. [CrossRef]
11. Baselga, J.; Albanell, J.; Ruiz, A.; Lluch, A.; Gascon, P.; Gonzalez, S.; Guillen, V.; Sauleda, S.; Averbuch, S.; Rojo, F. Phase II and tumor pharmacodynamic study of gefitinib (ZD1839) in patients with advanced breast cancer. *J. Clin. Oncol.* **2005**, *23*, 5323–5333. [CrossRef]
12. Zhang, X.; Zhang, B.; Liu, J.; Liu, J.; Li, C.; Dong, W.; Fang, S.; Li, M.; Song, B.; Tang, B.; et al. Mechanisms of Gefitinib-mediated reversal of tamoxifen resistance in MCF-7 breast cancer cells by inducing ERα re-expression. *Sci. Rep.* **2015**, *5*, 7835. [CrossRef] [PubMed]
13. Taurin, S.; Rosengren, R.J. Raloxifene potentiates the effect of gefitinib in triple-negative breast cancer cell lines. *Med. Oncol.* **2022**, *40*, 45. [CrossRef]
14. Engebraaten, O.; Edvardsen, H.; Løkkevik, E.; Naume, B.; Kristensen, V.; Ottestad, L.; Natarajan, V. Gefitinib in Combination with Weekly Docetaxel in Patients with Metastatic Breast Cancer Caused Unexpected Toxicity: Results from a Randomized Phase II Clinical Trial. *ISRN Oncol.* **2012**, *2012*, 176789. [CrossRef] [PubMed]
15. Hu, Y.; Zhang, J.; Hu, H.; Xu, S.; Xu, L.; Chen, E. Gefitinib encapsulation based on nano-liposomes for enhancing the curative effect of lung cancer. *Cell Cycle* **2020**, *19*, 3581–3594. [CrossRef]
16. Gupta, M.; Marwaha, R.K.; Dureja, H. Development and Characterization of Gefitinib Loaded Polymeric Nanoparticles by Ionic Gelation Method. *Pharm. Nanotechnol.* **2017**, *5*, 301–309. [CrossRef] [PubMed]
17. Sherif, A.Y.; Harisa, G.I.; Alanazi, F.K.; Nasr, F.A.; Alqahtani, A.S. PEGylated SLN as a Promising Approach for Lymphatic Delivery of Gefitinib to Lung Cancer. *Int. J. Nanomed.* **2022**, *17*, 3287–3311. [CrossRef]
18. Huang, X.; Huang, J.; Leng, D.; Yang, S.; Yao, Q.; Sun, J.; Hu, J. Gefitinib-loaded DSPE-PEG2000 nanomicelles with CD133 aptamers target lung cancer stem cells. *World J. Surg. Oncol.* **2017**, *15*, 167. [CrossRef]
19. Moon, D.O.; Kim, M.O.; Heo, M.S.; Lee, J.D.; Choi, Y.H.; Kim, G.Y. Gefitinib induces apoptosis and decreases telomerase activity in MDA-MB-231 human breast cancer cells. *Arch. Pharm. Res.* **2009**, *32*, 1351–1360. [CrossRef]
20. LeFevre, M.E.; Olivo, R.; Vanderhoff, J.W.; Joel, D.D. Accumulation of latex in Peyer's patches and its subsequent appearance in villi and mesenteric lymph nodes. *Proc. Soc. Exp. Biol. Med.* **1978**, *159*, 298–302. [CrossRef]
21. Savic, R.; Luo, L.; Eisenberg, A.; Maysinger, D. Micellar nanocontainers distribute to defined cytoplasmic organelles. *Science* **2003**, *300*, 615–618. [CrossRef]
22. Imran, M.; Iqubal, M.K.; Imtiyaz, K.; Saleem, S.; Mittal, S.; Rizvi, M.M.A.; Ali, J.; Baboota, S. Topical nanostructured lipid carrier gel of quercetin and resveratrol: Formulation, optimization, in vitro and ex vivo study for the treatment of skin cancer. *Int. J. Pharm.* **2020**, *587*, 119705. [CrossRef]
23. Gidwani, B.; Vyas, A.; Kaur, C.D. Investigation of inclusion behaviour of gefitinib with epichlorohydrin-β-cyclodextrin polymer: Preparation of binary complex, stoichiometric determination and characterization. *J. Pharm. Biomed. Anal.* **2018**, *160*, 31–37. [CrossRef]
24. Alshetaili, A.S. Gefitinib loaded PLGA and chitosan coated PLGA nanoparticles with magnified cytotoxicity against A549 lung cancer cell lines. *Saudi J. Biol. Sci.* **2021**, *28*, 5065–5073. [CrossRef]
25. Hasan, N.; Imran, M.; Kesharwani, P.; Khanna, K.; Karwasra, R.; Sharma, N.; Rawat, S.; Sharma, D.; Ahmad, F.J.; Jain, G.K.; et al. Intranasal delivery of Naloxone-loaded solid lipid nanoparticles as a promising simple and non-invasive approach for the management of opioid overdose. *Int. J. Pharm.* **2021**, *599*, 120428. [CrossRef] [PubMed]
26. Olbrich, C.; Kayser, O.; Müller, R.H. Lipase degradation of Dynasan 114 and 116 solid lipid nanoparticles (SLN)—Effect of surfactants, storage time and crystallinity. *Int. J. Pharm.* **2002**, *237*, 119–128. [CrossRef]
27. Mohtar, N.; Khan, N.; Darwis, Y. Solid Lipid Nanoparticles of Atovaquone Based on 2(4) Full-Factorial Design. *IJPR* **2015**, *14*, 989–1000. [PubMed]
28. Wang, T.; Markham, A.; Thomas, S.J.; Wang, N.; Huang, L.; Clemens, M.; Rajagopalan, N. Solution Stability of Poloxamer 188 Under Stress Conditions. *J. Pharm. Sci.* **2019**, *108*, 1264–1271. [CrossRef]
29. Ramadhani, N.; Shabir, M.; McConville, C. Preparation and characterisation of Kolliphor®P 188 and P 237 solid dispersion oral tablets containing the poorly water soluble drug disulfiram. *Int. J. Pharm.* **2014**, *475*, 514–522. [CrossRef] [PubMed]
30. Sharma, A.; Arora, K.; Mohapatra, H.; Sindhu, R.K.; Bulzan, M.; Cavalu, S.; Paneshar, G.; Elansary, H.O.; El-Sabrout, A.M.; Mahmoud, E.A.; et al. Supersaturation-Based Drug Delivery Systems: Strategy for Bioavailability Enhancement of Poorly Water-Soluble Drugs. *Molecules* **2022**, *27*, 2969. [CrossRef] [PubMed]
31. Kushwaha, A.K.; Vuddanda, P.R.; Karunanidhi, P.; Singh, S.K.; Singh, S. Development and evaluation of solid lipid nanoparticles of raloxifene hydrochloride for enhanced bioavailability. *BioMed Res. Int.* **2013**, 584549. [CrossRef]

32. El Guerrab, A.; Bamdad, M.; Kwiatkowski, F.; Bignon, Y.J.; Penault-Llorca, F.; Aubel, C. Anti-EGFR monoclonal antibodies and EGFR tyrosine kinase inhibitors as combination therapy for triple-negative breast cancer. *Oncotarget* **2016**, *7*, 73618–73637. [CrossRef] [PubMed]

33. Wu, J.; Xiao, S.; Yuan, M.; Li, Q.; Xiao, G.; Wu, W.; Ouyang, Y.; Huang, L.; Yao, C. PARP inhibitor re-sensitizes Adriamycin resistant leukemia cells through DNA damage and apoptosis. *Mol. Med. Rep.* **2018**, *19*, 75–84. [CrossRef] [PubMed]

34. Ahmed, M.M.; Anwer, M.K.; Fatima, F.; Aldawsari, M.F.; Alalaiwe, A.; Alali, A.S.; Alharthi, A.I.; Kalam, M.A. Boosting the Anticancer Activity of Sunitinib Malate in Breast Cancer through Lipid Polymer Hybrid Nanoparticles Approach. *Polymers* **2022**, *14*, 2459. [CrossRef] [PubMed]

35. Wei, L.; Yang, Y.; Shi, K.; Wu, J.; Zhao, W.; Mo, J. Preparation and characterization of Loperamide-loaded Dynasan 114 Solid Lipid Nanoparticles for increased oral absorption in the treatment of diarrhea. *Front. Pharmacol.* **2016**, *7*, 332. [CrossRef] [PubMed]

36. Pooja, D.; Tunki, L.; Kulhari, H.; Reddy, B.B.; Sistla, R. Characterization, biorecognitive activity and stability of WGA grafted lipid nanostructures for the controlled delivery of Rifampicin. *Chem. Phys. Lipids* **2015**, *193*, 11–17. [CrossRef] [PubMed]

37. Anwer, M.K.; Ahmed, M.M.; Aldawsari, M.F.; Alshahrani, S.; Fatima, F.; Ansari, M.N.; Rehman, N.U.; Al-Shdefat, R.I. Eluxadoline Loaded Solid Lipid Nanoparticles for Improved Colon Targeting in Rat Model of Ulcerative Colitis. *Pharmaceuticals* **2020**, *13*, 255. [CrossRef] [PubMed]

38. Shi, Y.; Su, C.; Cui, W. Gefitinib loaded folate decorated bovine serum albumin conjugated carboxymethyl-beta-cyclodextrin nanoparticles enhance drug delivery and attenuate autophagy in folate receptor-positive cancer cells. *J. Nanobiotechnol.* **2014**, *12*, 43. [CrossRef]

39. Anwer, M.K.; Mohammad, M.; Ezzeldin, E.; Fatima, F.; Alalaiwe, A.; Iqbal, M. Preparation of sustained release apremilast-loaded PLGA nanoparticles: In vitro characterization and in vivo pharmacokinetic study in rats. *Int. J. Nanomed.* **2019**, *14*, 1587–1595. [CrossRef]

40. Peppas, N.A. A simple equation for description of solute release I. Fickian and non-fickian release from non-swellable devices in the form of slabs, spheres, cylinders or discs, 1987. *J. Control. Release* **1987**, *5*, 23–36.

41. Ritger, P.L.; Peppas, N.A. A simple equation for description of solute release II. Fickian and anomalous release from swellable devices. *J. Control. Release* **1987**, *5*, 37–42. [CrossRef]

42. Alali, A.S.; Kalam, M.A.; Ahmed, M.M.; Aboudzadeh, M.A.; Alhudaithi, S.S.; Anwer, M.K.; Fatima, F.; Iqbal, M. Nanocrystallization Improves the Solubilization and Cytotoxic Effect of a Poly (ADP-Ribose)-Polymerase-I Inhibitor. *Polymers* **2022**, *14*, 4827. [CrossRef]

43. Khan, Z.U.; Razzaq, A.; Khan, A.; Rehman, N.U.; Khan, H.; Khan, T.; Khan, A.U.; Althobaiti, N.A.; Menaa, F.; Iqbal, H.; et al. Physicochemical Characterizations and Pharmacokinetic Evaluation of Pentazocine Solid Lipid Nanoparticles against Inflammatory Pain Model. *Pharmaceutics* **2022**, *14*, 409. [CrossRef]

44. Gee, J.M.W.; Harper, M.E.; Hutcheson, I.R.; Madden, T.A.; Barrow, D.; Knowlden, J.M.; McClelland, R.A.; Jordan, N.; Wakeling, A.E.; Nicholson, R.I. The antiepidermal growth factor receptor agent gefitinib (ZD1839/Iressa) improves antihormone response and prevents development of resistance in breast cancer in vitro. *Endocrinology* **2003**, *144*, 5105–5117. [CrossRef]

45. Normanno, N.; Luca, A.D.; Maiello, M.R.; Campiglio, M.; Napolitano, M.; Mancino, M.; Carotenuto, A.; Viglietto, G.; Menard, S. The MEK/MAPK pathway is involved in the resistance of breast cancer cells to the EGFR tyrosine kinase inhibitor gefitinib. *J. Cell Physiol.* **2006**, *207*, 420–427. [CrossRef]

46. Tomankova, K.; Polakova, K.; Pizova, K.; Binder, S.; Kolarova, M.; Kriegova, E.; Zapletalova, J.; Malina, L.; Horakova, J.; Malohlava, J.; et al. In vitro cytotoxicity analysis of doxorubicin-loaded/superparamagnetic iron oxide colloidal nanoassemblies on MCF7 and NIH3T3 cell lines. *Int. J. Nanomed.* **2015**, *10*, 949–961. [CrossRef] [PubMed]

47. Pilco-Ferreto, N.; Calaf, G.M. Influence of doxorubicin on apoptosis and oxidative stress in breast cancer cell lines. *Int. J. Oncol.* **2016**, *49*, 753–762. [CrossRef] [PubMed]

48. Fu, L.; Wang, S.; Wang, X.; Wang, P.; Zheng, Y.; Yao, D.; Guo, M.; Zhang, L.; Ouyang, L. Crystal structure-based discovery of a novel synthesized PARP1 inhibitor (OL-1) with apoptosis-inducing mechanisms in triple-negative breast cancer. *Sci. Rep.* **2016**, *6*, 3. [CrossRef]

49. Md, S.; Alhakamy, N.A.; Alharbi, W.S.; Ahmad, J.; Shaik, R.A.; Ibrahim, I.M.; Ali, J. Development and Evaluation of Repurposed Etoricoxib Loaded Nanoemulsion for Improving Anticancer Activities against Lung Cancer Cells. *Int. J. Mol. Sci.* **2021**, *22*, 13284. [CrossRef] [PubMed]

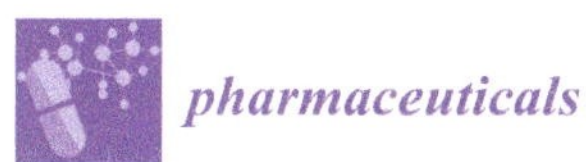

pharmaceuticals

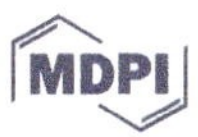

Article

Pharmacokinetics and Anti-Tumor Efficacy of PEGylated Liposomes Co-Loaded with Cisplatin and Mifepristone

Karen Ocaña-Arakachi [1,2], Julio Martínez-Herculano [1], Rafael Jurado [1], Monserrat Llaguno-Munive [1,3] and Patricia Garcia-Lopez [1,*]

[1] Laboratorio de Fármaco-Oncología, Subdirección de Investigación Básica, Instituto Nacional de Cancerología, Mexico City 14080, Mexico; arakachi_karendanahi@outlook.com (K.O.-A.); julenri_reiko@hotmail.com (J.M.-H.); fcojl@yahoo.com (R.J.); muniv1250@hotmail.com (M.L.-M.)

[2] Posgrado en Ciencias Biológicas, Universidad Nacional Autónoma de México, Mexico City 04510, Mexico

[3] Laboratorio de Física Médica, Subdirección de Investigación Básica, Instituto Nacional de Cancerología, Mexico City 14080, Mexico

* Correspondence: pgarcia_lopez@yahoo.com.mx; Tel.: +52-(55)-36935200 (ext. 223)

Abstract: Although cisplatin is an effective chemotherapy drug used against many types of cancer, it has poor bioavailability, produces severe adverse effects, and frequently leads to tumor resistance. Consequently, more effective formulations are needed. The co-administration of cisplatin with mifepristone, which counters an efflux pump drug-resistance mechanism in tumor cells, has shown important synergism, but without resolving the problem of poor bioavailability. Specificity to tumor tissue and bioavailability have been improved by co-encapsulating cisplatin and mifepristone in a liposomal formulation (L-Cis/MF), which needs further research to complete pre-clinical requirements. The aim of this current contribution was to conduct a pharmacokinetic study of cisplatin and mifepristone in male Wistar rats after administration of L-Cis/MF and the conventional (unencapsulated) formulation. Additionally, the capacity of L-Cis/MF to reduce tumor growth in male nude mice was evaluated following the implantation of xenografts of non-small-cell lung cancer. The better pharmacokinetics (higher plasma concentration) of cisplatin and mifepristone when injected in the liposomal versus the conventional formulation correlated with greater efficacy in controlling tumor growth. Future research on L-Cis/MF will characterize its molecular mechanisms and apply it to other types of cancer affected by the synergism of cisplatin and mifepristone.

Keywords: bioavailability; cisplatin; co-encapsulation; liposomes; mifepristone; pharmacokinetics; synergism

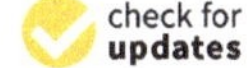

check for updates

Citation: Ocaña-Arakachi, K.; Martínez-Herculano, J.; Jurado, R.; Llaguno-Munive, M.; Garcia-Lopez, P. Pharmacokinetics and Anti-Tumor Efficacy of PEGylated Liposomes Co-Loaded with Cisplatin and Mifepristone. *Pharmaceuticals* **2023**, *16*, 1337. https://doi.org/10.3390/ph16101337

Academic Editors: Ana Catarina Silva, João Nuno Moreira and José Manuel Sousa Lobo

Received: 1 August 2023
Revised: 9 September 2023
Accepted: 19 September 2023
Published: 22 September 2023

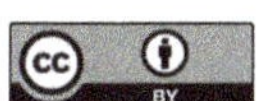

1. Introduction

Cisplatin is one of the most active anti-cancer drugs currently used in chemotherapy; it is applied to more than 50% of human cancers, including lung, head and neck, colon, bladder, ovarian, and cervical cancer. However, its lack of specificity to tumoral tissue leads to dose-dependent damage to normal tissue. Consequently, the administration of cisplatin is associated with significant adverse effects such as nephrotoxicity, neurotoxicity, ototoxicity, and myelotoxicity [1,2]. In addition to these adverse effects, another disadvantage of cisplatin treatment is the rapid development of resistance; thus, most patients experience therapy failure and relapse, resulting in a poor prognosis. Therefore, combining cisplatin with other agents has been investigated to improve the therapeutic response.

A common strategy in combination chemotherapy is the inclusion of a sensitizing agent, which has no direct cytotoxic effect on cancer cells but can improve the efficacy of the antineoplastic drug [3–5]. According to the evidence in the literature, one of the main mechanisms of action for a chemotherapy sensitizing agent is the inhibition of a drug-transport protein known as permeability glycoprotein (P-glycoprotein or P-gp) [6]. Since P-gp acts as an efflux pump in cells, its inhibition undermines the mechanism of multi-drug resistance. Many anticancer drugs, including cisplatin, are P-gp substrates. Hence, the administration of cisplatin with a P-gp inhibitor should increase its effectiveness.

Some groups have investigated treatments combining a cytotoxic drug with an anti-hormonal agent such as raloxifene, tamoxifen, or medroxyprogesterone [7]. However, the doses of these combinations in conventional formulations have not produced selectivity for tumor tissue. As a consequence, adverse effects have been triggered by the treatment schemes tested. Other research groups have demonstrated the efficacy of mifepristone (RU-486, an antiprogestin drug) as a chemosensitizer for improving cisplatin efficacy. In the last few years, our group has researched the effect of the antiprogestogen mifepristone as a possible sensitizing agent for chemotherapy with cisplatin, finding that it increases therapeutic efficacy [8,9]. Indeed, the addition of mifepristone to cisplatin produces an important synergism in chemo-radiotherapy for cervical cancer cells as well as cervix xenografts [8].

Despite the synergism between cisplatin and mifepristone, the chemical instability of cisplatin leads to limited bioavailability. That is, it does not reach an adequate concentration at the tumor site [10,11]. The biodistribution of cisplatin is limited by its binding to plasma proteins, which irreversibly inactivates more than 90% of the drug, leaving only a small percentage of the dose for cytotoxic activity. Additionally, there is evidence that tubular nephrotoxicity is related to the pharmacokinetic parameters of plasma cisplatin [12,13]. On the other hand, mifepristone is administered orally with an absorption rate of approximately 70% from the gut. Unfortunately, it undergoes a first-pass effect in the liver, which diminishes its bioavailability to 40% [14].

An improvement in the bioavailability of cancer chemotherapy agents has been achieved with the development of liposomal drug carriers, which provide increased activity and reduced side effects. Our group recently reported the development of a liposomal system to co-deliver cisplatin and mifepristone. After preparing the liposomes with a reverse-phase evaporation method, the physicochemical characterization revealed a particle size of around 109 nm, a uniform dispersion of particles with a polydispersity index (PDI) of 0.11, and a Zeta potential (mV) of −38. Drug release profiles (at room temperature) exhibited a maximum release of 15% for cisplatin and ~60% for mifepristone at 96 h, showing good stability in the formulation. The co-encapsulation efficiency was 18% for cisplatin and 25% for mifepristone [15].

The delivery of cisplatin and mifepristone by the liposomal formulation (denominated L-Cis/MF) produced notable cytotoxic activity against cervical cancer cells, an apoptotic effect in the same cells, and a significant decrease in tumor growth in mice with a xenotransplant of HeweLa cells La cells [15]. Hence, it is important to continue with the preclinical characterization of L-Cis/MF

The aim of the current contribution was to carry out a pharmacokinetic study of cisplatin and mifepristone in male Wistar rats post-administration of L-Cis/MF and the conventional (unencapsulated) formulation. Additionally, an evaluation was made of the capacity of L-Cis/MF (and the conventional formulation) to reduce tumor growth in male nude mice after implanting xenografts of non-small-cell lung cancer.

2. Results

The preparation of the liposomal formulation that co-encapsulated cisplatin and mifepristone (L-Cis/MF) was prepared and characterized as mentioned in our previous work [15]. We realized the characterization of the batch of L-Cis/MF used in this work and the results were a particle size of 116.8 nm, a polydispersity index (PDI) of 0.17, and a Zeta potential (mV) of −36. The co-encapsulation efficiency was 22% for cisplatin and 22% for mifepristone.

2.1. In Vitro Cisplatin and Mifepristone Release from L-Cis/MF

To quantify the cisplatin and mifepristone released from L-Cis/MF, the amount of each drug found by HPLC was compared to calibration curves with known concentrations.

The typical chromatograms obtained from the cisplatin standard solution spiked in blank liposomes show a retention time of 3.1 min for cisplatin and 4.0 min for nickel chloride, its internal standard (Figure 1A). The typical chromatograms of the mifepristone standard solution spiked in blank liposomes reveal a retention time of 3.4 min for mifepristone and 5.2 min for promegestone, its internal standard (Figure 1B).

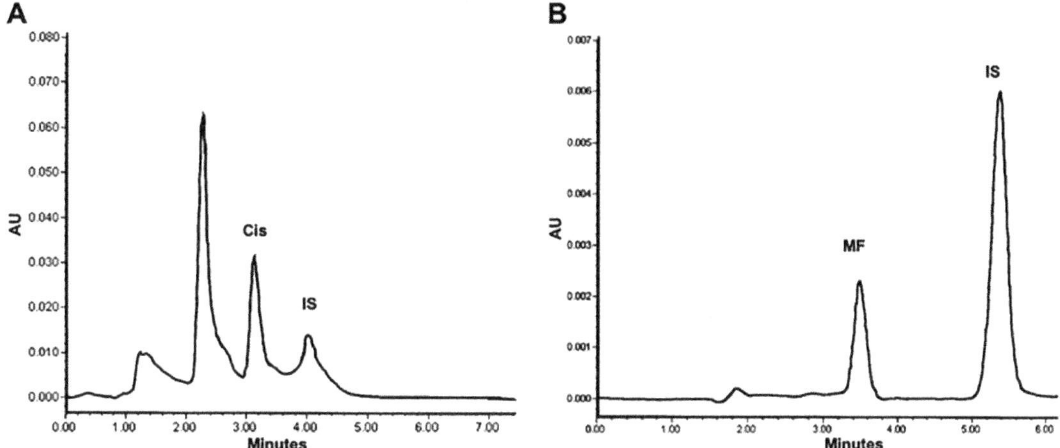

Figure 1. Chromatograms of liposomal cisplatin: (**A**) blank liposomes spiked with 5 µg/mL of cisplatin (Cis) and 50 µg/mL of nickel chloride, the internal standard (IS); (**B**) blank liposomes spiked with 1 µg/mL of mifepristone (MF) and 1 µg/mL of promegestone, the internal standard (IS).

Drug-release profiles of L-Cis/MF in human plasma (Figure 2) show a maximum release of 24% for cisplatin (Figure 2A) and 70% for mifepristone, both at the final reading (72 h) (Figure 2B).

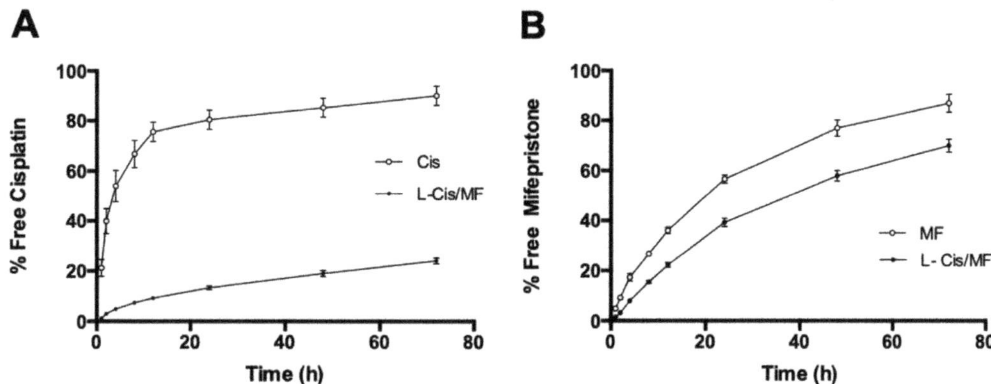

Figure 2. The percentage of cisplatin (**A**) and mifepristone (**B**) released from the L-Cis/MF formulation during 72 h of incubation at 37 °C in human plasma. Values are expressed as the mean ± SEM (n = 3).

The release profile is an important parameter that needs to be measured to evaluate the stability of the nanosystem. Drug release occurs as a function of membrane stability, so the drug release from liposomes can be attributed to the diffusion of the drug through the lipid layer and the disassembly of liposomes caused by various factors like the medium, pH, and temperature, among others [16]. The slow release of cisplatin from the liposome can be attributed to the rigidity of the liposomal membrane and the physicochemical characteristics of cisplatin. In contrast, the rate of mifepristone release from liposomes was the highest. The composition of the lipidic membrane and the lipophilicity of mifepristone strongly influence the dynamics of drug release. Furthermore, in vivo drug release from liposomes depends on several factors, like the interaction between lipid membranes with enzymatic degradation. Additionally, in vitro release experiments could not accurately predict the in vivo drug release. Therefore, pharmacokinetic and efficacy studies are necessary.

2.2. Pharmacokinetics of L-Cis/MF

The plasma concentration of cisplatin in the animals under study (Figure 3) was significantly higher post-administration of L-Cis/MF, versus the conventional (unencapsulated) formulation of cisplatin (both injected IV). The elevated plasma concentration of cisplatin generated by the L-Cis/MF treatment declined slowly and steadily but remained relatively high at 48 h. Contrarily, the plasma concentration of cisplatin derived from the conventional formulation dropped rapidly during the first 2 h. After analyzing the plasma concentration of cisplatin over time for the liposomal and conventional formulations, the results were fitted to a two-compartment model.

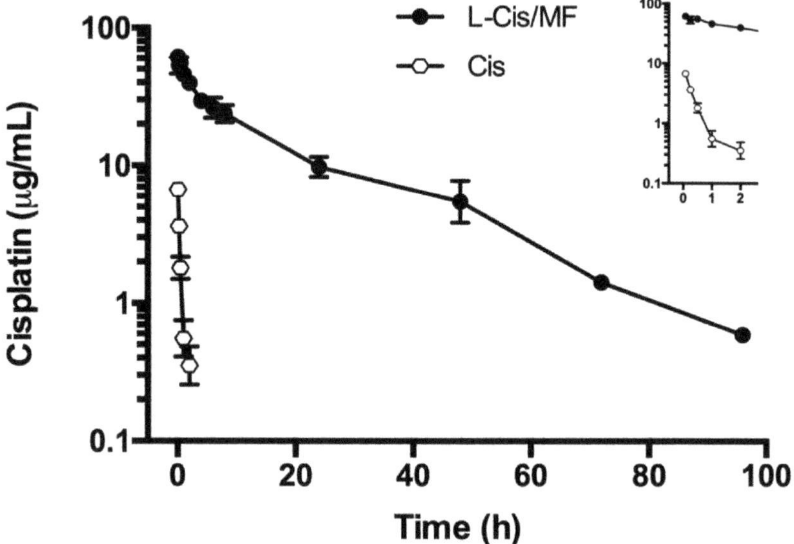

Figure 3. The plasma concentration of cisplatin in rats during the 96 h after the intravenous administration of cisplatin solution (Cis) or cisplatin-loaded liposomes (L-Cis/MF). In each case, the dose of cisplatin was 6 mg/kg. Each point represents the mean ± SEM (n = 6).

The corresponding pharmacokinetic parameters are listed in Table 1. The bioavailability of liposomal cisplatin, represented by AUC, was over 152-fold greater than that of conventional cisplatin. Furthermore, the Cmax and $t_{\frac{1}{2}}$ were approximately 6-fold and 3-fold higher, respectively, for liposomal versus conventional cisplatin; while the Vd and Cl were about 4-fold and 162-fold lower, respectively (Table 1). Figure 4 portrays typical chromatograms of cisplatin in plasma from blood samples drawn from the rats, one at 5 min post-injection of 6 mg/kg of conventional cisplatin and the other at 24 h post-injection of 6 mg/kg of liposomal cisplatin (L-Cis/MF), the latter diluted 1:10.

Table 1. Pharmacokinetic parameters of cisplatin after intravenous administration of conventional cisplatin (unencapsulated) or cisplatin-loaded liposomes (L-Cis/MF).

Parameter	Conventional Cisplatin	Liposomal Cisplatin
$AUC_{0 \to t}$ (µg·h/mL·kg)	5.27 ± 0.66	801.76 ± 77.88 *
$t_{1/2}$ (h)	5.73 ± 2.25	17.26 ± 3.73 *
C_{max} (µg/mL)	9.62 ± 0.66	61.17 ± 3.07 *
Vd (mL/kg)	636.73 ± 39.64	169.11 ± 16.35 *
Cl (mL/h)	1286.53 ± 248.37	7.95 ± 0.76 *

(*) Significant difference ($p < 0.05$) between conventional cisplatin and liposomal cisplatin (L-Cis/MF) based on Student's *t*-test. AUC, area under the curve; $t_{1/2}$, the elimination half-life; Cmax, plasma concentration at time zero; Vd, volume of distribution; and Cl, clearance. Values are expressed as the mean $\pm$ SEM (n = 6).

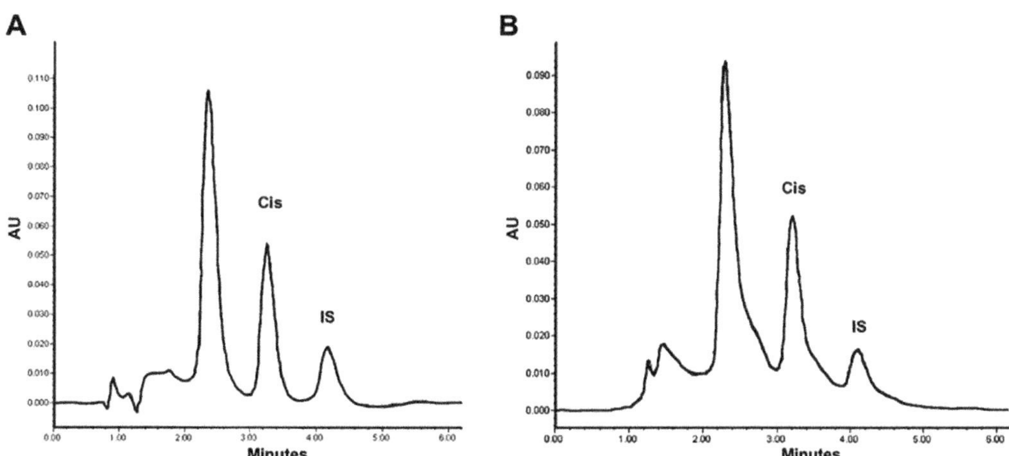

Figure 4. Chromatograms of cisplatin in plasma from blood samples drawn from rats: (**A**) at 5 min post-injection of 6 mg/kg of conventional cisplatin, and (**B**) at 1 h post-injection of 6 mg/kg of liposomal cisplatin; the samples were diluted 1:10 (**B**) and spiked with 50 µg/mL of internal standard (IS).

The pharmacokinetics of mifepristone were determined after administering the conventional and liposomal formulations (Figure 5). Analysis of the time course of the plasma concentration of mifepristone derived from the liposomal formulation was fitted to a two-compartment model. Whereas mifepristone was found in plasma for up to 4 h after the IV administration of L-Cis/MF, it was not detected at any sampling time post-injection of the conventional formulation (Figure 6). Since mifepristone administered conventionally was below the concentration quantifiable by the method of measurement used (0.05 µg/mL), the pharmacokinetic parameters of free mifepristone could not be determined (Table 2).

2.3. Tumor Growth Inhibition and Systemic Toxicity

An in vivo evaluation was made of the therapeutic efficacy of a 3-week treatment of tumor-bearing mice with the liposomal or conventional formulation of the cisplatin/mifepristone combination. The mice had received xenotransplants of A-549 cells of non-small-cell lung cancer (Figure 7). During the 6 weeks after initiating the treatments, tumor growth was better controlled by L-Cis/MF than the unencapsulated cisplatin/mifepristone combination. In relation to the initial tumor volume, the increase found was around 21-fold for the control group, 15-fold for the conventional formulation, and 7.5-fold for the liposomal nanosystem (Figure 7A,B). Regarding possible systemic toxicity, there was no significant change in animal body weight during the experiment and the general condition of the animals was normal (Figure 7C).

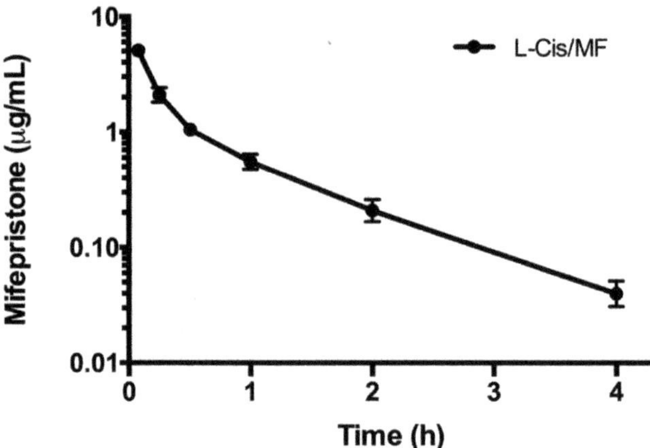

Figure 5. The plasma concentration of mifepristone in rats during the 4 h after intravenous injection of mifepristone-loaded liposomes (L-Cis/MF). The dose was 6.17 mg/kg of mifepristone. Each point represents the mean ± SEM (n = 6).

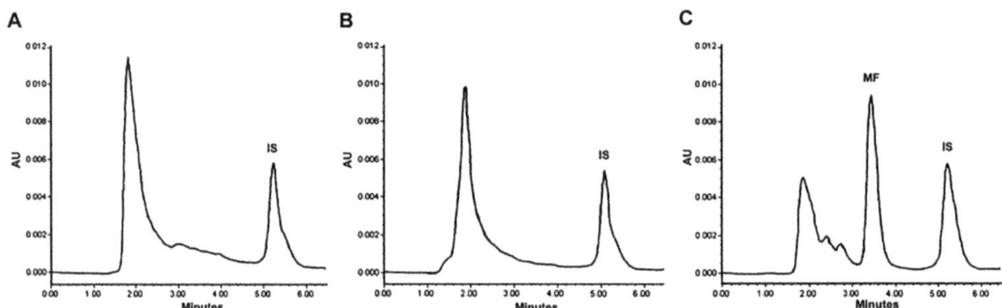

Figure 6. Chromatograms of the concentration of mifepristone in plasma from blood samples drawn from rats. Mifepristone was undetectable in samples (spiked with promegestone, the internal standard) taken at 5 min (**A**) and 1 h (**B**) after SC administration of a dose of 6.17 mg/kg of free mifepristone. Contrarily, mifepristone is clearly observed in a representative chromatogram of plasma from a blood sample drawn from a rat at 1 h (**C**) after a single intravenous injection of the same dose of mifepristone in the liposomal formulation (L-Cis/MF).

Table 2. Pharmacokinetic parameters of free mifepristone or mifepristone after the intravenous administration of L-Cis/MF.

Parameter	Conventional Mifepristone	Liposomal Mifepristone
$AUC_{0\rightarrow t}$ (μg·h/mL·kg)	Not detectable	2.03 ± 0.26
$t_{1/2}$ (h)	Not detectable	0.4 ± 0.16
C_{max} (μg/mL)	Not detectable	7.4 ± 1.01
Vd (mL/kg)	Not detectable	939.82 ± 105.40
Cl (mL/h)	Not detectable	3290.54 ± 351.22

AUC, area under the curve; $t_{1/2}$, the elimination half-life; Cmax, plasma concentration at time zero; Vd, volume of distribution; and Cl, clearance. Values are expressed as the mean ± SEM (n = 6).

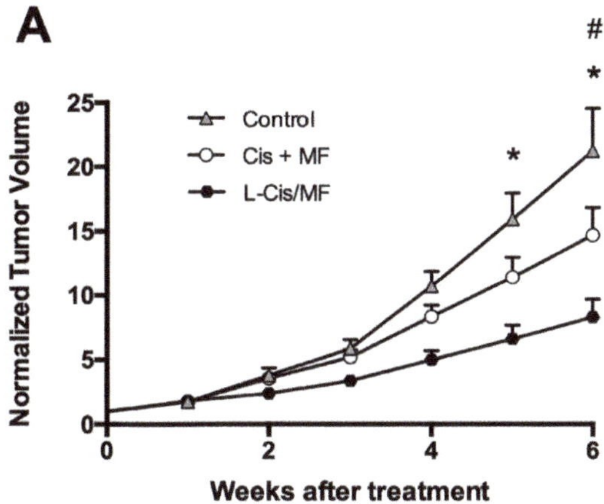

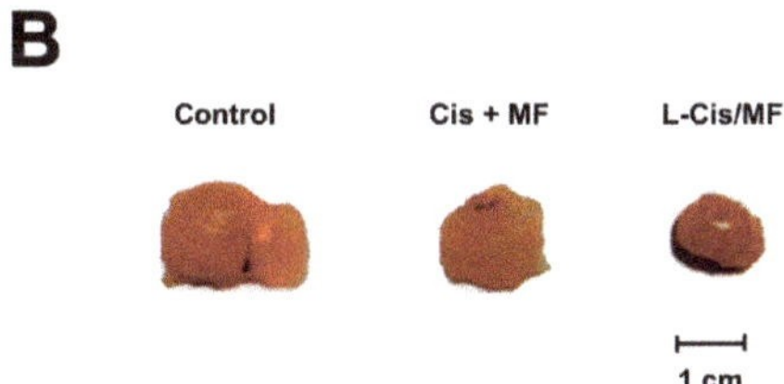

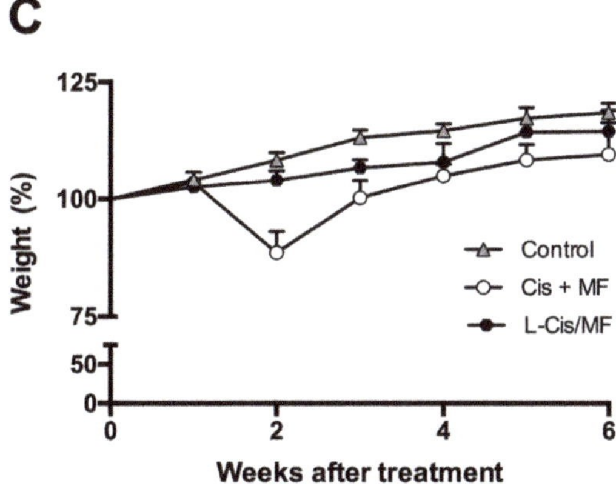

Figure 7. Efficacy of the 3-week treatments after subcutaneously implanting A-549 cell xenografts in the flank of nude mice. The treatments were initiated when the tumors reached ~70 mm^3 (day 0) and ended 3 weeks later. (**A**) Normalized tumor volume during 6 weeks after initiating the three treatments: the conventional (unencapsulated) formulation of cisplatin and mifepristone, the drug-loaded liposomes (L-Cis/MF), and empty liposomes (the control group). (**B**) Final tumor volume after 6 weeks of initiating the treatments. (**C**) Body weight of the mice in the different groups during the 6 weeks after initiating the treatments. Data are expressed as the mean ± SEM (n = 6), and significant differences ($p < 0.05$) were examined by analysis of variance (ANOVA). * Significant difference between L-Cis/MF and the control; # Significant difference between the conventional formulation and the control.

2.4. Quantitative Detection of VEGF in Tumors

Analysis of the tissue of the xenografts of non-small-cell lung cancer at the end of the study showed a slightly but not significantly lower protein level of VEGF for the L-Cis/MF treatment versus the control (Figure 8).

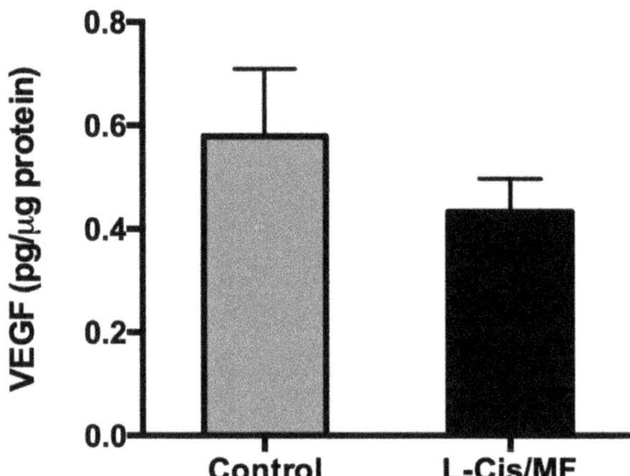

Figure 8. At the end of the study, analysis of the tissue of whole lysed tumors (A-540 xenografts) evidenced a slightly but not significantly lower level of the VEGF protein for the L-Cis/MF versus vehicle (control) treatment group.

3. Discussion

3.1. Strategies for Cancer Therapy with Cisplatin

Cancer is characterized by unspecific symptomology during the first stages of development. Consequently, the majority of patients are diagnosed in advanced stages of the disease and treated with chemotherapy. Although antineoplastic treatments have improved significantly over the last decade, they still leave much to be desired. For example, cisplatin is a chemotherapy drug with a widespread clinical use for various types of cancer due to its effectiveness in eliminating tumor tissue. Nevertheless, chemotherapy with this drug is associated with severe adverse effects, including nephrotoxicity, neurotoxicity, ototoxicity, and myelotoxicity [1,2]. Moreover, it frequently leads to the development of tumor resistance, causing most patients treated with cisplatin to experience failure and relapse and therefore to have a poor prognosis. As a result of all the aforementioned factors, nowadays the standard treatment for the majority of advanced-stage cancer treated with cisplatin consists of a combination of drugs [17]. The combination of cisplatin with mifepristone has shown synergistic effects, but the problem of low bioavailability in tumor tissue remains [9,18].

Nanotechnology has been employed to develop drug delivery systems in order to achieve greater systemic distribution and bioavailability of drugs, leading to an improved selectivity and efficacy of therapy as well as reduced adverse effects. Various systems of drug delivery exist, including solid lipidic nanoparticles, polymeric micelles, and liposomes [19]. Recently, the co-delivery of antineoplastic drugs in a single nanosystem has been described [20–22]. In tests carried out with various formulations of nanoparticles containing a cytotoxic drug and a sensitizing agent, synergism has been found in the treatment of cancer [23].

Our group has reported the co-encapsulation of cisplatin and mifepristone by a nanosystem (L-Cis/MF) with a lipidic membrane made of HSPC, cholesterol, and DSPE-mPEG2000 [15]. In vitro assays have revealed the dynamics of drug release from the encapsulated formulation. Meanwhile, in vivo assays utilizing xenotransplants of cervical cancer have demonstrated that the liposomal co-encapsulation of cisplatin and mifepristone affords a significantly greater inhibition of tumor growth than the conventional (unencapsulated) formulation of the same combination [15]. Encapsulation is an interesting way to efficiently deposit both drugs at the tumor site. It achieves a better synergistic response than that observed with the conventional application of the same drugs.

Defining the pharmacokinetics of the L-Cis/MF nanosystem is an essential part of its preclinical characterization, as is the evaluation of the therapeutic efficacy of this nanosystem in distinct experimental animal models. One such model is the implantation of xenografts of non-small-cell lung cancer, for which cisplatin constitutes part of the standard treatment. These steps of preclinical characterization may facilitate clinical trials of the L-Cis/MF nanosystem in the future.

3.2. Profile of the Release of Cisplatin and Mifepristone from L-Cis/MF

The good stability of the present liposomal nanosystem in human plasma at 37 °C led to prolonged release of the two drugs. The percentage of release of cisplatin was 19% (Figure 2A). The current results correlate with previous publications describing a slow rate of release of hydrophilic chemotherapy agents co-encapsulated with sensitizing agents in liposomal systems [24,25].

Mendes et al. (2014) reported the co-encapsulation of genistein and paclitaxel in a multicompartmental nanostructured system. Genistein was entrapped in the external phospholipid bilayer of the polymeric nanoparticle and was released quickly (85% during the first 48 h). Paclitaxel, on the other hand, was encapsulated in the internal compartment of the polymeric core and showed a gradual and sustained release constituting only 10% of the compound [25]. A similar outcome was found with the present liposomal nanosystem. Cisplatin was encapsulated in the center of the formulation and was slowly and gradually released, leading to a low overall delivery.

Some studies on liposomal systems containing cisplatin have described elevated rates of the release of this drug (up to 50% at 24 h) [26–28]. Contrarily, the current formulation (L-Cis/MF) released 13% of the cisplatin in 24 h, possibly indicating the greater stability of the co-encapsulation of drugs in the same liposomal system. The slow release of cisplatin from the liposomal formulation could stem from various factors including the rigidity of the liposomal membrane and the physicochemical characteristics of the encapsulated drug. The mechanisms of release may involve transport by means of the polymer and/or the dissolution of the polymeric capsule. Accordingly, the release of the drugs encapsulated in the core of the liposomal formulation can be explained by slowly occurring processes, such as diffusion, hydration of the polymers, swelling, and degradation [25].

In contrast, the external envelope (the phospholipid bilayer) undergoes a dynamic and more rapid process, accounting for the more rapid release of mifepristone than cisplatin from L-Cis/MF, reaching 70% at 72 h (Figure 2B). Mifepristone is characterized by high lipophilicity, which favors its location in the external lipidic bilayer.

The location of drugs within the phospholipid membranes depends on their solubility as well as the hydrogen bonds or Van der Waals interactions between a hydrophobic drug and the hydrophobic chains of phospholipids in the bilayer. The composition of the lipidic membrane and the lipophilicity of the drug strongly influence the dynamics of drug release [29]. Hence, the percentage of release of mifepristone from the L-Cis/MF formulation is likely due in part to the dynamics of the lipids in the membrane [30,31].

3.3. Pharmacokinetics of L-Cis/MF

The pharmacokinetics of the release of cisplatin into the bloodstream was evaluated for the liposomal and conventional formulations. When comparing the administration of L-Cis/MF and free cisplatin, the former led to a higher plasma concentration of cisplatin over time, resulting in a significantly higher AUC, a lower rate of clearance, and a smaller volume of distribution (Figure 3, Table 1). In the liposomal formulation, as can be appreciated, there was a substantial increase in bioavailability and a slower rate of elimination of cisplatin, as well as a more limited distribution in tissues (probably greater specificity for tumor tissue).

This may be due to the modification of the liposomal system by attaching polyethylene glycol (PEG)-units to the bilayer, leading to pegylated (stealth) liposomes. The latter prolongs systemic circulation in the bloodstream through a reduction in recognition by the mononuclear phagocytic system, and also through a decrease in interaction with plasma opsonins. As a consequence, stealth liposomes enhance the stability of encapsulated drugs, diminish their toxicity, increase their half-life, and decrease their clearance and immunogenicity [32,33].

Only a small percentage of conventional antineoplastic drugs in systemic circulation reach tumor tissue. These drugs leave the intravascular space by crossing the capillary wall to the interstitium through a process called extravasation. Subsequently, the free drugs are taken up by tumor cells by means of passive diffusion [34,35]. In contrast, PEGylated liposomes are usually internalized by endocytosis. They have the potential for improved drug targeting, and for controlled release from the nanosystem by passive targeting through a phenomenon known as the enhanced permeability and retention (EPR) effect in solid tumors. Due to the difference in vascular structure between tumor tissue and normal tissue, and to the nanoparticle size, the EPR effect favors a greater accumulation of liposomes in tumor cells [36].

When the tumor reaches a certain size, the original vessels are insufficient to supply the necessary oxygen and nutrients. Thus, cancer cells begin to develop a necrotic core, leading to the secretion of growth factors that trigger cell proliferation and angiogenesis, which in turn facilitate the rapid development of new blood vessels. Since these vessels have a discontinuous epithelium and lack a basement membrane, they contain spaces called fenestrae between endothelial cells, which makes it easier for the liposomes to reach tumor tissue [31].

Several studies have demonstrated that the pharmacokinetic profile of encapsulated drugs is modified significantly by the use of PEGylated liposomes [32]. The present results correlate with the data reported in the literature for liposomal formulations utilized clinically, such as PEGylated liposomal doxorubicin, commonly administered for the treatment of breast cancer. There is a significantly different pharmacokinetic profile for doxorubicin (a higher plasma concentration) with the application of the PEGylated liposomal versus the conventional (unencapsulated) formulation [37]. PEGylation offers a great advantage for anticancer drugs by decreasing immunogenicity, while increasing the time of systemic circulation and the serum half-life.

The in vitro assays evidenced a more rapid release of mifepristone than cisplatin, which may influence its rate of distribution and consequently its pharmacokinetic parameters. The pharmacokinetic evaluation showed a plasma concentration of mifepristone of 7.4 µg/mL following treatment with L-Cis/MF, with an AUC of 2.03 µg·h/mL·kg and a Vd of 939.82 mL/kg. The undetectable plasma level of mifepristone after administering the conventional formulation did not allow for the determination of the pharmacokinetic parameters.

Compared to the current results, a significantly lower plasma concentration of mifepristone was found in a previous study after rats were orally administered 10 mg/kg of mifepristone. The maximum plasma concentration was 0.167 µg/mL, with an AUC of 0.338 µg·h/mL·kg and a Vd of 1470 mL/kg [38]. This suggests that the use of liposome-based vectors to deliver drugs significantly modifies the pharmacokinetics of the encapsulated active agents, causing an increased plasma concentration and bioavailability of the drug, thus favoring a higher concentration in tumor tissue. Another relevant factor capable of affecting the efficacy of mifepristone treatment is its low solubility. An important challenge for many insoluble drugs, or those with limited solubility, is the development of new nanoformulations with the aim of enhancing their pharmacological potential.

3.4. The Therapeutic Efficacy of L-Cis/MF In Vivo

The therapeutic response, herein evaluated as the inhibition of tumor growth, was significantly better in the animals that received the liposomal versus the conventional (unencapsulated) formulation of the cisplatin/mifepristone combination. A previous report from our group demonstrated significantly greater drug accumulation in tumor xenografts of the cervix after the injection of a liposomal nanosystem containing cisplatin compared to the injection of unencapsulated free cisplatin [39]. The present comparison of the liposomal versus the conventional formulation reveals that the enhanced therapeutic response observed with L-Cis/MF correlates well with the increased bioavailability of the same (greater plasma concentration over time).

Overall, the better specificity of the liposomal formulation afforded superior cytotoxicity in tumor tissue as well as an absence of systemic toxicity (judging by the stability of animal weight). The pharmacokinetic characterization showed a significantly higher plasma concentration of both drugs in the animals that received L-Cis/MF versus the conventional (unencapsulated) formulation. Moreover, the distribution and elimination parameters were strongly modified, indicating a longer circulation time for both drugs. There was probably a higher concentration of the drugs in the tumor tissue. The hypothesis is that the co-encapsulated drugs were able to reach the tumor tissue more efficiently and accumulate there at a higher concentration than free drugs, resulting in a greater decrease in tumor growth. Further research on tissue distribution is needed to clearly define the mechanisms responsible for the inhibition of tumor growth stemming from treatment with L-Cis/MF.

Since the application of two or more drugs is a common practice in cancer treatment to achieve synergistic effects (and given our data about the better pharmacokinetics and greater efficacy of cisplatin and mifepristone co-loaded in liposomes), our work shows great prospects for designing new and better nanosystems of co-encapsulation, functionalized or conjugated with a variety of antibodies or ligands to target cancer cell receptors, enhancing drug delivery and internalization into tumor cells, and reducing drug distribution in normal tissue, so as to improve treatment outcomes in cancer therapy. The natural future step would be clinical trials on patients with cancer.

4. Materials and Methods

4.1. Drugs and Reagents

Cisplatin, mifepristone, trypsin, sodium chloride, nickel chloride, and sodium diethyl dithiocarbamate (DDTC) were supplied by Sigma–Aldrich Chemical Co. (St. Louis, MO, USA). Hydrogenated soybean L-α-phosphatidylcholine (HSPC), 1,2-distearoyl-sn-glycero-3-phosphoethanolamine-N-[methoxy(polyethyleneglycol)-2000] (DSPEm-PEG2000), and cholesterol were purchased from Avanti Polar Lipids (Birmingham, AL, USA). High-performance liquid chromatography (HPLC)-grade acetonitrile, chloroform, and methanol were acquired from Honeywell International, Inc. (Morristown, NJ, USA). Dulbecco's modified Eagle's medium (DMEM, Thermo Fisher Scientific Inc., Waltham, MA, USA), fetal calf serum (FCS, Thermo Fisher Scientific Inc., Waltham, MA, USA), ethylenediaminetetraacetic acid (EDTA, Thermo Fisher Scientific Inc., Waltham, MA, USA), Tris, and SDS were procured from GIBCO Inc. (Grand Island Biological Company, New York, NY, USA). High-quality water employed to prepare solutions was obtained with a Continental Milli-Q Reagent Water System (Millipore, El Paso, TX, USA).

4.2. Animals

Male Wistar rats (230–250 g, 6–7 weeks old) and male athymic Balb-C nu/nu mice (6–7 weeks old) were supplied by the Metropolitan Autonomous University (Universidad Autonoma Metropolitana, or UAM), Mexico City, Mexico. All animals were kept in a pathogen-free environment on a 12/12 h light/dark cycle and provided food and water ad libitum. Procedures for the care and handling of the animals were reviewed and approved by the Ethics Committee of the National Cancer Institute, Mexico City, Mexico (2020, with Ref. # 010/015/IBI-CB/619/10), and were in accordance with the Mexican Federal Regulation for Animal Experimentation and Care (NOM-062-ZOO-1999, Ministry of Agriculture, Mexico City, Mexico).

4.3. Preparation of Liposomes Co-Loaded with Cisplatin and Mifepristone

The liposomal formulation that co-encapsulated cisplatin and mifepristone (L-Cis/MF) was elaborated as described in Ledezma–Gallegos et al. (2020) [15]. Briefly, three lipids (HSPC, cholesterol, and DSPE-mPEG2000 at a molar ratio of 60:35:5) were dissolved in chloroform/methanol (2:1 v/v) and mixed with 5 mg of mifepristone. This mixture was deposited dropwise into a saturated cisplatin solution in sterile water (8 mg/mL) heated at 65 °C, maintaining a molar ratio of 1:12 for cisplatin and the phospholipids. The organic solvents were removed in a rotatory evaporator and the suspension was sonicated for 2 h to reduce and homogenize the size of the liposomes. Unencapsulated cisplatin was removed by dialysis using a 12,000 Da MWCO membrane (Spectrum Labs Inc., San Francisco, CA, USA), and unencapsulated mifepristone was removed by molecular exclusion chromatography on PD-10 columns packed with Sephadex-G-25 resin (GE Healthcare Inc., Chicago, IL, USA). Empty liposomes were prepared by following the same methodology but without adding any drugs. The liposomes were stored at 4 °C and protected from light. The amount of cisplatin and mifepristone co-encapsulated in the liposomes was measured, the former with HPLC based on the method described by our group [39], and the latter with another reported method [40].

Briefly, an aliquot of liposomes was transferred to a centrifuge tube, with promegestone serving as the internal standard (IS). After adding acetonitrile to disrupt the liposome and release the encapsulated mifepristone, the solution was centrifuged at 10,000 rpm and 4 °C. The supernatant was dried under an N_2 atmosphere and resuspended in the mobile phase (water/acetonitrile), and then the sample was injected into the HPLC system. The mobile phase was a water/acetonitrile mixture delivered at 0.8 mL/min, and the detection system was set at 302 nm.

4.4. In Vitro Assay to Evaluate the Release of Cisplatin and Mifepristone from L-Cis/MF

The release of cisplatin and mifepristone from L-Cis/MF was assessed by using Franz diffusion cells assembled with a polycarbonate membrane (with 0.05 μm pores) (Millipore Corporation, Burlington, MA, USA) at 37 °C in human serum. An aliquot of L-Cis/MF was placed into the donor cell compartment (1 mL) and tamped down to the polycarbonate membrane. At specific time intervals (1, 2, 4, 8, 12, 24, 48, 72, and 96 h), the whole receptor phase medium (5 mL) was removed and replaced with an equal volume of fresh medium. The receptor phase was a saline solution for cisplatin and 2% sodium lauryl sulfate for mifepristone. The amount of cisplatin and mifepristone released was determined by the aforementioned HPLC methods.

4.5. Pharmacokinetics of L-Cis/MF

Pharmacokinetic studies were conducted on male Wistar rats anesthetized with isoflurane (Baxter, Mexico City, Mexico). The jugular vein was cannulated for the intravenous (IV) injection of the drugs, and the caudal artery was cannulated for blood sampling. Animals were randomly divided into three groups (n = 6) and given one of three treatments: (a) free cisplatin (6 mg/kg, IV); (b) free mifepristone administered subcutaneously (SC) (6.17 mg/kg); or (c) cisplatin/mifepristone-loaded liposomes (L-Cis/MF) applied IV at the same doses. Blood samples (300 μL) were collected from the caudal artery at 0, 5, 15, and 30 min and at 1, 2, 4, 6, 8, 24, 48, 72, and 96 h.

The concentration of cisplatin and mifepristone in plasma was evaluated by HPLC as aforementioned. The plasma samples were handled as detailed hereafter. The concentration of free cisplatin was determined in plasma that was ultra-filtered at 4 °C through Amicon Centriflo cones (10,000 molecular weight cut-off) immediately after drawing the blood sample. To quantify liposomal cisplatin, the methodology described by Toro-Córdova et al. (2016) was used [39]. Briefly, acetonitrile was added to 100 μL of plasma, and the samples were vortexed and centrifuged at 10,000 rpm for for 10 min. The supernatant was transferred to an Eppendorf tube and dried under N2 atmosphere. The pellet was suspended in 0.9% sodium chloride; nickel chloride was used as internal standard. After the samples were derivatized with DDTC in NaOH and incubated at 37 °C for 30 min, cisplatin was extracted with 100 µL of chloroform. Finally, 20 µL of the chloroform layer was injected into the chromatographic system, which consisted of a Waters 650E solvent delivery (Waters Assoc., Milford, MA, USA), a 20-µL loop injector (Rheodyne, Cotati, CA, USA) and a UV detector 486. Separation was carried out at 23 °C on a 150×3.9 mm ID Symmetry C18 column of 4 µm particle size. The mobile phase was a mixture of water, methanol, and acetonitrile. Detection was performed at 254 nm.

To quantify mifepristone, acetonitrile was added to an aliquot of plasma, and the mixture was centrifuged at 10,000 rpm. The resulting supernatant was dried and resuspended, and mifepristone was isolated with Oasis-HLB 3cc columns (Waters, Milford, MA, USA). The amount of mifepristone was established by utilizing the aforementioned method.

Plasma concentrations of cisplatin and mifepristone were plotted against time, and the following pharmacokinetic parameters were obtained on WinNonlin® Proffesional Edition Version 2.0 software (Certara, Princeton, NJ, USA): the area under the concentration-time curve (AUC), the elimination half-life ($t_{1/2}$), clearance (Cl), the volume of distribution (Vd), and the plasma concentration at time zero (Cmax).

4.6. Tumor Xenografts and Systemic Toxicity

Athymic (nu/nu) male nude mice (6–7 weeks of age) were inoculated SC in the back with 5×10^6 A549 (ATCC® CCL185TM) cells, a model for non-small-cell lung cancer. Tumor growth was monitored weekly by measuring two perpendicular diameters with a caliper. Tumor volume was calculated with the following equation: $V = \pi/6 \times$ (large diameter $\times$ [small diameter]/2). Once the tumor volume reached approximately 70 mm^3, the animals were randomly divided into three groups (n = 6) to initiate treatment: (1) empty liposomes (L-Control); (2) free cisplatin (5 mg/kg/week) plus free mifepristone (9.7 mg/kg/week); and (3) liposomes loaded with cisplatin (at 5 mg/kg/week) and mifepristone (at 9.7 mg/kg/week) (L-Cis/MF). All treatments were administered for three cycles (3 weeks), with an intraperitoneal injection of all drugs, except for an SC injection of free mifepristone.

A weekly evaluation was made (for 6 weeks as of the beginning of the treatments) of the therapeutic efficacy and systemic toxicity by determining the tumor volume and recording animal weight (as well as by observing the general condition of the animals). The growth rate of tumors was analyzed with a graph by plotting normalized tumor volume against the number of days after initiating treatment. Normalized tumor volume (VNi) was calculated as VNi = Vi/V0, where Vi is the volume on a specific day i, and V0 is its initial volume on day 0 [41]. Systemic toxicity was considered at 20% of weight loss. At the end of the experiment, the mice were euthanized under anesthesia (isoflurane/oxygen 3%).

4.7. Quantitative Determination of VEGF in Tumors

The level of vascular endothelial growth factor (VEGF) in the tissue of the xeno-transplants of non-small-cell lung cancer was assessed at the end of the study with an ultra-sensitive ELISA kit (ENZO Life Sciences, Farmingdale, NY, USA). Briefly, whole tumors were lysed, and the total protein content was isolated. Samples of each treatment were assayed according to the manufacturer's protocol. Optical density was measured at a wavelength of 450 nm on a Multiskan Microplate Reader (Thermo Fisher Scientific, Waltham, MA, USA). The results, calculated by using a calibration curve, were expressed as pg VEGF/g of tissue.

4.8. Statistical Analysis

Data are expressed as the mean $\pm$ standard error of the mean (SEM). Significant differences between groups (considered at $p < 0.05$) were established by one-way analysis of variance (ANOVA) followed by the Bonferroni test. These tests were processed on SPSS 20.0 software (SPSS Inc., Chicago, IL, USA).

5. Conclusions

Novel anti-cancer therapeutic strategies now exist based on nanomedicine. They represent a promising approach due to their capability for overcoming the lack of specificity in conventional chemotherapeutic delivery systems, a problem responsible for an inadequate concentration of drugs at the tumor site and toxicity for normal cells. To increase the pharmacological effect through synergism, nanoparticle delivery systems can be loaded with two drugs possessing different mechanisms of action, such as the present case of combining a chemotherapy agent (cisplatin) with a sensitizing agent (mifepristone) that counters the drug resistance mechanism of tumors. The co-encapsulation of these two drugs in a liposomal nanosystem (L-Cis/MF) led to better pharmacokinetics (i.e., a higher concentration in blood plasma over a longer period of time), correlating with greater efficacy in the control of the growth of tumors resulting from the growth of xenografts of non-small-cell lung cancer. In future research, in vitro and in vivo assays will be used to characterize the molecular mechanisms of L-Cis/MF. Additionally, this liposomal nanosystem will be applied to other types of cancer that are likely to be affected by the synergism of cisplatin and mifepristone.

Author Contributions: Conceptualization, P.G.-L.; methodology, K.O.-A.; validation, K.O.-A. and J.M.-H.; formal analysis, R.J.; investigation, M.L.-M.; data curation, R.J.; writing—original draft preparation, P.G.-L.; writing—review and editing, P.G.-L. All authors have read and agreed to the published version of the manuscript.

Funding: This research was partially funded by CONAHCYT (Mexico) through grant CF-2023-I-2771.

Institutional Review Board Statement: The animal study protocol was approved by the Ethics Committee of the National Cancer Institute, Mexico City, Mexico (2020, with Ref. # 010/015/IBI-CB/619/10).

Informed Consent Statement: Not applicable.

Data Availability Statement: Data is contained within the article.

Acknowledgments: We thank Bruce Allan Larsen for proofreading the manuscript.

Conflicts of Interest: The authors declare no conflict of interest.

References

1. Brown, A.; Kumar, S.; Tchounwou, P.B. Cisplatin-Based Chemotherapy of Human Cancers. *J. Cancer Sci. Ther.* **2019**, *11*, 97.
2. Ranasinghe, R.; Mathai, M.L.; Zulli, A. Cisplatin for cancer therapy and overcoming chemoresistance. *Heliyon* **2022**, *8*, e10608. [CrossRef]
3. Chi, R.A.; van der Watt, P.; Wei, W.; Birrer, M.J.; Leaner, V.D. Inhibition of Kpnbeta1 mediated nuclear import enhances cisplatin chemosensitivity in cervical cancer. *BMC Cancer* **2021**, *21*, 106. [CrossRef]
4. Aktepe, O.H.; Sahin, T.K.; Guner, G.; Arik, Z.; Yalcin, S. Lycopene sensitizes the cervical cancer cells to cisplatin via targeting nuclear factor- kappa B (NF-kappaB) pathway. *Turk. J. Med. Sci.* **2021**, *51*, 368–374. [CrossRef] [PubMed]
5. Li, H.; Zhang, Y.; Lan, X.; Yu, J.; Yang, C.; Sun, Z.; Kang, P.; Han, Y.; Yu, D. Halofuginone Sensitizes Lung Cancer Organoids to Cisplatin via Suppressing PI3K/AKT and MAPK Signaling Pathways. *Front. Cell Dev. Biol.* **2021**, *9*, 773048. [CrossRef]
6. Nanayakkara, A.K.; Follit, C.A.; Chen, G.; Williams, N.S.; Vogel, P.D.; Wise, J.G. Targeted inhibitors of P-glycoprotein increase chemotherapeutic-induced mortality of multidrug resistant tumor cells. *Sci. Rep.* **2018**, *8*, 967. [CrossRef]
7. Yardley, D.A. Drug resistance and the role of combination chemotherapy in improving patient outcomes. *Int. J. Breast Cancer* **2013**, *2013*, 137414. [CrossRef]
8. Segovia-Mendoza, M.; Jurado, R.; Mir, R.; Medina, L.A.; Prado-Garcia, H.; Garcia-Lopez, P. Antihormonal agents as a strategy to improve the effect of chemo-radiation in cervical cancer: In vitro and in vivo study. *BMC Cancer* **2015**, *15*, 21. [CrossRef]
9. Jurado, R.; Lopez-Flores, A.; Alvarez, A.; Garcia-Lopez, P. Cisplatin cytotoxicity is increased by mifepristone in cervical carcinoma: An in vitro and in vivo study. *Oncol. Rep.* **2009**, *22*, 1237–1245. [CrossRef]
10. Zamboni, W.C.; Gervais, A.C.; Egorin, M.J.; Schellens, J.H.; Hamburger, D.R.; Delauter, B.J.; Grim, A.; Zuhowski, E.G.; Joseph, E.; Pluim, D.; et al. Inter- and intratumoral disposition of platinum in solid tumors after administration of cisplatin. *Clin. Cancer Res.* **2002**, *8*, 2992–2999.
11. Ramon-Lopez, A.; Escudero-Ortiz, V.; Carbonell, V.; Perez-Ruixo, J.J.; Valenzuela, B. Population pharmacokinetics applied to optimising cisplatin doses in cancer patients. *Farm. Hosp.* **2012**, *36*, 392–402. [CrossRef] [PubMed]
12. Karasawa, T.; Sibrian-Vazquez, M.; Strongin, R.M.; Steyger, P.S. Identification of cisplatin-binding proteins using agarose conjugates of platinum compounds. *PLoS ONE* **2013**, *8*, e66220. [CrossRef] [PubMed]

13. Chang, Q.; Ornatsky, O.I.; Siddiqui, I.; Straus, R.; Baranov, V.I.; Hedley, D.W. Biodistribution of cisplatin revealed by imaging mass cytometry identifies extensive collagen binding in tumor and normal tissues. *Sci. Rep.* **2016**, *6*, 36641. [CrossRef] [PubMed]
14. Sarkar, N.N. Mifepristone: Bioavailability, pharmacokinetics and use-effectiveness. *Eur. J. Obstet. Gynecol. Reprod. Biol.* **2002**, *101*, 113–120. [CrossRef] [PubMed]
15. Ledezma-Gallegos, F.; Jurado, R.; Mir, R.; Medina, L.A.; Mondragon-Fuentes, L.; Garcia-Lopez, P. Liposomes Co-Encapsulating Cisplatin/Mifepristone Improve the Effect on Cervical Cancer: In Vitro and In Vivo Assessment. *Pharmaceutics* **2020**, *12*, 897. [CrossRef]
16. Novais, M.V.M.; Gomes, E.R.; Miranda, M.C.; Silva, J.O.; Gomes, D.A.; Braga, F.C.; Pádua, R.M.; Oliveira, M.C. Liposomes co-encapsulating doxorubicin and glucoevatromonoside derivative induce synergic cytotoxic response against breast cancer cell lines. *Biomed. Pharmacother.* **2021**, *136*, 111123. [CrossRef]
17. Dasari, S.; Tchounwou, P.B. Cisplatin in cancer therapy: Molecular mechanisms of action. *Eur. J. Pharmacol.* **2014**, *740*, 364–378. [CrossRef]
18. Kapperman, H.E.; Goyeneche, A.A.; Telleria, C.M. Mifepristone inhibits non-small cell lung carcinoma cellular escape from DNA damaging cisplatin. *Cancer Cell Int.* **2018**, *18*, 185. [CrossRef]
19. Rosenblum, D.; Joshi, N.; Tao, W.; Karp, J.M.; Peer, D. Progress and challenges towards targeted delivery of cancer therapeutics. *Nat. Commun.* **2018**, *9*, 1410. [CrossRef]
20. Fumoto, S.; Nishida, K. Co-delivery Systems of Multiple Drugs Using Nanotechnology for Future Cancer Therapy. *Chem Pharm Bull* **2020**, *68*, 603–612. [CrossRef]
21. Al Bostami, R.D.; Abuwatfa, W.H.; Husseini, G.A. Recent Advances in Nanoparticle-Based Co-Delivery Systems for Cancer Therapy. *Nanomaterials* **2022**, *12*, 2672. [CrossRef]
22. Yang, J.; Jin, R.M.; Wang, S.Y.; Xie, X.T.; Hu, W.; Tang, H.F.; Liu, B. Co-delivery of paclitaxel and doxorubicin using polypeptide-engineered nanogels for combination therapy of tumor. *Nanotechnology* **2022**, *33*. [CrossRef] [PubMed]
23. Qi, S.S.; Sun, J.H.; Yu, H.H.; Yu, S.Q. Co-delivery nanoparticles of anti-cancer drugs for improving chemotherapy efficacy. *Drug Deliv.* **2017**, *24*, 1909–1926. [CrossRef] [PubMed]
24. Sun, C.; Wang, X.; Zheng, Z.; Chen, D.; Wang, X.; Shi, F.; Yu, D.; Wu, H. A single dose of dexamethasone encapsulated in polyethylene glycol-coated polylactic acid nanoparticles attenuates cisplatin-induced hearing loss following round window membrane administration. *Int. J. Nanomed.* **2015**, *10*, 3567–3579. [CrossRef]
25. Mendes, L.P.; Gaeti, M.P.; de Avila, P.H.; de Sousa Vieira, M.; Dos Santos Rodrigues, B.; de Avila Marcelino, R.I.; Dos Santos, L.C.; Valadares, M.C.; Lima, E.M. Multicompartimental nanoparticles for co-encapsulation and multimodal drug delivery to tumor cells and neovasculature. *Pharm. Res.* **2014**, *31*, 1106–1119. [CrossRef] [PubMed]
26. Dhar, S.; Gu, F.X.; Langer, R.; Farokhzad, O.C.; Lippard, S.J. Targeted delivery of cisplatin to prostate cancer cells by aptamer functionalized Pt(IV) prodrug-PLGA-PEG nanoparticles. *Proc. Natl. Acad. Sci. USA* **2008**, *105*, 17356–17361. [CrossRef] [PubMed]
27. Das, S.; Jagan, L.; Isiah, R.; Rajesh, B.; Backianathan, S.; Subhashini, J. Nanotechnology in oncology: Characterization and in vitro release kinetics of cisplatin-loaded albumin nanoparticles: Implications in anticancer drug delivery. *Indian. J. Pharmacol.* **2011**, *43*, 409–413. [CrossRef]
28. Yücel, Ç.; Değim, Z.; Yilmaz, Ş. Development of Cisplatin-loaded Liposome and Evaluation of Transport Prop-596 erties Through Caco-2 Cell Line. *Turk. J. Pharm. Sci.* **2016**, *13*, 95–108. [CrossRef]
29. Nsairat, H.; Khater, D.; Sayed, U.; Odeh, F.; Al Bawab, A.; Alshaer, W. Liposomes: Structure, composition, types, and clinical applications. *Heliyon* **2022**, *8*, e09394. [CrossRef]
30. Gupta, S.; De Mel, J.U.; Schneider, G.J. Dynamics of liposomes in the fluid phase. *Curr. Opin. Colloid. Interface Sci.* **2019**, *42*, 121–136. [CrossRef]
31. Liu, P.; Chen, G.; Zhang, J. A Review of Liposomes as a Drug Delivery System: Current Status of Approved Products, Regulatory Environments, and Future Perspectives. *Molecules* **2022**, *27*, 1372. [CrossRef] [PubMed]
32. Salmaso, S.; Caliceti, P. Stealth properties to improve therapeutic efficacy of drug nanocarriers. *J. Drug Deliv.* **2013**, *2013*, 374252. [CrossRef] [PubMed]
33. Papini, E.; Tavano, R.; Mancin, F. Opsonins and Dysopsonins of Nanoparticles: Facts, Concepts, and Methodological Guidelines. *Front. Immunol.* **2020**, *11*, 567365. [CrossRef] [PubMed]
34. Yao, Y.; Zhou, Y.; Liu, L.; Xu, Y.; Chen, Q.; Wang, Y.; Wu, S.; Deng, Y.; Zhang, J.; Shao, A. Nanoparticle-Based Drug Delivery in Cancer Therapy and Its Role in Overcoming Drug Resistance. *Front. Mol. Biosci.* **2020**, *7*, 193. [CrossRef] [PubMed]
35. Li, Y.; Wang, J.; Wientjes, M.G.; Au, J.L. Delivery of nanomedicines to extracellular and intracellular compartments of a solid tumor. *Adv. Drug Deliv. Rev.* **2012**, *64*, 29–39. [CrossRef]
36. Subhan, M.A.; Yalamarty, S.S.K.; Filipczak, N.; Parveen, F.; Torchilin, V.P. Recent Advances in Tumor Targeting via EPR Effect for Cancer Treatment. *J. Pers. Med.* **2021**, *11*, 571. [CrossRef]
37. Dadpour, S.; Mehrabian, A.; Arabsalmani, M.; Mirhadi, E.; Askarizadeh, A.; Mashreghi, M.; Jaafari, M.R. The role of size in PEGylated liposomal doxorubicin biodistribution and anti-tumour activity. *IET Nanobiotechnol.* **2022**, *16*, 259–272. [CrossRef]
38. Heikinheimo, O.; Pesonen, U.; Huupponen, R.; Koulu, M.; Lahteenmaki, P. Hepatic metabolism and distribution of mifepristone and its metabolites in rats. *Hum. Reprod.* **1994**, *9* (Suppl. 1), 40–46. [CrossRef]

39. Toro-Cordova, A.; Ledezma-Gallegos, F.; Mondragon-Fuentes, L.; Jurado, R.; Medina, L.A.; Perez-Rojas, J.M.; Garcia-Lopez, P. Determination of Liposomal Cisplatin by High-Performance Liquid Chromatography and Its Application in Pharmacokinetic Studies. *J. Chromatogr. Sci.* **2016**, *54*, 1016–1021. [CrossRef]
40. Guo, Z.; Wang, S.; Wei, D.; Zhai, J. Development of a high-performance liquid chromatographic method for the determination of mifepristone in human plasma using norethisterone as an internal standard: Application to pharmacokinetic study. *Contraception* **2007**, *76*, 228–232. [CrossRef]
41. Medina, L.A.; Herrera-Penilla, B.I.; Castro-Morales, M.A.; Garcia-Lopez, P.; Jurado, R.; Perez-Cardenas, E.; Chanona-Vilchis, J.; Brandan, M.E. Use of an orthovoltage X-ray treatment unit as a radiation research system in a small-animal cancer model. *J. Exp. Clin. Cancer Res.* **2008**, *27*, 57. [CrossRef] [PubMed]

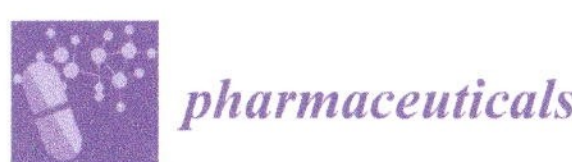

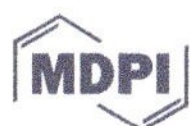

pharmaceuticals

Article

Enhanced Antidepressant Activity of Nanostructured Lipid Carriers Containing Levosulpiride in Behavioral Despair Tests in Mice

Sadia Tabassam Arif [1], Muhammad Ayub Khan [1], Shahiq uz Zaman [1], Hafiz Shoaib Sarwar [2], Abida Raza [3], Muhammad Sarfraz [4], Yousef A. Bin Jardan [5], Muhammad Umair Amin [6] and Muhammad Farhan Sohail [7,*]

[1] Riphah Institute of Pharmaceutical Sciences, Riphah International University, Islamabad 44000, Pakistan; tabassamsadia96@yahoo.com (S.T.A.); mayubkhan73@yahoo.com (M.A.K.); shahiq.zaman@riphah.edu.pk (S.u.Z.)
[2] Faculty of Pharmaceutical Sciences, University of Central Punjab, Lahore 54000, Pakistan; shoaib.sarwar@ucp.edu.pk
[3] Nanomedicine Research Laboratory, National Institute of Lasers and Optronics (NILOP), PIEAS, Islamabad 45650, Pakistan; abida_rao@yahoo.com
[4] College of Pharmacy, Al Ain University, Al Ain 64141, United Arab Emirates; muhammad.sarfraz@aau.ac.ae
[5] Department of Pharmaceutics, College of Pharmacy, King Saud University, Riyadh 11451, Saudi Arabia; ybinjardan@ksu.edu.sa
[6] Department of Pharmaceutics and Biopharmaceutics, University of Marburg, 35032 Marburg, Germany; umairami@staff.uni-marburg.de
[7] Riphah Institute of Pharmaceutical Sciences, Riphah International University Lahore Campus, Lahore 54000, Pakistan
*   Correspondence: farmacist.pk@gmail.com

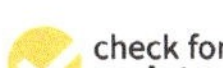

Citation: Arif, S.T.; Khan, M.A.; Zaman, S.u.; Sarwar, H.S.; Raza, A.; Sarfraz, M.; Bin Jardan, Y.A.; Amin, M.U.; Sohail, M.F. Enhanced Antidepressant Activity of Nanostructured Lipid Carriers Containing Levosulpiride in Behavioral Despair Tests in Mice. *Pharmaceuticals* **2023**, *16*, 1220. https://doi.org/10.3390/ph16091220

Academic Editors: José Manuel Sousa Lobo, João Nuno Moreira, Ana Catarina Silva and Guendalina Zuccari

Received: 25 July 2023
Revised: 12 August 2023
Accepted: 20 August 2023
Published: 29 August 2023

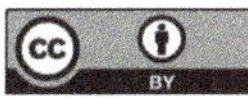

Abstract: The potential of levosulpiride-loaded nanostructured lipid carriers (LSP-NLCs) for enhanced antidepressant and anxiolytic effects was evaluated in the current study. A forced swim test (FST) and tail suspension test (TST) were carried out to determine the antidepressant effect whereas anxiolytic activity was investigated using light–dark box and open field tests. Behavioral changes were evaluated in lipopolysaccharide-induced depressed animals. The access of LSP to the brain to produce therapeutic effects was estimated qualitatively by using fluorescently labeled LSP-NLCs. The distribution of LSP-NLCs was analyzed using ex vivo imaging of major organs after oral and intraperitoneal administration. Acute toxicity studies were carried out to assess the safety of LSP-NLCs in vivo. An improved antidepressant effect of LSP-NLCs on LPS-induced depression showed an increase in swimming time (237 ± 51 s) and struggling time (226 ± 15 s) with a reduction in floating (123 ± 51 s) and immobility time (134 ± 15 s) in FST and TST. The anxiolytic activity in the light–dark box and open field tests exhibited superiority over LSP dispersion. Near-infrared images of fluorescently labeled LSP-NLCs demonstrated the presence of coumarin dye in the brain after 1 h of administration. An acute toxicity study revealed no significant changes in organ-to-body weight ratio, serum biochemistry or tissue histology of major organs. It can be concluded that nanostructured lipid carriers can efficiently deliver LSP to the brain for improved therapeutic efficacy.

Keywords: levosulpiride; antidepressant; nanostructured lipid carriers; acute toxicity; in vivo imaging

1. Introduction

Mental and behavioral disorders affect approximately one billion people globally, as reported by the World Health Organization (WHO). According to an estimate, 12 billion workdays are lost every year because of depression and anxiety, which costs the global economy USD 1 trillion [1]. Among these psychiatric diseases, depression is the second highest threatening mental health illness, resulting in an increased economic burden worldwide [2]. Depression and anxiety are comorbid conditions with prominent features that include lack of motivation, emotional instability, sleep distress, loss of interest in social activities and a higher incidence of suicidal tendencies [3]. Disturbance in transmission from presynaptic to postsynaptic neurons of major neurotransmitters like dopamine, serotonin and norepinephrine is the leading cause of depression [4]. The therapeutic response of depressed, anxious patients to available treatments is disappointing despite the adherence. The continuous presence of antidepressants at the site of action for a prolonged period is necessary for their efficacy. Route of administration plays a pivotal role in delivering therapeutically effective drugs to the brain. The blood-brain barrier, efflux transporters and blood-cerebrospinal fluid barrier portray major hindrances for orally administered drugs circulating in the blood after absorption [5].

An efficient drug delivery system that can maximize drug concentration in the brain should possess prominent features of prolonged-release rate, improved bioavailability and enhanced permeability [6]. The administration of antidepressant drugs through lipid nanocarriers satisfies these assumptions [7]. Nanostructured lipid carriers (NLCs) purport to be a promising formulation to deliver lipophilic drugs to the brain. Being a lipid-based formulation, it has the advantage of bioacceptability and rapid uptake by the brain. Nanostructured lipid carriers are the second generation of lipid nanoparticles that overcome the limitation of other lipid formulations including larger particle size, instability, drug expulsion, inability to target brain tissues and problems in scaling up [8]. These lipid nanoparticles have improved the transport of drugs to the brain by offering high drug entrapment, improved biological physical stability, reduced toxicity, and loading of both hydrophilic and lipophilic drugs [9,10]. The imperfections created by liquid lipids prevent the polymorphic transitions of solid lipids to a highly ordered crystal structure leading to the conception of NLCs which are solid, but not crystalline. This is derived from the fact that the crystallization process itself causes the expulsion of the drug, as evident in first generation counterparts composed of solid lipid alone [11]. By using binary mixtures of solid lipids and liquid lipids, the particles become solid after cooling but do not crystallize. NLC has easily stabilized with the minimum possible concentration of surfactants along with the best results of stability, entrapment, and release [12].

Levosulpiride (Figure 1A) is a benzamide derivative with antipsychotic, antidepressant and prokinetic activity. It inhibits the dopamine D_2 receptors at the trigger zone in the central and peripheral nervous system [13]. Due to the high selectivity of D_2 inhibition, LSP has a low sedation and hypotensive effect. Levosulpiride has low bioavailability (20–30%) at the dosage range of 100–200 mg after oral administration. The time to reach peak plasma concentration is 3 h with a half-life of approximately 6 h depending on the dose and route of administration. Being less soluble with low permeability, levosulpiride has difficulty penetrating the blood-brain barrier after oral administration [13].

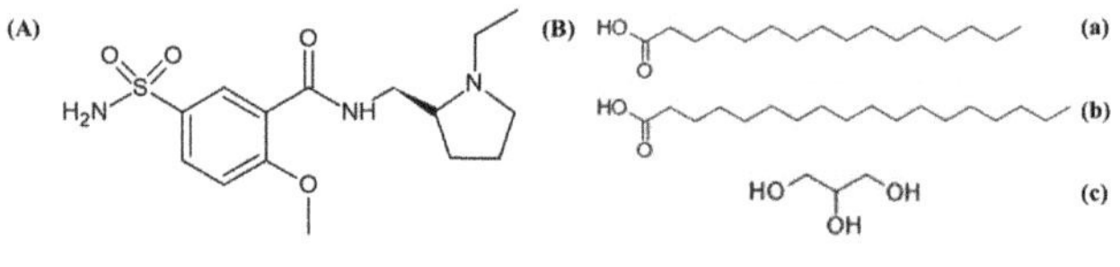

Figure 1. Chemical structure depiction of (**A**) levosulpiride and (**B**) component compounds of Precirol ATO 5. (a) Palmitic Acid, (b) Stearic Acid and (c) Glycerin.

In a previous study, we developed, optimized and characterized LSP-loaded NLCs which significantly increased bioavailability and enhanced the prokinetic efficacy of LSP after oral administration, but the antipsychotic and antidepressant effect of LSP-NLCs was not determined. Our current study aims to investigate the antipsychotic and antidepressant efficacy of LSP when administered through NLCs. Near-infrared fluorescence (NIRF) imaging was performed to determine the biodistribution of LSP-NLCs after administration. An acute toxicity study of LSP was carried out in rats.

2. Results and Discussion

2.1. Particle Characterization and Entrapment Efficiency

The developed optimized LSP-NLCs were subjected to particle size analysis, and PDI value and zeta potential were also measured. Optimized LSP-NLCs showed a mean particle size of 151.2 $\pm$ 1.06 nm in terms of % intensity (Figure 2). The obtained PDI value of LSP-NLCs was 0.25 $\pm$ 0.02, showing a narrow size and uniformly homogeneous distribution. The literature suggests that nanoparticles with a size of less than 200 nm show efficient absorption in the intestine and have a tendency to bypass uptake by the reticuloendothelial system and hepatocytes. These characteristics anticipate an enhanced LSP bioavailability with extended blood circulation and effective transport of LSP-NLCs to the brain to attain the desired therapeutic levels [14,15]. LSP-NLCs showed a zeta potential value of -23.17 ± 3.37 mV. Previously, it was reported that Tween 80 and Labrasol were responsible for the steric stabilization of the nano-formulation. In the presence of steric stabilization along with electrostatic stabilization, the lipid nano-formulations exhibited adequate physical stability at a zeta potential value of -20 mV. A zeta potential value of -23.17 ± 3.37 mV on the surface of LSP-NLCs demonstrated the LSP orientation within the lipid matrix and the prospects for physical stability of LSP-NLC formulation. Moreover, the highly negatively charged nanoparticles were reported to be more favorable for brain drug delivery than positively charged nanoparticles as they may compromise the blood-brain barrier integrity [16,17]. The LSP-NLCs showed a high incorporation efficiency of $86 \pm 3.1\%$, which could be due to the addition of the liquid lipid in the lipid matrix.

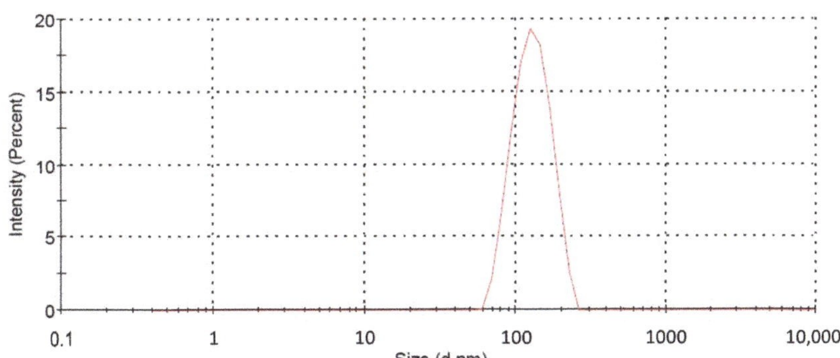

Figure 2. Particle size distribution curve.

2.2. Biodistribution Study

LSP-NLCs were physically tagged with coumarin 6 to make them fluorescent to track the biodistribution after subjecting them to NIRF imaging. The movement of F-NLCs in the GIT was tracked by harvesting the stomach, intestine and colon after oral administration at 0.5 h, 1 h, 2 h and 4 h. Ex vivo imaging studies were examined in excised organs (brain, heart, liver, kidneys) to identify the relative fluorescent signal at the abovementioned time points after an I.P. injection. The reason for the selection of the I.P route to determine the biodistribution of LSP-NLCs in different organs other than the GIT system was to avoid the digestion of NLCs in the small intestine as the coumarin-6 was physically tagged within the F-NLCs. The results in Figure 3A show ex vivo optical imaging in GIT to confirm the F-NLC movement. At the initial time point (0.5 h), a strong fluorescent signal was observed in the stomach which decreased with the increasing time intervals showing the gastric emptying of the stomach. Subsequently, the fluorescent signal in the initial part of the intestine was observed at the time point of 1 h after oral administration. A drop in florescent intensity with the movement to the lower portion of the intestine was translated as the absorption of F-NLCs in the intestine and GIT movements [18]. The fluorescence that appeared in the colon after 2 h was consistent throughout the colon and disappeared after 4 h, demonstrating no absorption in the colon. It is assumed that the florescent dye was disassociated from F-NLCs after the digestion process in the intestine and the luminal content was a mixture of unabsorbed coumarin and lipid digests. The ex vivo images exhibited in Figure 3B show that the signal for fluorescence intensity was increased in a time-dependent manner in the obtained organs, which indicates that the F-NLCs were absorbed from the peritoneal cavity and were available in the blood circulation from which they were distributed to different organs. The brain was the main organ of interest to study the biodistribution of NLCs as the concentration of LSP in the brain determines the therapeutic efficacy of the LSP in depression and anxiety treatments along with the role of NLCs in brain drug delivery. The fluorescent images of the brain showed a low intensity of fluorescence after 30 min of I.P injection whereas the maximum brain accumulation was observed after 1 h. Afterward, a decrease in fluorescence was detected. The strong fluorescence signal in the brain established the fact that LSP-NLCs have the tendency to pass the blood-brain barrier and increase the bioavailability of LSP in the brain. The possible mechanisms behind this phenomenon could be smaller particle size, which enhances permeability due to lipid nature [19,20], membrane fluidization due to the presence of surfactants, efflux pumps blocking the brain endothelial cells [21,22], and possible endocytosis or cytopempsis of the NLCs [23]. Furthermore, previously it was reported that low molecular weight and lipophilicity of the drug also play a role in the passive diffusion of the drug molecule which could also be a factor in enhanced brain delivery of LSP. Fewer signals in the liver and kidneys showed little accumulation of F-NLCs in the liver and the kidneys. The ex vivo images of the heart also presented a faint signal showing an insufficient amount of F-NLCs [13,24].

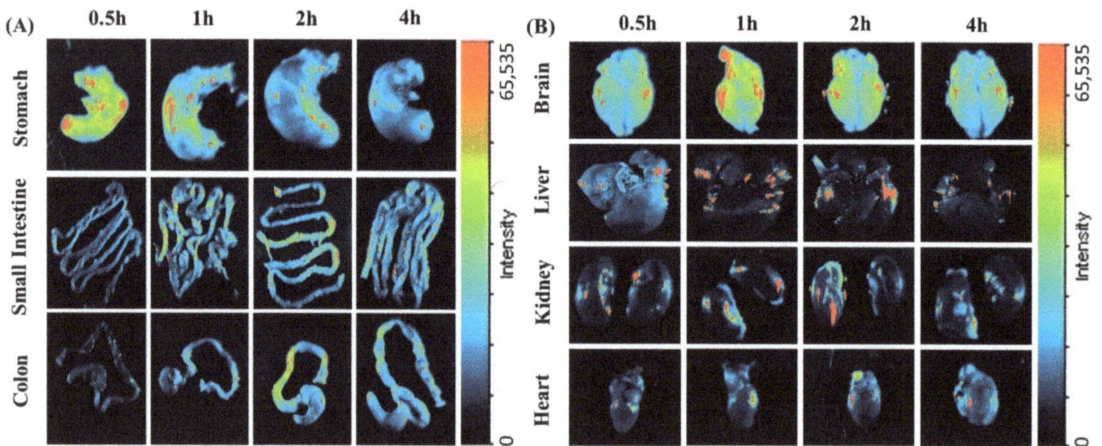

Figure 3. Fluorescent images of excised mice organs (**A**) stomach, small intestine and colon after oral administration (**B**) brain, liver, kidneys and heart after I.P injection of coumarin-6 labeled NLCs.

2.3. Antidepressant and Anxiolytic Activity

In an attempt to elucidate the treatment response to underlying psychiatric illness, complementary behavioral tests were performed to assess LPS-induced antidepressant and anxiolytic effects. LPS has been extensively used to induce behavioral changes in rodents which mimic depression and anxiety symptoms. These symptoms exhibit as behavioral despair, disturbance in the expression of inflammatory markers and alteration in neurotropic transmission. The antidepressant and anxiolytic effect of LSP-NLCs and LSP-DPN was evaluated in an LPS-induced depression and anxiety model after oral delivery. Struggling and immobility time in the forced swim test and tail suspension test were taken as a measure of the efficacy of the optimized LSP-NLCs. The LPS injection significantly reduced the swimming time of mice (142 ± 30 s) in the negative control group to which no treatment was given, indicating the induction of depression as compared to the P-Control group (260 ± 27 s). When LSP-NLCs and LSP dispersion were administered orally there was increased swimming time (237 ± 51 s & 157 ± 36 s) and reduced immobility (123 ± 51 s & 203 ± 35.6 s) as compared to the N-Control group (Figure 4A,B). The tail suspension test showed similar results to those from the FST. The obtained results (Figure 4C,D) suggest that LSP-NLCs substantially increased the struggling time to 226 ± 15 s and reduced immobility time to 134 ± 15 s, which was greater than that of LSP-DPN administered orally (212 ± 31, 148 ± 30.8 s). The results mentioned in Table 1 show a significant increase (119 ± 10 s) in the time spent and number of entries (7 ± 2) in the lightbox as compared to LPS-induced anxious mice. Similarly, the mouse group treated with LSP-NLCs showed an increase in the time spent in the central compartment and the number of compartments crossed (Table 1). Results from the pharmacodynamics studies (behavioral despair) revealed the effective delivery of levosulpiride loaded in NLCs through the oral pathway. Levosulpiride delivery in the form of NLCs enhanced the bioavailability of the LSP in systemic circulation ultimately leading to augmented brain delivery when compared with an equivalent dose of dispersion. The behavioral changes revealed in the pharmacodynamics studies in mice can be explained by the antagonist effect of LSP on D_2 receptors. The selective blockade of the D_2 receptor at presynaptic and postsynaptic neurons increases the behavioral response in depressed and anxious mice by controlling the synthesis and release of dopamine [25,26].

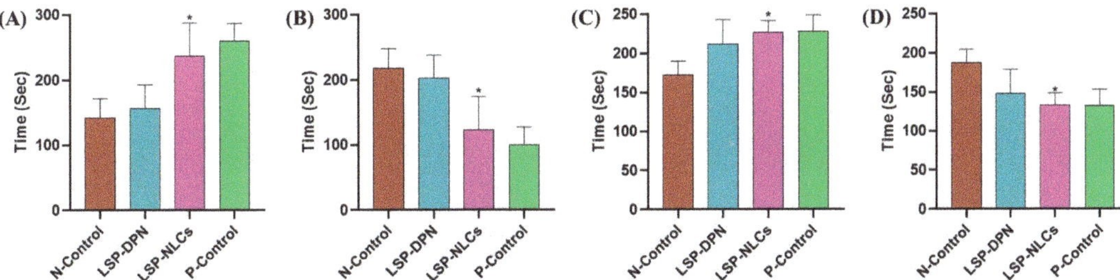

Figure 4. The effect of LSP dispersion (LSP-DPN) and LSP-NLCs on the (**A**) swimming time, (**B**) floating time in the forced swim test, (**C**) struggle time and (**D**) immobility time in the tail suspension test in LPS-induced depressed mice. The data are presented as mean ± S.D (n = 3). Data were analyzed by one-way ANOVA followed by Dunnett's test. * $p < 0.05$ compared to the negative control (LPS only) group.

Table 1. Comparison of the results of light–dark box model (time spent and number of entries into lightbox) and open field test (number of quadrants invaded and central compartment resting time) among the different treated and control groups.

Groups	Light Dark Box Model		Open Field Test	
	Time Spent in Light Box	**Number of Entries in the Lightbox**	**Number of Quadrant Invasion**	**Central Compartment Resting Time**
Positive control	144 ± 73	5 ± 2	76 ± 19	11 ± 9
Negative control	52 ± 34	2 ± 2	19 ± 5	2 ± 2
LSP dispersion	76 ± 32	4 ± 1	44 ± 12	3 ± 2
LSP-NLCs	119 ± 10 *	7 ± 2 *	75 ± 22 **	6 ± 2 *

Data are presented as mean ± S.D (n = 3). Data were analyzed by one-way ANOVA followed by Dunnett's test. * $p < 0.05$, ** $p < 0.01$ among treated vs. negative control.

2.4. Acute Oral Toxicity Study

2.4.1. Body Weight Measurements, Observation of Clinical Signs and Food Consumption

In vivo toxic effects of LSP and LSP-NLCs were evaluated at a comparatively higher concentration of 50 mg/kg of LSP. The treatments were orally administered to each mouse in the treated groups whereas normal saline was given to the control group. After the administration of specific treatment, the mice were monitored for 48 h for specific parameters (any change in the behavior pattern, physical appearance, occurrence of clinical or toxicological symptoms, feed consumption, and mortality) and after that were observed daily to check the occurrence of any toxic event macroscopically. No animal mortality or prominent exterior signs of toxicity were recorded. All the experimental animals showed normal patterns of physical condition and behavior. The body weights of the animals at day 0 and day 14 are given in Figure 5A. No significant change in body weight among the control and treated groups was noted throughout the duration of the study. On day 14, before the utilization of the mice to collect different organs for further study, the blood samples were taken from all mice individually and hematology and serum biochemistry analyses were performed.

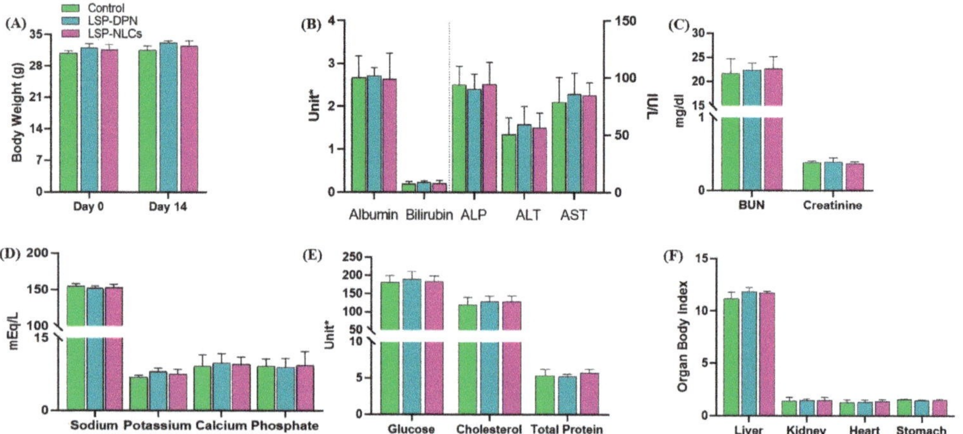

Figure 5. Evaluation of acute oral toxicity through analysis of (**A**) body weight comparison, serum biochemical analysis of blood, (**B**) liver function tests, (**C**) renal function tests, (**D**) serum electrolytes, (**E**) glucose, cholesterol, total protein and (**F**) organ body index after treatment with LSP dispersion (LSP-DPN) and LSP-NLCs. Data are represented as mean ± S.D (n = 3). Unit = Albumin (g/dL), Bilirubin (mg/dL), ALP (IU/L), ALT (IU/L), AST (IU/L), Glucose (mg/dL), Cholesterol (mg/dL), Total protein (g/dL).

2.4.2. Hematology Analysis

For a drug nanocarrier system, the most critical task is to ensure compatibility with the blood to avoid any unwanted inflammatory response which mostly occurs due to incompatibility with blood components. The hematological data results in Table 2 exhibit that no statistically significant differences were present among the treatment-exposed groups and the control group. The complete blood count results of all treated mice showed normal levels of total red blood cells, white blood cells, hemoglobin, and platelet count as well as packed cell volume, hematocrit, mean corpuscular volume and mean corpuscular hemoglobin in the peripheral blood and the results of treated groups remained in close proximity to the results for the control group.

Table 2. Hematological analysis of mice blood in acute toxicity studies after 14 days of oral administration of LSP dispersion (LSP-DPN) and LSP-NLCs.

Group	WBC ($\times 10^9$/L)	RBC ($\times 10^{12}$/L)	HCT %	Hb (g/dL)	MCV (fL)	MCH (pg)	PCV (%)	Platelets ($\times 10^9$/L)
Control	8.7 ± 2.3	8.4 ± 2.5	39.0 ± 2.9	14.5 ± 1.6	47.2 ± 3.1	14.4 ± 2.7	50.4 ± 7.4	762.3 ± 30.6
LSP-DPN	9.2 ± 2.5	9.4 ± 3.6	42.0 ± 2.5	15.1 ± 2.9	49.2 ± 1.9	15.0 ± 2.8	48.2 ± 5.1	755.1 ± 41.0
LSP-NLCs	8.9 ± 2.9	8.6 ± 2.8	40.3 ± 3.0	15.2 ± 2.2	48.8 ± 3.7	16.1 ± 2.4	48.8 ± 5.5	752.9 ± 52.5

Data are presented as mean ± S.D (n = 3).

2.4.3. Serum Biochemistry

Serum biochemistry parameters were analyzed to check for any abnormal effect of the LSP suspension and LSP-NLCs on the integrity and functions of the liver and kidneys. Liver function test parameters are shown in Figure 5B. The functionality of liver cells is described by the albumin levels which were not affected by the LSP dispersion or LSP-NLCs treatment. An insignificant difference in the level of alanine aminotransferase and alkaline phosphate was observed with LSP-DPN and LSP-NLCs compared to that of the controls and the values fall within the acceptable limits. Cellular integrity of the liver cells is portrayed through alanine aminotransferase and alkaline phosphate which are produced as indicators of the function of liver cells. An increased alanine aminotransferase level specifies cell damage or necrosis due to the outflow of this enzyme from liver cells to the blood. Elevated alkaline phosphate levels also illustrate cholestatic liver disease with liver cell damage connected with the bile duct. Normal aspartate aminotransferase values of the treated groups with an insignificant difference from the control show the integrity of the vital organs. A high aspartate aminotransferase level is a sign of organ damage. The liver is also the main production site for serum proteins and any variation in the total protein content shows liver abnormality. No significant changes were observed in the total bilirubin level. However, the total protein levels were unaffected by LSP-DPN and LSP-NLC treatment. The influence of LSP-NLCs on liver function tests was insignificant ($p > 0.05$). To evaluate the consequence of LSP-NLC treatment on the kidneys, renal function tests (RFTs) were performed. The outcomes in Figure 5C disclose no significant variation from the RFTs reference values among the treated and untreated control groups. All the treatments did not affect the creatinine and BUN levels. For further toxicity assessment induced by LSP-NLC treatment, serum electrolytes (Na, K, Ca, and P) were assessed. The results (Figure 5D) revealed no changes in serum Na and K levels in the case of LSP-NLCs compared to the control. No changes were observed in the levels of Ca and P compared with the control. The results in Figure 5E present no alteration in glucose levels and cholesterol levels were also unchanged in all groups compared to the control [27,28].

2.4.4. Organ to Body Ratio

The weights of the vital organs are considered a good parameter for the evaluation of in vivo toxicity. After 14 days of treatment exposure, the organ-to-body ratio of the vital organs including the liver, kidneys, heart and stomach was calculated. The organ-to-body index results (Figure 5F) exhibited no significant changes for all test organs from the treated groups when compared to the control.

2.4.5. Histopathology of Vital Organs

The macroscopic inspection of the heart, kidneys, liver and stomach did not display any observable variations or lesions on these organs. For further investigation, tissue histology studies were executed on the slides prepared from test organs, as presented in Figure 6. The normal morphological architecture was observed in microphotographs of tissue slides of all the vital organs from the control and treated groups. The macroscopic inspection of the heart, kidneys, liver and stomach did not display any observable variations or lesions on these organs. A normal arrangement of cardiac myofibrils and myocytes was observed without any structural change. Also, no signs of cardiac damage, necrosis, infiltration, inflammation, hemorrhage, vacuolization, or myocardial infarction were observed in all treated groups. Figure 6 shows that no morphological change occurred in the kidneys of the treated groups. The glomerular structure presented a regular appearance in the treated groups, which was similar to the control groups, without any interstitial and intraglomerular congestion or tubular atrophies. All the nephrons appeared to be normal without any degeneration or necrosis. In the microscopic examination of the liver slides, the hepatocytes displayed normal morphology with no signs of fatty accumulation, injury, or necrosis. These findings support the outcomes obtained from liver function tests and renal function tests demonstrating the safety of LSP-NLCs. Similarly, no signs of disruption were seen in the microscopic images of the stomach among the control and treated groups. The gastric mucosa appeared to be intact with a typical histological architecture and normal epithelium and glands.

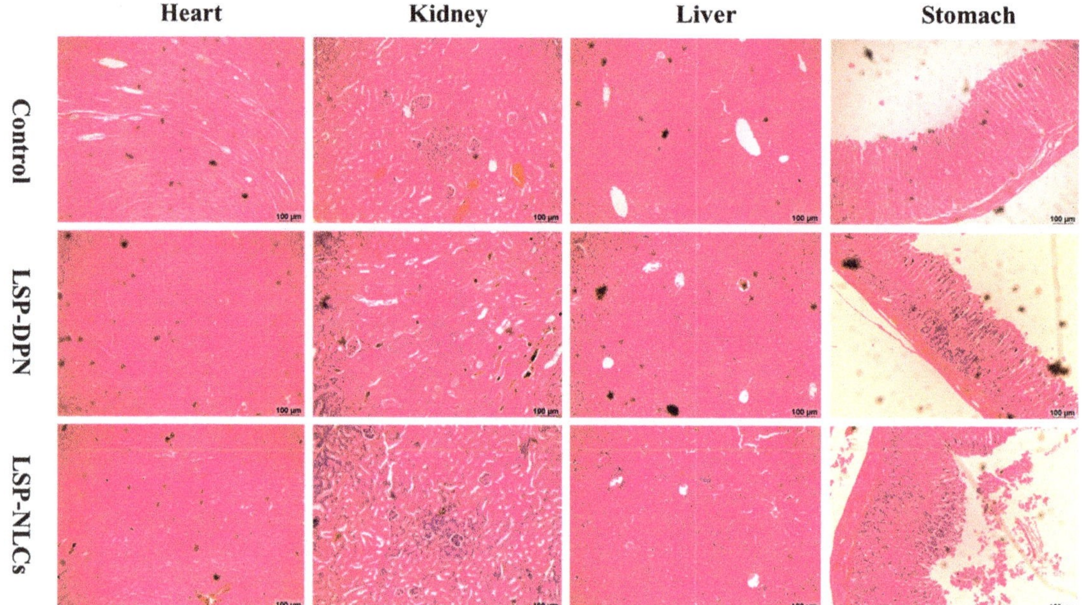

Figure 6. Histological microscopic images of vital organs of heart, kidneys, liver and stomach of mice on day 14 after treatment with LSP dispersion (LSP-DPN) and LSP-NLCs.

3. Materials and Methods

3.1. Materials

Levosulpiride was a kind gift from Bio-Lab Pvt. Ltd., Islamabad, Pakistan. Precirol® ATO5 (Glyceryl palmitostearate, Figure 1B) and Labrasol® (Caprylocaproyl Polyoxyl-8 glycerides) were generous gift by Gattefossé (Cedex, France). Coumarin, Tween 80 (polyoxyethylenesorbitan monooleate) and Span 80 (Sorbitan Monooleate) were purchased from Sigma-Aldrich (St. Louis, MO, USA). Methanol, acetonitrile and chloroform of HPLC grade were purchased from Merck (Hohenbrunn, Germany). All other chemicals were of analytical grade and were used without further purification.

3.2. Preparation of LSP-NLCs

LSP-NLCs were prepared using a hot homogenization ultrasonication technique. For this purpose, solid and liquid lipids and Span 80 were weighed and put into a glass vial. To obtain lipid melt, the glass vial was maintained at 70 °C in a water bath. Then, a definite amount of LSP was added to the melted lipids and mixed well in the molten lipids to completely dissolve the drug. For the preparation of an aqueous phase, surfactant Tween 80 was dissolved in distilled water in a separate vial and heated up to 70 °C. Then, this hot aqueous phase was poured into the lipid phase and homogenized using a homogenizer (HG-15D, DAIHAN Scientific, Wonju, Republic of Korea at 15,000 rpm for 5 min. The temperature of the system was maintained at 70 °C. A coarse o/w emulsion was obtained which was further sonicated for 3 min at an amplitude of 50% and power of 100 W using a probe sonicator (Vibracell™ VCX750; Sonics and Materials Inc., Newtown, CT, USA). The obtained nano-emulsion was rapidly cooled down in a glass jar filled with ice to obtain LSP-NLCs.

In our previous study, an initial screening was carried out to select the suitable solid, liquid lipid and surfactant. Precirol ATO 5 was selected as the solid lipid and Labrasol was chosen as the liquid lipid. The preferred surfactants used were Span 80 and Tween 80. The selection of the lipids was based on the solubility of levosulpiride in different lipids, whereas the selection of the surfactants was determined by the homogeneity and stability of the formulation. The LSP-loaded NLCs were optimized based on particle size, PDI value and entrapment efficiency. Design-Expert software (version 13, Stat-Ease Inc., Minneapolis, MN, USA) was used to find the optimal mixture composition of lipids and surfactants. Numerical optimization with desirability function was carried out to obtain the optimal formulation. The composition of the optimized formulation was 80.55% Precirol$^{®®}$ ATO 5, 19.45% Labrasol and 5% Tween 80/Span 80 mixture. The detailed results of the preliminary study have been described in Sadia et al. [29].

3.3. Particle Size, PDI and Zeta Potential Measurement

The mean particle size and PDI value for optimized LSP-NLCs were determined by a dynamic light scattering technique using a Zetasizer Nano ZSP (Malvern Instruments, Worcestershire, UK), whereas the zeta potential was measured using a phase analysis light scattering approach. The formulation was properly diluted with ultrapure water before measurements were taken and the analysis was carried out in triplicates [30].

3.4. Entrapment Efficiency

The entrapment efficiency (*EE*) of LSP-NLCs was calculated according to Equation (1). The untrapped drug and free lipids were separated by centrifugation of 1 mL of the LSP-NLCs formulation at 4 °C and 12,000 rpm for 15 min. The obtained LSP-NLCs were reconstituted with 1 mL of methanol and the concentration of the LSP incorporated in the NLCs was determined spectrophotometrically at 237 nm.

$$EE\ (\%) = \frac{Amount\ of\ LSP\ in\ NLCs}{Total\ amount\ of\ LSP\ added} \times 100 \tag{1}$$

3.5. In Vivo Studies

Experimental Animals

Assessment of the antidepressant and anxiolytic efficacy of LSP-NLCs via biodistribution and acute toxicity studies was carried out on albino mice (30 ± 5 g). All the experimental animals were obtained from the animal house of Riphah International University, Islamabad Pakistan. To acclimatize the animals to the lab environment, standard conditions were maintained. All animal studies were in accordance with the National Institute of Health policies, in line with the animal welfare act, and approved by the Research and Ethics Committee of Riphah Institute of Pharmaceutical Sciences (Approval# REC/RIPS/2019/015).

3.6. Biodistribution Study

The biodistribution of LSP through NLCs was carried out by performing a qualitative analysis using fluorescent-labeled NLCs (F-NLCs). F-NLCs were developed by mixing coumarin-6 (0.5% *w/w*) in the lipid melt during the preparation of NLCs before the addition of the aqueous phase. To separate the F-NLCs from the unentrapped coumarine-6 and free lipids, centrifugation was performed at 12,000 rpm for 15 min. In order to determine the fate of LSP-NLCs in the gastrointestinal tract (GIT), F-NLCs were given orally and to examine the LSP uptake in the brain and different organs, an intraperitoneal (I.P) injection equivalent to the oral dose was administered. Twenty-four male albino mice were divided into eight groups, four groups for the oral route and four groups for the I.P route (one group for each time point). Ex vivo imaging of different organs collected from sacrificed mice was performed at the predetermined time intervals of 0.5 h, 1 h, 2 h and 4 h after administration. Fluorescence imaging was performed using I-Box Explorer^2 (iBox$^®$ Explorer^2 Imaging

Microscope, UVP Ltd., Cambridge, UK) equipped with an automated BioLite™ Multi-Spectral Light Source, and the system excitation and emission filter were set at 535/45 and 605/50, respectively. A 3.2 MP OptiChemi 695 camera was used to capture the images and the images were captured at $0.17\times$ magnification. The recorded images were interpreted using Vision Works® LS Acquisition software [18,31].

3.7. Anti-Depressant and Anxiolytic Activity

The antidepressant and anxiolytic activity of LSP-loaded NLCs was investigated using a lipopolysaccharide (LPS)-induced depression and anxiety model in mice. Twelve experimental animals were divided into four groups (three mice in each group). Group-1 served as a positive control (P-Control) and was administered with 0.5 mL normal saline daily whereas group-2 was selected as negative control (N-Control) and was given LPS only to induce depression and anxiety. Group-3 and group-4 were treated groups and received individual LSP-DPN and LSP-NLCs daily at a dose equivalent to 5 mg/kg of LSP. Water was used as a vehicle to disperse the free LSP. The N-control group and treated groups also received intraperitoneal injections of LPS (500 µg/kg) on alternate days for 7 days. A pretest was conducted on day 8 of treatment followed by actual behavioral tests on day 9. The pictorial illustration of the LPS-induced depression and anxiety model is shown in Figure 7.

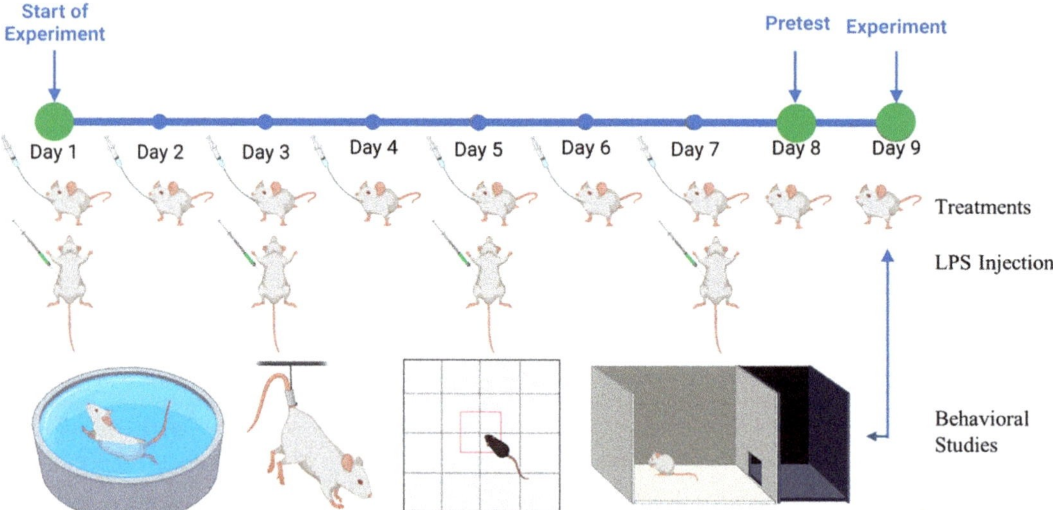

Figure 7. The pictorial illustration of LPS-induced depression and anxiety model (created with BioRender.com, accessed on 23 July 2023).

3.7.1. Behavioral Studies

To analyze the antidepressant activity of the LSP-NLCs, forced swim and tail suspension tests were carried out. Whereas, light–dark box and open field tests were performed to evaluate the anxiolytic behavior.

Forced Swim Test

The forced swim test, known as Porsolt's test, was carried out by gently placing the mice in a transparent glass cylinder measuring $50 \times 21 \times 21$ cm, filled with water up to 35 cm. The water was maintained at room temperature $25 + 2\ ^\circ$C and replaced with fresh water after each test to avoid the influence of contaminated water. The struggling motions of mice were recorded for 6 min. The struggling and immobility times were recorded for all mice. Immobility was considered as a loss of struggling effort to escape the container.

Swimming time was registered as a measure of mobility. Swimming was considered when forelimbs or hindlimbs moved in a paddling manner. The mice were removed from the water at the end of the experiment, dried with a towel and placed in a separate cage [6].

Tail Suspension Test

The tail suspension test was conducted by suspending the mice at a height of 50 cm by their tails and the tails were held away from the body with climb stoppers. Struggling and immobility time was videotaped for 6 min. Immobility was measured by the absence of any movements [32].

Light and Dark Box Test

For the light and dark experiment, a rectangular wooden box with dimensions of $44 \times 21 \times 21$ cm, divided into two compartments separated by a wooden board with an opening in its base for the movement of mice from one to another compartment, was used. The larger light compartment was painted white in color and lit up with a bulb and the smaller compartment was painted black. Each mouse was placed in the light compartment and the time it spent in each compartment and the number of entries were recorded for 6 min [33].

Open Field Test

The open field test was used to determine the effect of LSP-NLCs on the locomotor activity of the mice. For this purpose, the mice were separately positioned in the center of a box ($40 \times 60 \times 50$ cm) to which they were not habituated before the test. The locomotor activity of the animals was observed immediately up to 6 min. Time spent in the central compartment and the number of line crossings were the parameters considered for the activity. The apparatus was cleaned after each mouse activity [34].

3.8. Acute Oral Toxicity Study

The acute oral toxicity of LSP and LSP-NLCs in mice was evaluated after a single oral dose for a period of 14 days. Mice were divided into 3 groups (n = 3) and retained under accustomed conditions of food and water. Group-1 was given LSP dispersion, group-2 was given LSP-NLCs, and group-3 served as control and was given normal saline. A dose of (50 mg/kg) was given orally through gavage [27].

3.8.1. Body Weight Measurements and Observation of Clinical Signs and Food Consumption

The body weight of all the mice was measured on day 1 before dosing and after treatment on day 14. The experimental animals were visually observed initially for 48 h and then daily for 14 days for any change in behavior pattern, physical appearance, occurrence of clinical or toxicological symptoms, feed consumption, and mortality [35].

3.8.2. Hematology Analysis

On day 14, blood samples of mice were collected from tail veins in EDTA vacuumed blood collection tubes and were analyzed by an automatic hematology analyzer (Sysmex KX-21, Sysmex Corporation, Kobe, Japan) for red blood cell counts (RBCs), total white blood cells (WBCs), hemoglobin (Hb) levels and total number of platelets in each sample. Packed cell volume (PCV) was measured manually by using capillary microhematocrit tubes [27,36].

3.8.3. Serum Biochemistry

The serum was separated from the blood samples collected from tail veins and kept at -80 °C until further analysis. The renal and liver function test parameters and the concentration of serum enzymes, bilirubin, proteins and electrolytes were determined by using a semi-automated biochemistry analyzer (HumaLyzer 3500, Human Diagnostics, Wiesbaden, Germany) [28,37].

3.8.4. Organ to Body Ratio

Upon completion of the study duration, the mice were euthanized and the heart, kidneys, liver and stomach were removed. After washing, the weight of all the organs was measured individually and treated groups were equated with the organ weight of the control group. Organ-body weight index was calculated by using the formula below [38].

$$\text{Organ body weight index} = \text{Organ weight (g)}/\text{Body weight (g)} \times 100$$

3.8.5. Histopathology of Vital Organs

A macroscopic examination of all the previously removed and washed organs was carried out to check for any abnormality or lesion formation against the control. The tissue histology slides of the heart, kidneys, liver and stomach were cautiously prepared by fixing the organs in paraffin and cross-sections of tissues of 0.5 μm in size were carefully cut using a microtome. The tissue sections were fixed onto glass slides, stained with H&E stain and examined microscopically (Olympus CX43) for structural changes and signs of toxicity [39,40].

3.9. Statistical Analysis

GraphPad Prism 8 software (version 8.0.2, San Diego, CA, USA) was used for statistical analysis of the data and results were presented as mean $\pm$ S.D. Statistical significance between the treated groups and controls was determined by comparing their mean values using one-way ANOVA followed by Dunnett's test. The significance level was $p < 0.05$.

4. Conclusions

In this study, the antidepressant and anxiolytic performance of LSP-NLCs was investigated in vivo to reflect their therapeutic potential. LSP-NLCs significantly reduced depressive behavior in the animal model. Furthermore, F-NLCs show enhanced accessibility to brain tissues after intraperitoneal injection in biodistribution studies using ex vivo imaging analysis. However, LSP-NLCs were found to be safe after in vivo administration at higher doses and showed no signs of toxicity. These results suggest that LSP-NLCs could be a promising carrier system for the effective delivery of LSP to the brain for the treatment of depression.

Author Contributions: Methodology, M.A.K.; Formal analysis, S.T.A.; Investigation, H.S.S. and Y.A.B.J.; Resources, A.R. and M.S.; Writing—review & editing, M.U.A.; Supervision, M.F.S.; Project administration, S.u.Z. All authors have read and agreed to the published version of the manuscript.

Funding: This research was funded by King Saudi University Riyadh, Saudi Arabia, project grant number RSP2023R457. This study is also financially supported by Higher Education Commission (HEC) through the indigenous scholarship scheme grant number: 17-6/HEC/HRD/IS-II-5/2018 by awarding a Ph.D. fellowship to Sadia Tabassam Arif (PIN#518-86589-2MD5-025). The authors also acknowledge Al Ain University for their kind assistance in the provision of necessary resources.

Institutional Review Board Statement: All the animal studies were in accordance with the NIH policies, in line with the animal welfare act and approved by the Research and Ethics Committee of Riphah Institute of Pharmaceutical Sciences (Approval# REC/RIPS/2019/015).

Data Availability Statement: Data is contained within the article.

Conflicts of Interest: The authors declare no conflict of interest.

References

1. WHO. WHO and ILO Call for New Measures to Tackle Mental Health Issues at Work. Available online: https://www.who.int/news/item/28-09-2022-who-and-ilo-call-for-new-measures-to-tackle-mental-health-issues-at-work (accessed on 22 July 2023).
2. Alam, M.; Najmi, A.K.; Ahmad, I.; Ahmad, F.J.; Akhtar, M.J.; Imam, S.S.; Akhtar, M. Formulation and evaluation of nano lipid formulation containing CNS acting drug: Molecular docking, in-vitro assessment and bioactivity detail in rats. *Artif. Cells Nanomed. Biotechnol.* **2018**, *46*, 46–57. [CrossRef] [PubMed]
3. Kalin, N.H. The Critical Relationship Between Anxiety and Depression. *Am. J. Psychiatry* **2020**, *177*, 365–367. [CrossRef] [PubMed]

4. Pandey, Y.R.; Kumar, S.; Gupta, B.K.; Ali, J.; Baboota, S. Intranasal delivery of paroxetine nanoemulsion via the olfactory region for the management of depression: Formulation, behavioural and biochemical estimation. *Nanotechnology* **2016**, *27*, 025102. [CrossRef] [PubMed]
5. Yasir, M.; Sara, U.V.S.; Chauhan, I.; Gaur, P.K.; Singh, A.P.; Puri, D.; Ameeduzzafar. Solid lipid nanoparticles for nose to brain delivery of donepezil: Formulation, optimization by Box–Behnken design, in vitro and in vivo evaluation. *Artif. Cells Nanomed. Biotechnol.* **2018**, *46*, 1838–1851. [CrossRef]
6. Vitorino, C.; Silva, S.; Gouveia, F.; Bicker, J.; Falcão, A.; Fortuna, A. QbD-driven development of intranasal lipid nanoparticles for depression treatment. *Eur. J. Pharm. Biopharm.* **2020**, *153*, 106–120. [CrossRef]
7. Alam, M.I.; Baboota, S.; Ahuja, A.; Ali, M.; Ali, J.; Sahni, J.K.; Bhatnagar, A. Pharmacoscintigraphic evaluation of potential of lipid nanocarriers for nose-to-brain delivery of antidepressant drug. *Int. J. Pharm.* **2014**, *470*, 99–106. [CrossRef]
8. Costa, C.P.; Barreiro, S.; Moreira, J.N.; Silva, R.; Almeida, H.; Sousa Lobo, J.M.; Silva, A.C. In Vitro Studies on Nasal Formulations of Nanostructured Lipid Carriers (NLC) and Solid Lipid Nanoparticles (SLN). *Pharmaceuticals* **2021**, *14*, 711. [CrossRef]
9. Costa, C.; Moreira, J.N.; Amaral, M.H.; Sousa Lobo, J.M.; Silva, A.C. Nose-to-brain delivery of lipid-based nanosystems for epileptic seizures and anxiety crisis. *J. Control. Release* **2019**, *295*, 187–200. [CrossRef]
10. Cunha, S.; Almeida, H.; Amaral, M.H.; Lobo, S.J.M.; Silva, A.C. Intranasal Lipid Nanoparticles for the Treatment of Neurodegenerative Diseases. *Curr. Pharm. Des.* **2017**, *23*, 6553–6562. [CrossRef]
11. Wissing, S.A.; Müller, R.H. The influence of the crystallinity of lipid nanoparticles on their occlusive properties. *Int. J. Pharm.* **2002**, *242*, 377–379. [CrossRef]
12. Jaiswal, P.; Gidwani, B.; Vyas, A. Nanostructured lipid carriers and their current application in targeted drug delivery. *Artif. Cells Nanomed. Biotechnol.* **2016**, *44*, 27–40. [CrossRef] [PubMed]
13. Cho, H.-Y.; Lee, Y.-B. Improvement and validation of a liquid chromatographic method for the determination of levosulpiride in human serum and urine. *J. Chromatogr. B* **2003**, *796*, 243–251. [CrossRef] [PubMed]
14. Salunkhe, S.S.; Bhatia, N.M.; Bhatia, M.S. Implications of formulation design on lipid-based nanostructured carrier system for drug delivery to brain. *Drug Deliv.* **2016**, *23*, 1306–1316. [CrossRef] [PubMed]
15. Yousaf, R.; Khan, M.I.; Akhtar, M.F.; Madni, A.; Sohail, M.F.; Saleem, A.; Irshad, K.; Sharif, A.; Rana, M. Development and in-vitro evaluation of chitosan and glyceryl monostearate based matrix lipid polymer hybrid nanoparticles (LPHNPs) for oral delivery of itraconazole. *Heliyon* **2023**, *9*, e14281. [CrossRef]
16. Salunkhe, S.S.; Bhatia, N.M.; Thorat, J.D.; Choudhari, P.B.; Bhatia, M.S. Formulation, development and evaluation of ibuprofen loaded nanoemulsion prepared by nanoprecipitation technique: Use of factorial design approach as a tool of optimization methodology. *J. Pharm. Investig.* **2014**, *44*, 273–290. [CrossRef]
17. Jacobs, C.; Müller, R.H. Production and Characterization of a Budesonide Nanosuspension for Pulmonary Administration. *Pharm. Res.* **2002**, *19*, 189–194. [CrossRef]
18. Wang, K.; Cheng, F.; Pan, X.; Zhou, T.; Liu, X.; Zheng, Z.; Luo, L.; Zhang, Y. Investigation of the transport and absorption of Angelica sinensis polysaccharide through gastrointestinal tract both in vitro and in vivo. *Drug Deliv.* **2017**, *24*, 1360–1371. [CrossRef]
19. He, X.; Zhu, Y.; Wang, M.; Jing, G.; Zhu, R.; Wang, S. Antidepressant effects of curcumin and HU-211 coencapsulated solid lipid nanoparticles against corticosterone-induced cellular and animal models of major depression. *Int. J. Nanomed.* **2016**, *11*, 4975–4990. [CrossRef] [PubMed]
20. Mallipeddi, R.; Rohan, L.C. Progress in antiretroviral drug delivery using nanotechnology. *Int. J. Nanomed.* **2010**, *5*, 533–547.
21. Kaur, I.P.; Bhandari, R.; Bhandari, S.; Kakkar, V. Potential of solid lipid nanoparticles in brain targeting. *J. Control. Release* **2008**, *127*, 97–109. [CrossRef]
22. Blasi, P.; Giovagnoli, S.; Schoubben, A.; Ricci, M.; Rossi, C. Solid lipid nanoparticles for targeted brain drug delivery. *Adv. Drug Deliv. Rev.* **2007**, *59*, 454–477. [CrossRef]
23. Saraiva, C.; Praça, C.; Ferreira, R.; Santos, T.; Ferreira, L.; Bernardino, L. Nanoparticle-mediated brain drug delivery: Overcoming blood–brain barrier to treat neurodegenerative diseases. *J. Control. Release* **2016**, *235*, 34–47. [CrossRef] [PubMed]
24. Takano, H.; Ito, S.; Zhang, X.; Ito, H.; Zhang, M.-R.; Suzuki, H.; Maeda, K.; Kusuhara, H.; Suhara, T.; Sugiyama, Y. Possible Role of Organic Cation Transporters in the Distribution of [^{11}C]Sulpiride, a Dopamine D_2 Receptor Antagonist. *J. Pharm. Sci.* **2017**, *106*, 2558–2565. [CrossRef]
25. Ford, C.P. The role of D2-autoreceptors in regulating dopamine neuron activity and transmission. *Neuroscience* **2014**, *282*, 13–22. [CrossRef]
26. Singh, S.; Kamal, S.S.; Sharma, A.; Kaur, D.; Katual, M.K.; Kumar, R. Formulation and in-vitro evaluation of solid lipid nanoparticles containing Levosulpiride. *Open Nanomed. J.* **2017**, *4*, 17–29. [CrossRef]
27. Sohail, M.F.; Hussain, S.Z.; Saeed, H.; Javed, I.; Sarwar, H.S.; Nadhman, A.; Huma, Z.E.; Rehman, M.; Jahan, S.; Hussain, I.; et al. Polymeric nanocapsules embedded with ultra-small silver nanoclusters for synergistic pharmacology and improved oral delivery of Docetaxel. *Sci. Rep.* **2018**, *8*, 13304. [CrossRef]
28. Singh, T.; Sinha, N.; Singh, A. Biochemical and histopathological effects on liver due to acute oral toxicity of aqueous leaf extract of Ecliptaalba on female Swiss albino mice. *Indian J. Pharmacol.* **2013**, *45*, 61–65. [CrossRef] [PubMed]
29. Arif, S.T.; Zaman, S.u.; Khan, M.A.; Tabish, T.A.; Sohail, M.F.; Arshad, R.; Kim, J.-K.; Zeb, A. Augmented Oral Bioavailability and Prokinetic Activity of Levosulpiride Delivered in Nanostructured Lipid Carriers. *Pharmaceutics* **2022**, *14*, 2347. [CrossRef]

30. Khan, M.A.; Ansari, M.M.; Arif, S.T.; Raza, A.; Choi, H.-I.; Lim, C.-W.; Noh, H.-Y.; Noh, J.-S.; Akram, S.; Nawaz, H.A.; et al. Eplerenone nanocrystals engineered by controlled crystallization for enhanced oral bioavailability. *Drug Deliv.* **2021**, *28*, 2510–2524. [CrossRef]

31. Sabzichi, M.; Mohammadian, J.; Mohammadi, M.; Jahanfar, F.; Movassagh Pour, A.A.; Hamishehkar, H.; Ostad-Rahimi, A. Vitamin D-Loaded Nanostructured Lipid Carrier (NLC): A New Strategy for Enhancing Efficacy of Doxorubicin in Breast Cancer Treatment. *Nutr. Cancer* **2017**, *69*, 840–848. [CrossRef] [PubMed]

32. Jangra, A.; Kwatra, M.; Singh, T.; Pant, R.; Kushwah, P.; Sharma, Y.; Saroha, B.; Datusalia, A.K.; Bezbaruah, B.K. Piperine Augments the Protective Effect of Curcumin Against Lipopolysaccharide-Induced Neurobehavioral and Neurochemical Deficits in Mice. *Inflammation* **2016**, *39*, 1025–1038. [CrossRef]

33. Es-safi, I.; Mechchate, H.; Amaghnouje, A.; Elbouzidi, A.; Bouhrim, M.; Bencheikh, N.; Hano, C.; Bousta, D. Assessment of Antidepressant-like, Anxiolytic Effects and Impact on Memory of *Pimpinella anisum* L. Total Extract on Swiss Albino Mice. *Plants* **2021**, *10*, 1573. [CrossRef]

34. Liao, J.-C.; Tsai, J.-C.; Liu, C.-Y.; Huang, H.-C.; Wu, L.-Y.; Peng, W.-H. Antidepressant-like activity of turmerone in behavioral despair tests in mice. *BMC Complement. Altern. Med.* **2013**, *13*, 299. [CrossRef]

35. Saleem, U.; Ahmad, B.; Ahmad, M.; Erum, A.; Hussain, K.; Irfan Bukhari, N. Is folklore use of Euphorbia helioscopia devoid of toxic effects? *Drug Chem. Toxicol.* **2016**, *39*, 233–237. [CrossRef] [PubMed]

36. Tariq, I.; Ali, M.Y.; Sohail, M.F.; Amin, M.U.; Ali, S.; Bukhari, N.I.; Raza, A.; Pinnapireddy, S.R.; Schäfer, J.; Bakowsky, U. Lipodendriplexes mediated enhanced gene delivery: A cellular to pre-clinical investigation. *Sci. Rep.* **2020**, *10*, 21446. [CrossRef]

37. Ali, M.Y.; Tariq, I.; Farhan Sohail, M.; Amin, M.U.; Ali, S.; Pinnapireddy, S.R.; Ali, A.; Schäfer, J.; Bakowsky, U. Selective anti-ErbB3 aptamer modified sorafenib microparticles: In vitro and in vivo toxicity assessment. *Eur. J. Pharm. Biopharm.* **2019**, *145*, 42–53. [CrossRef] [PubMed]

38. Sarwar, H.S.; Sohail, M.F.; Saljoughian, N.; Rehman, A.U.; Akhtar, S.; Nadhman, A.; Yasinzai, M.; Gendelman, H.E.; Satoskar, A.R.; Shahnaz, G. Design of mannosylated oral amphotericin B nanoformulation: Efficacy and safety in visceral leishmaniasis. *Artif. Cells Nanomed. Biotechnol.* **2018**, *46*, 521–531. [CrossRef] [PubMed]

39. Sohail, M.F.; Sarwar, H.S.; Javed, I.; Nadhman, A.; Hussain, S.Z.; Saeed, H.; Raza, A.; Irfan Bukhari, N.; Hussain, I.; Shahnaz, G. Cell to rodent: Toxicological profiling of folate grafted thiomer enveloped nanoliposomes. *Toxicol. Res.* **2017**, *6*, 814–821. [CrossRef]

40. Ali, S.; Amin, M.U.; Tariq, I.; Sohail, M.F.; Ali, M.Y.; Preis, E.; Ambreen, G.; Pinnapireddy, S.R.; Jedelská, J.; Schäfer, J.; et al. Lipoparticles for Synergistic Chemo-Photodynamic Therapy to Ovarian Carcinoma Cells: In vitro and in vivo Assessments. *Int. J. Nanomed.* **2021**, *16*, 951–976. [CrossRef] [PubMed]

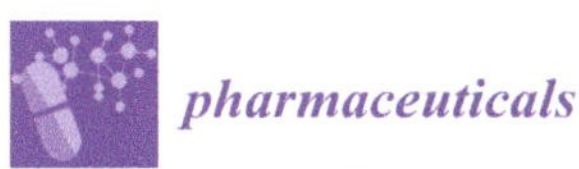 *pharmaceuticals*

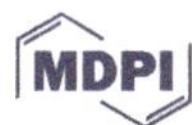

Article

Formulation and Evaluation of Plumbagin-Loaded Niosomes for an Antidiabetic Study: Optimization and In Vitro Evaluation

Rama Tyagi [1]**, Ayesha Waheed** [2]**, Neeraj Kumar** [3]**, Abdul Ahad** [4]**, Yousef A. Bin Jardan** [4]**, Mohd. Mujeeb** [3]**, Ashok Kumar** [5]**, Tanveer Naved** [1] **and Swati Madan** [1,*]

[1] Amity Institute of Pharmacy, Amity University, Noida 201303, Uttar Pradesh, India
[2] Department of Pharmaceutics, School of Pharmaceutical Education and Research, Jamia Hamdard, M. B. Road, New Delhi 110062, India
[3] Department of Pharmacognosy & Phytochemistry, School of Pharmaceutical Education and Research, Jamia Hamdard, M. B. Road, New Delhi 110062, India
[4] Department of Pharmaceutics, College of Pharmacy, King Saud University, Riyadh 11451, Saudi Arabia; aahad@ksu.edu.sa or
[5] Department of Internal Medicine, University of Kansas Medical Centre, Kansas City, KS 66160, USA
* Correspondence: smadan3@amity.edu

Abstract: Diabetes treatment requires focused administration with quality systemic circulation to determine the optimal therapeutic window. Intestinal distribution through oral administration with nanoformulation provides several benefits. Therefore, the purpose of this study is to create plumbagin enclosed within niosomes using the quality by design (QbD) strategy for efficient penetration and increased bioavailability. The formulation and optimization of plumbagin-loaded niosomes (P-Ns-Opt) involved the use of a Box–Behnken Design. The particle size (PDI) and entrapment efficiency of the optimized P-Ns-Opt were 133.6 nm, 0.150, and 75.6%, respectively. TEM, DSC, and FTIR were used to analyze the morphology and compatibility of the optimized P-Ns-Opt. Studies conducted in vitro revealed a controlled release system. P-Ns-Opt's antioxidant activity, α-amylase, and α-glucosidase were evaluated, and the results revealed a dose-dependent efficacy with $60.68 \pm 0.02\%, 90.69 \pm 2.9\%$, and $88.43 \pm 0.89\%$, respectively. In summary, the created P-Ns-Opt demonstrate remarkable potential for antidiabetic activity by inhibiting oxygen radicals, α-amylase, and α-glucosidase enzymes and are, therefore, a promising drug delivery nanocarrier in the management and treatment of diabetes.

Keywords: quality by design; plumbagin; diabetes; in vitro; niosomes

Citation: Tyagi, R.; Waheed, A.; Kumar, N.; Ahad, A.; Bin Jardan, Y.A.; Mujeeb, M.; Kumar, A.; Naved, T.; Madan, S. Formulation and Evaluation of Plumbagin-Loaded Niosomes for an Antidiabetic Study: Optimization and In Vitro Evaluation. *Pharmaceuticals* **2023**, *16*, 1169. https://doi.org/10.3390/ph16081169

Academic Editors: Ana Catarina Silva, João Nuno Moreira and José Manuel Sousa Lobo

Received: 26 July 2023
Revised: 10 August 2023
Accepted: 11 August 2023
Published: 17 August 2023

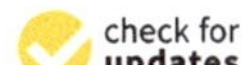

1. Introduction

1,4-naphthoquinones are a class of phytoconstituents that have been extracted from natural resources over the past few decades, and these compounds have a wide range of biological attributes and regulate a number of pharmacological functions, making them promising new targets for various illnesses [1]. A naturally occurring naphthoquinone called plumbagin (5-hydroxy-2-methyl-1,4-napthoquinone, PLB) has been identified in the roots of the traditional medicine plant *Plumbago zeylanica* L. Plumbagin has been shown to have a variety of biological effects, including anti-inflammatory, anti-cancer, antioxidant, antibacterial, antifungal, anti-atherosclerosis, and analgesic actions. It is a pro-oxidant and a vitamin K3 analog [2]. Plumbagin is known to inhibit diabetes by enhancing GLUT4 translocation and glucose homeostasis [3]. According to research, plumbagin exhibits restricted biopharmaceutical qualities, including high lipophilicity, insolubility in water, a short biological half-life, and a low melting point, which result in it having bioavailability of only 39% upon oral administration [4]. Using an alternative and correct dosage form, plumbagin can be utilized to deal with issues related to its biopharmaceutical properties.

Switching from conventional form to nanoformulation-loaded natural compounds can tackle the challenges caused by solubility, penetration, toxicity, bioavailability, etc.

Niosomes are vesicular systems comprising nonionic surfactants, and they have a unique structure that enables the integration and distribution of hydrophobic and hydrophilic medicinal molecules, respectively. Niosomes are also osmotically responsive, nontoxic, immune suppressive, biocompatible, and biodegradable. Niosomes have been studied as a potential drug carrier system with a number of administration methods, including oral, parenteral, dermal/transdermal, ophthalmic, and pulmonary [5]. The findings revealed that encapsulating curcumin in niosomal nanoparticles would enhance anti-tumor results of curcumin on glioblastoma [6].According to an in vitro study, utilizing niosomes to encapsulate Law can dramatically boost the formulation's anticancer activity in the MCF-7 cell line. Niosomes are a potentially useful delivery mechanism for phytochemical substances, since they have low solubility in bodily fluids [7]. Various niosomes have been synthesized to overcome the limitations of phytoconstituents [8].

The investigation was designed to encapsulate the plumbagin into niosomes by optimizing three independent variables: cholesterol (X1), span 20 (X2), and sonication time (X3). Vesicle size (Y1), entrapment effectiveness (Y2), and PDI (Y3) were used as dependent variables to optimize the niosomes. The antioxidant activity (DPPH assay) and invitro diabetic assay of the optimized formulation were also assessed.

2. Results and Discussion

2.1. Independent Variables Impact on Vesicle Size

The study revealed that cholesterol has a optimistic impact, while Span 20 and sonication time have a negative impact, on vesicle size, as shown in the equation below:

$$Y1 = +86.49583 + 1.26000X1 - 1.74125X2 + 5.69792X3 - 0.001500X1 \times X2 - 0.010000X1 \times X3 + 0.006250X2 \times X3 + 0.006635X12 + 0.018292X22 - 1.00521X32$$

The P-Ns formulation exhibited the lowest vesicles size of 106.4 nm (P-Ns-11), while the highest vesicles size of 204.4 nm was recorded for the P-Ns-15 formulation. The P-Ns-11 formulation presented minimum vesicles of 106.4 nm in size and composed of cholesterol (40 mg), Span 20 (30 mg), and sonication time (6.0 min), and the P-Ns-15 formulation presented maximum vesicles of 204.4 nm in size and composed of cholesterol (80 mg), Span 20 (20 mg), and sonication time (4 min) (Table 1). Our findings revealed that P-Ns' vesicles size increases as the concentration of cholesterol increases (Figure 1). It was noted that the formulations that contained 80 mg of cholesterol showed higher vesicles sizes, such as P-Ns-2 (196.8 nm), P-Ns-3 (185.1 nm), and P-Ns-4 (187.9 nm), while P-Ns-1, P-Ns-5, P-Ns-7, and P-Ns-11 formulations, which included 40 mg of cholesterol, produced vesicles with lower sizes of 110.3 nm, 133.6 nm, 116.5 nm, and 106.4 nm, respectively. Changes in vesicle size that augmented the cholesterol concentration could be attributed to various factors, such as strength, elasticity, membrane rigidity, and solubility [9]. It was noted that smaller vesicles might be produced by increasing the concentration of the surfactant (Span 20) [10]. As the Span 20 concentration increases from 20 to 40 mg, the sizes of vesicles decrease from 133.6 to 110.3 nm, 162.3 to 138.7 nm, and 150.9 to 106.4 nm, respectively, as can be observed in the P-Ns-5 and P-Ns-1, P-Ns-6 and P-Ns-10, and P-Ns-13 and P-Ns-11 formulations. Additionally, it was found that a longer sonication period results in smaller vesicles [11]. The P-Ns-2 formulation prepared with less sonication (2 min) displayed bigger vesicles size than the P-Ns-8 and P-Ns-10 (4 and 6 min) formulations (Figure 1A).

Table 1. Composition and optimization of P-Ns.

Formulation Codes	Independent Variables			Dependent Variables		
	Cholesterol (mg)	Span 20 (mg)	Sonication Time (min)	Vesicles Size (nm)	PDI	Entrapment Efficiency (%)
P-Ns-1	40	40	4	110.3	0.132	60.1
P-Ns-2	80	30	2	196.8	0.224	87.5
P-Ns-3	80	30	6	185.1	0.235	81.9
P-Ns-4	80	40	4	187.9	0.242	79.7
P-Ns-5	40	20	4	133.6	0.150	75.6
P-Ns-6	60	20	2	162.3	0.193	83.1
P-Ns-7	40	30	2	116.5	0.135	67.6
P-Ns-8	60	30	4	152.1	0.186	75.2
P-Ns-9	60	30	4	152.7	0.185	75.4
P-Ns-10	60	40	6	138.7	0.183	64.7
P-Ns-11	40	30	6	106.4	0.127	61.8
P-Ns-12	60	40	2	149.6	0.185	68.4
P-Ns-13	60	20	6	150.9	0.182	76.3
P-Ns-14	60	30	4	152.9	0.183	75.7
P-Ns-15	80	20	4	204.4	0.252	94.6

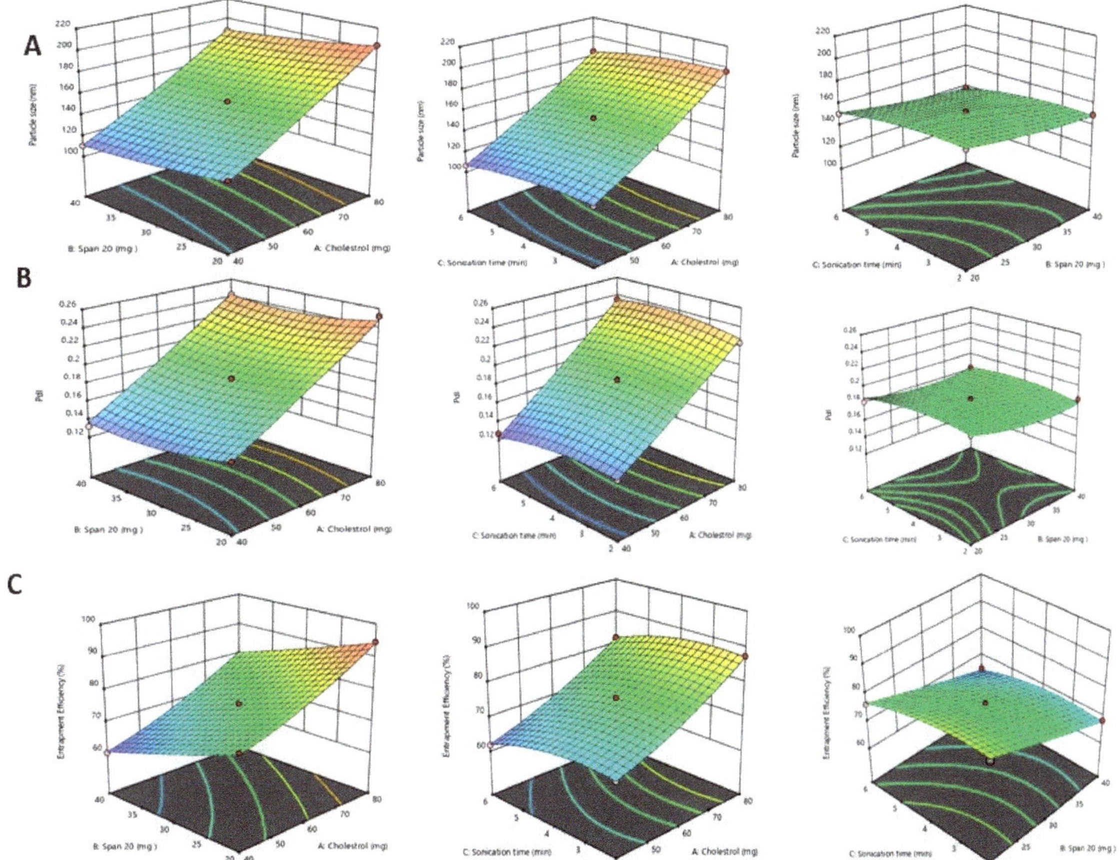

Figure 1. A 3D response surface plot showing the effect of independent variables on (**A**) vesicle size, (**B**) PDI, and (**C**) %EE.

2.2. Independent Variables Impact on PDI

The results of the trial suggest that the independent variables cholesterol and Span 20 have positive effects on PDI, as shown in the equation below.

$$Y2 = +0.165583 + 0.001206X1 - 0.005938X2 + 0.001542X3 + 0.000010X1 \times X2 + 0.000119X1 \times X3 + 0.000113X2 \times X3 + 4.79167 \times 10^{-6}X12 + 0.000074X22 - 0.001583X32$$

For the P-Ns-15 formulation, the maximum PDI was reported to be 0.252, while the minimum PDI was observed to be 0.127 (Figure 1B, Table 1). When the amount of cholesterol was increased from 40 to 80 mg, it was found that the PDI increased immediately from 0.132 (P-Ns-1) to 0.252 (P-Ns-15), while with Span 20, vesicle size decreased upon increasing the quantity from 20 to 40 mg (P-Ns-15 and P-Ns-10), and the sonication time was shown decrease in PDI (0.193, 0.150 and 0.127) as the duration of sonication increased from 2 to 4 and 6 min in formulations P-Ns-6, P-Ns-5, and P-Ns-11, respectively, maintaining the same values for the Span 20 (X2) and sonication time (X3). This finding indicates that Span 20 (X2) has a significant impact on PDI. In comparison, the P-Ns-1, P-Ns-8, and P-Ns-6 formulations, which had the highest to lowest concentrations of Span 20, exhibited lower to greater PDI.

2.3. Independent Variables Impact on Entrapment Efficiency%

In the current investigation, cholesterol had a favorable effect, while Span 20 had a detrimental impact on the effectiveness of entrapment of P-Ns vesicles, as mentioned in the equation below.

$$Y3 = +87.37917 - 0.082500X1 - 1.05625X2 + 2.50208X3 + 0.000750X1 \times X2 + 0.001250X1 \times X3 + 0.038750X2 \times X3 + 0.004552X12 + 0.002458X22 - 0.638542X32$$

P-Ns-15 and P-Ns-1 had the highest and lowest entrapment efficiencies, which were found to be 94.6% and 60.1%, respectively (Table 1). In contrast to Span 20, cholesterol (X1) had a favorable impact on %EE, while Span 20 (X2) had a negative impact (Figure 1C). It was shown that, as demonstrated in the P-Ns-11 and P-Ns-7, P-Ns-9 and P-Ns-6, and P-Ns-3 and P-Ns-15 formulations, an increase in the content of cholesterol (40 mg–80 mg) increased the %EE from 61.8 to 67.6%, 75.4 to 83.1%, and 81.9 to 94.6%, respectively. The EE% decreased in the P-Ns-15 and P-Ns-6, P-Ns-3 and P-Ns-8, and P-Ns-1 and P-Ns-11 formulations from 94.6 to 83.1%, 81.9 to 75.2%, and 61.8 to 60.1% when the concentration of Span 20 was increased from 20 to 40 mg. The %EE steadily dropped as the sonication period increased. Ultra-sonication of formulations not only aided in shrinking vesicles, but also had an impact on drug entrapment by breaking vesicles, which caused drug(s) to leak from vesicles and reduced drug entrapment. As seen in P-Ns-2 and P-Ns-6, P-Ns-4 and P-Ns-8, and P-Ns-13 and P-Ns-10 formulations, increasing the duration of the sonication time (2 min to 6 min) decreased the %EE from 87.5 to 83.1%, 79.2 to 75.2%, and 76.3 to 64.7%.

2.4. Point Prediction

For the purpose of choosing an optimum formulation and performing additional characterization, the point prediction approach was utilized. The optimized P-Ns-Opt formulation had cholesterol (40 mg), Span 20 (20 mg), and 4 min of sonication. The identification of the actual and predicted values of all of the dependent variables was also examined. PDI was 0.150, entrapment efficiency was 75.6%, and the actual vesicle size was 133.6 nm. According to the expected parameters, the vesicle was 152.56 nm in size, having a PDI of 0.150 and entrapment effectiveness of 75.43%.

2.5. Vesicle Dimensions and PDI

The optimized plumbagin-loaded niosomes had particles with a size of 133.6 nm, as determined using dynamic light scattering and a nano-zeta sizer. An extraordinarily low PDI of 0.150 for the particle size distribution was discovered (Figure 2A).

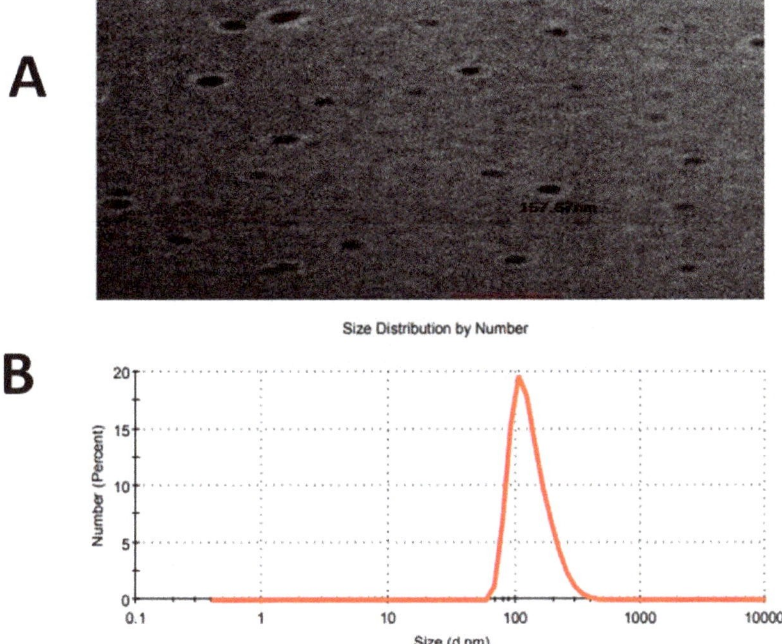

Figure 2. (**A**) TEM image of optimized formulation P-Ns-Opt and (**B**) vesicle size.

2.6. Morphological Study

The morphology and existence of the P-Ns-Opt formulation were verified using the TEM micrograph. The micrograph of the optimized P-Ns-Opt formulation (Figure 2B) showed a homogeneous distribution of sizes and spherical-shaped sealed formations.

2.7. Thermal Analysis

According to the supplier's certificate of analysis, plumbagin has a melting point between 76 and 78 °C. A strong endothermic peak at 79.752 °C was seen during the DSC analysis of pure plumbagin, confirming its purity (Figure 3A). The DSC of the lyophilized P-Ns-Opt (Figure 3B) showed a peak at 169.187 °C, which belonged to mannitol. Additionally, it was noted that there were no additional peaks of available free drug in the thermogram, suggesting that there had been no precipitation and the drug had been entirely enclosed in the vesicles. As a result, it can be inferred that cholesterol and Span 20 interact or combine with one another, and this finding verifies the production of plumbagin niosomes and the absence of the anticipated plumbagin leaking.

2.8. FTIR Analysis

To evaluate the compatibility with excipients, the FTIR was used to evaluate the plumbagin and P-Ns-Opt formulations (Figure 4). Peaks at 3293.59, 2966.65, 2144.94, 1984.84, 1903.32, 1805.45, 1664.64, 1452.46, 1263.43, 1112.97, 1030.03, 934.70, and 898.87 cm^{-1} were visible in the characteristic spectra of the plumbagin sample. Peaks at 3733.33, 2906.25, 2322.39, 2011.34, 1741.90, 1647.23, 1423.53, 1232.72, 1036.93, 1015.57, 923.76, and 877.65 cm^{-1} were shown by the P-Ns-Opt. The FTIR spectra showed the standard sample peak, which was also present in the spectra peaks of P-Ns-Opt, demonstrating the unaltered attachment of the plumbagin molecule derived from the optimized formulation to the excipients.

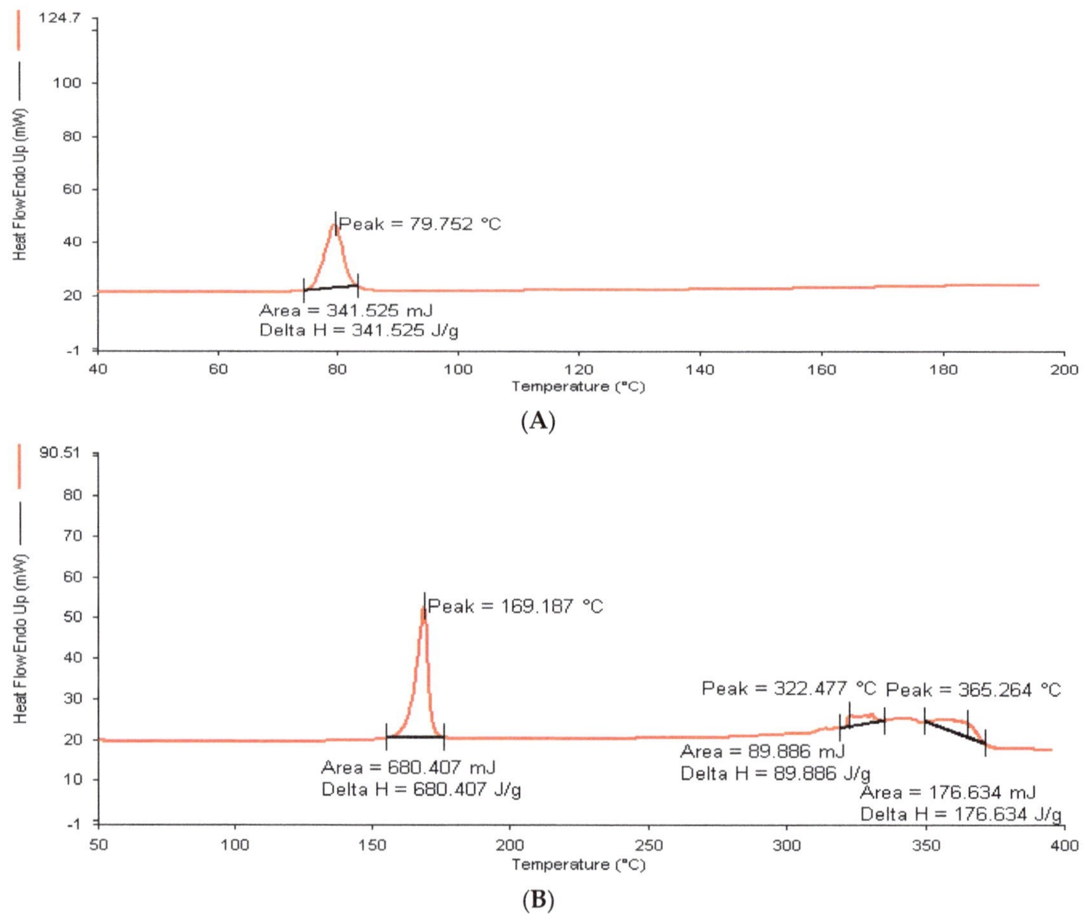

Figure 3. DSC image of (**A**) plumbagin and (**B**) P-Ns-Opt.

2.9. In Vitro Drug Release

P-Ns-Opt and plumbagin dispersion were compared on the basis of the drug release behavior (Figure 5). After 6 h of the trial, 36.6% of the cumulative release of plumbagin from the plumbagin suspension was seen to be rapidly released. After 24 h, a release rate of 66.17% was seen. While P-Ns-Opt demonstrated prolonged drug release, it also displayed an initial rapid release that might have been brought on by the unentrapped drug. Later, P-Ns-Opt displayed a plumbagin release rate of 88.19% at 12 h and a release rate of 93.04% at 24 h. The plumbagin was first released in bursts over a few hours, as shown in Figure 5, and the release was then continued for up to 24 h. By replenishing the receiver medium, the new buffer was employed to preserve the sink condition; however, this cannot entirely replicate the sink condition. As a result, it might not be able to completely remove pharmaceuticals from the matrix.

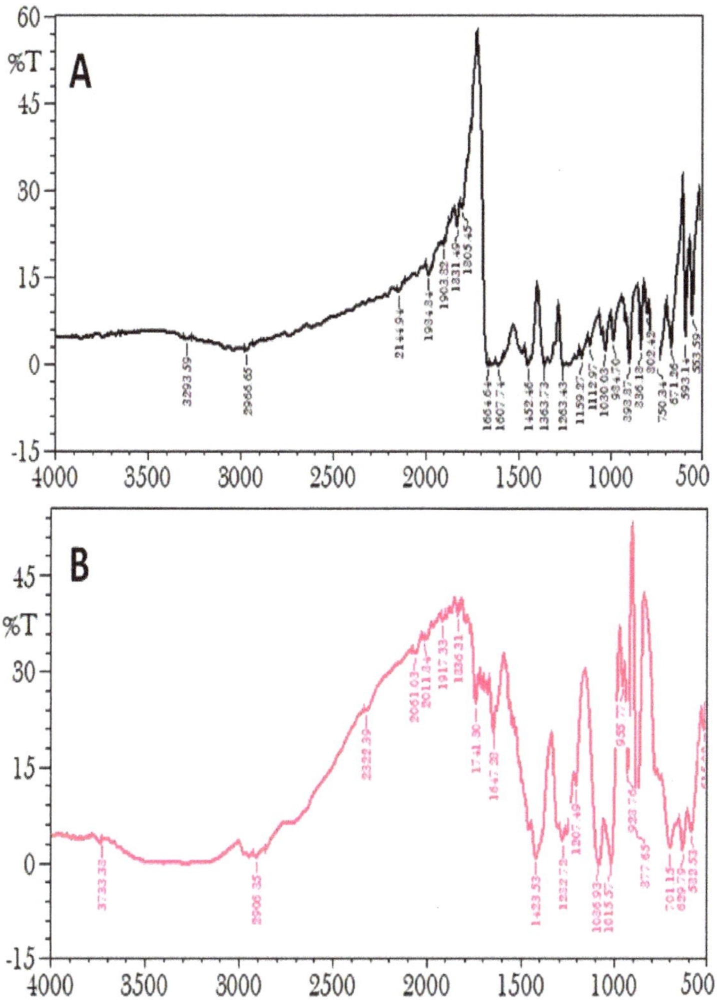

Figure 4. FT-IR spectra of (**A**) plumbagin and (**B**) P-Ns-Opt.

Several drug release kinetic models, including the Korsmeyer–Peppas, Higuchi, zero-order, and first-order models, were employed to assess the drug release data. The Korsmeyer–Peppas model had the greatest R2 value (0.971), the Higuchi model had R2 = 0.891, the first-order model had R2 = 0.488, and the zero-order model had the lowest R2 value (0.666). As a result, the release of plumbagin from P-NS-Opt showed the best-fitting model to be the Korsmeyer–Peppas model.

2.10. Antioxidant Study

To inhibit, oppose, or delay a reaction, antioxidants can bind with free oxygen radicals in a chemically synthesized or natural way. In this study, the antioxidant capabilities of the ascorbic acid, P-Ns-Opt, and plumbagin were evaluated using the DPPH method (Figure 6). Ascorbic acid, plumbagin, and P-Ns-Opt each had antioxidant activities of 77.86 ± 0.03%, 49.59 ± 0.06, and 60.68 ± 0.02%, respectively. Thus, it is clear that the produced ascorbic acid and P-Ns-Opt have greater potential than plumbagin to treat a variety of disorders linked to oxidative stress.

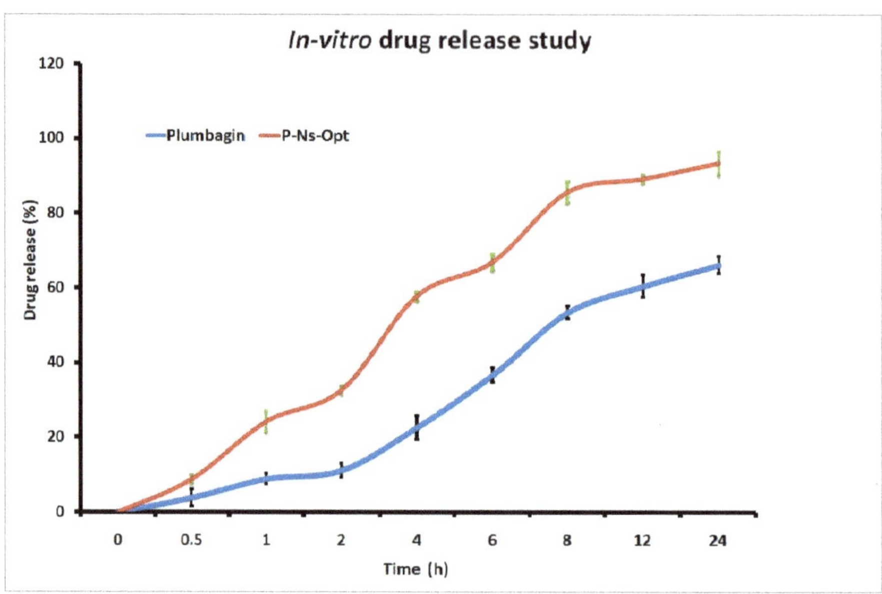

Figure 5. Comparative drug release of plumbagin and plumbagin-Ns-Opt.

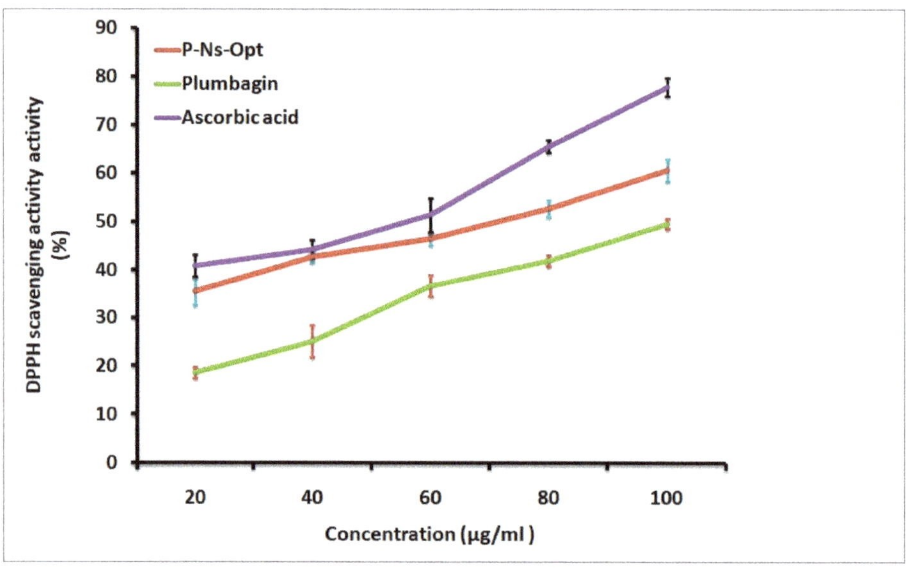

Figure 6. DPPH scavenging activity of Ascorbic acid, P-Ns-Opt, and plumbagin.

2.11. Inhibitory Assay of α-Amylase and α-Glucosidase Assay

The primary enzymes that assist in breaking apart glucose and speed up the way in which it is absorbed by the gastrointestinal tract are α-amylase and α-glucosidase, which result in higher level of sugar in blood and the suppression of the enzymes responsible for the digestion of carbohydrates, leading to the lowering of blood sugar levels. Figure 7 depicts the inhibitory effects of plumbagin, P-Ns-Opt, and acarbose. Standard (acarbose) suppressed α-amylase at the maximum level, followed by P-Ns-Opt and plumbagin at 93.71 ± 2.6%, 90.69 ± 2.9%, and 83.64 ± 3.5%, respectively. The results of the α-glucosidase inhibition assay showed that acarbose exhibited greater levels of inhibition effectiveness (93.16 ± 1.7%) than P-Ns-Opt (88.43 ± 0.89%) and plumbagin (81.07 ± 1.2%).

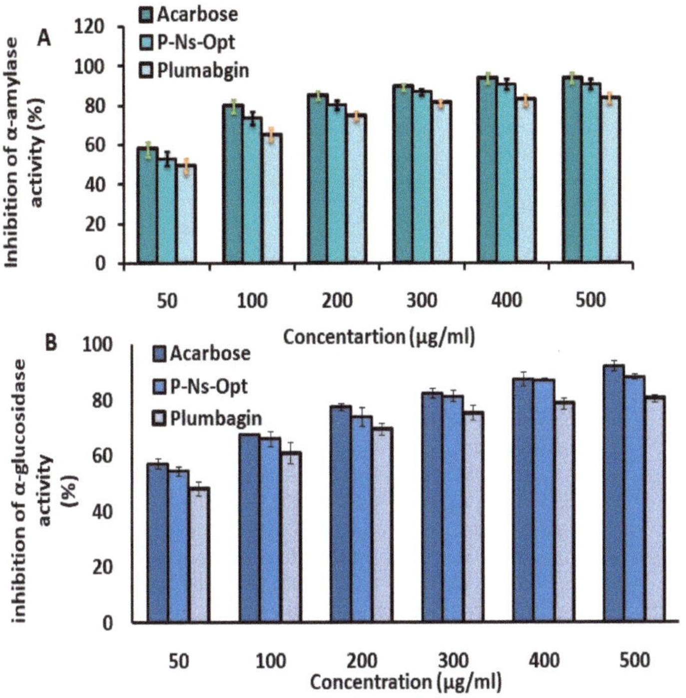

Figure 7. Inhibition of (**A**) α-amylase and (**B**) α-glucosidase activity of plumbagin and P-Ns-Opt.

2.12. Stability Study

The P-Ns-Opt formulation's stability studies were conducted to assess its durability during storage (8 weeks) and any medication degradation/loss stemming from niosomes (Table 2). At the conclusion of the first month, the EE% and vesicle size of the P-Ns-Opt formulation maintained at 4 °C/60 ± 5% RH were assessed. The measurements of EE% and vesicle size were 69.93 ± 2.1% and 166.56 ± 6.3 nm, respectively. The remaining medication was once more assessed after 8 weeks using the same technique as that used to assess the entrapment effectiveness and vesicle size. The findings indicated that the vesicles were stable under refrigeration and the EE% were 63.71 ± 2.7% and 180.96 ± 1.8 nm, respectively.

Table 2. Stability study of P-Ns-Opt at 4 ± 0.5 °C.

Observations	0 Days	30 Days	60 Days
Vesicle size	139.93 ± 6.77 nm	166.56 ± 6.35 nm	180.96 ± 1.89 nm
EE%	73.86 ± 4.1%	69.71 ± 1.5%	63.71 ± 2.7%

3. Materials and Methods

3.1. Materials

Span 20, cholesterol, disodium hydrogen phosphate, and potassium dihydrogen phosphate were procured from SD Fine chemicals, Mumbai, India. Plumbagin was purchased from Sigma-Aldrich. Methanol, ethanol, sulfuric acid, and HCl (LR grade and AR grade) were purchased from Merck, Mumbai, India.

3.2. Methods

3.2.1. Encapsulation of Niosomes Loaded with Plumbagin

The solvent evaporation method approach was used to manufacture P-Ns-Opt. The recipe used cholesterol, Span 20, and plumbagin as components. Each ingredient was measured out in the required amounts, before being dissolved in ethanol. For thorough mixing, samples underwent a 10-minutevortexing process. Separately for one hour at room temperature, a magnetic stirrer was used to continuously mix the surfactant solution at 800 rpm while the ethanolic lipid mixture was introduced using a syringe. The obtained dispersions were probe sonicated in the presence of ice after the ethanol had been completely removed in order to produce nano-sized niosomes (NNs). The niosomes were assessed for additional criteria.

3.2.2. Optimization of Plumbagin Niosomes Formulation using Response Surface Methodology (RSM)

The three factors found at three levels were applied to enable the optimization of P-NNs using Design–Expert software (Version 12, Stat-Ease, MN, USA). To ascertain their impacts on the particle size (Y1), PDI (Y2) and entrapment efficiency (Y3) of niosomes, the various process parameters—cholesterol concentration (X1), Span 20 (X2), and sonication time (X3)—were thoroughly studied. To obtain the ideal composition, independent variables were mentioned at low (−), medium (0), and high (+) concentrations (Table 3). To evaluate the impact of independent variables, we included 15 distinct composition formulation runs with three center points. Polynomial equations and response surface plots were used to assess the impacts of independent variables. The polynomial equation provided numerous models, including the quadratic and linear impacts of independent factors on dependent variables. The quadratic model was the best of all the models because the variables utilized showed both individual and combined impacts on the dependent variables.

Table 3. Independent variables used to prepare and optimize P-Ns via Box–Behnken design.

Variables	Low	High
Independent variables		
X1 = Cholesterol (mg)	40	80
X2 = Span 20 (mg)	20	40
X3 = Sonication time (min)	2	6
Dependent variables		
Y1 = Vesicles size(nm)		
Y2 = PDI		
Y3 = Entrapment (%)		

3.2.3. Characterization

Vesicles Size and Poly Dispersity Index (PdI)

The vesicle size and PDI of P-Ns-Opt were measured using a Malvern zeta sizer (Zeta sizer, Malvern Instruments Ltd., Malvern, UK). Using Milli-Q water, analysis was performed on samples that had been diluted up to 50 times while keeping the system's temperature at 25 °C and the scattering angle at 90°.

Assessment of Entrapment Efficiency

Utilizing the ultra-centrifugation method, the % entrapment efficiency was evaluated [12]. The centrifuge (Remi cooling centrifuge, Mumbai) was used to centrifuge a plumbagin-loaded niosome sample at a specified concentration for one hour at 4 °C. After appropriate dilution, the obtained supernatant was examined to determine the presence of free drugs, and quantification was carried out using the formula below.

$$\text{Entrapment Efficiency} = A1 - A2/A1 \times 100,$$

where A1 is the plumbagin concentration utilized in the loaded niosomes, and A2 is the plumbagin concentration assumed to be present in the supernatant.

Thermal Analysis

DSC (Perkin Elmer, Pyris 6 DSC, Shelton, CT, USA) was carried out for plumbagin and lyophilized optimized P-Ns-Opt to validate the entrapment and type of drug [13]. A tiny amount of the sample was placed in an enclosed in an aluminum pan. The instrument's temperature was set in arrange 40 to 400 °C. The rate of nitrogen flow was regulated at 60 mL/min while the heating rate increased by 10 °C/min. Mannitol was added as a cryoprotectant at a concentration of 5%, before the formulation was freeze-dried to enable lyophilization.

FTIR Analysis

The spectra of the prepared plumbagin niosomes and the individual plumbagin were obtained using an FTIR spectrophotometer (Perkin Elmer-spectrum RX-I, Lamba, Shelton, CT, USA) based on the KBr disc method under the influence of a hydraulic press employing 600 kg/cm^2 pressure. FTIR was utilized to examine sample structural characteristics, drug-ingredient interactions, and compatibility [14].

Transmission Electron Microscopy

The morphology of the P-Ns-Opt sample was investigated via transmission electron microscopy (JEOL; 120CX Microscope, Tokyo, Japan) [15].The dispersion was applied to a copper grid with carbon coating and allowed to attach to the carbon substrate for 1 min. Further, niosomes were stained with a drop of 1% phosphotungstic acid and placed on the grid, dried, scanned, and photographed, before being stored.

In Vitro Drug Release

The Franz diffusion cell was used to carry out the drug release investigation, and a (pre-treated) dialysis membrane was used. The donor and receiver chambers were then positioned on either side of the active membrane. The recipient chamber contained phosphate-buffered saline (PBS) with a pH of 5.5, was maintained at room temperature, and swirled at 100 rpm for 24 h [16]. P-Ns-Opt and plumbagin suspension (1 mg/mL) were placed in the donor compartments. At pre-determined intervals of 1, 2, 4, 6, 8, 12, and 24 h, 1-millilitersamples were taken. To equalize the sink conditions, fresh release medium was again simultaneously put in the receiver compartment. Using UV spectroscopy and the proper dilutions, the removed sample was further evaluated to determine drug presence.

$$\%CDR = \text{Conc.} \times \text{DF} \times \text{Vol. of release media}/\text{Amount of drug added} \times 100$$

where DF is the dilution factor, and Conc. is the drug concentration achieved at a certain time interval. Time vs. cumulative drug release % was shown on the X and Y axes of a release profile graph.

Different kinetic models, such as the Korsmeyer–Peppas, Higuchi, zero-order, and first-order models were used to study the drug release data derived from the P-Ns-Opt. The model with a value of R^2 nearer to 1 was selected as the model best suited to drug release.

DPPH Assay

The approach outlined, followed by with a few minor modifications, was used to estimate the DPPH's radical scavenging capacities [17]. Various dilutions of plumbagin and P-Ns-Opt sample were combined with DPPH solution and left at 37 ± 0.5 °C for 1 h (the time needed for reactions to maintain a plateau). To prepare a blank solution, methanol and DPPH were added to the control solution, sample, and DPPH solution. Ascorbic acid was used as a standard for the study. Then, its absorbance was evaluated at 517 nm. The DPPH antioxidant action was determined as a % of DPPH inhibition.

Inhibition of α-Amylase Activity

The starch was utilized as the substrate to analyze the inhibition of α-amylase activity using a protocol that was slightly modified [18]. Various concentrations of P and P-Ns-Opt (50 to 250 µg/mL) were prepared, and 500 µL of sodium phosphate buffer (0.02 M) with sodium chloride (6 mM) was added separately, before being stored at room temperature for 20 min. Test tubes were filled with each sample and the amylase solution, which were then incubated for 10 min at 25 °C. Following incubation, starch solution was added and incubated at 25 °C for an additional 10 min. Dinitrosalicylic acid (DNSA) color reagent was added to the reaction to stop it and further incubated via a boiling water bath at 100 °C for five minutes. After allowing the reaction mixture to reach room temperature, 3 mL of double-distilled water was added.

The absorbance was then measured at 540 nm via a microplate reader set to 25 °C using a 200-microliter aliquot of the reaction mixture. Each well had a blank reading (the addition of buffer to replace the enzyme) removed. The maltose equivalents emitted from starch at 540 nm were used to measure the enzyme activity. The same methodology was utilized to assess an artificial α-amylase inhibitor (acarbose), which served as a standard. The α-amylase inhibition percentage was calculated using the formula given below:

$$\text{Percentage of inhibition} = [(Ac - As)/Ac] \times 100$$

where Ac = absorbance of the controls, and As = absorbance of the sample.

Inhibition of α-Glucosidase Activity

50 µL of plumbagin and P-Ns-Opt were made at various concentrations and then stored for 20 min at room temperature with 10 mL of α-glucosidase (maltase) and 125 mL of 0.1-molarity phosphate buffer (pH 6.8) [19]. Next, 20 µL of 1-molarity 4-Nitrophenyl-D-glucopyranoside was mixed to begin the reaction, which was then incubated for 30 min. The reaction was stopped by adding 50 µL of 0.1-newton Na2CO3. In order to determine the optical density, a spectrophotometer was used at 405 nm. Acarbose served as a standard. All tests were conducted in triplicate.

The inhibition percentage of P-Ns-Opt was estimated using the following formula:

$$\text{Percentage of inhibition} = [(Ac - As)/Ac] \times 100$$

where Ac = absorbance of the controls, and As = absorbance of the sample.

Stability Study

The stability of the optimized P-Ns-Opt was evaluated while the formulation samples were kept at 25 °C and 4 °C for an 8-week period [20]. Samples were obtained at 0, 4, and 8 weeks to determine particle size and EE%, which were used as the stability parameters.

4. Conclusions

Plumbagin has the capacity to heal wounds, as well as having anti-diabetic, anti-inflammatory, anti-cancer, and immunosuppressive effects. Plumbagin has penetration-related issues due to the size of vesicles, solubility, and bioavailability. Such issues may be mitigated by developing nano-formulations, boosting bioavailability, including therapeutic activity, etc.

Niosomes are one drug delivery system which has the efficiency to carry the drug through various routes, like ophthalmic, nasal, parenteral, transdermal, and oral routes. A niosome is known as a "drug depot" because it has the potential to transfer the drug in a controlled or sustained manner to the targeted site. The improved version of a loaded drugs is enclosed in niosomes by enhancing solubility and biocompatibility. Niosomes have hydrophilic, amphiphilic, and lipophilic properties. So, diverse drugs with broad levels of solubility can be accommodated via the structure of a niosome. This fact is the reason that drugs loaded in niosomes can pass through the stomach without being degraded by the acid present in the stomach. Another problem with conventional drugs involves penetration through the intestine and reaching the bloodstream. Niosomes have the capability to enhance the bioavailability of loaded drugs and promote their efficiency. Niosomes are composed of nonionic surfactants and cholesterol. Cholesterol is the carrier of the lipophilic and amphiphilic drugs. Cholesterol prepares the bilayer system, which is rigid, helps to maintain stability, and results in less leaky and larger-sized niosomes. Meanwhile, the surfactant's HLB value shows an effect on the vesicle size. The higher the HLB value, the higher the surface energy, which will lead to a large vesicle size (higher hydrophilicity due to the higher uptake of water).

In this investigation, we have formulated P-Ns-Opt that improved in vitro performance related to diabetes. The optimized formulation generated vesicles with diameters of 133.6 nm, a PDI of 0.150, an entrapment efficiency of 75.6%, and a drug release of 93.04%. P-Ns-Opt's vesicle morphology was discovered to be in the appropriate spherical form. The complete entrapment of plumbagin in niosomes was validated via thermal analysis data, and excipient compatibility was established based on the absence of chemical reaction among the excipients of niosomes and plumbagin. The improved formulation, known as P-Ns-Opt, showed intense release at first, but thereafter showed sluggish drug release in the in vitro drug release assessment. The Korsmeyer–Peppas, Higuchi, zero-order, and first-order models were among those examined. Additionally, P-Ns-Opt's antioxidant activity was found to be $60.68 \pm 0.02\%$, which was comparable to those of ascorbic acid ($77.86 \pm 0.03\%$) and plumbagin (49.59 ± 0.06). The in vitro antidiabetic activity (α-amylase) was analyzed, and P-Ns-Opt ($90.69 \pm 2.9\%$) demonstrated improved results as compared to plumbagin ($83.64 \pm 3.5\%$). Similarly, α-glucosidase assay was performed, and P-Ns-Opt displayed an $88.43 \pm 0.89\%$ inhibition percentage compared to plumbagin, i.e., $81.07 \pm 1.2\%$, indicating that the developed formulation could effectively treat and manage diabetes.

The current study shows that the QbD technique may be used to manufacture plumbagin-loaded niosomes. BBD with a solvent evaporation procedure was applied to prepare and optimize the formulation. The expected and observed values were in agreement. The generated P-Ns-opts' particle sizes will be suitable for oral administration. DSC and FTIR studies demonstrated that the produced P-Ns-opt contained plumbagin while preserving the formulation. The improved P-Ns-opt demonstrated good stability and sustained release. A dose-dependent inhibitory impact was also seen in antioxidant activity, in vitro α-amylase and α-glucosidase study. This study represents the first report of P-Ns-Opt formulation that investigated antioxidant and in vitro antidiabetic activity. In conclusion, it was determined that plumbagin-loaded niosomes are a more effective form of delivery of plumbagin and a better strategy for managing diabetes mellitus. Further studies using experimental animal models will facilitate the utilization of this formulation as a potent antidiabetic therapeutic agent.

Author Contributions: Conceptualization, S.M., T.N., M.M. and A.K; Supervision, S.M., A.K. and M.M.; formal analysis, N.K., A.W., A.K. and T.N.; Writing—original draft, R.T., A.W. and N.K.; Writing—review and editing, R.T., Y.A.B.J., A.A., S.M., T.N., A.K. and M.M.; Funding, A.A.; Software, R.T., A.W. and A.A. All authors have read and agreed to the published version of the manuscript.

Funding: The authors extend their appreciation to the Deputyship for Research and Innovation, "Ministry of Education", in Saudi Arabia for funding this research (IFKSUOR3-130-1).

Data Availability Statement: Data are contained within this article.

Conflicts of Interest: The authors declare no conflict of interest.

References

1. Aminin, D.; Polonik, S. 1,4-Naphthoquinones: Some Biological Properties and Application. *Chem. Pharm. Bull.* **2020**, *68*, 46–57. [CrossRef] [PubMed]
2. Yin, Z.; Zhang, J.; Chen, L.; Guo, Q.; Yang, B.; Zhang, W.; Kang, W. Anticancer Effects and Mechanisms of Action of Plumbagin: Review of Research Advances. *BioMed Res. Int.* **2020**, *2020*, 6940953. [CrossRef] [PubMed]

3.	Sunil, C.; Duraipandiyan, V.; Agastian, P.; Ignacimuthu, S. Antidiabetic Effect of Plumbagin Isolated from *Plumbago zeylanica* L. Root and Its Effect on GLUT4 Translocation in Streptozotocin-Induced Diabetic Rats. *Food Chem. Toxicol.* **2012**, *50*, 4356–4363. [CrossRef] [PubMed]

4.	Rajalakshmi, S.; Vyawahare, N.; Pawar, A.; Mahaparale, P.; Chellampillai, B. Current Development in Novel Drug Delivery Systems of Bioactive Molecule Plumbagin. *Artif. Cells Nanomed. Biotechnol.* **2018**, *46*, 209–218. [CrossRef] [PubMed]

5.	Momekova, D.B.; Gugleva, V.E.; Petrov, P.D. Nanoarchitectonics of Multifunctional Niosomes for Advanced Drug Delivery. *ACS Omega* **2021**, *6*, 33265–33273. [CrossRef] [PubMed]

6.	Sahab-Negah, S.; Ariakia, F.; Jalili-Nik, M.; Afshari, A.R.; Salehi, S.; Samini, F.; Rajabzadeh, G.; Gorji, A. Curcumin Loaded in Niosomal Nanoparticles Improved the Anti-Tumor Effects of Free Curcumin on Glioblastoma Stem-like Cells: An In Vitro Study. *Mol. Neurobiol.* **2020**, *57*, 3391–3411. [CrossRef] [PubMed]

7.	Barani, M.; Mirzaei, M.; Torkzadeh-Mahani, M.; Nematollahi, M.H. Lawsone-Loaded Niosome and Its Antitumor Activity in MCF-7 Breast Cancer Cell Line: A Nano-Herbal Treatment for Cancer. *DARU J. Pharm. Sci.* **2018**, *26*, 11–17. [CrossRef]

8.	Han, H.S.; Koo, S.Y.; Choi, K.Y. Emerging Nanoformulation Strategies for Phytocompounds and Applications from Drug Delivery to Phototherapy to Imaging. *Bioact. Mater.* **2022**, *14*, 182–205. [CrossRef] [PubMed]

9.	Nakhaei, P.; Margiana, R.; Bokov, D.O.; Abdelbasset, W.K.; Jadidi Kouhbanani, M.A.; Varma, R.S.; Marofi, F.; Jarahian, M.; Beheshtkhoo, N. Liposomes: Structure, Biomedical Applications, and Stability Parameters With Emphasis on Cholesterol. *Front. Bioeng. Biotechnol.* **2021**, *9*, 705886. [CrossRef] [PubMed]

10.	Yeo, P.L.; Lim, C.L.; Chye, S.M.; Ling, A.P.K.; Koh, R.Y. Niosomes: A Review of Their Structure, Properties, Methods of Preparation, and Medical Applications. *Asian Biomed.* **2017**, *11*, 301–313. [CrossRef]

11.	Asthana, G.S.; Sharma, P.K.; Asthana, A. In Vitro and in Vivo Evaluation of Niosomal Formulation for Controlled Delivery of Clarithromycin. *Scientifica* **2016**, *2016*, 6492953. [CrossRef]

12.	Khan, D.H.; Bashir, S.; Khan, M.I.; Figueiredo, P.; Santos, H.A.; Peltonen, L. Formulation Optimization and in Vitro Characterization of Rifampicin and Ceftriaxone Dual Drug Loaded Niosomes with High Energy Probe Sonication Technique. *J. Drug Deliv. Sci. Technol.* **2020**, *58*, 101763. [CrossRef]

13.	Chen, J.; Qin, X.; Zhong, S.; Chen, S.; Su, W.; Liu, Y. Characterization of Curcumin/Cyclodextrin Polymer Inclusion Complex and Investigation on Its Antioxidant and Antiproliferative Activities. *Molecules* **2018**, *23*, 1179. [CrossRef] [PubMed]

14.	Afreen, U.; Fahelelbom, K.M.; Shah, S.N.H.; Ashames, A.; Almas, U.; Khan, S.A.; Yameen, M.A.; Nisar, N.; BinAsad, M.H.H.; Murtaza, G. Formulation and Evaluation of Niosomes-Based Chlorpheniramine Gel for the Treatment of Mild to Moderate Skin Allergy. *J. Exp. Nanosci.* **2022**, *17*, 467–495. [CrossRef]

15.	Judy, E.; Lopus, M.; Kishore, N. Mechanistic Insights into Encapsulation and Release of Drugs in Colloidal Niosomal Systems: Biophysical Aspects. *RSC Adv.* **2021**, *11*, 35110–35126. [CrossRef] [PubMed]

16.	Herdiana, Y.; Wathoni, N.; Shamsuddin, S.; Muchtaridi, M. Drug Release Study of the Chitosan-Based Nanoparticles. *Heliyon* **2022**, *8*, e08674. [CrossRef] [PubMed]

17.	Chen, X.; Liang, L.; Han, C. Borate Suppresses the Scavenging Activity of Gallic Acid and Plant Polyphenol Extracts on DPPH Radical: A Potential Interference to DPPH Assay. *Lwt* **2020**, *131*, 109769. [CrossRef]

18.	Awosika, T.O.; Aluko, R.E. Inhibition of the in Vitro Activities of α-Amylase, α-Glucosidase and Pancreatic Lipase by Yellow Field Pea (*Pisum sativum* L.) Protein Hydrolysates. *Int. J. Food Sci. Technol.* **2019**, *54*, 2021–2034. [CrossRef]

19.	Mechchate, H.; Es-Safi, I.; Louba, A.; Alqahtani, A.S.; Nasr, F.A.; Noman, O.M.; Farooq, M.; Alharbi, M.S.; Alqahtani, A.; Bari, A.; et al. In Vitro Alpha-Amylase and Alpha-Glucosidase Inhibitory Activity and in Vivo Antidiabetic Activity of *Withania frutescens* L. Foliar Extract. *Molecules* **2021**, *26*, 293. [CrossRef] [PubMed]

20.	Hnin, H.M.; Stefánsson, E.; Loftsson, T.; Asasutjarit, R.; Charnvanich, D.; Jansook, P. Physicochemical and Stability Evaluation of Topical Niosomal Encapsulating Fosinopril/γ-Cyclodextrin Complex for Ocular Delivery. *Pharmaceutics* **2022**, *14*, 1147. [CrossRef] [PubMed]

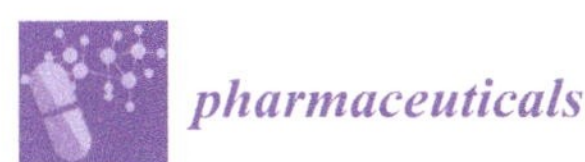
pharmaceuticals

Article

Mannose-Functionalized Isoniazid-Loaded Nanostructured Lipid Carriers for Pulmonary Delivery: In Vitro Prospects and In Vivo Therapeutic Efficacy Assessment

Shaveta Ahalwat [1,*], Dinesh Chandra Bhatt [2,*], Surbhi Rohilla [2], Vikas Jogpal [1], Kirti Sharma [1], Tarun Virmani [3], Girish Kumar [3], Abdulsalam Alhalmi [4], Ali S. Alqahtani [5], Omar M. Noman [5] and Marwan Almoiliqy [6]

[1] School of Medical and Allied Sciences, G. D. Goenka University, Gurugram 122103, India; vikas.jogpal@gdgu.org (V.J.); kirti.sharma@gdgu.org (K.S.)
[2] Department of Pharmaceutical Sciences, Guru Jambheshwar University of Science and Technology, Hisar 125001, India; surbhiraman.rohilla22@gmail.com
[3] School of Pharmaceutical Sciences, MVN University, Palwal 121105, India; tarun.virmani@mvn.edu.in (T.V.); girish.kumar@mvn.edu.in (G.K.)
[4] Department of Pharmaceutics, School of Pharmaceutical Education and Research, Jamia Hamdard, New Delhi 110062, India; asalamahmed5@gmail.com
[5] Department of Pharmacognosy, College of Pharmacy, King Saud University, P.O. Box 2457, Riyadh 11451, Saudi Arabia; alalqahtani@ksu.edu.sa (A.S.A.); onoman@ksu.edu.sa (O.M.N.)
[6] Department of Translational Molecular Pathology, The University of Texas MD Anderson Cancer Center, Houston, TX 77030, USA; msmohammed@mdanderson.org
* Correspondence: shaveta.ahalwat@gmail.com (S.A.); bhatt_2000@yahoo.com (D.C.B.)

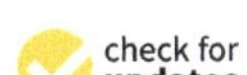
check for updates

Citation: Ahalwat, S.; Bhatt, D.C.; Rohilla, S.; Jogpal, V.; Sharma, K.; Virmani, T.; Kumar, G.; Alhalmi, A.; Alqahtani, A.S.; Noman, O.M.; et al. Mannose-Functionalized Isoniazid-Loaded Nanostructured Lipid Carriers for Pulmonary Delivery: In Vitro Prospects and In Vivo Therapeutic Efficacy Assessment. *Pharmaceuticals* **2023**, *16*, 1108. https://doi.org/10.3390/ph16081108

Academic Editors: Ana Catarina Silva, João Nuno Moreira and José Manuel Sousa Lobo

Received: 26 June 2023
Revised: 23 July 2023
Accepted: 1 August 2023
Published: 4 August 2023

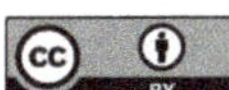

Abstract: Resistance to isoniazid (INH) is common and increases the possibility of acquiring multidrug-resistant tuberculosis. For this study, isoniazid-loaded nanostructured lipid carriers (INH-NLCs) were developed and effectively functionalized with mannose (Man) to enhance the residence time of the drug within the lungs via specific delivery and increase the therapeutic efficacy of the formulation. The mannose-functionalized isoniazid-loaded nanostructured lipid carrier (Man-INH-NLC) formulation was evaluated with respect to various formulation parameters, namely, encapsulation efficiency (EE), drug loading (DL), average particle size (PS), zeta potential (ZP), polydispersity index (PDI), in vitro drug release (DR), and release kinetics. The in vitro inhalation behavior of the developed formulation after nebulization was investigated using an Andersen cascade impactor via the estimation of the mass median aerosolized diameter (MMAD) and geometric aerodynamic diameter (GAD) and subsequently found to be suitable for effective lung delivery. An in vivo pharmacokinetic study was carried out in a guinea pig animal model, and it was demonstrated that Man-INH-NLC has a longer residence time in the lungs with improved pharmacokinetics when compared with unfunctionalized INH-NLC, indicating the enhanced therapeutic efficacy of the Man-INH-NLC formulation. Histopathological analysis led us to determine that the extent of tissue damage was more severe in the case of the pure drug solution of isoniazid compared to the Man-INH-NLC formulation after nebulization. Thus, the nebulization of Man-INH-NLC was found to be safe, forming a sound basis for enhancing the therapeutic efficacy of the drug for improved management in the treatment of pulmonary tuberculosis.

Keywords: isoniazid; nanostructured lipid carriers; in vivo pharmacokinetics; drug release profile; histopathological toxicity; mannosylation

1. Introduction

Tuberculosis is widely spread pandemic disease caused by the bacteria *Mycobacterium tuberculosis*, and it remains a common cause of death despite the availability of effective treatment [1,2]. The major drawback of the current drug treatments is the emergence of resistance, i.e., extensive drug-resistant (XDR) tuberculosis and multidrug-resistant (MDR) tuberculosis [3]. This occurs due to high doses and long-term treatment plans that trigger the natural process of spontaneous chromosomal mutations in mycobacteria linked to inadequate treatment outcomes, post-treatment relapse, and death [4,5]. To eradicate this life-threatening disease, drug doses and dosing frequencies must be considerably reduced to reduce resistance and increase the effectiveness of treatments [6,7].

Isoniazid is the safest first-line antitubercular drug, and it acts by suppressing mycolic acid synthesis (a basic unit of the bacterial cell wall) [8]. It comes under BCS class III (high solubility and limited permeability). It is rapidly absorbed and achieves peak plasma concentration within 1–3 h post-oral administration [9]. It has a very short half-life of 1–2 h and requires frequent dosing. The recommended dose for isoniazid ranges from 5 to 10 mg/kg/day. Although, a higher dose (up to 25 mg/kg/day) can also be prescribed in severe cases [10]. The bacteria quickly become resistant to INH due to patient non-adherence, which has hampered the effectiveness of the drug [11]. So, there is a need to redevelop the conventional formulations of isoniazid with an emphasis on targeting efficiency, decreasing dosage and dosing frequency, and increasing the therapeutic efficacy of treatment [12].

Passive and active targeting approaches are widely used to achieve targeted therapeutic delivery to the lungs for the successful treatment of tuberculosis [13]. Passive targeting can be achieved by maintaining an optimal mean particle diameter of 200 to 600 nm to deposit the particles deep into the lungs [14,15]. Active targeting can be achieved via mannose functionalization of the formulation as it is more capable of delivering a high drug payload to the target site and increasing the mean residence time in the lungs compared to conventional dosage forms [16–21].

Nanostructured lipid carriers have been exploited as drug delivery carriers and are enhanced versions of the solid lipid nanoparticles employed in the development of lipid nanocarrier formulations [22,23]. The inclusion of liquid lipids in the formation of nanostructured lipid carriers is crucial as it significantly enhances the properties of the formulation [24]. NLCs are advantageous as they are capable of overcoming the limitations of solid lipid nanoparticles, such as the poor drug loading of hydrophilic drugs, low physical stability, and degradation of the loaded bio-actives, and provide high drug loading capacity [25,26]. NLCs can incorporate both hydrophilic and lipophilic drugs, providing a sustained release effect with high in vivo tolerance and facilitating administration via various routes [27].

This work aimed to formulate isoniazid-loaded nanostructured lipid carriers using solid lipids, such as compritol 888 (COMP) and octadecyl amine (ODA); a liquid lipid, namely, linoleic acid (LA); and surfactants, namely, tween 80 and poloxamer 40. This formulation was functionalized using D-mannose to enhance the specificity and delivery of the nanocarrier formulation deep into the lungs. The developed Man-INH-NLC formulation was characterized for encapsulation efficiency, drug loading, average particle size, polydispersity index, and zeta potential. In vitro drug release was estimated for both INH-NLC and Man-INH-NLC in a suitable medium at different pH to simulate the different parts of the lungs. Surface morphology was observed via TEM photomicrographs. The in vitro behavior of the nebulized mist was also investigated by estimating the mass median aerosolized diameter and geometric aerodynamic diameter, output efficiency (OE), and respirable fraction (RF). Furthermore, an in vivo pharmacokinetic and bioavailability assessment was carried out using a guinea pig animal model. Histopathological studies were also conducted, and hepatotoxicity was investigated by assessing the toxicity of the formulation.

2. Results and Discussion

2.1. Investigation of Mannose-Functionalized NLC

The INH-NLC formulation was functionalized with mannose for specific delivery into the lungs. For this purpose, the mannose ring opening phenomenon was used. The acidic environment provided by the acetate buffer results in the opening of the mannose ring. A Schiff's base (–N=CH–) was formed due to the interaction between the aldehydic group of D-mannose and the octadecylamine amino group of the INH-NLC formulation. Figure 1 shows a characteristic absorption band of the aldehydic -C(H)=O mannose group at around 2850.11 cm^{-1}, whereas the absorption band at 3351.17 cm^{-1} represents the -NH$_2$ group of octadecylamine in the spectrum of INH-NLC formulation. An interaction between these two groups resulted in the constitution of Schiff's base, which was confirmed by an absorption band at around 1639.86 cm^{-1} in the FT-IR spectra of the Man-INH-NLC formulation. These observations were similar to that reported in the research work of Pinheiro M. et al., 2016 [28].

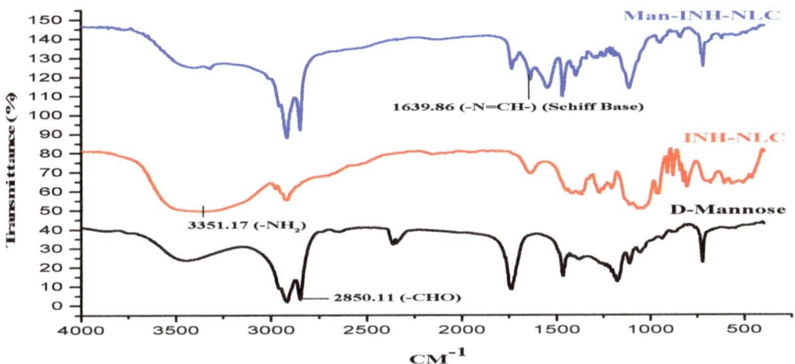

Figure 1. FT-IR spectra of INH–NLC and Man–INH–NLC for the detection of Schiff base (–N=CH–).

2.2. Encapsulation Efficiency and Drug Loading

The INH-NLC and Man-INH-NLC formulations were analyzed for EE and DL and found to be decreased insignificantly ($p > 0.05$) for Man-INH-NLC compared to INH-NLC (Table 1). This might be due to the diffusion of some surface-adsorbed drugs in a buffer medium during the process of mannosylation. This finding is consistent with earlier research [29].

Table 1. Investigation of INH-NLC and Man-INH-NLC formulations for %EE and %DL.

S. No.	Formulation	Encapsulation Efficiency (%EE)	Drug Loading (%DL)
1.	INH-NLC	82.09 ± 3.60 **	18.39 ± 0.81 **
2.	Man-INH-NLC	79.71 ± 1.65 **	17.86 ± 0.37 **

** $p > 0.05$. (One-way ANOVA, post-Dunnet test). Values are expressed as mean ± SD; $n = 3$.

2.3. Average Particle Size, Polydispersity Index, and Zeta Potential Measurements

The average particle size of INH-NLC and Man-INH-NLC formulations are presented in Table 2. The Mannosylation process resulted in a substantial increase in particle size due to mannose functionalization on the surface of INH-NL [30]. For effective passive targeting, the particle size should be in the range of 200 to 600 nm. The mannose-functionalized NLCs that have a mean diameter of 273 nm and are administered through the pulmonary route are likely to reach the deeper region of the lungs [14]. The PDI values for the INH-NLC and Man-INH-NLC formulations were estimated to be 0.289 ± 0.04 and 0.223 ± 0.02, respectively. A PDI value below 0.3 indicated the uniform dispersion of the particles (monodisperse) within the formulation. The INH-NLC formulation showed a positive zeta potential due to the positive amine group of octadecylamine. A significant decrease in zeta potential was observed for Man-INH-NLC after the process of mannosylation. This is because positively charged amine groups of octadecylamine reacted with the aldehyde group of D-mannose and caused shielding of the positive charge. This strongly suggests the successful mannosylation of the Man-INH-NLC formulation. Also, the positive charge of the mannosylated formulation enhances the cell internalization and intracellular accumulation of the drug within the infected cells, leading to an improvement in the anti-bacterial function of the drug [31,32]. Moreover, Man-INH-NLC was regarded as physically stable due to its steric stabilization and electrostatic repulsions between particles [33].

Table 2. Characterization of INH-NLC and Man-INH-NLC formulations in terms of average PS, PDI, and ZP.

S. No.	Formulation	Particle Size Analysis (nm)	The Polydispersity Index (PDI)	Zeta Potential (mV)
1.	INH-NLC	247.6 ± 4.05	0.289 ± 0.04	+42.48 ± 1.86
2.	Man-INH-NLC	273.4 ± 8.24	0.223 ± 0.02	+24.18 ± 2.26

Values are expressed as mean ± SD; $n = 3$.

2.4. In Vitro Drug Release Analysis

The in vitro drug release from Man-INH-NLC was evaluated at different pH conditions of phosphate-buffered saline and compared with unfunctionalized INH-NLC, and the results are shown in Figure 2. It was observed that drug release from Man-INH-NLC (72.35 ± 1.09%) is slower compared to INH-NLC (78.11 ± 1.27%) in phosphate-buffered saline pH 7.4. Drug release was also analyzed at other pH levels (PBS pH 6.2 and 5.0) to simulate the behavior of the nanocarrier formulations in different parts of the lungs, and drug release was found to be slightly slower for Man-INH-NLC compared to INH-NLC. This could be a result of the extra outer coating of mannose around nanocarriers, which acts as a barrier, significantly slowing the release of the drug. The drug release from Man-INH-NLC had slight differences at all pH values and was comparable to the others, as shown in Figure 2A. A similar kind of effect can be seen in Figure 2B for the INH-NLC formulation. This led us to conclude that the drug release of both formulations was independent of the pH values and that both could be suitable drug carriers for pulmonary administration.

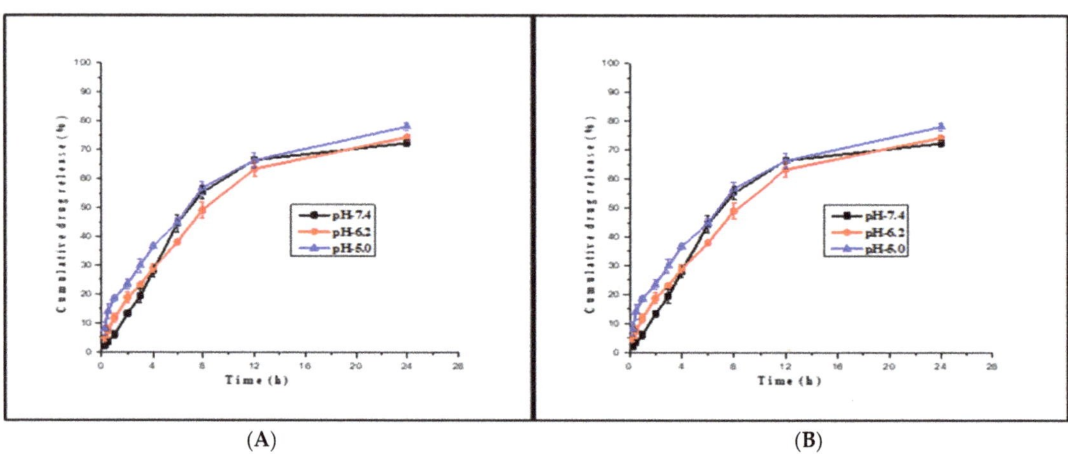

Figure 2. In vitro drug release studies of Man-INH-NLC (**A**) and INH-NLC (**B**) at pH 7.4 for lung fluid, pH 6.2 for phagosomes, and pH 5.0 for phagolysosomes (all the values are expressed as mean ± SD; $n = 3$).

2.5. In Vitro Release Kinetics

The behavior of drug release from the nanocarrier formulation was examined using numerous mathematical models. For INH-NLC and Man-INH-NLC, the plots of log time versus log percent drug release were shown to be linear, with the highest correlation coefficients being 0.9661 and 0.9717, respectively (Table 3). The %DR for both INH-NLC and Man-INH-NLC was determined according to the Korsmeyer–Peppas model, and it was found that the drug was released by a non-Fickian diffusion-controlled mechanism with *n* values of 0.8086 and 0.8788, respectively [34].

Table 3. Correlation coefficient (r^2) of various kinetic drug release models for different formulations.

S. No.	Formulation	Zero-Order	First-Order	Higuchi's Square Root Model	Korsmeyer–Peppas Model
1	INH-NLC	0.739	0.739	0.9019	0.9661
2	Man-INH-NLC	0.7881	0.7881	0.9298	0.9717

2.6. Transmission Electron Microscopy

TEM images of both INH-NLC and Man-INH-NLC showed spherical particles with uniform shapes and smooth surfaces. The coating around the INH-NLC nanocarriers can be seen in Figure 3B. The nanometric size of INH-NLC was increased after mannosylation. No evidence of particle agglomeration was found. As can be observed below, the morphologies of both the INH-NLC (Figure 3A) and Man-INH-NLC (Figure 3B) formulations are identical, showing that mannosylation does not affect particle shape and surface.

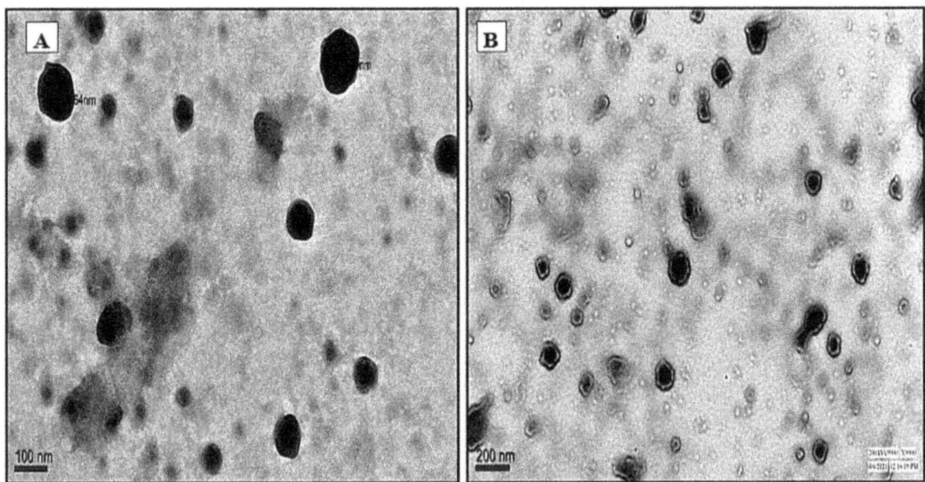

Figure 3. TEM micrographs of (**A**) INH-NLC and (**B**) Man-INH-NLC at $10\times$ magnification.

2.7. In Vitro Evaluation of Inhalation Behavior of Nebulized Mist

The Anderson cascade impactor was utilized to evaluate the in vitro inhalation properties of the mist formed from NLC dispersion produced by the nebulizer [35]. MMAD represents the value below which 50% of the particles are present in the respirable range. As per WHO guidelines, MMAD should be below 5.5 µm. MMAD of 2.3 ± 1.1 µm showed that 50% of the particles of the nebulized mist of the Man-INH-NLC dispersion were below the size of 2.3 ± 1.1 µm. GSD refers to the geographic mean of all aerosolized particles, which should be below 2.3 µm. A GSD value of 1.9 ± 0.2 µm showed that the geographic mean of all aerosolized particles was 1.9 ± 0.2 µm. The output efficiency represents the efficiency of the nebulizer in producing the mist of the nanoformulation, and it was found to be 95.24 ± 4.56%. Respirable fractions represent the inhalation characteristics of the formulation and provide the concentration of the formulation that reaches the lungs. The respirable fraction was found to be 87.33 ± 6.09% for the nebulizer. This study proved that the air jet nebulizer has high efficiency, provides good inhalation characteristics, and is suitable for the passive targeting of the Man-INH-NLC formulation. These values indicated the efficient delivery of nanocarrier-encapsulated drugs into deeper pulmonary regions [36].

2.8. In Vivo Pharmacokinetic Analysis

Pharmacokinetic parameters were analyzed for a comparative bioavailability assessment of the developed formulation. The results stated that, after a single nebulization, a very small amount of the drug was detected in the plasma for 4 h in the case of Man-INH-NLC formulation and 2 h in the case of the INH-NLC formulation, indicating its slow initial absorption (Figure 4). The delayed appearance of the drug in the blood was more notable for the Man-INH-NLC formulation in comparison to the INH-NLC formulation. The reason behind this is the effective coating of mannose and their affinity for mannose receptors, which increase the drug residence time in the lungs. The Man-INH-NLC and INH-NLC formulations remained in the therapeutic range for 48 h and 24 h, respectively. The longer stay of Man-INH-NLC is due to the encapsulation of the hydrophilic drug into a lipophilic matrix, and the additional mannose coating over it represents the greater sustained release effect of the drug compared to INH-NLC. In contrast, a relatively shorter stay of the parent drug in the lungs was observed after nebulization. The drug started to appear in plasma after one hour of pulmonary administration due to its highly hydrophilic nature and the non-availability of lipid encapsulation. The drug was not detected in the plasma as it was quickly eliminated from the blood after 12 h of nebulization due to very short $t_{1/2}$.

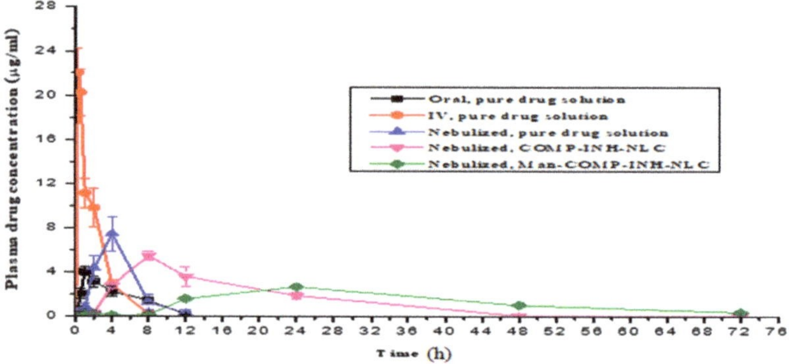

Figure 4. Plasma drug profile of isoniazid after single nebulization of Man-INH-NLC, INH-NLC, and parent drug. Values mean $\pm$ S.D.; $n = 6$ at each time point.

The pharmacokinetic parameters of isoniazid are given in Table 4. C_{max} represents the maximum drug concentration that usually reaches the plasma after its administration, whereas T_{max} is the time taken to achieve C_{max} within the same. Man-INH-NLC gives rise to a shorter peak plasma concentration (C_{max}) and takes a longer time to achieve it (T_{max}). Among the pulmonary administered formulations, the highest C_{max} ($p < 0.05$) was observed for the pure drug solution, followed by the INH-NLC formulation and, lastly, the Man-INH-NLC formulation, which resulted in the sustained release of the formulation due to its lipophilic nature. Additionally, the maximum C_{max} ($p < 0.05$) was found for the intravenously administered pure drug solution, followed by the orally administered pure drug solution, and the former gets quickly eliminated from the body. K_{el} represents the rate at which a drug is removed from the human system. A low elimination rate value (K_{el}) represented the extended $t_{1/2}$ of any formulation. Man-INH-NLC has a slower elimination rate compared to INH-NLC. Mean residence time (MRT) indicated the average time taken by a drug to reside in the body. The MRT of the INH-NLC and Man-INH-NLC formulations experienced significant three-fold and seven-fold increases, respectively, when compared with the nebulized pure drug solution and four-fold and eleven-fold when compared to the orally administered parent drug solution. The highest $AUC_{0-\infty}$ value was found for the Man-INH-NLC formulation, followed by the INH-NLC, which affected both relative and absolute bioavailability. Relative bioavailability (compared to oral) after nebulization increased four- and five-fold for INH-NLC and Man-INH-NLC, respectively. Absolute bioavailability (compared to i.v.) also increased by nearly two- and three-fold for INH-NLC and Man-INH-NLC, respectively.

Table 4. Salient pharmacokinetic parameters of isoniazid following a single nebulization of Man-INH-NLC compared with a free drug.

Formulations	C_{max}, mg/L	T_{max}, Hour	K_{el}	$t_{1/2}$, Hour	MRT, Hour	$AUC_{0-\infty}$ (mg.h/L)	Relative Bioavailability	Absolute Bioavailability
Pure drug solution, Oral	4.08 ± 0.42	1	0.16 ± 0.01	4.25 ± 0.34	4.87 ± 0.2	22.65 ± 2.55	1	0.49
Pure drug solution, IV	22.04 ± 2.21	0.25	0.66 ± 0.19	1.12 ± 0.3 **	1.88 ± 0.14	45.87 ± 3.97	ns	1
Pure drug solution, Nebulized	7.46 ± 1.55	4	0.093 ± 0.04 **	8.53 ± 3.33 **	7.43 ± 3.11 **	42.03 ± 9.70	1.86	0.92
INH-NLC, Nebulized	5.51 ± 0.4 **	8	0.027 ± 0.01	26.80 ± 6.39	18.81 ± 2.91	100.85 ± 3.83	4.45	2.10
Man-INH-NLC, Nebulized	2.72 ± 0.24 **	24	-0.0174 ± 0.001	40.06 ± 3.78	51.11 ± 2.46	118.61 ± 8.28	5.24	2.89

** $p > 0.05$. (One-way ANOVA, post-Dunnet with respect to the oral-free drug). Values are expressed as mean $\pm$ SD; $n = 6$; ns— not significant.

In vivo pharmacokinetic parameters bear important therapeutic implications and proved improved drug delivery with an enhanced residence time and improved pharmacokinetic profile with respect to the Man-INH-NLC formulation in the lungs as well as in blood compared to the unfunctionalized INH-NLC formulation and the pure drug solutions administered via oral and intravenous routes. This provided a better way to increase the therapeutic effect of isoniazid in the management of tuberculosis treatment [37].

2.9. Histological Evaluation

Histological analysis was carried out at high doses of isoniazid (40 mg/kg/day) and administered in different formulations via a different route of administration. The evaluation was carried out for any kind of allergic reaction and toxicity to the lungs and other body organs after repeated administration for a long time. Figure 5A–D show the untreated (control) lung, liver, brain, and kidney tissues of the experimental animals, respectively. After 4 weeks of the daily nebulization of the Man-INH-NLC and blank Man-NLC formulations, some minor changes were observed in the alveolar area of the lungs, which were not toxic when compared to the untreated control. The interalveolar spaces and interalveolar septum of the lungs were found to be normal for both formulations after nebulization (Figure 5E,I). No kind of inflammation or degenerative changes were observed in the liver (Figure 5F,J) and brain (Figure 5G,K), resulting in its safe use. After the nebulization of the pure drug solutions, the lungs of the treated animals showed edema in alveolar spaces (Figure 5M). Mild changes in hepatocytes and low-grade central congestion were observed in the liver of the animals compared to the group receiving Man-INH-NLC (Figure 5N). No kind of histological changes were found in any part of the brain among the treated animals (Figure 5O). Animals receiving a pure drug solution via nebulization showed higher inflammation in their lungs than those treated with pure drug solutions administered intravenously (Figure 5Q). Metabolic changes and an increased concentration of glial cells resulted in increased inflammation being observable in the liver and brain, respectively. (Figure 5R,S). In the case of the orally administered pure drug solution, thickening of the interalveolar septum and vascular degeneration to a small extent were found in the lungs and liver, respectively (Figure 5U,V), whereas a degenerated nucleus was found in the cerebrum of the brain of the treated animals (Figure 5W). No kind of changes or signs of toxicity were observed in the kidneys for all of the formulations administered via a different route of administration. Glomerular filtration and glomerular tubule appeared normal. The solution responsible for causing the most toxicity to the liver and brain was found to be the orally administered pure drug solution, while the nebulized pure drug solution facilitated large toxicity in the lungs in contrast to other organs. It was concluded that treatment with a high dose of blank mannosylated nanocarrier formulation (Man-COMP-NLC) and a drug-loaded mannosylated nanocarrier formulation (Man-INH-NLC) via nebulization appeared to be well tolerated by the animals, having been found safe during the entire period of study. No toxicity was observed for the blank Man-NLC and Man-INH-NLC formulations due to the encapsulation of the drug in biocompatible/physiological lipids and the provision of a sustained release effect for a large duration of time.

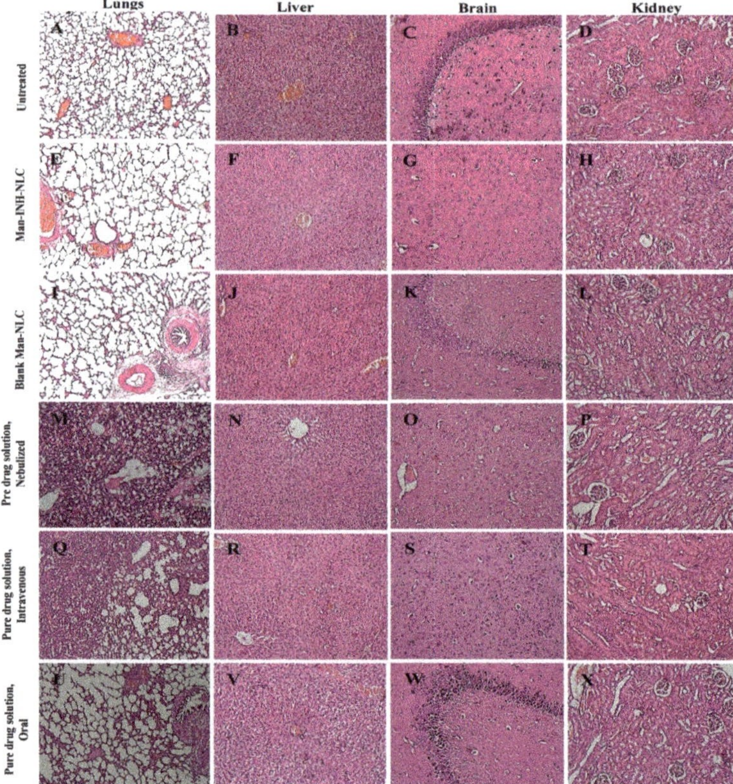

Figure 5. Histology of different organs (i.e., lung, liver, brain, and kidney) in each group of animals (guinea pig; *n* = 6) receiving different treatments viz. Untreated (**A–D**), Man-INH-NLC, Nebulized (**E–H**), Blank Man-NLC, Nebulized (**I–L**), Pure drug solution, Nebulized (**M–P**), Pure drug solution, Intravenous (**Q–T**), Pure drug solution, Oral (**U–X**). The generation of the images shown was facilitated by using a light microscope at 10× magnification.

2.10. Hepatotoxic and Nephrotoxic Evaluation

The parameters for hepato- and nephrotoxicity in serum were evaluated with respect to normal functioning of the liver and kidney, respectively. ALT/ALP/AST were used as indicators of liver function tests, and urea/creatinine/bilirubin were used as markers of kidney function tests. An increase in these parameters beyond normal values indicated the presence of toxicity or an allergic reaction in the respective organs. An evaluation of hepatotoxicity and nephrotoxicity was carried out for Man-INH-NLC, blank Man-NLC, and the pure drug solutions administered via different routes of administration, and the results are shown in Table 5. The results indicated a remarkable increase ($p < 0.05$) in serum ALT, ALP, and AST levels upon the administration of high doses of the pure drug solutions administered via oral, intravenous, and pulmonary routes in comparison with the untreated control group. Significant ($p < 0.05$) increases in serum ALT (38.64, 103.77, 97.06 IU/L), ALP (153.51, 379.99, 371.66 IU/L), and AST (34.71, 96.52, 103.68 IU/L) activities were found upon the administration of the pure drug solutions administered via the oral, intravenous, and pulmonary routes, respectively, indicating that a pure drug solution of isoniazid induces damage to hepatic cells possibly because the free drug was exposed to liver cells without any shielding effect to non-target cells, thereby leading to more toxic action. The administration of blank Man-NLC and Man-INH-NLC resulted in a slight increase of ALT, ALP, and AST to 39.78, 193.64, and 49.13 IU/L, respectively, which was found to be within the normal limits compared to the untreated control group because of the encapsulation of the drug in the biocompatible lipids and its sustained drug release effect from the lipid matrix. Furthermore, both blank and isoniazid-encapsulated Man-INH-NLC administered via the pulmonary route led to a slight increase in urea, bilirubin, and creatinine levels within normal ranges in serum compared to the untreated control. This may be due to the fact that the drug is directly targeted to the lungs, meaning that the drug's access to the kidney was minimal. A moderate increase in the same parameters was found in the case of pure drug solutions administered via the oral, intravenous, and pulmonary routes, and this increase was found to be within the normal ranges. These results indicate that both the pure isoniazid drug solution and the drug encapsulated in the lipid nanocarrier formulation had no harmful effect on the kidney and failed to induce any toxic effects in kidney cells. These results are in close agreement with the results obtained in the histological studies and point towards the safety of administering Man-INH-NLC through the pulmonary route using a nebulizer.

Table 5. Hepatotoxic and nephrotoxic evaluation in animals treated with a pure drug solution, blank Man-NLC, and Man-INH-NLC.

Formulation Code	Liver Function Test			Kidney Function Test		
	ALT (IU/L)	ALP (IU/L)	AST (IU/L)	Urea (mg/dL)	Bilirubin (mg/dL)	Creatinine (mg/dL)
Untreated control	38.64 ± 5.33	153.51 ± 10.29	34.71 ± 3.62	15.17 ± 1.36	0.39 ± 0.07	1.13 ± 0.09
The oral, pure drug solution	103.77 ± 7.21	379.99 ± 13.47	96.52 ± 10.72	25.63 ± 2.68	0.62 ± 0.16	1.65 ± 0.10
IV, the pure drug solution	97.058 ± 5.64	371.66 ± 14.75	103.68 ± 3.38	27.69 ± 3.36	0.68 ± 0.15	1.75 ± 0.13
The nebulized, pure drug solution	98.47 ± 8.61	359.25 ± 5.73	87.27 ± 7.39	23.71 ± 2.91	0.61 ± 0.17	2.01 ± 0.24
Nebulized, blank Man-NLC	53.64 ± 2.81 **	171.12 ± 10.75	42.77 ± 7.87	16.43 ± 1.13 **	0.48 ± 0.03 **	1.25 ± 0.12 **
Nebulized, Man-INH-NLC	39.78 ± 6.26	193.64 ± 5.81	49.13 ± 9.44 **	18.98 ± 0.67	0.43 ± 0.09 **	1.31 ± 0.12

Values are expressed as mean $\pm$ SD; $n = 6$. ** represents $p > 0.05$ (one-way ANOVA, post Dunnet) with respect to the untreated control. The normal ranges in guinea pigs—ALT: 10 to 90 IU/L; ALP: 80 to 350 IU/L; AST: 10 to 90; urea: 9 to 32 mg/dL; total bilirubin: 0.3 to 1.0 mg/dL; creatinine: 0.6 to 2.2 mg/dL.

3. Materials and Methods

3.1. Material and Components

Compritol 888 was procured as a gift sample from Gattefosse Pvt Ltd., Saint-Priest, France. Other chemicals, namely, isoniazid, octadecylamine, linoleic acid, tween 80, and poloxamer 407 were purchased from Merck, Burlington, MA, USA. All the chemicals and analytical reagent (AR) were of analytical grade. Double distilled water was used for all experiments.

3.2. Method of Preparation of NLC

The hot homogenization–ultrasonication technique was used to prepare the INH-NLC formulation. The concentrations of all of the lipids and drugs were optimized in our previous studies and used accordingly [38]. Briefly, all of the lipids (compritol-50.67 w/w, octadecyl amine-26.94 w/w, and linoleic acid-22.38 w/w), together with tween 80 (0.1 g), were heated to 80 °C under continuous stirring. The aqueous phase was constituted separately using poloxamer 407 (1%) in double-distilled water and heated at an identical temperature. This aqueous solution (1 mL) was used to dissolve the drug (INH- 239.82 mg), and this lipid melt was subsequently subjected to homogenization at 18,000 rpm (Heidolph, Schwabach, Germany) for 5 min to make w/o emulsion. A constant temperature was maintained throughout the entire procedure. The dropwise addition of a surfactant solution (aqueous phase) was carried out to obtain w/o/w emulsion and subjected to sonication by employing a probe sonicator (Q55, Sonica Sonicators, New York, NY, USA) at an amplitude of 80% for 5 min. This INH-NLC dispersion was subjected to cooling at room temperature to facilitate nanosuspension.

3.3. Mannosylation of Nanostructured Lipid Carriers

The mannose functionalization of INH-NLC was accomplished using a previously reported method with some modifications [17,39]. Firstly, a 50 Mm D-(+)-mannose solution was prepared in acetate buffer pH 4.0 and added to the INH-NLC dispersion till the concentration of octadecylamine remained at 0.02% w/v in the final INH-NLC dispersion. Secondly, this dispersion was subjected to continuous and gentle stirring for 48 h to obtain the completion of the reaction at room temperature. This dispersion was subjected to 70 °C temperature under vacuum to obtain a concentrated formulation. The removal of free mannose was achieved by exhibiting the Man-INH-NLC under extensive dialysis with double-distilled water for 45 min using an activated dialysis bag (molecular weight cut-off 12–14 k Da, Hi-Media, Mumbi, India). The resulting nanocarriers were freshly reconstituted in normal saline to facilitate nanosuspension [6]. The blank NLC formulation was formulated similarly, without the addition of INH.

3.4. Fourier-Transform Infrared Spectroscopy

FTIR spectroscopy was carried out to confirm the mannose coating on the Man-INH-NLC surface by analyzing the formation of Schiff's base. FTIR analysis of INH-NLC and Man-INH-NLC was performed via the KBr pellet method using an FTIR spectrophotometer (Spectrum BX, Perkin Almer, New York, NY, USA). Analysis was carried out in a frequency range ranging from 4500 cm^{-1} to 350 cm^{-1} at 4 cm^{-1} resolutions with a sample/KBr ratio of 1:10 [40].

3.5. Encapsulation Efficiency and Drug Loading Analysis

A UV spectrophotometer (UV-1800, Shimadzu, Tokyo, Japan) was used to evaluate the %EE and %DL of both INH-NLC and Man-INH-NLC at λ_{max} 262 nm. Centrifugation of NLC suspension was carried out at 18,000 rpm for 45 min at 4 °C to obtain the NLC pellet. The NLC pellet was separated, and the below aqueous phase was subjected to a suitable solvent extraction method to recover the drug. The obtained drug samples were sufficiently diluted with distilled water, filtered through 45 μm filter paper, and analyzed for drug content [41].

$$Entrapment\ efficiency\ (\%) = \frac{Wi - Wf}{Wi} \times 100 \qquad (1)$$

$$Drug\ Loading\ (\%) = \frac{Wi - Wf}{Wi - Wf + Wt} \times 100 \qquad (2)$$

where W_i = weight of drug added during NLC formation; W_f = weight of unentrapped drug; W_t = total weight of all lipids and drugs added to the NLC formulation [42].

3.6. Average Particle Size, Polydispersity Index, and Zeta Potential Analysis

The particle sizes of both the INH-NLC and Man-INH-NLC formulations were analyzed using a Zeta sizer (Nano ZS®, Malvern, UK) at 25 °C with backscattered light at 90°. This gives the average particle size as a z-average, also known as the average hydrodynamic diameter of a nanoformulation [43]. PDI represents the homogeneity of the dispersion, and its value ranges from 0 to 1. Values approaching 0 indicate relatively homogenous dispersion, while values larger than 0.5 indicate heterogeneous dispersion [44]. The zeta potential (ZP) indicates particle surface charge, and the Helmholtz–Smoluchowski equation was used to calculate particle electrophoretic mobility and convert it into zeta potential. Multiple scattering effects were prevented by making suitable dilutions with deionized water [45].

3.7. In Vitro Drug Release Analysis

The release of INH from both the INH-NLC and Man-INH-NLC formulations was investigated via the dialysis bag approach using an activated dialysis tube in phosphate-buffered saline (PBS) pH 7.4 for lung fluid, pH 6.2 for nasal fluid and phagosomes, and pH 5 for phagolysosomes to simulate the lung environment after pulmonary administration. The NLC dispersion was equivalent to 5 mg of INH and put into a double-folding dialysis bag that was carefully sealed on both sides and immersed in beakers carrying 250 mL of dissolution media. The stirring rate was set to 200 rpm, and the temperature was kept at 37 ± 0.5 °C. A parafilm was used to cover all the beakers to prevent solvent loss. The samples (5 mL) were withdrawn at different time points (0.25, 0.5, 1, 2, 3, 4, 6, 8, 12, and 24 h), and the same amount was substituted with fresh dissolution media after each withdrawal to maintain the sink condition. The amounts of INH released were analyzed spectrophotometrically [46].

3.8. In Vitro Drug Release Kinetics

Numerous release kinetic models (zero-order, first-order, Higuchi's square root, and Korsmeyer–Peppas) were employed to investigate the behavior of drug release from the optimized formulation. The model with the best fit was determined based on which had the highest correlation coefficient (R^2). The n-value indicated the behavior of drug release ($n < 0.5$ represents Fickian transport; $n = 0.5$ to 0.9 represents non-Fickian transport) in the Korsmeyer–Peppas model [34].

3.9. Transmission Electron Microscopy

TEM analyses of the INH-NLC and Man-INH-NLC formulations were performed to evaluate the particle sizes and internal morphologies of the formulations. A TEM instrument (Tecnai G2 F20 U-TWIN, Beijing, China) was used to capture the photomicrographs of the NLC formulation. A droplet of both INH-NLC and Man-INH-NLC dispersion was put on a copper grid (Boston Industries, Inc., Walpole, MA, USA). Filter paper was used to wipe off the excess droplets. After 60 s, uranyl acetate (2% w/v) was again put on the grid and subjected to drying. These samples were inserted and evaluated using TEM imaging analysis (TIA) software version 2 [47].

3.10. In Vitro Evaluation of Inhalation Behavior of Nebulized Mist

The air-jet nebulizer (OMRON Healthcare Inc., Kyoto, Japan) was used to nebulize the Man-INH-NLC dispersion, which was evaluated using an Andersen cascade impactor (AN-200, TISCH Environmental Inc., New York, NY, USA) with a throat-connecting tube. Cascade impactors may partially dry aqueous aerosol droplets due differences in temperature between the nebulizer outlet and the body of the impactor, resulting in the overestimation of the respirable fractions. So, the impactor was cooled for one hour before use to reduce the evaporation of aqueous aerosol droplets and increase the efficiency of the instrument [31]. A total of 5 mL of Man-INH-NLC dispersion was nebulized, and a vacuum was created in the system with an air stream of 28.3 L/min for 30 min. After complete nebulization, the formulation leftover in the nebulizer was measured. The NLCs deposited on the 0 to 6 stages of the instrument were washed out with 0.01 M hydrochloric acid (100 mL). The solution was diluted accordingly with the same. Also, 10 mL of the resultant solutions were centrifuged at 18,000 rpm for 45 min, and the aqueous phase was analyzed for drug content spectrophotometrically. The output efficiency and respirable fraction were established to express the spray and inhalation characteristics of the nebulizer (Equations (3) and (4)). MMAD is the diameter of the aerosol below which half of the particles are enclosed, and GSD is the geometric mean of all the aerosolized particles that were also evaluated [36].

$$Output\ efficiency\ (\%OE) = \frac{INH\ loaded\ in\ the\ system - INH\ remained\ in\ the\ nebulizer}{INH\ loaded\ into\ the\ system} \times 100 \tag{3}$$

$$Respirable\ fraction\ (\%RF) = \frac{INH\ deposited\ on\ stages\ 2\ to\ 6}{INH\ loaded\ into\ the\ system} \times 100 \tag{4}$$

3.11. Experimental Animal Model

3.11.1. Animals

Dunkin Hartley male guinea pigs (400–500 g) were acquired from Chaudhary Charan Singh Haryana Agricultural University, Hisar, (India), and used for the present study. This animal protocol was approved with the letter minutes of IAEC/2020/10-18/01 by the Animal Ethics Committee of the institute, Guru Jambheshwar University of Science and Technology, Hisar. The animals were housed as per CPCSEA guidelines and fed on green vegetable-based diets, and water was supplied ad libitum. The animals were subjected to fasting for 24 h before study [48].

3.11.2. Nebulization Conditions

An air jet nebulizer system (250 kPa pressure; airflow 5.5 L/min) was employed. Treatments were given to the animals according to the protocol. The sterilized isotonic solution was used to prepare a pure drug solution. The inhalable dose of NLC dispersion was calculated based on the percent respirable fraction. The formulation was exposed for 3–4 min per animal using a nebulizer with the help of an appropriate face mask. A nebulizer spacer was attached in between the nebulizer and face mask to keep the medicated mist within the spacer for a sufficiently long time and prevent environmental loss. The animals were exposed to NLC dispersion (2 mL) for 3–4 min/animal. Instead of the duration of administration, the size of the dose was determined by the volume of sterile isotonic solution used [49].

3.11.3. In Vivo Pharmacokinetic Analysis

The guinea pigs were divided into six groups, each with six animals: Group 1, INH-NLC, administered via a nebulizer; Group 2, Man-INH-NLC, administered via a nebulizer; Group 3, blank Man-NLC, administered via a nebulizer; Group 4, pure drug solution, administered orally; Group 5, pure drug solution, administered intravenously (iv); Group 6: pure drug solution, administered via a nebulizer. An isoniazid dose equivalent to 10 mg/kg/day was used for this study. Upon drug administration, 0.5 mL of blood was withdrawn at appropriate time points (0.25, 0.5, 1, 2, 4, 8, 12-, 24-, 48-, and 72-h) following administration and collected in pre-heparinized microcentrifuge tubes. The whole blood was centrifuged at 5000 rpm for 10 min at 4 °C; the supernatant plasma was separated and stored at -20 °C until it was required for analysis. Drug content in the plasma was analyzed using ultra-sensitive high-performance liquid chromatography (U-HPLC) [37].

Pharmacokinetic parameters were estimated by using the plasma concentration–time isoniazid curve. Peak plasma concentration (C_{max}) and the time taken to achieve C_{max} (T_{max}) were estimated directly from this curve. The elimination rate constant (K_{el}) was estimated via regression analysis and half-life elimination ($t_{1/2}$) was derived using $0.693/K_{el}$. The trapezoidal method was used to estimate the area under the concentration–time curve (AUC_{0-t}). The terminal $AUC_{t-\infty}$ was obtained by dividing the last measurable plasma drug concentration by K_{el}. The mean residence time (MRT) was estimated by dividing the area under the moment curve (AUMC) by the area under the curve (AUC). Both relative and absolute bioavailability were calculated using Equations (5) and (6) [50].

$$Absolute\ bioavailability = \frac{AUC\ nebulizer}{AUC\ i.v.} \times \frac{Dose\ i.v.}{Dose\ nebulizer} \tag{5}$$

$$Relative\ bioavailability = \frac{AUC\ nebulizer}{AUC\ oral} \times \frac{Dose\ oral}{Dose\ nebulizer} \tag{6}$$

3.12. Reverse-Phase High-Performance Liquid Chromatographic Condition

A previously reported simple, sensitive, and reliable RP-HPLC method was used to evaluate isoniazid (INH) content in blood plasma [51]. The HPLC system (Nexera X2, Shimadzu Corporation, Kyoto, Japan) consisted of a gradient pump, an online degasser, and an ultraviolet DAD detector, and an autosampler was used. Chromatographic separation was carried out using the reverse-phase column C-18 (250 mm $\times$ 4.6 mm; 3–5 µm particle size). Nicotinamide was used as an internal standard. The mobile phase consisted of water and methanol in an initial composition of 95:05 v/v at a flow rate of 1.5 mL/min for 12 min, followed by a composition change to 20:80 v/v for 23 min. At 23 min composition was again changed to the 95:05 v/v for 3 to 5 min before the next injection. The injection volume used was 100 µL, and the estimation was carried out at 262 nm for both INH and NA.

3.13. Method Validation and Preparation of Calibration Curve

Stock solutions (1.00 mg/mL) of both the drug and internal standard were prepared in water. Appropriate concentrations were prepared using different volumes of this stock solution and diluting them with water. Calibration standards of 0.5, 1.0, 2.5, 5.0, 10.0, and 20.0 µg/mL of INH were constructed by adding 45 µL of the standard and 5 µL of the internal standard solution to 150 µL of a blank plasma. Three quality control (QC) samples of isoniazid were prepared using blank plasma: low (2.0 µg/mL), middle (5.0 µg/mL), and high (12.0 µg/mL). The lower limit of quantification (LLOQ) and limit of detection (LOD) were also calculated. LLOQ is the lowest concentration on the calibration curve (estimated with an accuracy of above 80% with precision below 20%). LOQ is defined as a signal-to-noise ratio (S/N) of 3:1.

3.14. Preparation of Plasma Samples

The plasma samples were prepared by adding 195 µL of plasma and 5 µL of internal standard solution and subsequently thawed either fresh or at room temperature. Afterwards, 40 µL of acetonitrile, 160 µL of zinc sulfate (10% in water), and 5 µL of ammonia (25%) were added separately and vortexed for 1 min after each addition. The samples were centrifuged at 14,000 rpm for 15 min at 5 °C. The clear supernatants were stored at 5 °C, and each sample was removed from the cooling system 5 min before injection. The samples were then injected (100 µL) into the HPLC system.

3.15. Histological Evaluation

For the histological studies, the Man-INH-NLC formulation was evaluated for any kind of allergic reaction and toxicity to lung tissue. For this, the animals were divided into six groups (n = 6), and a high dose of isoniazid (40 mg/kg/day) was administered to each animal. The details of the groups were as follows: Group 1—high dose of pure drug solution, oral; Group 2—high dose of pure drug solution, i.v.; Group 3—high dose of pure drug solution, nebulizer; Group 4—high dose of Man-INH-NLC, nebulizer; Group 5—blank Man-NLC, nebulizer; Group 6—untreated control. The treatments were administered for 4 weeks once daily to simulate the long-term treatment of isoniazid. The next day of the last dosage administration, the animals were euthanized after an overdose of pentobarbitone sodium injection. The lungs, liver, kidney, and brain were recovered and preserved in a 10% buffered formalin solution. Sections of 5 μm were cut using a microtome and embedded in paraffin. The tissues were stained using hematoxylin-eosin (H&E), and the sections were investigated for granulomas, gross lesions or inflammation, and the degree of necrosis was determined by a certified pathologist who was completely oblivious to the treatment group [28,52].

3.16. Hepatotoxic and Nephrotoxic Evaluation

Hepatotoxicity and nephrotoxicity were evaluated simultaneously with histological evaluation. After 4 weeks of treatment, 1 mL of blood was withdrawn from each animal and subjected to a liver function test and kidney function test to evaluate any toxic effects and allergic reactions to the liver and kidney tissues, respectively. The blood samples were immediately processed by a certified pathologist to analyze total urea; bilirubin; creatinine for hepatotoxic evaluation; and alanine aminotransferase (ALT), alkaline phosphatase (ALP), and aspartate transaminase (AST) for evaluating nephrotoxicity in the animal groups. The normal range of these parameters was evaluated via the control group [50].

3.17. Statistical Analysis

Statistical data were analyzed using Prism 8.4.0® software. Analysis of variance was carried out via one-way ANOVA–post-Dunnett to differentiate two or more experimental groups. The data were considered statistically significant at $p < 0.05$. All values are displayed as the mean and standard deviation (mean $\pm$ SD where n = 3 or 6).

4. Conclusions

The isoniazid-loaded NLC formulation was formulated and successfully functionalized with D-mannose. The Man-INH-NLC formulation was found to have an encapsulation efficiency of 79.71 $\pm$ 1.65% with an average particle size of 273.4 $\pm$ 8.24 nm. In vitro release studies showed the non-Fickian pH-independent sustained release of drugs from the nanocarrier formulation. The majority of the nebulized nanoparticles were found in the respirable range for delivering the encapsulated drug deep into the lungs. In vivo studies revealed that the Man-INH-NLC formulation increased the mean residence time of the drug into the lungs compared to the non-functionalized INH-NLC formulation. The other pharmacokinetic parameters (relative bioavailability, half-life, AUC, T_{max}, C_{max}) of Man-INH-NLC were also improved after encapsulating isoniazid into lipid nanocarriers when compared with pure drug solution administered via different routes of administration. Furthermore, no toxicity was observed for both blank Man-NLC and the drug-loaded Man-INH-NLC formulations after repeated nebulization during the entire study period, as revealed following biochemical hepatotoxicity evaluation and histopathological evaluation. From the results, it can be concluded that the Man-INH-NLC formulation can safely improve the dosage regimen and substitute the conventional formulations for better therapeutic efficacy in the management of tuberculosis.

Future Prospects

The pulmonary route is a growing alternative to the oral or injectable administration of anti-tubercular drugs as it provides targeted drug delivery, reduces systemic side effects, and improves patient compliance. Tuberculosis treatment often involves a combination of multiple drugs to combat drug resistance and improve treatment outcomes. So, combination drug therapy can be applied to this research work to deliver therapeutics directly to the lungs to achieve the synergistic effect and enhance treatment effectiveness. Personalized medicine approaches and optimized drug delivery strategies can also be applied to allow for tailored treatment regimens.

Author Contributions: Conceptualization, S.A. and D.C.B.; methodology, S.A. and S.R.; software, S.R. and V.J.; validation, S.A., S.R. and T.V.; formal analysis, D.C.B. and G.K.; investigation, S.A. and G.K.; resources, S.A. and K.S.; data curation, S.A. and D.C.B.; writing—original draft preparation, S.A. and D.C.B.; writing—review and editing, S.A., A.S.A., A.A. and D.C.B.; visualization, A.A. and V.J.; supervision, D.C.B. and T.V.; project administration, S.A.; funding acquisition, A.S.A., O.M.N. and M.A. All authors have read and agreed to the published version of the manuscript.

Funding: This research was funded by the Researchers Supporting Project number (RSP2023R132), King Saud University, Riyadh, Saudi Arabia.

Institutional Review Board Statement: Approval for the animal studies protocol was given by the Institutional Animal Ethical Committee of Guru Jambheshwar University of Science and Technology, Hisar, India (approval no. IAEC/2020/10-18/01).

Informed Consent Statement: Not applicable.

Data Availability Statement: Data is contained within the article.

Acknowledgments: The authors are thankful to the Researchers Supporting Project number (RSP2023R132), King Saud University, Riyadh, Saudi Arabia. Also, the authors are thankful to Deepika Lather, Associate professor and certified Pathologist, Department of animal biotechnology, Lala Lajpat Rai University of Veterinary and Animal Sciences for their help in the histological and hepatological analysis of the blood and tissue samples of the tested animals.

Conflicts of Interest: The authors declare no conflict of interest.

References

1. Fogel, N. Tuberculosis: A Disease without Boundaries. *Tuberculosis* **2015**, *95*, 527–531. [CrossRef] [PubMed]
2. Miggiano, R.; Rizzi, M.; Ferraris, D.M. *Mycobacterium tuberculosis* Pathogenesis, Infection Prevention and Treatment. *Pathogens* **2020**, *9*, 385. [CrossRef] [PubMed]
3. Seung, K.J.; Keshavjee, S.; Rich, M.L. Multidrug-Resistant Tuberculosis and Extensively Drug-Resistant Tuberculosis. *Cold Spring Harb. Perspect. Med.* **2015**, *5*, a017863. [CrossRef]
4. Kebede, B. Tuberculosis Epidemiology, Pathogenesis, Drugs and Drug Resistance Development: A Review. *J. Biomed. Sci.* **2019**, *8*, 1–10.
5. Agyeman, A.A.; Ofori-Asenso, R. Tuberculosis—An Overview. *J. Public Health Emerg.* **2017**, *1*, 7. [CrossRef]
6. Zumla, A.; Nahid, P.; Cole, S.T. Advances in the Development of New Tuberculosis Drugs and Treatment Regimens. *Nat. Rev. Drug Discov.* **2013**, *12*, 388–404. [CrossRef]
7. Franzblau, S.G.; DeGroote, M.A.; Cho, S.H.; Andries, K.; Nuermberger, E.; Orme, I.M.; Mdluli, K.; Angulo-Barturen, I.; Dick, T.; Dartois, V.; et al. Comprehensive Analysis of Methods Used for the Evaluation of Compounds against *Mycobacterium tuberculosis*. *Tuberculosis* **2012**, *92*, 453–488. [CrossRef]
8. Timmins, G.S.; Deretic, V. Mechanisms of Action of Isoniazid. *Mol. Microbiol.* **2006**, *62*, 1220–1227. [CrossRef]
9. Khatak, S.; Mehta, M.; Awasthi, R.; Paudel, K.R.; Singh, S.K.; Gulati, M.; Hansbro, N.G.; Hansbro, P.M.; Dua, K.; Dureja, H. Solid Lipid Nanoparticles Containing Anti-Tubercular Drugs Attenuate the *Mycobacterium marinum* Infection. *Tuberculosis* **2020**, *125*, 102008. [CrossRef]
10. Weber, W.W.; Hein, D.W. Clinical Pharmacokinetics of Isoniazid. *Clin. Pharmacokinet.* **1979**, *4*, 401–422. [CrossRef]
11. Diallo, T.; Adjobimey, M.; Ruslami, R.; Trajman, A.; Sow, O.; Obeng Baah, J.; Marks, G.B.; Long, R.; Elwood, K.; Zielinski, D.; et al. Safety and Side Effects of Rifampin versus Isoniazid in Children. *N. Engl. J. Med.* **2018**, *379*, 454–463. [CrossRef] [PubMed]
12. Stagg, H.R.; Lipman, M.C.; Mchugh, T.D.; Jenkins, H.E. Isoniazid-Resistant Tuberculosis: A Cause for Concern? *Int. J. Tuberc. Lung Dis.* **2017**, *21*, 129–139. [CrossRef]
13. Pardeshi, C.V.; Agnihotri, V.V.; Patil, K.Y.; Pardeshi, S.R.; Surana, S.J. Mannose-Anchored N,N,N-Trimethyl Chitosan Nanoparticles for Pulmonary Administration of Etofylline. *Int. J. Biol. Macromol.* **2020**, *165*, 445–459. [CrossRef] [PubMed]

14. Patil, T.S.; Deshpande, A.S. Mannosylated Nanocarriers Mediated Site-Specific Drug Delivery for the Treatment of Cancer and Other Infectious Diseases: A State of the Art Review. *J. Control. Release* **2020**, *320*, 239–252. [CrossRef] [PubMed]

15. Rojanarat, W.; Nakpheng, T.; Thawithong, E.; Yanyium, N.; Srichana, T. Inhaled Pyrazinamide Proliposome for Targeting Alveolar Macrophages. *Drug Deliv.* **2012**, *19*, 334–345. [CrossRef]

16. Wijagkanalan, W.; Kawakami, S.; Takenaga, M.; Igarashi, R.; Yamashita, F.; Hashida, M. Efficient Targeting to Alveolar Macrophages by Intratracheal Administration of Mannosylated Liposomes in Rats. *J. Control. Release* **2008**, *125*, 121–130. [CrossRef]

17. Saraogi, G.K.; Sharma, B.; Joshi, B.; Gupta, P.; Gupta, U.D.; Jain, N.K.; Agrawal, G.P. Mannosylated Gelatin Nanoparticles Bearing Isoniazid for Effective Management of Tuberculosis. *J. Drug Target.* **2011**, *19*, 219–227. [CrossRef]

18. Filatova, L.Y.; Klyachko, N.L.; Kudryashova, E.V. Targeted Delivery of Anti-Tuberculosis Drugs to Macrophages: Targeting Mannose Receptors. *Russ. Chem. Rev.* **2018**, *87*, 374. [CrossRef]

19. Tiwari, S.; Chaturvedi, A.P.; Tripathi, Y.B.; Mishra, B. Macrophage-Specific Targeting of Isoniazid Through Mannosylated Gelatin Microspheres. *AAPS PharmSciTech* **2011**, *12*, 900–908. [CrossRef]

20. Virmani, T.; Kumar, G.; Sharma, A.; Pathak, K.; Akhtar, M.S.; Afzal, O.; Altamimi, A.S.A. Amelioration of Cancer Employing Chitosan, Its Derivatives, and Chitosan-Based Nanoparticles: Recent Updates. *Polymers* **2023**, *15*, 2928. [CrossRef]

21. Alhalmi, A.; Beg, S.; Almalki, W.H.; Alghamdi, S.; Kohli, K. Recent Advances in Nanotechnology-Based Targeted Therapeutics for Breast Cancer Management. *Curr. Drug Metab.* **2022**, *14*, 35657282. [CrossRef]

22. Nandvikar, N.Y.; Lala, R.R.; Shinde, A.S. Nanostructured Lipid Carrier: The Advanced Lipid Carriers. *Int. J. Pharm. Sci. Res.* **2019**, *10*, 5252–5265. [CrossRef]

23. Virmani, T.; Kumar, G.; Virmani, R.; Sharma, A.; Pathak, K. Nanocarrier-Based Approaches to Combat Chronic Obstructive Pulmonary Disease. *Nanomedicine* **2022**, *17*, 1833–1854. [CrossRef] [PubMed]

24. Kumar, G.; Virmani, T.; Sharma, A.; Pathak, K. Codelivery of Phytochemicals with Conventional Anticancer Drugs in Form of Nanocarriers. *Pharmaceutics* **2023**, *15*, 889. [CrossRef]

25. Vieira, R.; Severino, P.; Nalone, L.A.; Souto, S.B.; Silva, A.M.; Lucarini, M.; Durazzo, A.; Santini, A.; Souto, E.B. Sucupira Oil-Loaded Nanostructured Lipid Carriers (NLC): Lipid Screening, Factorial Design, Release Profile, and Cytotoxicity. *Molecules* **2020**, *25*, 685. [CrossRef]

26. Subramaniam, B.; Siddik, Z.H.; Nagoor, N.H. Optimization of Nanostructured Lipid Carriers: Understanding the Types, Designs, and Parameters in the Process of Formulations. *J. Nanoparticle Res.* **2020**, *22*, 141. [CrossRef]

27. Haider, M.; Abdin, S.M.; Kamal, L.; Orive, G. Nanostructured Lipid Carriers for Delivery of Chemotherapeutics: A Review. *Pharmaceutics* **2020**, *12*, 288. [CrossRef]

28. Pinheiro, M.; Ribeiro, R.; Vieira, A.; Andrade, F.; Reis, S. Design of a Nanostructured Lipid Carrier Intended to Improve the Treatment of Tuberculosis. *Drug Des. Devel. Ther.* **2016**, *10*, 2467–2475. [CrossRef]

29. Sahu, P.K.; Mishra, D.K.; Jain, N.; Rajoriya, V.; Jain, A.K. Mannosylated Solid Lipid Nanoparticles for Lung-Targeted Delivery of Paclitaxel. *Drug Dev. Ind. Pharm.* **2015**, *41*, 640–649. [CrossRef]

30. Jain, A.; Agarwal, A.; Majumder, S.; Lariya, N.; Khaya, A.; Agrawal, H.; Majumdar, S.; Agrawal, G.P. Mannosylated Solid Lipid Nanoparticles as Vectors for Site-Specific Delivery of an Anti-Cancer Drug. *J. Control. Release* **2010**, *148*, 359–367. [CrossRef]

31. Sharma, P.R.; Dravid, A.A.; Kalapala, Y.C.; Gupta, V.K.; Jeyasankar, S.; Goswami, A.; Agarwal, R. Cationic Inhalable Particles for Enhanced Drug Delivery to *M. tuberculosis* Infected Macrophages. *Biomater. Adv.* **2022**, *133*, 112612. [CrossRef]

32. Vieira, A.C.C.; Magalhães, J.; Rocha, S.; Cardoso, M.S.; Santos, S.G.; Borges, M.; Pinheiro, M.; Reis, S. Targeted Macrophages Delivery of Rifampicin-Loaded Lipid Nanoparticles to Improve Tuberculosis Treatment. *Nanomedicine* **2017**, *12*, 2721–2736. [CrossRef] [PubMed]

33. Zainab; Ahmad, S.; Khan, I.; Saeed, K.; Ahmad, H.; Alam, A.; Almehmadi, M.; Alsaiari, A.A.; Haitao, Y.; Ahmad, M. A Study on Green Synthesis, Characterization of Chromium Oxide Nanoparticles and Their Enzyme Inhibitory Potential. *Front. Pharmacol.* **2022**, *13*, 1008182. [CrossRef]

34. Kumar, G.; Virmani, T.; Pathak, K.; Al Kamaly, O.; Saleh, A. Central Composite Design Implemented Azilsartan Medoxomil Loaded Nanoemulsion to Improve Its Aqueous Solubility and Intestinal Permeability: In Vitro and Ex Vivo Evaluation. *Pharmaceuticals* **2022**, *15*, 1343. [CrossRef]

35. Zhou, Y.; Ahuja, A.; Irvin, C.M.; Kracko, D.A.; McDonald, J.D.; Cheng, Y.-S. Medical Nebulizer Performance: Effects of Cascade Impactor Temperature. *Respir. Care* **2005**, *50*, 1077–1082.

36. Al Ayoub, Y.; Gopalan, R.C.; Najafzadeh, M.; Mohammad, M.A.; Anderson, D.; Paradkar, A.; Assi, K.H. Development and Evaluation of Nanoemulsion and Microsuspension Formulations of Curcuminoids for Lung Delivery with a Novel Approach to Understanding the Aerosol Performance of Nanoparticles. *Int. J. Pharm.* **2019**, *557*, 254–263. [CrossRef]

37. Sharma, A.; Sharma, S.; Khuller, G.K. Lectin-Functionalized Poly (Lactide-Co-Glycolide) Nanoparticles as Oral/Aerosolized Antitubercular Drug Carriers for Treatment of Tuberculosis. *J. Antimicrob. Chemother.* **2004**, *54*, 761–766. [CrossRef]

38. Alhalmi, A.; Amin, S.; Beg, S.; Al-Salahi, R.; Mir, S.R.; Kohli, K. Formulation and Optimization of Naringin Loaded Nanostructured Lipid Carriers Using Box-Behnken Based Design: *In Vitro* and *Ex Vivo* Evaluation. *J. Drug Deliv. Sci. Technol.* **2022**, *74*, 103590. [CrossRef]

39. Patil, T.S.; Deshpande, A.S. Design, Development, and Characterisation of Clofazimine-Loaded Mannosylated Nanostructured Lipid Carriers: 33-Box-Behnken Design Approach. *Mater. Technol.* **2021**, *36*, 460–475. [CrossRef]

40. Alhalmi, A.; Amin, S.; Khan, Z.; Beg, S.; Al, O.; Saleh, A.; Kohli, K. Nanostructured Lipid Carrier-Based Codelivery of Raloxifene and Naringin: Formulation, Optimization, In Vitro, Ex Vivo, In Vivo Assessment, and Acute Toxicity Studies. *Pharmaceutics* **2022**, *14*, 1771. [CrossRef]
41. Shah, N.V.; Seth, A.K.; Balaraman, R.; Aundhia, C.J.; Maheshwari, R.A.; Parmar, G.R. Nanostructured Lipid Carriers for Oral Bioavailability Enhancement of Raloxifene: Design and in Vivo Study. *J. Adv. Res.* **2016**, *7*, 423–434. [CrossRef] [PubMed]
42. Rahman, M.; Almalki, W.H.; Afzal, O.; Altamimi, A.S.A.; Kazmi, I.; Al-Abbasi, F.A.; Choudhry, H.; Alenezi, S.K.; Barkat, M.A.; Beg, S.; et al. Cationic Solid Lipid Nanoparticles of Resveratrol for Hepatocellular Carcinoma Treatment: Systematic Optimization, in Vitro Characterization and Preclinical Investigation. *Int. J. Nanomed.* **2020**, *15*, 9283–9299. [CrossRef] [PubMed]
43. Patil-Gadhe, A.; Pokharkar, V. Montelukast-Loaded Nanostructured Lipid Carriers: Part I Oral Bioavailability Improvement. *Eur. J. Pharm. Biopharm.* **2014**, *88*, 160–168. [CrossRef] [PubMed]
44. Fernandes, A.V.; Pydi, C.R.; Verma, R.; Jose, J.; Kumar, L. Design, Preparation and In Vitro Characterizations of Fluconazole Loaded Nanostructured Lipid Carriers. *Braz. J. Pharm. Sci.* **2020**, *56*, e18069. [CrossRef]
45. Czajkowska-Kośnik, A.; Szymańska, E.; Czarnomysy, R.; Jacyna, J.; Markuszewski, M.; Basa, A.; Winnicka, K. Nanostructured Lipid Carriers Engineered as Topical Delivery of Etodolac: Optimization and Cytotoxicity Studies. *Materials* **2021**, *14*, 596. [CrossRef]
46. Velmurugan, R.; Selvamuthukumar, S. Development and Optimization of Ifosfamide Nanostructured Lipid Carriers for Oral Delivery Using Response Surface Methodology. *Appl. Nanosci.* **2016**, *6*, 159–173. [CrossRef]
47. Tyagi, N.; Gupta, P.; Khan, Z.; Neupane, Y.R.; Mangla, B.; Mehra, N.; Ralli, T.; Alhalmi, A.; Ali, A.; Al Kamaly, O. Superparamagnetic Iron-Oxide Nanoparticles Synthesized via Green Chemistry for the Potential Treatment of Breast Cancer. *Molecules* **2023**, *28*, 2343. [CrossRef]
48. Yamamoto, H.; Kuno, Y.; Sugimoto, S.; Takeuchi, H.; Kawashima, Y. Surface-Modified PLGA Nanosphere with Chitosan Improved Pulmonary Delivery of Calcitonin by Mucoadhesion and Opening of the Intercellular Tight Junctions. *J. Control. Release* **2005**, *102*, 373–381. [CrossRef]
49. Pandey, R.; Khuller, G.K. Solid Lipid Particle-Based Inhalable Sustained Drug Delivery System against Experimental Tuberculosis. *Tuberculosis* **2005**, *85*, 227–234. [CrossRef]
50. Pandey, R.; Sharma, A.; Zahoor, A.; Sharma, S.; Khuller, G.K.; Prasad, B. Poly (Dl-Lactide-Co-Glycolide) Nanoparticle-Based Inhalable Sustained Drug Delivery System for Experimental Tuberculosis. *J. Antimicrob. Chemother.* **2003**, *52*, 981–986. [CrossRef]
51. Dasht Bozorg, B.; Goodarzi, A.; Fahimi, F.; Tabarsi, P.; Shahsavari, N.; Kobarfard, F.; Dastan, F. Simultaneous Determination of Isoniazid, Pyrazinamide and Rifampin in Human Plasma by High-Performance Liquid Chromatography and UV Detection. *Iran. J. Pharm. Res. IJPR* **2019**, *18*, e124712. [CrossRef]
52. Kar, R.; Nangpal, P.; Mathur, S.; Singh, S.; Tyagi, A.K. BioA Mutant of *Mycobacterium tuberculosis* Shows Severe Growth Defect and Imparts Protection against Tuberculosis in Guinea Pigs. *PLoS ONE* **2017**, *12*, e0179513. [CrossRef] [PubMed]

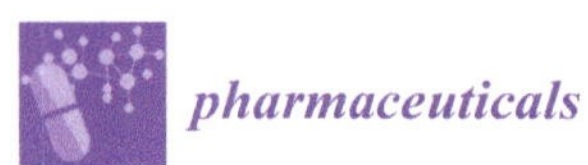 *pharmaceuticals*

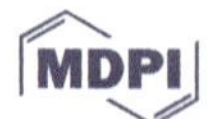

Article

Enhancing Oral Bioavailability and Brain Biodistribution of Perillyl Alcohol Using Nanostructured Lipid Carriers

Samila Horst Peczek [1], Ana Paula Santos Tartari [1], Isabella Camargo Zittlau [1], Camila Diedrich [1], Christiane Schineider Machado [1] and Rubiana Mara Mainardes [1,2,*]

[1] Laboratory of Nanostructured Formulations, Universidade Estadual do Centro-Oeste, Alameda Élio Antonio Dalla Vecchia St., 838, Guarapuava 85040-167, PR, Brazil; samylahp@hotmail.com (S.H.P.); ap.tartari@hotmail.com (A.P.S.T.); isazittlau99@gmail.com (I.C.Z.); camiladiedrich@hotmail.com (C.D.); chrischineider@outlook.com (C.S.M.)

[2] Department of Pharmacy, Universidade Estadual do Centro-Oeste, Alameda Élio Antonio Dalla Vecchia St., 838, Guarapuava 85040-167, PR, Brazil

* Correspondence: mainardes@unicentro.br; Tel.: +55-42-3629-8160

Abstract: Perillyl alcohol (POH), a bioactive monoterpenoid derived from limonene, shows promise as an antitumor agent for brain tumor treatment. However, its limited oral bioavailability and inadequate brain distribution hinder its efficacy. To address these challenges, this study developed nanostructured lipid carriers (NLCs) loaded with POH to improve its brain biodistribution. The NLCs prepared using hot homogenization exhibited an average diameter of 287 nm and a spherical morphology with a polydispersity index of 0.143. High encapsulation efficiency of 99.68% was achieved. X-ray diffraction analyses confirmed the semicrystalline state of POH-loaded NLCs. In vitro release studies demonstrated a biphasic release profile. Stability studies in simulated gastric and intestinal fluids confirmed their ability to withstand pH variations and digestive enzymes. In vivo pharmacokinetic studies in rats revealed significantly enhanced oral bioavailability of POH when encapsulated in the NLCs. Biodistribution studies showed increased POH concentration in brain tissue with NLCs compared with free POH, which was distributed more in non-target tissues such as the liver, lungs, kidneys, and spleen. These findings underscore the potential of NLCs as effective delivery systems for enhancing oral bioavailability and brain biodistribution of POH, providing a potential therapeutic strategy for brain tumor treatment.

Keywords: lipid nanoparticles; perillyl acid; pharmacokinetics; biodistribution

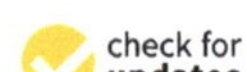 **check for updates**

Citation: Peczek, S.H.; Tartari, A.P.S.; Zittlau, I.C.; Diedrich, C.; Machado, C.S.; Mainardes, R.M. Enhancing Oral Bioavailability and Brain Biodistribution of Perillyl Alcohol Using Nanostructured Lipid Carriers. *Pharmaceuticals* **2023**, *16*, 1055. https://doi.org/10.3390/ph16081055

Academic Editors: Ana Catarina Silva, João Nuno Moreira and José Manuel Sousa Lobo

Received: 25 June 2023
Revised: 15 July 2023
Accepted: 19 July 2023
Published: 25 July 2023

1. Introduction

Perillyl alcohol (POH; IUPAC name: [4-(prop-1-en-2-yl)cyclohex-1-en-1-yl]methanol) is a natural compound belonging to the monocyclic terpene group, which can be found in the essential oils of various plants and citrus fruits, including mint, cherries, lavender, lemongrass, celery seeds, ginger, and sage, among others [1]. Regarding its pharmacokinetics, POH exhibits a relatively short half-life, necessitating frequent dosing to maintain therapeutic plasma concentrations. After oral administration, the compound is rapidly absorbed, although its bioavailability may be limited due to extensive first-pass metabolism in the liver [2,3]. Notably, POH undergoes significant hepatic metabolism, leading to the formation of perilaldehyde, perillyl acid, and dihydroperillic acid. These metabolites are subsequently subjected to glucuronidation and primarily eliminated through the renal system, with a minor fraction excreted through the bile. These factors contribute to the pharmacokinetic limitations of POH [4–6].

Over the past few decades, there has been a substantial increase in the interest surrounding the medicinal properties of POH, driven by the discovery of its potent antitumor activity. Numerous in vitro and in vivo studies have demonstrated the chemopreventive effects of POH against various types of cancer, including lung [7], skin [8], liver [9], pancreas [10], colon [11], breast [12], leukemia cells [13], and glioblastomas [14]. Although the precise mechanisms by which POH exerts its antitumor effects are not fully elucidated, several significant mechanisms have been reported. These include the inhibition of Ras protein isoprenylation [15–17], modulation of AP-1 (activator protein-1) activity, induction of early G1 arrest and apoptosis, negative regulation of cyclin proteins, and targeting of various other cellular factors such as telomerase reverse transcriptase (hTERT), eukaryotic translation initiation factors eIF4E and eIF4G, sodium/potassium adenosine triphosphatase (Na/K-ATPase), Notch, nuclear factor kappa B (NF-κB), mammalian target of rapamycin (mTORC), M6P/IGF-II receptor genes, and transforming growth factor beta (TGFβ) [16–18].

Given its potential as an antitumor agent, POH has undergone a series of phase I and II clinical trials in patients with glioblastoma multiforme (GBM), a highly malignant grade IV astrocytic lineage glioma according to the WHO classification of CNS tumors [19]. While it demonstrated disease stabilization, oral administration of POH was associated with gastrointestinal toxicities. Increased side effects were reported with the use of high and frequent doses required to maintain the plasma concentration of POH and its metabolites at levels sufficient to induce the desired therapeutic effect [5,20,21].

Within this context, nanotechnology emerges as a compelling alternative for drug delivery, offering the capability to manipulate properties such as toxicological profiles, controlled release mechanisms, and targeted delivery to specific sites. In the field of oncology, the rapid advancements in nanotechnology have propelled nano-oncology as a promising approach for cancer therapy. The escalating interest in the application of nanotechnology in oncology primarily stems from the remarkable ability of nanomedicines to modify pharmacokinetic parameters and improve drug distribution at tumor sites, while concurrently reducing concentrations in healthy tissues. Consequently, these advancements have the potential to minimize undesirable side effects and address the limitations associated with conventional cancer treatments [22,23]. Our research group has successfully developed a nanoemulsion containing POH, which exhibited enhanced bioavailability and brain targeting when administered intranasally in rats [24]. However, we are now eager to explore an alternative nanoparticle system for the same purpose, with a specific focus on oral administration. This novel approach aims to overcome the limitations of intranasal delivery and provide a more convenient and patient-friendly route for the effective delivery of POH.

Among the various nanoparticulate drug delivery systems, lipid-based systems have emerged as a prominent field of research, with nanostructured lipid carriers (NLCs) receiving significant attention in recent decades. The supramolecular structure of NLCs is characterized by the arrangement of lipids in a nanostructured pattern. NLCs are comprised of a blend of solid and liquid lipids, exhibiting a core–shell structure. The composition of NLCs allows the incorporation of various lipids with diverse physicochemical properties, such as triglycerides, phospholipids, and fatty acids. This versatility enables the encapsulation of a wide range of hydrophobic and hydrophilic drugs, making NLCs suitable for delivering diverse therapeutic agents [25,26]. They contribute to the stability of the carriers, protect the encapsulated drugs from degradation, and facilitate controlled-release kinetics. Additionally, the supramolecular organization of NLCs influences their interactions with biological membranes and cellular uptake mechanisms, affecting their overall performance as drug delivery systems. Furthermore, NLCs exhibit scalability, enabling large-scale production to meet the demands of the pharmaceutical industry. Moreover, they possess sterilization potential, ensuring the maintenance of product quality and safety. These collective attributes make NLCs a versatile and promising platform for advanced drug delivery systems [27,28].

In this study, it was hypothesized that NLCs could enhance the oral bioavailability and brain biodistribution of POH, aiming to develop an effective oral formulation with reduced adverse effects for the treatment of glioblastoma. NLCs containing POH were synthesized and characterized, and their in vitro release properties were evaluated. Furthermore, the pharmacokinetic parameters and biodistribution were assessed following single oral administration in rats, providing valuable insights into the absorption, distribution, metabolism, and excretion of POH when encapsulated within NLCs. These comprehensive evaluations contribute to the understanding of the potential benefits of NLCs as a drug delivery system for improving the therapeutic outcomes of POH in glioblastoma treatment.

2. Results and Discussion

2.1. Preparation and Characterization of NLCs Containing POH

The NLCs-POH were successfully obtained using the hot homogenization method. The methodology proved to be effective for NLCs' production, as they exhibited appropriate size for oral delivery, low polydispersity, and excellent incorporation of POH (see Table 1), which served both as a structural component, being the liquid lipid of NLCs, and as the drug. SEM images (Figure 1A,B) revealed a relatively spherical morphology of the POH-loaded NLCs. Also, some aggregation was observed, however that may be attributed to drying processes involved in SEM sample preparation, which may not accurately represent the state of the particles in their dispersed form.

Table 1. Characteristics of NLCs incorporating POH.

Characteristic	Result (Mean $\pm$ SD)
Mean particle size (nm)	288 ± 23
Polydispersity index	0.143 ± 0.040
Zeta potential (mV)	-32.5 ± 1.4
Entrapment efficiency (%)	99.6 ± 0.4

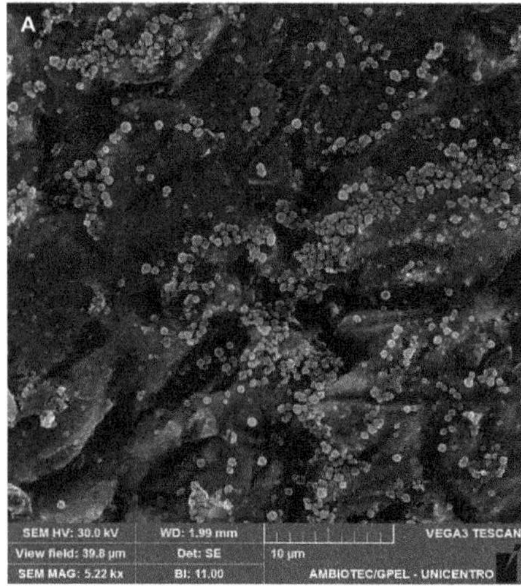

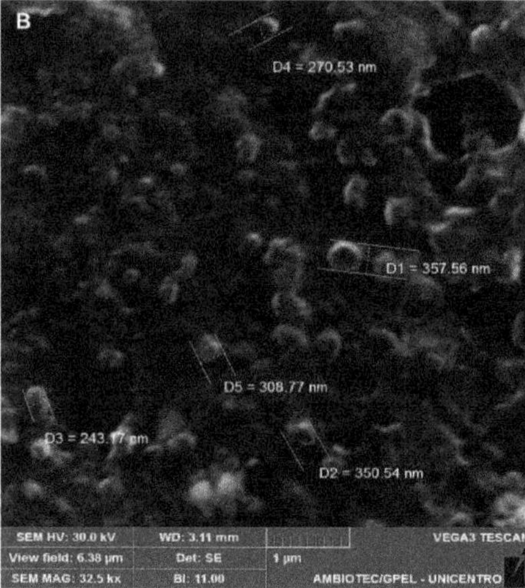

Figure 1. SEM images of POH-loaded NLCs at different magnification (**A**) 5.22 Kx and (**B**) 32.5 Kx.

The mean diameter of the obtained NLCs was below 300 nm. Considering that tumor tissue vasculature has pores ranging from 200 to 1200 nm [29], the size of the NLCs is ideal for entering the fenestrations of tumor tissue neovasculature, while being unable to enter the narrow fenestrations of normal endothelium (10 to 50 nm), contributing to the enhanced permeability and retention (EPR) effect, leading to nanoparticle accumulation at the tumor site through passive targeting [30,31]. Furthermore, particles with a size $\leq$ 300 nm are more suitable for oral drug administration, as they are preferentially internalized by enterocytes and M cells and demonstrate increased intestinal transport compared with larger particles [32,33]. The choice of lipids with different physicochemical properties, such as chain length, degree of saturation, and melting point, can affect the lipid matrix arrangement and ultimately influence the size of the NLCs. Lipids with a higher melting point result in larger particle sizes due to the increased fusion viscosity in the system, consequently reducing the efficiency of the homogenization step for size reduction [34,35]. Studies have shown that NLCs prepared with Gelucire® 43/01 exhibit smaller particle size compared with glyceryl tripalmitate [36], glyceryl behenate, and glyceryl monostearate [37], due to its relatively lower melting point. Moreover, the chemical composition of Gelucire® 43/01, which contains mono- and diglycerides along with polyethylene glycol esters of fatty acids, provides certain emulsifying properties, facilitating emulsification and assisting in the formation of NLCs with smaller particle size [35–37].

The polydispersity index (PDI) serves as a measure of the uniformity in the size distribution of particles, reflecting the homogeneity or heterogeneity of the sample. It is a numerical value ranging from 0.0 (indicating a perfectly uniform sample) to 1.0 (representing a highly polydisperse sample with various particle sizes). Ideally, PDI values ≤ 0.2 indicate a more homogeneous size distribution, highlighting a desirable characteristic for nanoparticle formulations [38]. In the context of this study, the obtained NLCs exhibited a PDI value < 0.15 (see Table 1), falling within the desired range and indicating a relatively uniform particle size distribution. The achievement of such low PDI values can be attributed to the careful selection and combination of surfactants, which play a crucial role in stabilizing the NLCs and controlling their size and PDI. In this investigation, polysorbate 80 and soybean lecithin were employed as surfactant combination. It has been demonstrated in previous studies that utilizing a mixture of surfactants can lead to a reduction in PDI compared with using a single surfactant, thereby improving the overall stability of the NLC system [35,39]. Furthermore, the inclusion of non-ionic surfactants, such as polysorbate 80, has been shown to contribute to lower PDI values compared with anionic or cationic surfactants. This can be attributed to the ability of polysorbate 80 to decrease particle size and minimize aggregation tendencies, ultimately leading to a more uniform particle size distribution [40,41].

The obtained NLCs showed a zeta potential of −32.5 mV, indicating excellent predictability of formulation stability. This highly negative value suggests strong repulsive forces among the particles, effectively preventing internal phase aggregation [42]. The anionic nature of the solid lipid Gelucire® 43/01 is responsible for conferring the negative charge, which contributes to the zeta potential observed. Encouragingly, similar zeta potential values (<−30 mV) have been reported in other investigations utilizing Gelucire® 43/01 as the solid lipid for NLCs' development [37,43]. The zeta potential not only ensures the stability and dispersion of NLCs, but also has implications for their interaction with biological systems. The electrostatic repulsion between NLC particles with such a significant negative charge can inhibit particle aggregation, enhance their colloidal stability, and promote their prolonged circulation time in biological fluids [44].

The entrapment efficiency (EE) of POH in NLCs was remarkably high, reaching almost 100%. The exceptional EE observed in this study can be attributed to the distinctive dual functionality of POH, as both a pharmacological agent and a structural element within the NLCs. As an oil, POH obviates the need for an additional liquid lipid component to form the supramolecular structure of the NLCs, ensuring its efficient encapsulation.

The diffractograms of the samples, including soybean lecithin, Gelucire® 43/01, NLCs -POH, and blank nanoparticles (without POH), are presented in Figure 1. The XRD pattern of solid lipid Gelucire® 43/01 (Figure 2A) exhibited characteristic peaks at 2θ: 20.9 and 23.1°, indicating its semicrystalline nature [45]. In contrast, the XRD pattern of soybean lecithin (Figure 2B) displayed a broad band at 20.3°, suggesting a completely amorphous profile with the absence of well-defined peaks [46]. The diffractograms of the blank NLCs (Figure 2C) and POH-loaded NLCs (Figure 2D) exhibited similar patterns, with a partial overlap of the characteristic Gelucire® peaks at 2θ: 20.9 and 23.1°, although less distinct, and a broad base attributed to the lecithin's broad band. This characterization indicates a semicrystalline profile of NLCs, which is anticipated to contribute to faster dissolution rates, improved absorption, and enhanced bioavailability [47].

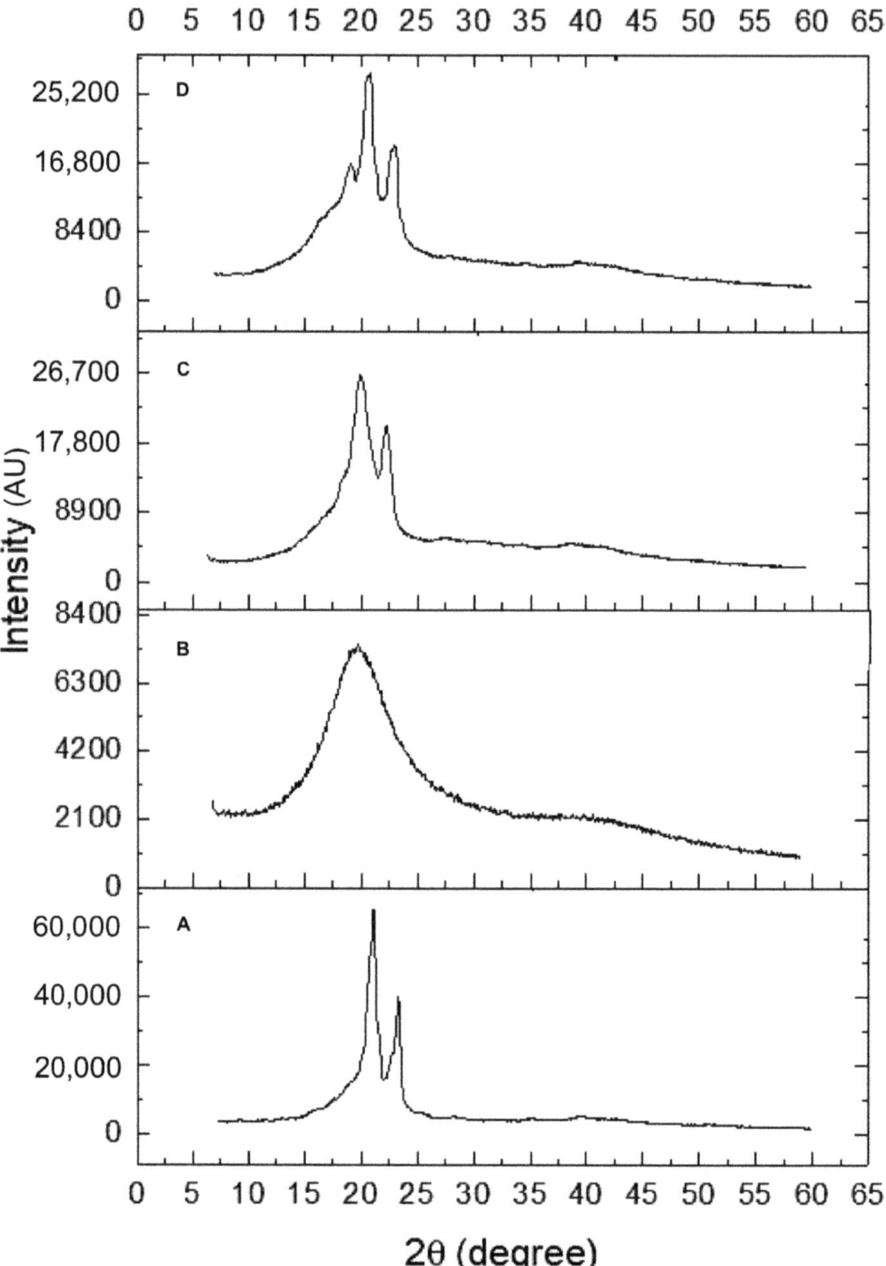

Figure 2. Diffractograms of: (**A**) Gelucire® 43/01, (**B**) soybean lecithin, (**C**) blank NLCs, and (**D**) POH-loaded NLCs.

2.2. In Vitro Release Profile

Figure 3 shows the in vitro release profile of POH from NLCs over a 48 h assay period. A prolonged release characterized by a biphasic profile was observed. An initial rapid release, known as the burst effect, was observed at 8 h, during which approximately 25% of

POH was released from the NLCs. After this time, the release continued at a constant and slower rate, resulting in a cumulative release of 29% at the end of 48 h. The release profile obtained for POH was very similar to the one reported in the study by Zielińska et al. [48], using the same methodology, where the release of different monoterpenes, including limonene, a precursor of POH, was evaluated. Mathematical models were applied to the release data (Table 2), and the results showed that the best-fitted model (r = 0.922) was the Weibull model. This model suggests a drug release mechanism involving dissolution, diffusion, and mixed dissolution–diffusion rate-limited processes. The application of the semi-empirical Korsmeyer–Peppas model resulted in a release exponent of $n = 0.40$, indicating that drug release occurred through diffusion within the lipid matrix [49]. Thus, the initial burst release effect is attributed to the fraction of drug adsorbed on the NLCs' surfaces, while Fickian diffusion drives sustained release curves according to the Weibull and Korsmeyer–Peppas models. Due to the inherent limitations of conducting in vitro release experiments with the physically oily nature of POH, it is expected that the release under in vivo conditions will exhibit a faster rate. Obviously, the pharmacokinetic assays will provide a comprehensive understanding of POH's pharmacokinetic behavior that cannot be fully captured by in vitro experiments alone.

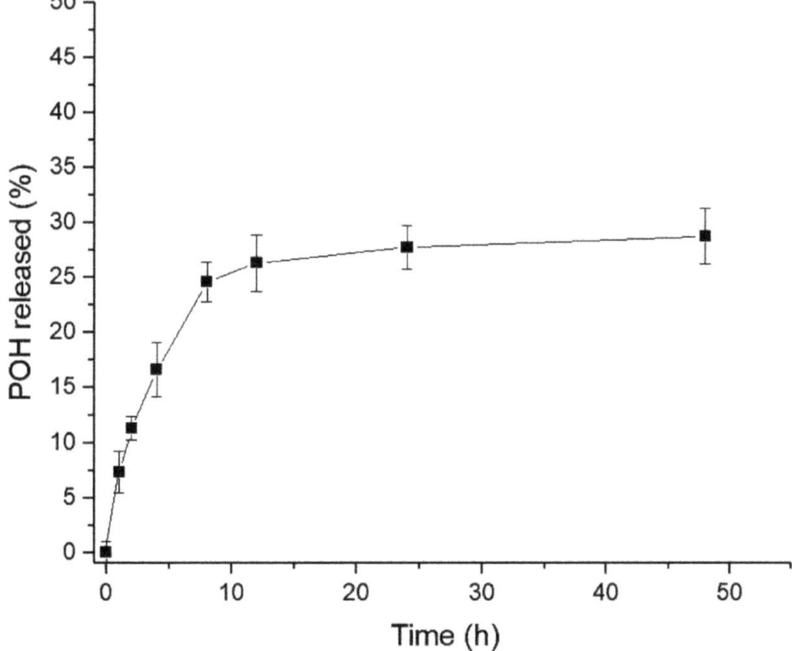

Figure 3. In vitro release of POH from NLCs in PBS pH 7.4, 37 °C (*n* = 3).

The release assay in simulated gastric fluid (SGF) and simulated intestinal fluids (SIF) was conducted to assess the suitability of the NLCs for oral administration. The study was conducted for 2 h in SGF pH 1.2, followed by a medium change to SIF pH 6.8 for 4 h. The release profile of POH from NLCs is presented in Figure 4. The NLCs showed low release of POH in both fluids, with a total of 12.4% released at the end of 6 h, suggesting excellent incorporation of the drug within the lipid matrix. These results indicate that the NLCs used for oral administration of POH demonstrated good stability, maintaining their integrity in the face of different pH variations and the presence of digestive enzymes. Therefore, the results suggest that the main content of POH incorporated in NLCs could be absorbed by intestinal cells and enter the bloodstream for sustained release in vivo. Moreover, this result is promising, considering that the oral administration of free-form POH caused significant gastrointestinal side effects in glioblastoma patients [20,21].

Table 2. Kinetic analysis of POH release from NLCs in 50 mM PBS solution, pH 7.4, 37 °C.

Kinetic Model	*r* (Correlation Coefficient)
Zero order	0.554
First order	0.449
Second order	0.337
Third order	0.247
Higuchi	0.277
Korsmeyer–Peppas	0.916
Weibull	0.922
Hickson–Crowell	0.486

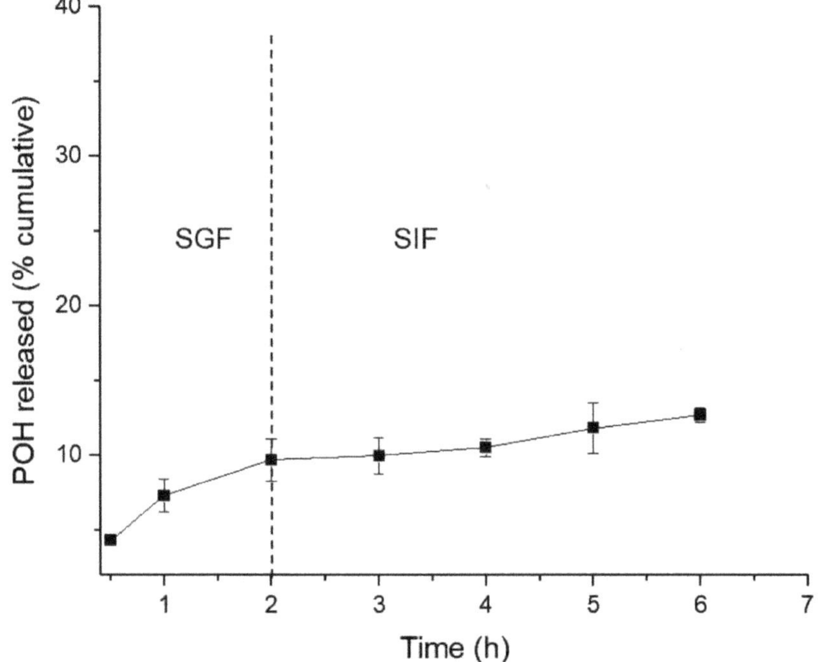

Figure 4. In vitro release of POH from NLCs in simulated gastric fluid (SGF) pH 1.2 and simulated intestinal fluid (SIF) pH 6.8, 37 °C (*n* = 3).

2.3. Pharmacokinetic Study

The pharmacokinetic study was conducted in rats to evaluate whether NLCs can alter the pharmacokinetic profile of POH. The absorption, bioavailability, and elimination profiles of orally administered POH-loaded NLCs were assessed in a single-dose study and compared with the pharmacokinetic profile obtained for free-form POH. Considering the properties of POH, such as low water solubility and low polarity, which pose challenges for its determination by ESI in the UPLC/MS-MS method, a decision was made to quantify the perillyl acid (PA), a metabolite of POH. Furthermore, due to the rapid metabolism of POH to PA, the levels of PA in plasma and brain were quantified instead [24,50].

The mean plasma and brain concentration–time curves of PA following oral administration of 500 mg/kg of free-form POH and the equivalent of 500 mg/kg of POH in the

NLCs are shown in Figures 5 and 6, and the pharmacokinetic parameters are presented in Tables 3 and 4.

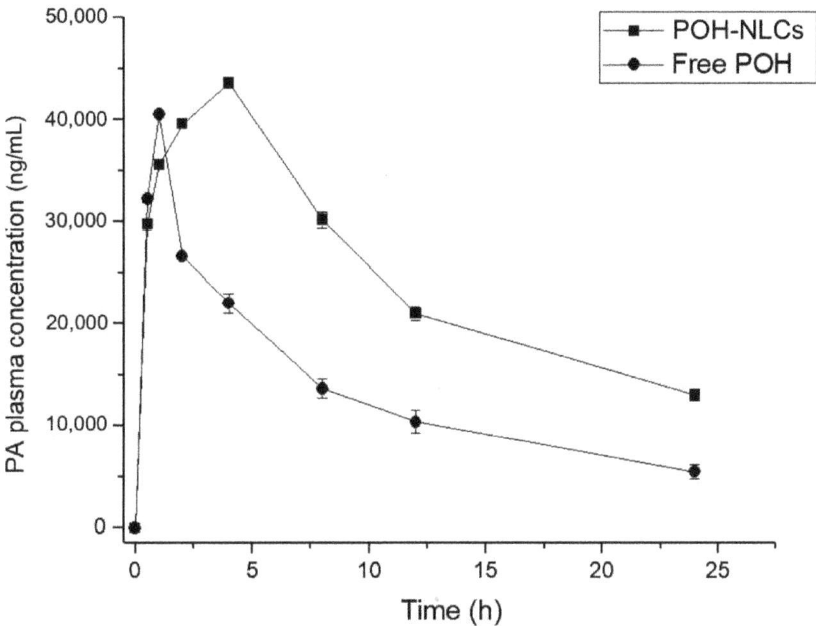

Figure 5. Plasma concentration–time curves of perillyl acid (PA) obtained after single oral administration of 500 mg/kg of POH in rats, using NLCs and in its free form.

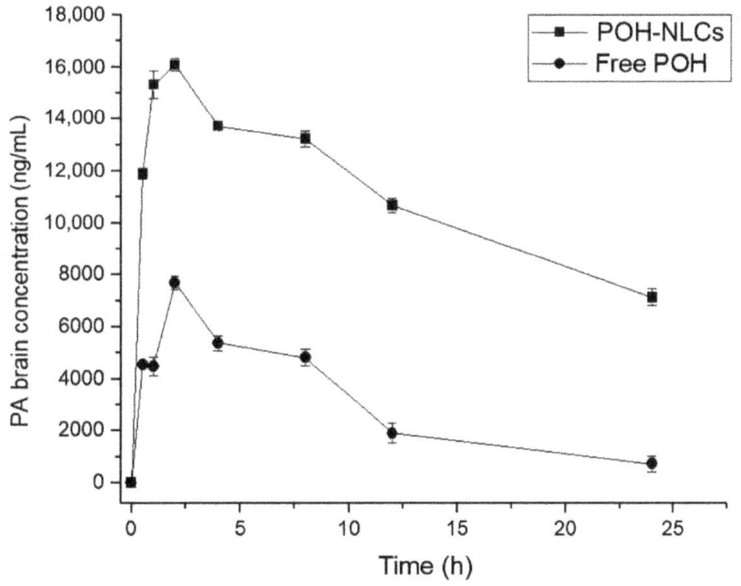

Figure 6. Brain concentration–time curves of perillyl acid (PA) obtained after single oral administration of 500 mg/kg of POH in rats, using NLCs and in its free form.

Table 3. Pharmacokinetic plasma parameters of perillyl acid, following oral administration of a single dose of 500 mg/kg of free POH and POH-loaded NLCs.

Parameter	Free POH	POH-Loaded NLCs
C_{max} (ng·mL^{-1})	40,507.18	43,552.17
T_{max} (h)	1	4
AUC_{0-24h} (ng·h/mL)	322,833.78	598,139.18
$T_{\frac{1}{2}}$ (h)	8.65	11.90
Kel (1/h)	0.080	0.058
Cl (L/h)	0.0015	0.0008
Vd (L)	0.0193	0.0143

C_{max}: maximum concentration; T_{max}: time to reach maximum concentration; AUC_{0-24h}: area under the plasma concentration–time curve; $T_{\frac{1}{2}}$: half-life; Kel: elimination rate constant; Vd: apparent volume of distribution; Cl: clearance.

Table 4. Pharmacokinetic tissues parameters of perillyl acid, following oral administration of a single dose of 500 mg/kg of free POH and POH-loaded NLCs.

Treatment	Tissue	C_{max} (ng·mL^{-1})	T_{max} (h)	AUC_{0-24h} (ng·h/mL)	$T_{\frac{1}{2}}$ (h)	Kel (1/h)
Free POH	Brain	7694.15	2	72,104.51	6.40	0.108
	Lung	41,265.63	2	442,244.37	8.63	0.080
	Kidney	34,245.26	2	437,725.63	12.92	0.053
	Liver	40,490.68	4	678,190.26	29.11	0.023
	Spleen	13,022.72	4	225,678.26	8.68	0.079
POH-loaded NLCs	Brain	16,085.07	2	263,771.20	19.35	0.035
	Lung	19,067.11	1	192,494.69	12.15	0.057
	Kidney	23,873.44	1	228,540.18	10.10	0.068
	Liver	28,884.92	2	320,092.07	19.74	0.035
	Spleen	10,662.32	1	75,687.80	5.52	0.125

C_{max}: maximum concentration; T_{max}: time to reach maximum concentration; AUC_{0-24h}: area under the tissue concentration–time curve; $T_{\frac{1}{2}}$: half-life; Kel: elimination rate.

Upon conducting an analysis of the plasma profile (Figure 5), it was evident that the oral administration of the free POH resulted in rapid absorption, with a maximum plasma concentration (C_{max}) of 40,507.18 ng/mL observed at 1 h, followed by a decline to 5480.12 ng/mL after 24 h. In contrast, the NLCs exhibited a slower absorption rate, with a C_{max} of 43,552.17 ng/mL observed at 4 h and a sustained concentration of 12,999.93 ng/mL at the end of 24 h. This indicates a prolonged absorption period and sustained presence of the drug in the bloodstream when it is encapsulated in NLCs. Unlike the free drug, which is readily available for absorption, the drug encapsulated in the nanostructured delivery system undergoes lipid matrix dissociation, gradually releasing into the bloodstream. The oral bioavailability was enhanced two-fold ($p < 0.05$) with the utilization of NLCs in comparison to free-form POH treatment, as demonstrated by the increased AUC_{0-24h}. Moreover, the half-life of the drug was prolonged from 8 to 11 h, indicating a reduced clearance rate and sustained presence in the systemic circulation.

The administration of NLCs significantly increased the brain concentration of PA compared to free-form POH treatment (Figure 6). This finding demonstrates that NLCs enhanced the absorption of POH, reaching a maximum concentration of PA (C_{max}) of 16,085.07 ng/mL, which was approximately two times higher than the C_{max} of the free drug (7694.15 ng/mL) ($p < 0.05$). Furthermore, the prolonged duration of PA in the brain was evident, with a concentration of 7126.73 ng/mL at the end of 24 h, whereas the free-form POH had a PA final concentration of approximately 719.71 ng/mL. Analysis of the AUC_{0-24h} (Table 4) revealed a remarkable enhancement in the brain bioavailability of PA when the treatment was with NLCs, as its AUC_{0-24h} was increased 3.6-fold compared with the free drug. The efficacy of brain delivery can also be assessed by evaluating the AUCbrain/AUCplasma ratio of POH-loaded NLCs in comparison to free POH. The results revealed a ratio of 2, indicating that NLCs enhanced brain distribution by two-fold compared with the free drug. This ratio is correlated with a proportional improvement in bioavailability, also doubled, demonstrating the enhanced drug concentration in the brain. These results highlight the superior performance of NLCs in enhancing the brain uptake of PA and increasing its bioavailability in the brain.

In contrast, the distribution of free POH to organs such as the lungs, kidneys, liver, and spleen was more pronounced, indicating that NLCs displayed enhanced selectivity for brain delivery. This was evidenced by the AUC results (Table 4), where NLCs exhibited a higher accumulation of the drug in the brain while the free drug showed higher distribution to non-target tissues, such as liver, lungs, kidneys, and spleen. Furthermore, the plasma and brain half-life ($T\frac{1}{2}$) was prolonged in animals treated with NLCs, reinforcing the notion of sustained release mediated by these nanostructures and suggesting a prolonged therapeutic effect. These findings underscore the advantageous characteristics of NLCs in terms of improved tissue selectivity, extended drug release, and potential for enhanced therapeutic outcomes.

The precise mechanism underlying the transport of drugs across the blood–brain barrier (BBB) mediated by nanoparticles remains to be fully elucidated. Several potential mechanisms have been proposed to account for this phenomenon. These include the small size of nanoparticles, which provides a large surface area, as well as the lipophilic nature of NLCs. These factors enhance the interaction and prolonged contact time between the particles and the BBB, facilitating the transport of drugs to the brain by establishing a concentration gradient. The lipophilic properties of lipid nanoparticles enable their passage across the BBB through various transport pathways, such as paracellular, transcellular, transcytosis, and receptor-mediated endocytosis [51,52]. Further investigations are needed to gain a comprehensive understanding of the intricate mechanisms involved in lipid nanoparticle-mediated drug delivery to the brain.

Several studies have highlighted the role of polysorbate-80 in brain targeting, as it exerts specific effects on membrane fluidity, enhances interaction with the BBB, and inhibits efflux pumps like P-glycoprotein (P-gp) expressed in brain endothelial cells. These actions contribute to increased brain delivery of nanoparticles. Another significant mechanism involves the covalent association of polysorbate-80 with apolipoprotein E in the bloodstream. Apolipoprotein E is essential for the transportation of low-density lipoprotein (LDL) to the brain. By binding to the nanoparticle surface, polysorbate-80 enables the nanoparticles to mimic LDL particles, facilitating their interaction with LDL receptors. This interaction promotes the uptake of nanoparticles by cerebral capillary endothelial cells and enhances drug distribution within the brain compared with the free drug solution [53,54]. In this study, the presence of polysorbate-80 on the surface of NLCs indicates that the enhanced brain bioavailability may be attributed to its role in facilitating nanoparticle uptake via endocytosis, in addition to the previously discussed factors such as improved plasma bioavailability and prolonged release properties.

The findings of this study provide valuable insights into the pharmacokinetic behavior of the NLCs encapsulating the drug POH. The observed differences in the absorption, biodistribution, and elimination profiles between the POH-loaded NLCs and the free drug highlight the potential of nanotechnology in modulating drug pharmacokinetics for improved therapeutic outcomes. The sustained release, improved bioavailability, and enhanced brain bioavailability observed with NLCs offer promising prospects for improving the treatment of brain-related diseases. In the case of POH, a candidate for the treatment of glioblastoma multiforme, providing patients with an alternative that minimizes the frequency of administration and enhances action in the affected organ is of great importance. This increased selectivity of NLCs for brain delivery can help minimize potential adverse effects in non-target organs and improve the overall safety profile of the drug. Continued research and development in this field hold great potential for advancing therapeutic strategies and addressing the challenges associated with drug delivery to the brain.

3. Materials and Methods

3.1. Materials

Gelucire® 43/01 (a mixture of mono-, di-, and triglyceride esters of fatty acids) and soy lecithin were kindly donated by Prati-Donaduzzi pharmaceutical company (Toledo, Brazil). Formic acid (98–100% purity), perillyl acid (PA, 95% purity), perillyl alcohol (POH, ≥95% purity), L-carvone (96% purity), pancreatin (99%), Pepsin (99%), and Tween 80—polysorbate 80 were obtained from Sigma-Aldrich® (St. Louis, MO, USA). Potassium chloride (99%), sodium chloride (99%), and anhydrous monobasic sodium phosphate (99%) were acquired from Biotec® (São José dos Pinhais, Brazil). HPLC-grade acetonitrile was purchased from Honeywell® (NJ, USA). Dibasic sodium phosphate (99%) was obtained from Synth® (São Paulo, Brazil). Purified water was obtained using a Milli-Q Plus system (Millipore Corporation, Bedford, MA, USA) with a conductivity of 18 MΩ.

3.2. Preparation of Nanostructured Lipid Carriers (NLCs) Containing POH

The NLCs containing POH were obtained using the hot homogenization method, according to Zhuang et al. (2010) [55], with modifications. It is noteworthy that POH, in addition to being the drug, also served a structural function as the liquid lipid component of the NLCs. In brief, the oily phase composed of POH (700 μL) and the solid lipid Gelucire® 43/01 (1.3 g) was heated to 53 °C (10 °C above the melting temperature of the solid lipid) for 10 min. Separately, 10 mL of an aqueous solution containing polysorbate 80 (1%) and soy lecithin (1%) was heated to the same temperature and added to the melted oily phase, followed by agitation using an Ultra Turrax homogenizer (Dremel®, 300, São Paulo, Brazil) at 33,000 RPM for 2 min. The obtained pre-emulsion was subjected to sonication using an ultrasonic sonicator (Eco-Sonics®, Indaiatuba, Brasil) for 2 cycles of 1 min each, at a power of 90 Watts, and subsequently cooled (2–8 °C) for 5 min to allow the formation of the NLCs. Afterwards, NLCs underwent ultracentrifugation at 25,240× g and 4 °C for 20 min (Hermle—Z36HKl centrifuge, Wehingen, Germany). Subsequently, the resulting precipitate was redispersed in ultrapure water, while the supernatant was retained for subsequent analysis.

3.3. Physicochemical Characterization

The mean size and polydispersity index (PDI) of the NLCs were determined using dynamic light scattering (BIC 90 plus, Brookhaven Inst. Corp., Holtsville, NY, USA). The samples were diluted in ultrapure water and subjected to analysis using a scattering angle of 90 degrees and a laser beam with a wavelength of 695 nm. The zeta potential was measured based on the electrophoretic mobility of the nanoparticles (Zetasizer ZS, Malvern, UK). The morphological features were evaluated using a scanning electron microscope (SEM) operated at an acceleration voltage of 30 kV (VEGA3, Tescan Orsay Holding, Brno, Czech Republic). X-ray diffraction (XRD) analysis was performed using an X-ray diffractometer (D2 Phaser, Bruker, Mannheim, Germany) equipped with Cu Kα radiation (λ = 1.5418 Å) at 30 kV voltage and 10 mA current. The samples were placed on a glass support and analyzed in the 2θ open-angle range of 5 to 60°.

3.4. Entrapment Efficiency Determination

The entrapment efficiency (EE) was determined indirectly by quantifying the amount of POH present in the supernatant obtained after the NLCs' ultracentrifugation. This was achieved using a validated high-performance liquid chromatography (HPLC) method. A sample of the supernatant was taken and diluted in the mobile phase before being filtered through a 0.22 μm pore-size filter. The HPLC analysis was conducted using a Waters® 600 Alliance system with a diode array detector (DAD) model 2696. A C18 column (5 μm, 4.6 mm × 250 mm—AtlantisTM) was utilized. The chromatographic conditions involved a mobile phase composition of acetonitrile:acidified water (0.5% formic acid) (60:40, v/v). The separation was performed using isocratic elution at a flow rate of 1.0 mL/min, with the detection wavelength set at 193 nm for POH. Subsequently, the EE% was calculated according to Equation (1):

$$EE\ (\%) = (POHi - POHs)/POHi \times 100 \tag{1}$$

where initial POHi represents the initial quantity of the POH incorporated into the NCLs, and POHs refers to the portion of the POH that remains unincorporated in the supernatant of NLCs.

3.5. In Vitro Release Profile

The in vitro release of POH from NLCs was assessed using Franz diffusion cells (Hanson Corp., Chatsworth, CA, USA). The receptor medium, phosphate-buffered saline (PBS, 50 mM, pH 7.4), was maintained at a temperature of 37 ± 0.5 °C with continuous stirring at 400 rpm. A cellulose acetate membrane with a pore-size cutoff of 0.22 μm was interposed between the donor and receptor compartments. A 20 μL suspension of NLCs-POH, ensuring sink conditions, was applied onto the membrane. At predetermined time intervals (0.5, 1, 2, 4, 8, 12, 24, and 48 h), 1.0 mL aliquots were collected and subsequently analyzed using HPLC.

Furthermore, the in vitro release of POH was evaluated in simulated gastric fluid (SGF) and simulated intestinal fluid (SIF), utilizing the dialysis membrane technique. In this experiment, a 500 μL aliquot of the loaded POH was placed inside a dialysis bag (MWCO 14,000, INLAB®, São Paulo, Brazil) and dispersed in 2 mL of pH 7.4 PBS. The bag was immersed in reservoirs containing 60 mL of pH 1.2 SGF supplemented with pepsin for a period of 2 h. Subsequently, the medium was replaced with pH 6.8 simulated SIF containing pancreatin and incubated for an additional 4 h. The release media were maintained at 37 ± 0.5 °C with magnetic stirring at 500 rpm. At specific time points (0.5, 1, 2, 3, 4, 5, and 6 h), aliquots were collected, and the withdrawn volume was replenished with fresh SGF or SIF. The collected samples were filtered through 0.22 μm PVDF membranes and subjected to analysis using HPLC.

3.6. Pharmacokinetic Study

3.6.1. UPLC-MS/MS Analysis

Ultra-performance liquid chromatography (UPLC) coupled with a triple quadrupole mass spectrometer (XEVO-TQD, Waters®, Milford, MA, USA) equipped with a electrospray ionization source (Waters®, Milford, MA, USA) was employed to determine and quantify the presence of perillyl acid (PA, a metabolite of POH) in rat plasma and organs following treatment. The chromatographic conditions included a reverse-phase C18 column (100 mm × 2.1 mm) with a mobile phase composed of acetonitrile (ACN) and acidified water (0.1% formic acid) in a ratio of 70:30 (v/v). The mobile phase was delivered isocratically at a flow rate of 0.3 mL/min, and a 2 μL injection volume was used. The total run time was 3 min, with retention times of 1.14 min for PA and 1.31 min for the internal standard (IS), carvone. The column oven was maintained at 40 °C, while the samples were kept at 10 °C in the autosampler. Electrospray ionization in positive mode (ESI+) was employed for mass spectrometric detection of the analytes. The MS conditions were as follows: capillary voltage at 4 kV, source temperature at 150 °C, desolvation temperature at 500 °C, and desolvation gas flow rate at 800 L/h. Quantification was performed using multiple reaction monitoring (MRM) mode, with m/z 167 → 92.97 for PA and m/z 151.01 → 122.98 for the IS. The optimized collision energies were 16 eV for PA and 8 eV for the IS. Instrument control, data acquisition, and processing were carried out using MassLynx™ 4.1 software (Milford, MA, USA).

3.6.2. Treatment

The pharmacokinetic study was approved by the Animal Ethics Committee of the Universidade Estadual do Centro-Oeste, Brazil (registration number 025/2021). It used adult male Wistar rats weighing between 200 and 300 g. The animals were housed in cages with ad libitum access to water and food, following a 12 h light/dark cycle. To minimize the influence of food, a fasting period of 12 h was implemented prior to drug administration in all rats. However, unrestricted access to water was provided throughout the study. The animal subjects were allocated into two distinct groups: Group A, which received free POH, and Group B, which received a suspension of NLCs encapsulating POH. In both groups, POH was administered orally via gavage as a single dose equivalent to 500 mg/kg. After the designated treatment duration, the animals were anesthetized (using Ketamine at a dose of 75 mg/kg and Xylazine at a dose of 10 mg/kg, administered intraperitoneally) and euthanized by decapitation at predefined time points (0.5, 1, 2, 4, 8, 12, and 24 h). Each of the seven time intervals in Groups A and B involved the use of six animals. Subsequent to euthanasia, blood samples were collected, and the following organs were extracted from the animals: brain, lungs, kidneys, spleen, and liver.

3.6.3. Sample Preparation

The collected blood samples were transferred to heparinized microtubes and centrifuged at 5000 rpm, 4 °C for 15 min to extract the plasma. Subsequently, liquid–liquid extraction with acetonitrile was performed. For this purpose, a 50 μL aliquot of plasma sample was added to 250 μL of acetonitrile containing the IS carvone (100 ng/mL). The tubes were then centrifuged at 15,000 rpm for 10 min at 4 °C. The supernatant was filtered through 0.22 μm syringe filters (Filtrilo, PVDF, São Paulo, Brazil) and transferred to an injection vial.

The organ homogenates were obtained by adding 5 mL of PBS (pH 7.4) to each 1 g of tissue, followed by homogenization at 33,000 rpm for 1 min for 2 cycles. A 250 μL aliquot of the homogenate was taken, and 750 μL of acetonitrile with the internal standard (100 ng/mL) was added. The samples were then centrifuged at 5000 rpm for 10 min at 4 °C and subsequently filtered through a 0.22 μm PVDF filter and analyzed using UPLC-MS/MS.

3.6.4. Data Analysis

The pharmacokinetic parameters analyzed included peak plasma concentration (C_{max}), time to reach peak plasma concentration (T_{max}), area under the plasma concentration versus time curve (AUC_{0-24h}), elimination half-life ($T_{\frac{1}{2}}$), elimination rate constant (Kel), apparent volume of distribution (Vd), and clearance (Cl).

3.7. Statistical Analysis

Data of all the experiments were expressed as the mean value $\pm$ SD. One-way ANOVA with Tukey test was used to compare means at the statistical significance level of 95% level of confidence, $p < 0.05$ (Statistica v. 12 StatSoft Inc., Tulsa, OK, USA).

4. Conclusions

This study investigated the pharmacokinetic profile of a nanostructured drug delivery system consisting of NLCs encapsulating the drug POH. The findings demonstrate notable advantages of the formulation compared with the free drug form. Specifically, the NLCs exhibited prolonged absorption time and elevated drug concentration in the bloodstream, indicating enhanced systemic exposure. Moreover, the NLCs demonstrated enhanced selectivity for brain delivery, leading to significantly higher levels of the drug in the brain compared with the free drug. This represents a significant advantage over the free drug, which exhibits faster clearance and distribution to non-target tissues. This increased brain bioavailability of POH-loaded NLCs offers promising prospects for the treatment of glioblastoma multiforme, where efficient drug delivery to the brain is crucial. Looking ahead, several perspectives emerge from this study. Firstly, further investigations are warranted to elucidate the underlying mechanisms responsible for the enhanced brain delivery observed with the NLC formulation. Understanding the specific interactions between the NLCs and the blood–brain barrier can offer valuable insights into optimizing and tailoring the delivery system for improved efficacy. Additionally, exploring the therapeutic efficacy of the POH-loaded NLCs in preclinical and clinical studies, particularly in glioblastoma models, would provide essential evidence for their potential as a viable treatment strategy. Lastly, investigating the long-term stability, scalability, and manufacturing feasibility of the NLC formulation will be crucial for its future translation into clinical applications.

Author Contributions: Conceptualization, R.M.M.; methodology, S.H.P., A.P.S.T., C.D., I.C.Z. and C.S.M.; data curation, S.H.P. and C.S.M.; writing—original draft preparation, S.H.P.; writing—review and editing, S.H.P. and R.M.M.; supervision, R.M.M.; project administration, R.M.M.; funding acquisition, R.M.M. All authors have read and agreed to the published version of the manuscript.

Funding: This research was partially funded by Coordenação de Aperfeiçoamento de Pessoal de Nível Superior—Brazil (CAPES)—Finance Code 001, as a scholarship for S. H. Peczek, and Financiadora de Estudos e Projetos (Finep)-Brazil.

Institutional Review Board Statement: The animal study protocol was approved by the Animal Ethics Committee of the Universidade Estadual do Centro-Oeste, Brazil (registration number 025/2021).

Informed Consent Statement: Not applicable.

Data Availability Statement: The data presented in this study are available on request from the corresponding author.

Acknowledgments: The authors would like to thank Coordenação de Aperfeiçoamento de Pessoal de Nível Superior—Brazil (CAPES)—Finance Code 001 for the scholarship for S. H. Peczek, and Financiadora de Estudos e Projetos (Finep).

Conflicts of Interest: The authors declare no conflict of interest.

References

1. Shojaei, S.; Kiumarsi, A.; Moghadam, A.R.; Alizadeh, J.; Marzban, H.; Ghavami, S. Perillyl Alcohol (Monoterpene Alcohol), Limonene. In *Enzymes*, 1st ed.; Elsevier Inc.: Amsterdam, The Netherlands, 2014; Volume 36, pp. 7–32. [CrossRef]
2. Hernandez, O.; Cenis, J.L.; Ferragut, J.A.; Seco, E.M. Antitumor Effects of Perillyl Alcohol in the Malignant Cells Derived from Glioblastoma Multiforme: An In Vitro and In Vivo Preclinical Study. *Investig. New Drugs* **2011**, *29*, 518–526. [CrossRef]
3. de Lima, D.C.; Rodrigues, S.V.; Boaventura, G.T.; Cho, H.-Y.; Chen, T.C.; Chonthal, A.H.; Da Fonseca, C.O. Simultaneous measurement of perillyl alcohol and its metabolite perillic acid in plasma and lung after inhalational administration in Wistar rats. *Drug Test. Anal.* **2020**, *12*, 268–279. [CrossRef] [PubMed]
4. Chen, T.C.; Da Fonseca, C.O.; Schönthal, A.H. Intranasal Perillyl Alcohol for Glioma Therapy: Molecular Mechanisms and Clinical Development. *Int. J. Mol. Sci.* **2018**, *19*, 3905. [CrossRef] [PubMed]
5. Chen, T.C.; Da Fonseca, C.O.; Schönthal, A.H. Preclinical development and clinical use of perillyl alcohol for chemoprevention and cancer therapy. *Am. J. Cancer Res.* **2015**, *5*, 1580–1593. [PubMed]
6. Hudes, G.R.; Szarka, C.E.; Adams, A.; Ranganathan, S.; McCauley, R.A.; Weiner, L.M.; Langer, C.J.; Litwin, S.; Yeslow, G.; Halberr, T.; et al. Phase I pharmacokinetic trial of perillyl alcohol (NSC 641066) in patients with refractory solid malignancies. *Clin. Cancer Res.* **2000**, *6*, 3071–3080.
7. Xu, M.; Floyd, H.S.; Greth, S.M.; Chang, W.-C.L.; Lohman, K.; Stoyanova, R.; Kucera, G.L.; Kute, T.E.; Willingham, M.C.; Miller, M.S. Perillyl alcohol-mediated inhibition of lung cancer cell line proliferation: Potential mechanisms for its chemotherapeutic effects. *Toxicol. Appl. Pharmacol.* **2004**, *195*, 232–246. [CrossRef]
8. Barthelman, M.; Chen, W.; Gensler, H.L.; Huang, C.; Dong, Z.; Bowden, G.T. Inhibitory effects of perillyl alcohol on UVB-induced murine skin cancer and AP-1 transactivation. *Cancer Res.* **1998**, *58*, 711–716.
9. Mills, J.J.; Chari, R.S.; Boyer, I.J.; Gould, M.N.; Jirtle, R.L. Induction of apoptosis in liver tumors by the monoterpene perillyl alcohol. *Cancer Res.* **1995**, *55*, 979–983.
10. Stark, M.; Burke, Y.D.; McKinzie, J.H.; Ayoubi, A.; Crowell, P.L. Chemotherapy of pancreatic cancer with the monoterpene perillyl alcohol. *Cancer Lett.* **1995**, *96*, 15–21. [CrossRef]
11. Reddy, B.S.; Wang, C.X.; Samaha, H.; Lubet, R.; Steele, V.E.; Kelloff, G.J.; Rao, C.V. Chemoprevention of colon carcinogenesis by dietary perillyl alcohol. *Cancer Res.* **1997**, *57*, 420–425.
12. Yuri, T.; Danbara, N.; Tsujita-Kyutoku, M.; Kiyozuka, Y.; Senzaki, H.; Shikata, N.; Kanzaki, H.; Tsubura, A. Perillyl Alcohol Inhibits Human Breast Cancer Cell Growth in vitro and in vivo. *Breast Cancer Res. Treat.* **2004**, *84*, 251–260. [CrossRef]
13. Clark, S.S.; Zhong, L.; Filiault, D.; Perman, S.; Ren, Z.; Gould, M.; Yang, X. Anti-leukemia effect of perillyl alcohol in Bcr/Abl-transformed cells indirectly inhibits signaling through Mek in a Ras- and Raf-independent fashion. *Clin. Cancer Res.* **2003**, *9*, 4494–4504. [PubMed]
14. da Fonseca, C.O.; Simão, M.; Lins, I.R.; Caetano, R.O.; Futuro, D.; Quirico-Santos, T. Efficacy of monoterpene perillyl alcohol upon the survival rate of patients with recurrent glioblastoma. *J. Cancer Res. Clin. Oncol.* **2011**, *137*, 287–293. [CrossRef] [PubMed]

15. Crowell, P.L.; Ren, Z.; Lin, S.; Vedejs, E.; Gould, M.N. Structure-activity relationships among monoterpene inhibitors of protein isoprenylation and cell proliferation. *Biochem. Pharmacol.* **1994**, *47*, 1405–1415. [CrossRef] [PubMed]

16. da Fonseca, C.O.; Landeiro, J.A.; Clark, S.S.; Quirico-Santos, T.; Carvalho, M.d.G.d.C.; Gattass, C.R. Recent advances in the molecular genetics of malignant gliomas disclose targets for antitumor agent perillyl alcohol. *Surg. Neurol.* **2006**, *65* (Suppl. S1), S2–S8. [CrossRef] [PubMed]

17. da Fonseca, C.O.; Santos, T.Q.; Fernandes, J.; da Costa Carvalho MD, G.; Gatass, C.R. Biologia molecular dos glioblastomas: Perspectivas terapêuticas do monoterpeno álcool perílico. *J. Bras. Neurocir.* **2003**, *14*, 46–54.

18. Chen, T.C.; da Fonseca, C.O.; Levin, D.; Schönthal, A.H. The Monoterpenoid Perillyl Alcohol: Anticancer Agent and Medium to Overcome Biological Barriers. *Pharmaceutics* **2021**, *13*, 2167. [CrossRef]

19. Louis, D.N.; Perry, A.; Reifenberger, G.; Von Deimling, A.; Figarella-Branger, D.; Cavenee, W.K.; Ohgaki, H.; Wiestler, O.D.; Kleihues, P.; Ellison, D.W. The 2016 World Health Organization Classification of Tumors of the Central Nervous System: A summary. *Acta Neuropathol.* **2016**, *131*, 803–820. [CrossRef]

20. Bailey, H.H.; Wilding, G.; Tutsch, K.D.; Arzoomanian, R.Z.; Alberti, D.; Feierabend, C.; Simon, K.; Marnocha, R.; Holstein, S.A.; Stewart, J.; et al. A phase I trial of perillyl alcohol administered four times daily for 14 days out of 28 days. *Cancer Chemother. Pharmacol.* **2004**, *54*, 368–376. [CrossRef]

21. Bailey, H.H.; Levy, D.; Harris, L.S.; Schink, J.C.; Foss, F.; Beatty, P.; Wadler, S. A Phase II Trial of Daily Perillyl Alcohol in Patients with Advanced Ovarian Cancer: Eastern Cooperative Oncology Group Study E2E96. *Gynecol. Oncol.* **2002**, *85*, 464–468. [CrossRef]

22. Chaturvedi, V.K.; Singh, A.; Singh, V.K.; Singh, M.P. Cancer Nanotechnology: A New Revolution for Cancer Diagnosis and Therapy. *Curr. Drug Metab.* **2018**, *20*, 416–429. [CrossRef]

23. Diedrich, C.; Zittlau, I.C.; Machado, C.S.; Fin, M.T.; Khalil, N.M.; Badea, I.; Mainardes, R.M. Mucoadhesive nanoemulsion enhances brain bioavailability of luteolin after intranasal administration and induces apoptosis to SH-SY5Y neuroblastoma cells. *Int. J. Pharm.* **2022**, *626*, 122142. [CrossRef] [PubMed]

24. Santos, J.D.S.; Diedrich, C.; Machado, C.S.; da Fonseca, C.O.; Khalil, N.M.; Mainardes, R.M. Intranasal administration of perillyl alcohol–loaded nanoemulsion and pharmacokinetic study of its metabolite perillic acid in plasma and brain of rats using ultra-performance liquid chromatography/tandem mass spectrometry. *Biomed. Chromatogr.* **2021**, *35*, e5037. [CrossRef]

25. Khosa, A.; Reddi, S.; Saha, R.N. Nanostructured lipid carriers for site-specific drug delivery. *Biomed. Pharmacother.* **2018**, *103*, 598–613. [CrossRef] [PubMed]

26. Tapeinos, C.; Battaglini, M.; Ciofani, G. Advances in the design of solid lipid nanoparticles and nanostructured lipid carriers for targeting brain diseases. *J. Control. Release* **2017**, *264*, 306–332. [CrossRef] [PubMed]

27. Müller, R.H.; Mäder, K.; Gohla, S. Solid lipid nanoparticles (SLN) for controlled drug delivery: A review of the state of the art. *Eur. J. Pharm. Biopharm.* **2000**, *50*, 161–177. [CrossRef] [PubMed]

28. Mehnert, W.; Mäder, K. Solid lipid nanoparticles: Production, characterization and applications. *Adv. Drug Deliv. Rev.* **2001**, *47*, 165–196. [CrossRef]

29. Aslan, B.; Ozpolat, B.; Sood, A.K.; Lopez-Berestein, G. Nanotechnology in cancer therapy. *J. Drug Target* **2013**, *21*, 26–27. [CrossRef]

30. Maeda, H.; Greish, K.; Fang, J. The EPR Effect and Polymeric Drugs: A Paradigm Shift for Cancer Chemotherapy in the 21st Century. *Adv. Polym. Sci.* **2006**, *193*, 103–121. [CrossRef]

31. Antonio, E.; Dos Reis Antunes Junior, O.; Marcano, R.; Diedrich, C.; da Silva Santos, J.; Machado, C.; Khalil, N.; Mainardes, R. Chitosan modified poly (lactic acid) nanoparticles increased the ursolic acid oral bioavailability. *Int. J. Biol. Macromol.* **2021**, *172*, 133–142. [CrossRef]

32. He, C.; Yin, L.; Tang, C.; Yin, C. Size-dependent absorption mechanism of polymeric nanoparticles for oral delivery of protein drugs. *Biomaterials* **2012**, *33*, 8569–8578. [CrossRef]

33. Banerjee, A.; Qi, J.; Gogoi, R.; Wong, J.; Mitragotri, S. Role of nanoparticle size, shape and surface chemistry in oral drug delivery. *J. Control. Release* **2016**, *238*, 176–185. [CrossRef]

34. Lasoń, E.; Sikora, E.; Ogonowski, J. Influence of process parameters on properties of Nanostructured Lipid Carriers (NLC) formulation. *Acta Biochim. Pol.* **1970**, *60*, 773–777. [CrossRef]

35. Subramaniam, B.; Siddik, Z.H.; Nagoor, N.H. Optimization of nanostructured lipid carriers: Understanding the types, designs, and parameters in the process of formulations. *J. Nanoparticle Res.* **2020**, *22*, 141. [CrossRef]

36. Fatouh, A.M.; Elshafeey, A.H.; Abdelbary, A. Intranasal agomelatine solid lipid nanoparticles to enhance brain delivery: Formulation, optimization and in vivo pharmacokinetics. *Drug Des. Dev. Ther.* **2017**, *11*, 1815–1825. [CrossRef] [PubMed]

37. Elmowafy, M.; Ibrahim, H.M.; Ahmed, M.A.; Shalaby, K.; Salama, A.; Hefesha, H. Atorvastatin-loaded nanostructured lipid carriers (NLCs): Strategy to overcome oral delivery drawbacks. *Drug Deliv.* **2017**, *24*, 932–941. [CrossRef] [PubMed]

38. Danaei, M.; Dehghankhold, M.; Ataei, S.; Hasanzadeh Davarani, F.; Javanmard, R.; Dokhani, A.; Khorasani, S.; Mozafari, M.R. Impact of Particle Size and Polydispersity Index on the Clinical Applications of Lipidic Nanocarrier Systems. *Pharmaceutics* **2018**, *10*, 57. [CrossRef]

39. Han, F.; Li, S.; Yin, R.; Liu, H.; Xu, L. Effect of surfactants on the formation and characterization of a new type of colloidal drug delivery system: Nanostructured lipid carriers. *Colloids Surfaces A: Physicochem. Eng. Asp.* **2008**, *315*, 210–216. [CrossRef]

40. Kovačević, A.B.; Müller, R.H.; Savić, S.D.; Vuleta, G.M.; Keck, C.M. Solid lipid nanoparticles (SLN) stabilized with polyhydroxy surfactants: Preparation, characterization and physical stability investigation. *Colloids Surf. A Physicochem. Eng. Asp.* **2014**, *444*, 15–25. [CrossRef]

41. Bhadra, A.; Karmakar, G.; Nahak, P.; Chettri, P.; Roy, B.; Guha, P.; Mandal, A.; Nath, R.; Panda, A. Impact of detergents on the physiochemical behavior of itraconazole loaded nanostructured lipid carriers. *Colloids Surf. A Physicochem. Eng. Asp.* **2017**, *516*, 63–71. [CrossRef]
42. Penteado, L.; Lopes, V.F.; Karam, T.K.; Nakamura, C.V.; Khalil, N.M.; Mainardes, R.M. Chitosan-coated poly(ε-caprolactone) nanocapsules for mucoadhesive applications of perillyl alcohol. *Soft Mater.* **2021**, *20*, 1–11. [CrossRef]
43. Nnamani, P.O.; Hansen, S.; Windbergs, M.; Lehr, C.-M. Development of artemether-loaded nanostructured lipid carrier (NLC) formulation for topical application. *Int. J. Pharm.* **2014**, *477*, 208–217. [CrossRef]
44. Wissing, S.; Müller, R. Solid lipid nanoparticles as carrier for sunscreens: In vitro release and in vivo skin penetration. *J. Control. Release* **2002**, *81*, 225–233. [CrossRef] [PubMed]
45. Notario-Pérez, F.; Cazorla-Luna, R.; Martín-Illana, A.; Ruiz-Caro, R.; Peña, J.; Veiga, M.-D. Tenofovir Hot-Melt Granulation using Gelucire® to Develop Sustained-Release Vaginal Systems for Weekly Protection against Sexual Transmission of HIV. *Pharmaceutics* **2019**, *11*, 137. [CrossRef] [PubMed]
46. Wang, X.; Luo, Z.; Xiao, Z. Preparation, characterization, and thermal stability of β-cyclodextrin/soybean lecithin inclusion complex. *Carbohydr. Polym.* **2014**, *101*, 1027–1032. [CrossRef]
47. Hu, F.Q.; Jiang, S.P.; Du, Y.Z.; Yuan, H.; Ye, Y.Q.; Zeng, S. Nanostructured Lipid Carriers: A Potential Oral Drug Delivery System for Improving Drug Bioavailability. *Pharmaceutics* **2018**, *10*, 34. [CrossRef]
48. Zielińska, A.; Ferreira, N.R.; Feliczak-Guzik, A.; Nowak, I.; Souto, E.B. Loading, release profile and accelerated stability assessment of monoterpenes-loaded solid lipid nanoparticles (SLN). *Pharm. Dev. Technol.* **2020**, *25*, 832–844. [CrossRef]
49. Son, G.-H.; Lee, B.-J.; Cho, C.-W. Mechanisms of drug release from advanced drug formulations such as polymeric-based drug-delivery systems and lipid nanoparticles. *J. Pharm. Investig.* **2017**, *47*, 287–296. [CrossRef]
50. Ripple, G.H.; Gould, M.N.; Arzoomanian, R.Z.; Alberti, D.; Feierabend, C.; Simon, K.; Binger, K.; Tutsch, K.D.; Pomplun, M.; Wahamaki, A.; et al. Phase I clinical and pharmacokinetic study of perillyl alcohol administered four times a day. *Clin. Cancer Res.* **2000**, *6*, 390–396.
51. Khan, N.; Shah, F.A.; Rana, I.; Ansari, M.M.; Din, F.U.; Rizvi, S.Z.H.; Aman, W.; Lee, G.-Y.; Lee, E.-S.; Kim, J.-K.; et al. Nanostructured lipid carriers-mediated brain delivery of carbamazepine for improved in vivo anticonvulsant and anxiolytic activity. *Int. J. Pharm.* **2020**, *577*, 119033. [CrossRef]
52. Saeedi, M.; Eslamifar, M.; Khezri, K.; Dizaj, S.M. Applications of nanotechnology in drug delivery to the central nervous system. *Biomed. Pharmacother.* **2019**, *111*, 666–675. [CrossRef] [PubMed]
53. Zhang, Q.; Jiang, X. Recent advances in nanotechnology-based drug delivery systems for enhanced drug penetration into the central nervous system. *Nano Today* **2020**, *35*, 100968. [CrossRef]
54. Chaves, L.L.; Cevolani, D.; Cavalcante, R.S. Role of Polysorbate 80 on brain drug delivery: Evidence and advances. *Eur. J. Pharm. Sci.* **2021**, *164*, 105964. [CrossRef]
55. Zhuang, C.Y.; Li, N.; Wang, M.; Zhang, X.N.; Pan, W.S.; Peng, J.J.; Pan, Y.-S.; Tang, X. Preparation and characterization of vinpocetine loaded nanostructured lipid carriers (NLC) for improved oral bioavailability. *Int. J. Pharm.* **2010**, *394*, 179–185. [CrossRef]

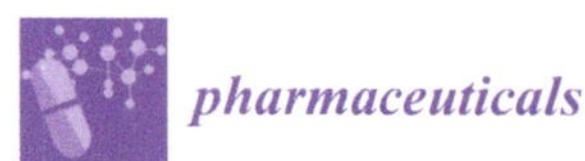

pharmaceuticals

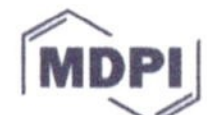

Article

Ocular Delivery of Bimatoprost-Loaded Solid Lipid Nanoparticles for Effective Management of Glaucoma

Sandeep Divate Satyanarayana [1], Amr Selim Abu Lila [2,3], Afrasim Moin [3], Ehssan H. Moglad [4,5], El-Sayed Khafagy [4,6], Hadil Faris Alotaibi [7], Ahmad J. Obaidullah [8] and Rompicherla Narayana Charyulu [1,*]

[1] Department of Pharmaceutics, NGSM Institute of Pharmaceutical Sciences, Nitte (Deemed to be University), Mangalore 575018, India; sandypharama@nitte.edu.in
[2] Department of Pharmaceutics and Industrial Pharmacy, Faculty of Pharmacy, Zagazig University, Zagazig 44519, Egypt; a.abulila@uoh.edu.sa
[3] Department of Pharmaceutics, College of Pharmacy, University of Hail, Hail 81442, Saudi Arabia; a.moinuddin@uoh.edu.sa
[4] Department of Pharmaceutics, College of Pharmacy, Prince Sattam Bin Abdulaziz University, Al-kharj 11942, Saudi Arabia; e.moglad@psau.edu.sa (E.H.M.); e.khafagy@psau.edu.sa (E.-S.K.)
[5] Department of Microbiology and Parasitology, Medicinal and Aromatic Plants Research Institute, National Center for Research, Khartoum 2404, Sudan
[6] Department of Pharmaceutics and Industrial Pharmacy, Faculty of Pharmacy, Suez Canal University, Ismailia 41522, Egypt
[7] Department of Pharmaceutical Sciences, College of Pharmacy, Princess Nourah Bint Abdul Rahman University, Riyadh 11671, Saudi Arabia; hfalotaibi@pnu.edu.sa
[8] Department of Pharmaceutical Chemistry, College of Pharmacy, King Saud University, Riyadh 11451, Saudi Arabia; aobaidullah@ksu.edu.sa
* Correspondence: narayana@nitte.edu.in

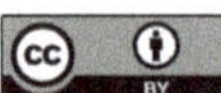

Citation: Satyanarayana, S.D.; Abu Lila, A.S.; Moin, A.; Moglad, E.H.; Khafagy, E.-S.; Alotaibi, H.F.; Obaidullah, A.J.; Charyulu, R.N. Ocular Delivery of Bimatoprost-Loaded Solid Lipid Nanoparticles for Effective Management of Glaucoma. *Pharmaceuticals* **2023**, *16*, 1001. https://doi.org/10.3390/ph16071001

Academic Editors: Ana Catarina Silva, João Nuno Moreira and José Manuel Sousa Lobo

Received: 6 June 2023
Revised: 7 July 2023
Accepted: 11 July 2023
Published: 13 July 2023

Abstract: Glaucoma is a progressive optic neuropathy characterized by a rise in the intraocular pressure (IOP) leading to optic nerve damage. Bimatoprost is a prostaglandin analogue used to reduce the elevated IOP in patients with glaucoma. The currently available dosage forms for Bimatoprost suffer from relatively low ocular bioavailability. The objective of this study was to fabricate and optimize solid lipid nanoparticles (SLNs) containing Bimatoprost for ocular administration for the management of glaucoma. Bimatoprost-loaded SLNs were fabricated by solvent evaporation/ultrasonication technique. Glyceryl Monostearate (GMS) was adopted as solid lipid and poloxamer 407 as surfactant. Optimization of SLNs was conducted by central composite design. The optimized formulation was assessed for average particle size, entrapment efficiency (%), zeta potential, surface morphology, drug release study, sterility test, isotonicity test, Hen's egg test-chorioallantoic membrane (HET-CAM) test and histopathology studies. The optimized Bimatoprost-loaded SLNs formulation had an average size of 183.3 ± 13.3 nm, zeta potential of -9.96 ± 1.2 mV, and encapsulation efficiency percentage of $71.8 \pm 1.1\%$. Transmission electron microscopy (TEM) study revealed the nearly smooth surface of formulated particles with a nano-scale size range. In addition, SLNs significantly sustained Bimatoprost release for up to 12 h, compared to free drug ($p < 005$). Most importantly, HET-CAM test nullified the irritancy of the formulation was verified its tolerability upon ocular use, as manifested by a significant reduction in mean irritation score, compared to positive control (1% sodium dodecyl sulfate; $p < 0.001$). Histopathology study inferred the absence of any signs of cornea tissue damage upon treatment with Bimatoprost optimized formulation. Collectively, it was concluded that SLNs might represent a viable vehicle for enhancing the corneal permeation and ocular bioavailability of Bimatoprost for the management of glaucoma.

Keywords: bimatoprost; central composite design; glaucoma; HET-CAM test; solid lipid nanoparticles (SLNs)

1. Introduction

Glaucoma is a progressive ocular neuropathy that is distinguished by an increment in the intraocular pressure (IOP) predisposing damage to the optic nerve [1]. Glaucoma has been called the silent killer of sight as it begins with minor symptoms and if it left untreated, permanent vision loss can occur. Worldwide, glaucoma is the second leading cause of blindness [2]. Currently, various drugs are available for the treatment of glaucoma.

Prostaglandins are considered the first-line treatment option for glaucoma. Bimatoprost is a prostaglandin analogue adopted to reduce the elevated intra ocular pressure (IOP) in patients suffering from glaucoma [3]. It is also used for reducing the ocular hypertension [4]. It was officially approved by FDA in the year 2001 for ocular hypertension [5] and later in 2008 for hypotricosis [6]. Bimatoprost has been reported to reduce the increased IOP in patients by boosting the aqueous humor outflow through trabecular meshwork and the uveoscleral pathway [7]. It also increases the production of aqueous humor in the eye that prevents the damage to optic nerve [8]. Bimatoprost has good corneal absorption; it reaches the plasma peak concentration after 10 min and then gets reduced after 1.5 h. Nevertheless, conventional Bimatoprost dosage forms, such as eye drops, show limitations such as lower bioavailability and shorter precorneal residence time. In addition, the commercial formulation of Bimatoprost (Lumigan^{TM}) contains benzalkonium chloride, which exerts adverse effects such as eye edema, discomfort, burning, or itching [9]. Furthermore, despite the efficacy of recently adopted approaches, such as nanosponge [10], ocular inserts [11], and intracameral implants [12], in enhancing Bimatoprost corneal accessibility, these treatment strategies usually need a surgical procedure, which might be problematic for patients.

Ocular drug delivery is considered one of the most difficult tasks confronting pharmaceutical scientists. The poor intraocular bioavailability of conventional ocular delivery systems, caused by high rates of drug dilution and elimination, along with, limited corneal permeability [13,14], usually demand either increased frequency of administration or higher drug levels in the formulation, which may result in problems with patient compliance or potential overdosing. To overcome these problems, novel delivery systems have been introduced, including ocular implants [12], liposomes [15], nanoparticles [16], or in situ gels [17]. Among them, solid lipid nanoparticles (SLNs) have evolved as a viable ocular drug delivery vehicle because of their potential to enhance corneal drug permeation [18].

Solid lipid nanoparticle (SLN) are minute colloidal carrier systems with particle size range of 10–1000 nm. Solid lipid nanoparticles represent a viable option for ocular delivery for its inherent properties such as biocompatibility, non-toxicity, and higher stability [19]. In addition, the nanosize range of SLN bestows them with prolonged pre-corneal residence time, controlled drug delivery, enhanced corneal absorption, and thereby, enhanced drug bioavailability. Several studies have addressed the ability of drug-loaded SLNs to effectively cross the corneal epithelium due to its lipophilic properties [19–21]. Furthermore, SLN offers the advantages of the ability to encapsulate both hydrophilic and lipophilic drugs, high drug loading efficiency, and ease of large-scale production [22,23].

In this study, Bimatoprost-loaded SLNs were formulated to improve the therapeutic effectiveness of drug for the management of glaucoma. Central composite design (CCD) was adopted for the optimization of Bimatoprost-loaded SLNs investigating the impact of two independent factor, drug: lipid ratio (*w:w*) and sonication time (min) on two product responses; particle size and entrapment efficiency. Further, the optimized Bimatoprost-loaded SLNs was subjected for evaluation parameters such as mean particle size, zeta potential, TEM analysis, drug release study, sterility test, isotonicity test, HET-CAM test and histopathology studies.

2. Results and Discussion

2.1. Preformulation Studies

FTIR studies were carried out to assess the compatibility of drug with lipid used for preparing the Bimatoprost-loaded SLNs. The FTIR spectra of pure Bimatoprost, glyceryl monostearate (GMS) and physical mixture of drug and GMS are depicted in Figure 1. The

FTIR spectrum of Bimatoprost showed characteristic peaks at 3324, 1618, 3427 and 3023 cm^{-1} corresponding to O-H stretching, N-C=O (amide) stretching, N-H (secondary amine) stretching and aliphatic C-H (stretching) groups. For GMS, the FTIR spectrum showed absorption peaks at 1218, 1730, 2951 and 3310 cm^{-1} demonstrating the characteristic function groups of C-O-C (ether) stretching, C=O (carbonyl), aliphatic C-H stretching and O-H (hydroxyl) groups, respectively. Of interest, the FTIR spectrum obtained for physical mixture of Bimatoprost and GMS exhibited prominent peaks at 3306, 1637, and 2915 cm^{-1} corresponding to the O-H (alcohol) stretching, N-C=O (amide) stretching, aliphatic C-H stretching functional groups. From the FTIR interpretation, it was evident that there was no interaction between the drug and lipid. Therefore, this study claimed that Bimatoprost was compatible with GMS.

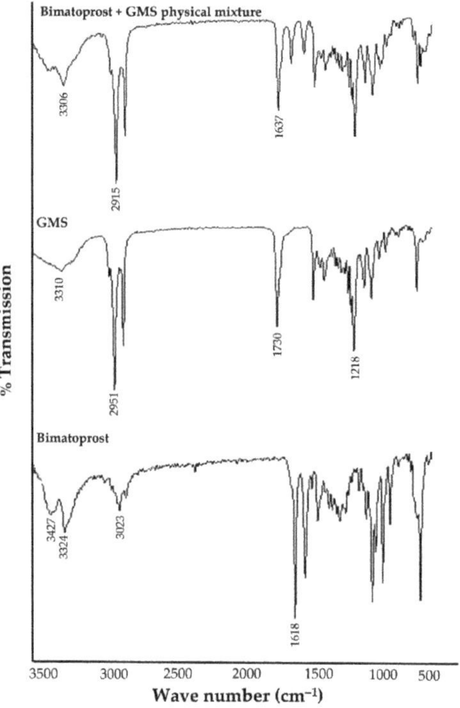

Figure 1. FTIR spectra of Bimatoprost, GMS, and their physical mixture.

2.2. Preparation of Bimatoprost-Loaded SLNs

A central composite statistical approach was adopted for the formulation of Bimatoprost-loaded SLNs and to study the impact of two independent factors; namely drug:lipid ratio and sonication time, on product characteristics. The influence of these factors on particle size and entrapment efficiency (%) was investigated as depicted by the 3D surface plots. Considering these two factors, a total of 13 formulation trials at different levels of independent factors were prepared. All the fabricated formulation trials were then evaluated for particle size and entrapment efficiency (%). The optimization was aimed at minimizing the particle size and maximizing the entrapment efficiency (%). The central composite design generated trails with variable particle sizes and entrapment efficiency (%) illustrated in the Table 1.

Table 1. Central composite design batches with results of dependent factors for Bimatoprost SLNs.

Formula	A: Drug:Lipid Ratio (*w:w*)	B: Sonication Time (min)	R_1: Particle Size (nm)	R_2: Entrapment Efficiency (%)
1	0	0	184.7 ± 11.4	72.7 ± 2.4
2	−1	−1	269.8 ± 18.2	61.4 ± 1.9
3	−1	1	244.3 ± 13.7	68.5 ± 1.1
4	0	0	188.6 ± 9.5	71.4 ± 2.1
5	0	0	185.5 ± 7.6	72.8 ± 1.8
6	0	0	192.8 ± 11.1	70.4 ± 1.6
7	0	0	198.4 ± 12.4	72.6 ± 1.9
8	0	−1.41421	248.2 ± 18.6	69.7 ± 0.9
9	0	1.41421	178.6 ± 9.3	78.6 ± 1.3
10	1	−1	310.6 ± 19.5	70.4 ± 2.5
11	1	1	232.6 ± 11.6	72.3 ± 1.7
12	1.41421	0	322.3 ± 17.6	69.3 ± 0.8
13	−1.41421	0	272.8 ± 12.3	60.8 ± 1.1

2.2.1. Effect of Formulation Variables on Particle Size

Generally, nanoparticles having an average particle size smaller than 200 nm are thought to be optimum for ocular delivery because of their enhanced penetration through the corneal barriers [24]. In this study, the particle size of all Bimatoprost-loaded SLNs was ranging from 178.6 ± 9.3 to 322.3 ± 17.6 nm. The data for particle size (R_1) were fitted into several polynomial models. ANOVA analysis (Table S1) revealed that R_1 was best fitted in a quadratic response surface model (Equation (1)).

$$\text{Particle size } (R_1) = +190.00 + 12.39\,A - 25.24\,B - 13.12\,AB + 55.99\,A^2 + 13.91\,B^2 \qquad (1)$$

The impact of independent variables on particle size was analyzed by the 3D surface plot obtained from the data of study with the Design Expert software (Figure 2A). The surface plots obtained with particle size showed a synergistic effect of drug:lipid ratio on SLNs particle size. Increasing lipid ratio from 1:1 to 1:5 resulted in a significant increase of particle size. By fixing the sonication time, the particle size of SLNs prepared with a drug:lipid ratio of 1:5 (F10; 310.6 ± 19.5 nm) was remarkably higher than that prepared at 1:1 drug:lipid ratio (F2; 269.8 ± 18.2 nm). This effect might be ascribed to the increase in the viscosity of the organic phase at higher polymer concentrations, which in turn, would increase the tendency of the lipid to coalesce, leading to the formation of larger nanoparticles. Similar results were obtained by Tiwari et al. [25] who reported the positive effect of increasing lipid content on the particle size of terbinafine hydrochloride-loaded SLNs.

Sonication energy played a crucial role in formation of the emulsion, and thus significantly affected the particle size of SLNs. The sonication energy was varied by altering the sonication period (5 to 15 min) while maintaining a constant power. Herein, sonication time was found to exert an antagonistic effect on particle size of SLNs. At fixed drug:lipid ratio, the particle size of Bimatoprost-loaded SLNs dramatically decreased from 310.6 ± 19.5 nm (F10) to 232.6 ± 11.6 nm (F11) as the sonication time increased from 5 min to 15 min. Collectively, these results revealed the pronounced effects of formulation variables on particle size.

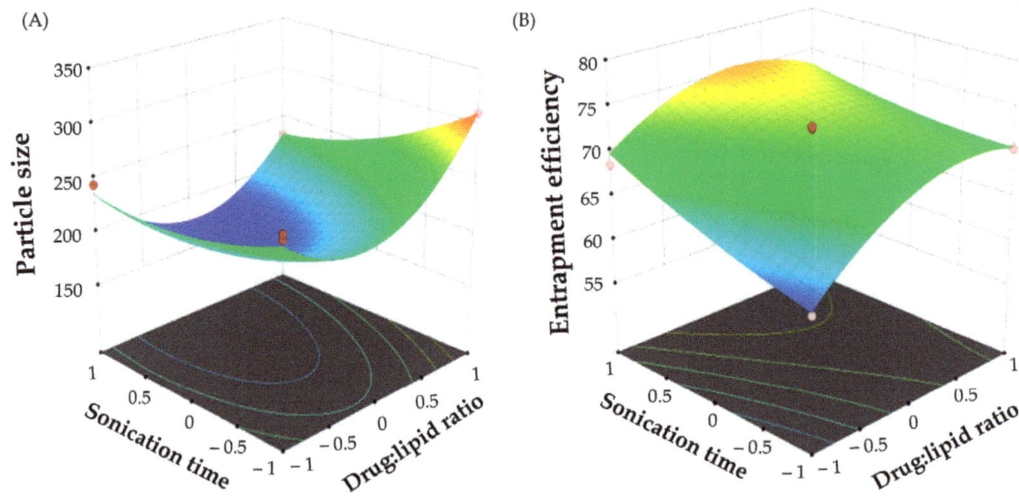

Figure 2. 3D surface plot of (**A**) Particle size, and (**B**) entrapment efficiency percentage.

2.2.2. Effect of Formulation Variables on Entrapment Efficiency Percentage

Entrapment efficiency is a crucial measure for characterizing solid lipid nanoparticles. In order to obtain an optimum encapsulation efficiency, several factors, including drug:lipid ratio and sonication time, were varied, and the entrapment efficiency was calculated. As depicted in Table 2, the percentage entrapment efficiency fluctuated from 60.8 ± 1.1 to $78.6 \pm 1.3\%$. The data for entrapment efficiency (R_2) were fitted into several polynomial models. ANOVA analysis (Table S1) revealed that R_2 was best fitted in a quadratic response surface model (Equation (2)).

$$\text{Entrapment efficiency (\%) } (R_2) = +71.98 + 3.10\ A - 2.70\ B - 1.30\ AB - 3.83\ A^2 + 0.72\ B^2 \tag{2}$$

Table 2. Sterility test results for optimized formulation.

Test Microorganism	Positive Control	Negative Control	Optimized Formulation
Staphylococcous aureus	+	−	−
Bacilus subtilus	+	−	−
Candida albicans	+	−	−
Asperges brasiliensis	+	−	−

where: + sign indicates microbial growth, while − sign indicates no microbial growth.

In addition, the influence of independent variables on entrapment efficiency was represented by the 3D surface plot (Figure 2B). It was evident that drug:lipid ratio exerted a positive effect on drug entrapment within SLNs. The entrapment efficiency rose from $61.4 \pm 1.9\%$ (F2) to $72.3 \pm 1.7\%$ (F10) when the drug-to-lipid weight ratio was changed from 1:1 to 1:5, indicating that the greater the lipid ratio, the higher the entrapment efficiency. This pattern was consistent with previous literature [26,27]. This synergistic effect of lipid content on drug entrapment efficiency might be explained, on the one hand, to the availability of higher space to accommodate more drug at higher lipid content [28], and on the other hand, to the elevated viscosity of the medium at higher lipid content, which result in rapid solidification of the nanoparticles, and thereby, constrain the leakage of drug to the external medium [29].

Similarly, sonication time has been verified to exert a synergistic effect on drug entrapment within SLNs. At fixed drug:lipid ratio, the entrapment efficiency percentage was increased as the sonication time increased from 5 min to 15 min. A higher entrapment efficiency (68.5 ± 1.1%; F3) was achieved when Bimatoprost-loaded SNLs dispersion was processed by probe-sonication for 20 min, compared to those sonicated for 5 min (F2; 61.4 ± 1.9%). This effect might be ascribed to the increased drug solubility in the lipid core upon increasing sonication time, which in turn, would increase the entrapment efficiency [21]. Similar findings were reported by Nair et al. who emphasized the positive effect of increasing sonication time on the entrapment of clarithromycin within solid lipid nanoparticles [30].

2.2.3. Numerical Optimization of Bimatoprost-Loaded SLNs

In order to obtain an optimized Bimatoprost-loaded SLN formulation, a numerical optimization analysis was carried out using Design-Expert® software employing the desirability function. The suggested formulation variables for the fabrication of the optimized Bimatoprost-loaded SLN formulation, obtained at a desirability of 0.936, was drug:lipid ratio of 1:3, and a sonication time of 20 min. The prepared optimized Bimatoprost-loaded SLNs was found to fulfill the requisites of a minimum particle size and maximum entrapment efficiency set by the design constrains for an optimum formulation. The estimated vesicle size was 183.3 ± 13.3 nm, and the % EE was 71.8 ± 1.1%, which were comparable to the predicted values for vesicle size and % EE (178.7 nm, and 75.4%, respectively).

2.3. Evaluation of Optimized Formulation of Bimatoprost SLNs

2.3.1. Particle Size and PDI

The average particle size of optimized Bimatoprost-loaded SLNs was found to be 183.3 ± 13.3 nm (Figure 3A), which is considered within the optimum size range (<200 nm) for ocular administration [24]. Polydispersity index (PDI) is another important parameter for characterizing nanodispersions. PDI is considered a measure of the heterogeneity of a sample based on size. Generally, colloidal particles with PDIs values less than 0.3 denotes homogenous size distribution. In this study, the PDI of optimized Bimatoprost-loaded SLNs was 0.205, indicating high particle homogeneity [31].

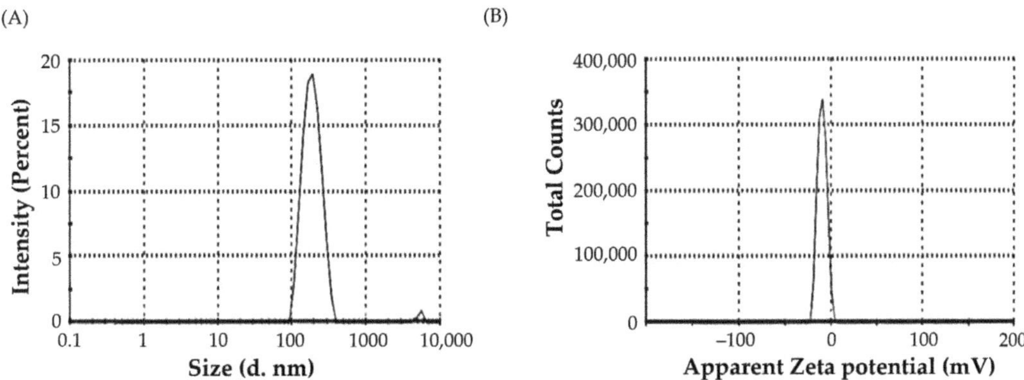

Figure 3. (**A**) Particle size, and (**B**) Zeta potential of optimized Bimatoprost-loaded SLNs.

2.3.2. Zeta Potential

The magnitude of the zeta potential of colloidal particles provides an indication of their physical stability. Colloidal particles with either large positive or negative zeta potential tend to repel each other, and thereby, enhance the overall stability of the colloidal system [32]. The zeta potential of optimized Bimatoprost-loaded SLNs was found to be −9.96 ± 1.2 mV (Figure 3B). This relatively negatively charged surface of the prepared

SLNs, along with the lower PDI value, is assumed to participate to the physical stability of formulated SLNs.

2.3.3. TEM Study

The surface morphology and particle size distribution of optimized formulation were evaluated by TEM analysis. As depicted in Figure 4, the optimized drug-loaded SLNs exerted a discrete structure with a nearly smooth surface. In addition, particle size of the optimized SLNs determined by TEM was in the range of 150–200 nm, which is close to that determined by dynamic light scattering technique.

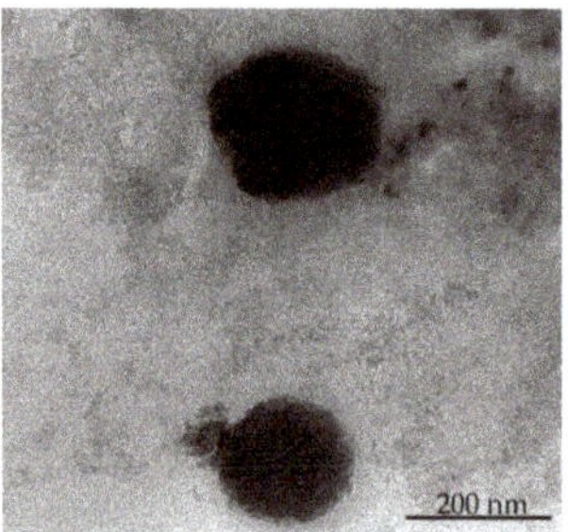

Figure 4. TEM analysis of optimized Bimatoprost-loaded SLNs.

2.4. In Vitro Drug Release Study

The in vitro dissolution/release profiles of both free Bimatoprost and optimized drug-loaded SLNs were illustrated in Figure 5. The study was conducted using simulated tear fluid (STF) as dissolution media using Franz diffusion cell. As shown in Figure 5, free Bimatoprost was released immediately from Bimatoprost solution with more than 95% of the drug released within the first 4 h. On the other hand, entrapment of Bimatoprost within SLNs remarkably prolonged the drug release for up to 12 h. Of interest, Bimatoprost-loaded SLNs showed a biphasic release pattern, with more than 25% of entrapped Bimatoprost was released from the SLNs during the first 3 h, followed by a sustained release over 12 h, with up to 60% of drug released at the end of release study. The initial rapid drug release from SLNs might be accounted for the ready dissolution of drug molecules adsorbed at the surface of SLNs, while the subsequent sustained drug release might be ascribed to the increase in the diffusion pathlength for drug molecules that are efficiently entrapped within the inner core of SLNs.

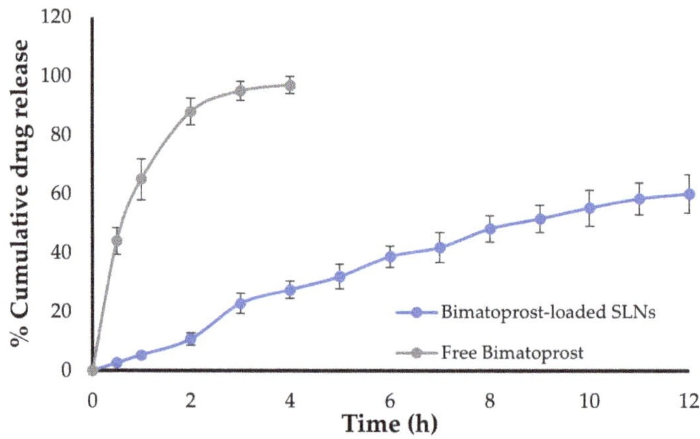

Figure 5. Drug release profile of optimized Bimatoprost SLNs.

The in vitro release profile of the optimized Bimatoprost-loaded SLNs was fitted to various kinetics models, i.e., zero order, first order, Highuchi release and Kores-peppas models. Fitting the release data into these release kinetic models demonstrated that Bimatoprost release from SLNs followed the Higuchi kinetics, indicating a diffusion-controlled mechanism (Table S2).

2.5. Stability Studies

The stability of colloidal dispersions is considered a crucial parameter for ensuring their satisfactory use. The stability data for optimized Bimatoprost-loaded SLNs are summarized in Table S3. The optimized formula was found to be stable upon storage as manifested by slight changes in the particle size, zeta potential and percentage drug entrapment at 8 weeks post storage compared to fresh samples.

2.6. Sterility Test

Generally, all ophthalmic preparations must fulfill a variety of safety and effectiveness standards, including product sterility. Sterility is defined as the lack of live microbial contamination, which if present in such formulations, might result in eye infections with potentially serious consequences. As summarized in Table 2, sterility testing confirmed the absence of any signs of either bacterial or fungal growth with the optimized formulation when compared with positive control. These results that optimized Bimatoprost SLNs formulation meets the criterion of sterility required for ophthalmic preparations.

2.7. Isotonicity Test

Isotonicity is another important feature of ophthalmic products. Isotonicity must be maintained to avoid tissue damage or eye discomfort [33]. Isotonic solutions keep blood cells intact, whereas hypotonic solutions cause cell bulging and hypertonic solutions cause cell shrinkage. As shown in Figure 6, microscopical examination of red blood cells (RBCs) upon treatment with few drops of optimized Bimatoprost-loaded SLNs revealed the absence of any alteration in RBCs shape, and the effect of drug-loaded SLNs on RBCs was comparable to that of marketed eye drops on RBCs. These results confirmed the safety of drug-loaded SLNs for ophthalmic application.

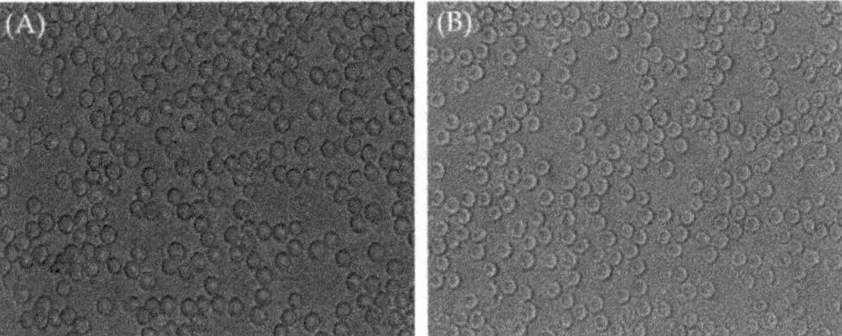

Figure 6. Microscopical images of RBCs treated with (**A**) marketed eye drops and (**B**) optimized Bimatoprost-loaded SLNs. Magnification 400x.

2.8. Ocular Irritation (HET-CAM) Test

In this study, the Hen's Egg Test on the ChorioAllantoic Membrane (HET-CAM) has been adopted as an alternative method to animal (Draize eye test) experimentation to evaluate the possible ocular irritation elicited by Bimatoprost-loaded SLNs [34]. In HET-CAM test, the optimized SLNs formulation was tested on chorioallantonic membrane, which mimics the structure of ocular membrane. The potential ocular irritancy of test formulation was investigated visually via recording the morphological changes in the CAM such as vascular lysis, coagulation and hemorrhage [35]. The mean irritation scores of test formulation, positive and negative controls were represented in Table 3. As illustrated in Table 3, the negative control (0.9% NaCl solution) had mean irritation score of ~ 0 with no signs of any ocular irritation (Figure 7A). On the other hand, the mean irritation score of positive control (1% SDS) was found to be 15.68, reflecting the induction of severe irritation as manifested by blood vessel lysis and severe hemorrhage in the CAM (Figure 7B). Of interest, the optimized formulation showed a mean irritation score of 0.02 with no signs of any ocular irritation in the CAM when compared with positive control (Figure 7C). Therefore, the study claimed that Bimatoprost-loaded SLNs were safe for ocular administration since it induced no signs of ocular irritation.

Table 3. Mean irritation scores of HET-CAM test.

Test Compound	Mean Irritation Score	Inference
Negative control (0.9% NaCl)	0.01 ± 0.01	No irritation
Optimized Bimatoprost SLNs	0.02 ± 0.01	No irritation
Positive control (1% SDS)	15.68 ± 0.78	Severe irritation

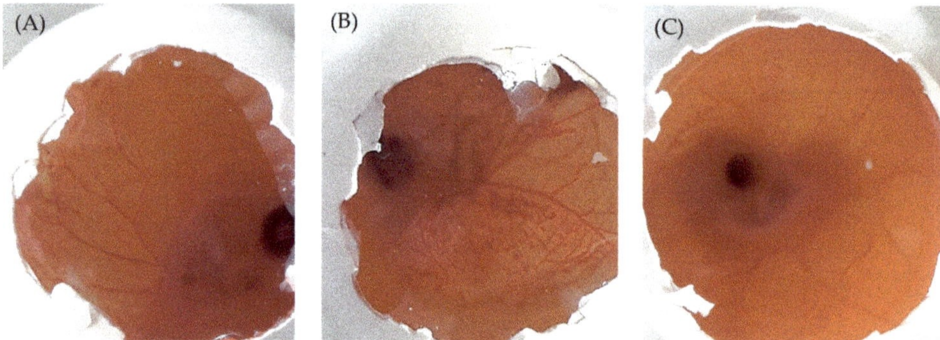

Figure 7. HET-CAM images after application of (**A**) 0.9% saline solution, (**B**) 1% sodium dodecyl sulfate, and (**C**) Optimized formulation. Magnification 10x.

2.9. Ex Vivo Histopathology Study

Histopathology studies were performed to address the occurrence of any changes or damage to corneal tissue upon optimized formula application. The histopathology images were depicted in Figure 8. The cornea treated with 0.9% sodium chloride solution (negative control) exhibited no signs of tissue injury (Figure 8A). Interestingly, cornea treated with optimized Bimatoprost-loaded SLNs showed no detrimental impact on corneal epithelium, endothelium, or stroma, indicating no or mild corneal toxicity. The corneal epithelium was intact and was found to be attached to Bowman's membrane (Figure 8B). These findings confirmed that the optimized formulation was non-toxic to the corneal membrane.

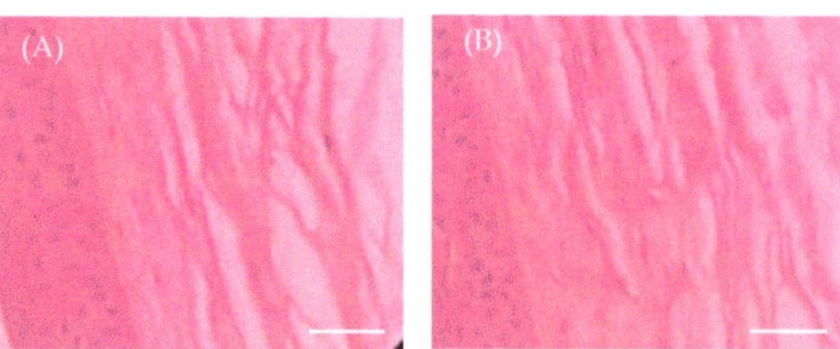

Figure 8. Ex vivo histopathology images of corneal membrane treated with (**A**) 0.9 NaCl solution and (**B**) optimized Bimatoprost-loaded SLNs. Scale bare 25 μm.

3. Materials and Methods

3.1. Materials

Bimatoprost was obtained from Dr. Pradeep Reddy Laboratories (Hyderabad, India). Glyceryl monostearate (GMS), chloroform, dimethyl sulfoxide (DMSO), sodium chloride, dibasic sodium phosphate and benzalkonium chloride were procured from Loba Chemie (Mumbai, India).

3.2. Drug-Lipid Compatibility by FTIR (Fourier Transform Infrared) Spectroscopy

For preparing Bimatoprost-loaded SLNs, glyceryl monostearate (GMS) was selected as lipid carrier and its compatibility with the drug was assessed by FTIR spectroscopy using IR spectrophotometer (Bruker, Billerica, MA, USA) [36]. The study involved getting the IR peaks of drug, lipid and their physical mixture and the obtained peaks were referred with standards and interpretation was done to confirm whether the drug and lipid used in the study are compatible with one another or not.

3.3. Preparation of Bimatoprost-Loaded SLNs

Bimatoprost-loaded SLNs were fabricated by solvent evaporation method and ultra-sonication technique using probe sonicator [37]. Briefly, accurately weighed amount of the drug and GMS were dissolved in chloroform/dimethyl sulfoxide mixture (1:1 v/v). In another beaker, 5% of poloxamer 407 was dissolved in 15 mL of distilled water by magnetic stirring. To this surfactant solution, the organic solvents containing drug and GMS mixture was slowly added drop by drop and the mixture was heated at 60–70 °C to evaporate the organic solvents followed by magnetic stirring. The SLNs dispersion was stirred for time period of 5 h. Finally, SLNs dispersion was subjected to probe sonication for further particle size reduction. The resultant dispersion was sterilized by filtering through a 0.22 μm pore size membrane and kept under refrigeration (2–8 °C) until use.

3.4. Optimization of Bimatoprost-Loaded SLNs

A central composite design (CCD) was used for optimization of Bimatoprost-loaded SLNs by varying drug:lipid ratio and sonication time as independent factors. The dependent factors considered were particle size (R_1) and percentage entrapment efficiency (R_2). The impact of independent formulation variables on dependent responses was investigated from three-dimensional (3D) surface plots constructed from the design study. Optimization study was done with Design Expert® software (Version 12; Stat-Ease, Inc., Minneapolis, MN, USA) which provided 13 experimental runs at different drug:lipid ratios and sonication times (low, medium and high). All the 13 formulations were evaluated for the particle size and entrapment efficiency (%) and these data were analyzed for final optimization. The dependent and independent factors with actual levels of factorial design were represented in Table 4.

Table 4. Central composite design with coded values of factors.

Factors	Levels, Actual (Coded)		
Independent Factors	**−1** **(Low)**	**0** **(Medium)**	**+1** **(High)**
A = Drug:lipid ratio ($w{:}w$)	1:1	1:3	1:5
B = Sonication time (in)	5	10	15
Dependent factors			
Particle size (nm) (R_1) Entrapment efficiency % (R_2)			

3.5. Evaluation of Bimatoprost-Loaded SLNs

3.5.1. Particle Size, Polydispersity Index (PDI) and Zeta-Potential

Particle size and PDI of all the SLNs were measured with zeta sizer (Malvern Instruments Ltd., Worcestershire, UK). Few drops of the formulation were placed in a cuvette cell and exposed to the laser beam. The intensity of scattered light were adopted to estimate the particle sizes of the samples [38].

The zeta potential was measured for the optimized formulation with zeta sizer (Malvern Instruments Ltd., Worcestershire, UK) [39].

3.5.2. Entrapment Efficiency (%)

Entrapment efficiency (%) gives information about the percentage of drug encapsulated within the lipid nanoparticles. The entrapment efficiency (%) of Bimatoprost-loaded SLNs was estimated indirectly by separating Bimatoprost-loaded SLNs from the supernatant containing free Bimatoprost by centrifugation at 15,000 rpm for about 30 min. The concentration of free drug in supernatant was quantified spectrophotometrically at 294 nm. The entrapment efficiency (%) was calculated using the following formula [40]:

$$\%EE = \frac{\text{Total initial amount of drug} - \text{Free drug}}{\text{Total initial amount of drug}}$$

3.5.3. Transmission Electron Microscopy (TEM) Study

The surface morphology, particle size range and the particle size distribution of optimized formulation was determined by TEM study. For this purpose, few drops of formulation were placed on 300 mesh copper grid (copper coated film) and allowed to air dry for 10 min. For staining the sample, 2% *w/v* of phosphotungstic acid was applied for about 2 min, and excess of liquid was dried with filter paper the sample was subsequently placed in transmission electron microscope. Later, TEM photographs were taken and examined for size distribution analysis [41].

3.6. Stability Study

The stability study of optimized formulation was carried out by storing SLNs at $4 \pm 1\ °C$ in glass vials for 2 months. The alteration in particle size, zeta potential and/or entrapment efficiency was assessed at entrapment efficiency at 0, 4, and 8-weeks following storage [42].

3.7. In Vitro Drug Release Study

The in vitro drug release from optimized formulation was conducted using modified Franz diffusion cell at $37 \pm 0.5\ °C$ under stirring at 50 rpm. Briefly, a dialysis membrane, previously soaked in the simulated tear fluid (STF) for overnight, was fitted in-between the receptor and donor compartments of diffusion cell. The receptor compartment was filled with 25 mL of freshly prepared STF (pH 7.4). A definite weight of formulation (containing 2 mg of drug) was placed in the donor compartment. Drug release study was lasted for 12 h during which aliquot samples (1 mL) from receptor compartment were taken at scheduled time points and were replaced with same amounts of STF to maintain sink condition. The samples were diluted with STF and their absorbances were measured at 294 nm using spectrophotometer. The obtained data was further converted to percentage cumulative drug release (% CDR).

Finally, drug release data of optimized formulation was fitted into different drug release kinetic models such as zero order, first order, Highuchi release and Kores-peppas release studies. The best kinetic model was predicted with that highest regression value (R^2) obtained [43].

3.8. Sterility Test

Sterility is one of the vital characteristic features of ophthalmic formulation. Sterility of optimized formulation was evaluated by following the direct inoculation method. The procedure of the method was described in Indian Pharmacopoeia (IP). The formulation was tested against two species of bacteria (*Staphylococcous aureus* and *Bacilus subtilus*) and two fungi species (*Candida albicans* and *Asperges brasiliensis*) inoculated in fluid thioglycolate medium for bacteria and soyabean casein digest medium for fungi in test tubes. The inoculated test tubes were incubated for a period of 7 days. After 7 days of incubation, the samples were tested for sterility by comparing the test sample with positive and negative controls [44].

3.9. Isotonicity Test

Isotonicity is one of the important characteristics of ophthalmic formulation. The formulation should be isotonic with blood for safe administration. Isotonicity of the formulation was checked with human blood. Few drops of optimized formulation were mixed with human blood and microscopically examined for the physical appearance of RBCs. The study was compared with the marketed eye drops of Bimatoprost to check if there is any variation in the RBCs shape and also to visualize any shrinkage and bulginess of RBCs [45].

3.10. Ocular Irritancy by HET-CAM Test

The ocular irritancy of the optimized formulation was examined by Hen's egg test-chorioallantoic membrane (HET-CAM). The chorioallantoic membrane (CAM) was developed in freshly collected fertile eggs. The eggs were kept on a tray and incubated at 37 ± 0.5 °C and at relative humidity of $55 \pm 5\%$ for a period of 5 days. Each day, the eggs were rotated manually 5 times for complete fertilization. After 5 days, the eggs were examined for the growth of embryo by candling them under flashlight. The non-viable eggs were discarded, while the viable eggs were further incubated till day 10. On the 10th day, all the eggs were removed from the incubator, the eggshell was broken with a blade without harming the embryo (CAM) present inside the egg. CAM of eggs was treated with 0.3 mL of optimized formulation, 0.3 mL of Sodium dodecyl sulfate (1%) as positive control and 0.3 mL of 0.9% Sodium chloride (NaCl) as negative control. CAM of eggs was observed visually for a time period of 5 min for the irritation signs like lysis of blood vessels, coagulation and hemorrhage. The mean irritation scores of all respective samples were determined and based on the irritation score value, the irritancy level was determined [46]. The irritation score was estimated using the following formula [9] and the level of irritancy with standard score range is represented in Table 5.

$$\text{Irritation score(IS)} = \frac{301 - \text{Hemorrhage}}{300} \times 5 + \frac{301 - \text{lysis}}{300} \times 7 + \frac{301 - \text{coagulation}}{300} \times 9$$

where, all the values of coagulation, lysis and hemorrhage are recorded in seconds.

Table 5. HET-CAM test irritation score chart.

Irritation Score	Mean Score Value	Level of Irritation
0–0.9	0	No irritation
1–4.9	1	Slight irritation
5–8.9	2	Moderate irritation
9–21	3	Severe irritation

3.11. Ex Vivo Histopathology Study

Histopathology study was carried out to evaluate the effect of formulation on the corneal tissue and its integrity. Goat corneas were isolated from the whole goat eyes that are procured from the slaughterhouse. Corneal layer with sclera tissue was carefully removed by using sterile scissors and preserved in normal saline to retain the tissue consistency. The corneas were treated with optimized formulation (Test). For comparison purpose, untreated cornea was used as negative control. All the corneas were immersed in 8% formalin and left for about 8 h. Later, the corneas were hydrated by washing with ethyl alcohol and distilled water. The corneal tissue was stained with hematoxylin and eosin and the images of all the corneas were taken and the assessment was to check any morphological changes found in corneas treated with test sample [47].

3.12. Statistical Analysis

All values were expressed as mean ± standard deviation. An unpaired Student's *t*-test and one-way ANOVA (GraphPad Software, Version 6, San Diego, CA, USA) were used for statistical analysis. A *p* value less than 0.05 implies a significant difference.

4. Conclusions

In this study, Bimatoprost-loaded SLNs were developed and optimized for ocular administration. The prepared drug loaded SLNs exhibited smooth surfaces with nano-scale size range. In vitro drug release study revealed the sustained release properties of optimized formulation. Sterility test confirmed the sterile nature of formulation with no signs of any microbial growth. Most importantly, HET-CAM test nullified the irritancy potential of optimized formulation against chorioallantonic membrane, claiming the non-irritant nature of the formulation. In addition, histopathology study verified the tolerability of test formulation by corneal tissue as manifested by the absence of any signs of corneal tissue damage. Collectively, it was concluded that Bimatoprost-loaded SLNs might represent a potential and promising ocular drug delivery approach for the effective management of glaucoma.

Supplementary Materials: The following supporting information can be downloaded at: https://www.mdpi.com/article/10.3390/ph16071001/s1, Table S1: Results of statistical analysis of all dependent variables R_1 and R_2; Table S2: In vitro release kinetics data of optimized Bimatoprost-loaded SLNs; Table S3: Stability study for optimized Bimatoprost-loaded SLNs.

Author Contributions: Conceptualization, A.M. and R.N.C.; methodology, S.D.S., A.M. and R.N.C.; software, H.F.A. and A.J.O.; validation, H.F.A. and A.J.O.; formal analysis, E.H.M. and E.-S.K.; investigation, S.D.S. and A.M.; resources, E.-S.K., H.F.A. and A.J.O.; writing—original draft preparation, S.D.S. and A.S.A.L.; writing—review and editing, A.S.A.L., H.F.A. and A.J.O.; supervision, R.N.C.; funding acquisition, E.-S.K., H.F.A. and A.J.O. All authors have read and agreed to the published version of the manuscript.

Funding: This study is supported via funding from Prince Sattam Bin Abdulaziz University project number (PSAU/2023/R/1444). This work was supported by Princess Nourah bint Abdulrahman University researchers supporting project number (PNURSP2023R205), Princess Nourah bint Abdulrahman University, Riyadh, Saudi Arabia. This work was also supported by the Researchers Supporting Project number (RSPD2023R620), King Saud University, Riyadh, Saudi Arabia.

Institutional Review Board Statement: Not applicable.

Informed Consent Statement: Not applicable.

Data Availability Statement: Data is contained within the article and Supplementary Material.

Acknowledgments: This study is supported via funding from Prince Sattam Bin Abdulaziz University project number (PSAU/2023/R/1444). The authors extend their appreciation to the Researchers Supporting Project number (RSPD2023R620), King Saud University, Riyadh, Saudi Arabia. Additionally, the authors extend their appreciation to Princess Nourah bint Abdulrahman University, Riyadh, Saudi Arabia for funding this work under researcher supporting project number (PNURSP2023R205).

Conflicts of Interest: The authors declare no conflict of interest.

References

1. Januleviciene, I.; Siaudvytyte, L.; Barsauskaite, R. Ophthalmic drug delivery in glaucoma—A review. *Pharmaceutics* **2012**, *4*, 243–251. [CrossRef] [PubMed]
2. Weinreb, R.N.; Aung, T.; Medeiros, F.A. The pathophysiology and treatment of glaucoma: A review. *JAMA* **2014**, *311*, 1901–1911. [CrossRef] [PubMed]
3. Plosker, G.L.; Keam, S.J. Bimatoprost: A pharmacoeconomic review of its use in open-angle glaucoma and ocular hypertension. *Pharmacoeconomics* **2006**, *24*, 297–314. [CrossRef] [PubMed]
4. Lee, D.; Mantravadi, A.V.; Myers, J.S. Patient considerations in ocular hypertension: Role of bimatoprost ophthalmic solution. *Clin. Ophthalmol.* **2017**, *11*, 1273–1280. [CrossRef]
5. Cantor, L.B. Bimatoprost: A member of a new class of agents, the prostamides, for glaucoma management. *Expert. Opin. Investig. Drugs* **2001**, *10*, 721–731. [CrossRef]
6. Jha, A.K.; Sarkar, R.; Udayan, U.K.; Roy, P.K.; Chaudhary, R.K.P. Bimatoprost in Dermatology. *Indian Dermatol. Online J.* **2018**, *9*, 224–228. [CrossRef]
7. Brubaker, R.F. Mechanism of Action of Bimatoprost (Lumigan™). *Surv. Ophthalmol.* **2001**, *45*, S347–S351. [CrossRef]
8. Patil, A.J.; Vajaranant, T.S.; Edward, D.P. Bimatoprost—A review. *Expert. Opin. Pharmacother.* **2009**, *10*, 2759–2768. [CrossRef]
9. Wadetwar, R.N.; Agrawal, A.R.; Kanojiya, P.S. In situ gel containing Bimatoprost solid lipid nanoparticles for ocular delivery: In-vitro and ex-vivo evaluation. *J. Drug Deliv. Sci. Technol.* **2020**, *56*, 101575. [CrossRef]
10. Lambert, W.S.; Carlson, B.J.; van der Ende, A.E.; Shih, G.; Dobish, J.N.; Calkins, D.J.; Harth, E.A. Nanosponge-Mediated Drug Delivery Lowers Intraocular Pressure. *Transl. Vis. Sci. Technol.* **2015**, *4*, 1. [CrossRef]
11. Franca, J.R.; Foureaux, G.; Fuscaldi, L.L.; Ribeiro, T.G.; Rodrigues, L.B.; Bravo, R.; Castilho, R.O.; Yoshida, M.I.; Cardoso, V.N.; Fernandes, S.O.; et al. Bimatoprost-loaded ocular inserts as sustained release drug delivery systems for glaucoma treatment: In vitro and in vivo evaluation. *PLoS ONE* **2014**, *9*, e95461. [CrossRef]
12. Seal, J.R.; Robinson, M.R.; Burke, J.; Bejanian, M.; Coote, M.; Attar, M. Intracameral Sustained-Release Bimatoprost Implant Delivers Bimatoprost to Target Tissues with Reduced Drug Exposure to Off-Target Tissues. *J. Ocul. Pharmacol. Ther.* **2019**, *35*, 50–57. [CrossRef]
13. Gaudana, R.; Ananthula, H.K.; Parenky, A.; Mitra, A.K. Ocular drug delivery. *AAPS J.* **2010**, *12*, 348–360. [CrossRef]
14. Agrahari, V.; Mandal, A.; Trinh, H.M.; Joseph, M.; Ray, A.; Hadji, H.; Mitra, R.; Pal, D.; Mitra, A.K. A comprehensive insight on ocular pharmacokinetics. *Drug Deliv. Transl. Res.* **2016**, *6*, 735–754. [CrossRef]
15. Tasharrofi, N.; Nourozi, M.; Marzban, A. How liposomes pave the way for ocular drug delivery after topical administration. *J. Drug Deliv. Sci. Technol.* **2022**, *67*, 103045. [CrossRef]
16. Omerović, N.; Vranić, E. Application of nanoparticles in ocular drug delivery systems. *Health Technol.* **2020**, *10*, 61–78. [CrossRef]
17. Wu, Y.; Liu, Y.; Li, X.; Kebebe, D.; Zhang, B.; Ren, J.; Lu, J.; Li, J.; Du, S.; Liu, Z. Research progress of in-situ gelling ophthalmic drug delivery system. *Asian J. Pharm. Sci.* **2019**, *14*, 1–15. [CrossRef]
18. Seyfoddin, A.; Shaw, J.; Al-Kassas, R. Solid lipid nanoparticles for ocular drug delivery. *Drug Deliv.* **2010**, *17*, 467–489. [CrossRef]
19. Seyfoddin, A.; Al-Kassas, R. Development of solid lipid nanoparticles and nanostructured lipid carriers for improving ocular delivery of acyclovir. *Drug. Dev. Ind. Pharm.* **2013**, *39*, 508–519. [CrossRef]
20. Battaglia, L.; Serpe, L.; Foglietta, F.; Muntoni, E.; Gallarate, M.; Del Pozo Rodriguez, A.; Solinis, M.A. Application of lipid nanoparticles to ocular drug delivery. *Expert Opin. Drug. Deliv.* **2016**, *13*, 1743–1757. [CrossRef]
21. Khames, A.; Khaleel, M.A.; El-Badawy, M.F.; El-Nezhawy, A.O.H. Natamycin solid lipid nanoparticles—Sustained ocular delivery system of higher corneal penetration against deep fungal keratitis: Preparation and optimization. *Int. J. Nanomed.* **2019**, *14*, 2515–2531. [CrossRef] [PubMed]
22. Kaur, I.P.; Kanwar, M. Ocular preparations: The formulation approach. *Drug Dev. Ind. Pharm.* **2002**, *28*, 473–493. [CrossRef] [PubMed]
23. Dong, Y.; Ng, W.K.; Shen, S.; Kim, S.; Tan, R.B.H. Solid lipid nanoparticles: Continuous and potential large-scale nanoprecipitation production in static mixers. *Colloids Surf. B Biointerfaces* **2012**, *94*, 68–72. [CrossRef] [PubMed]
24. Jiang, S.; Franco, Y.L.; Zhou, Y.; Chen, J. Nanotechnology in retinal drug delivery. *Int. J. Ophthalmol.* **2018**, *11*, 1038–1044. [CrossRef] [PubMed]
25. Tiwari, S.; Mistry, P.K.; Patel, V. SLNs Based on Co-Processed Lipids for Topical Delivery of Terbinafine Hydrochloride. *J. Pharm. Drug Dev.* **2014**, *2*, 604.
26. Reddy, L.H.; Vivek, K.; Bakshi, N.; Murthy, R.S. Tamoxifen citrate loaded solid lipid nanoparticles (SLN): Preparation, characterization, in vitro drug release, and pharmacokinetic evaluation. *Pharm. Dev. Technol.* **2006**, *11*, 167–177. [CrossRef]
27. Emami, J.; Mohiti, H.; Hamishehkar, H.; Varshosaz, J. Formulation and optimization of solid lipid nanoparticle formulation for pulmonary delivery of budesonide using Taguchi and Box-Behnken design. *Res. Pharm. Sci.* **2015**, *10*, 17–33.
28. Shah, M.; Pathak, K. Development and statistical optimization of solid lipid nanoparticles of simvastatin by using 2(3) full-factorial design. *AAPS PharmSciTech* **2010**, *11*, 489–496. [CrossRef]
29. Yang, Y.Y.; Chung, T.S.; Bai, X.-L.; Chan, W.K. Effect of preparation conditions on morphology and release profiles of biodegradable polymeric microspheres containing protein fabricated by double-emulsion method. *Chem. Eng. Sci.* **2000**, *55*, 2223–2236. [CrossRef]

30. Nair, A.B.; Shah, J.; Al-Dhubiab, B.E.; Jacob, S.; Patel, S.S.; Venugopala, K.N.; Morsy, M.A.; Gupta, S.; Attimarad, M.; Sreeharsha, N.; et al. Clarithromycin Solid Lipid Nanoparticles for Topical Ocular Therapy: Optimization, Evaluation and In Vivo Studies. *Pharmaceutics* **2021**, *13*, 523. [CrossRef]

31. Araújo, J.; Gonzalez-Mira, E.; Egea, M.A.; Garcia, M.L.; Souto, E.B. Optimization and physicochemical characterization of a triamcinolone acetonide-loaded NLC for ocular antiangiogenic applications. *Int. J. Pharm.* **2010**, *393*, 167–175. [CrossRef]

32. Al Hagbani, T.; Rizvi, S.M.D.; Hussain, T.; Mehmood, K.; Rafi, Z.; Moin, A.; Abu Lila, A.S.; Alshammari, F.; Khafagy, E.S.; Rahamathulla, M.; et al. Cefotaxime Mediated Synthesis of Gold Nanoparticles: Characterization and Antibacterial Activity. *Polymers* **2022**, *14*, 771. [CrossRef]

33. Baranowski, P.; Karolewicz, B.; Gajda, M.; Pluta, J. Ophthalmic drug dosage forms: Characterisation and research methods. *Sci. World J.* **2014**, *2014*, 861904. [CrossRef]

34. Vinardell, M.P.; Macián, M. Comparative study of the HET-CAM test and the Draize eye test for assessment of irritancy potential. *Toxicol. Vitr.* **1994**, *8*, 467–470. [CrossRef]

35. Tavaszi, J.; Budai, P. The use of HET-CAM test in detecting the ocular irritation. *Commun. Agric. Appl. Biol. Sci.* **2007**, *72*, 137–141.

36. Moin, A.; Wani, S.U.D.; Osmani, R.A.; Abu Lila, A.S.; Khafagy, E.S.; Arab, H.H.; Gangadharappa, H.V.; Allam, A.N. Formulation, characterization, and cellular toxicity assessment of tamoxifen-loaded silk fibroin nanoparticles in breast cancer. *Drug Deliv.* **2021**, *28*, 1626–1636. [CrossRef]

37. Duong, V.A.; Nguyen, T.T.; Maeng, H.J. Preparation of Solid Lipid Nanoparticles and Nanostructured Lipid Carriers for Drug Delivery and the Effects of Preparation Parameters of Solvent Injection Method. *Molecules* **2020**, *25*, 4781. [CrossRef]

38. Küçüktürkmen, B.; Öz, U.C.; Bozkir, A. In Situ Hydrogel Formulation for Intra-Articular Application of Diclofenac Sodium-Loaded Polymeric Nanoparticles. *Turk. J. Pharm. Sci.* **2017**, *14*, 56–64. [CrossRef]

39. Dorraj, G.; Moghimi, H.R. Preparation of SLN-containing Thermoresponsive In-Situ Forming Gel as a Controlled Nanoparticle Delivery System and Investigating its Rheological, Thermal and Erosion Behavior. *Iran. J. Pharm. Res.* **2015**, *14*, 347–358.

40. Abu Lila, A.S.; Amran, M.; Tantawy, M.A.; Moglad, E.H.; Gad, S.; Alotaibi, H.F.; Obaidullah, A.J.; Khafagy, E.-S. In Vitro Cytotoxicity and In Vivo Antitumor Activity of Lipid Nanocapsules Loaded with Novel Pyridine Derivatives. *Pharmaceutics* **2023**, *15*, 1755. [CrossRef]

41. Khafagy, E.S.; Abu Lila, A.S.; Sallam, N.M.; Sanad, R.A.; Ahmed, M.M.; Ghorab, M.M.; Alotaibi, H.F.; Alalaiwe, A.; Aldawsari, M.F.; Alshahrani, S.M.; et al. Preparation and Characterization of a Novel Mucoadhesive Carvedilol Nanosponge: A Promising Platform for Buccal Anti-Hypertensive Delivery. *Gels* **2022**, *8*, 235. [CrossRef] [PubMed]

42. Aldawsari, M.F.; Khafagy, E.S.; Alotaibi, H.F.; Abu Lila, A.S. Vardenafil-Loaded Bilosomal Mucoadhesive Sponge for Buccal Delivery: Optimization, Characterization, and In Vivo Evaluation. *Polymers* **2022**, *14*, 4184. [CrossRef] [PubMed]

43. Khalil, R.M.; Abd-Elbary, A.; Kassem, M.A.; Ghorab, M.M.; Basha, M. Nanostructured lipid carriers (NLCs) versus solid lipid nanoparticles (SLNs) for topical delivery of meloxicam. *Pharm. Dev. Technol.* **2014**, *19*, 304–314. [CrossRef] [PubMed]

44. Shanmugam, S.; Valarmathi, S.; Kumars, S. Sterility Testing Procedure of Ophthalmic Ocusert Aciclovir Used for Treating Herpes Simplex Virus. *Asian J. Pharm. Clin. Res.* **2017**, *10*, 344–346.

45. Kurniawansyah, I.S.; Rusdiana, T.; Abnaz, Z.D.; Sopyan, I.; Subarnas, A. Study of Isotonicity and Ocular Irritation of Chloramphenicol in situ Gel. *Int. J. Appl. Pharm.* **2021**, *13*, 103–107. [CrossRef]

46. Wilson, S.L.; Ahearne, M.; Hopkinson, A. An overview of current techniques for ocular toxicity testing. *Toxicology* **2015**, *327*, 32–46. [CrossRef]

47. Zubairu, Y.; Negi, L.M.; Iqbal, Z.; Talegaonkar, S. Design and development of novel bioadhesive niosomal formulation for the transcorneal delivery of anti-infective agent: In-vitro and ex-vivo investigations. *Asian J. Pharm. Sci.* **2015**, *10*, 322–330. [CrossRef]

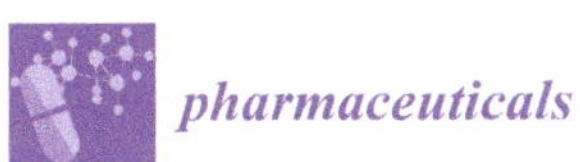
pharmaceuticals

Article

Baricitinib Lipid-Based Nanosystems as a Topical Alternative for Atopic Dermatitis Treatment

Núria Garrós [1,2], Paola Bustos-Salgados [1], Òscar Domènech [1,2], María José Rodríguez-Lagunas [3], Negar Beirampour [1], Roya Mohammadi-Meyabadi [1,2], Mireia Mallandrich [1,2,*], Ana C. Calpena [1,2] and Helena Colom [1]

[1] Departament de Farmàcia i Tecnologia Farmacèutica, i Fisicoquímica, Facultat de Farmàcia i Ciències de l'Alimentació, Universitat de Barcelona (UB), 08028 Barcelona, Spain; ngarroar50@alumnes.ub.edu (N.G.)

[2] Institut de Nanociència i Nanotecnologia, Universitat de Barcelona (UB), 645 Diagonal Avenue, 08028 Barcelona, Spain

[3] Departament de Bioquímica i Fisiologia, Facultat de Farmàcia i Ciències de l'Alimentació, Universitat de Barcelona (UB), Av. Joan XXIII, 08028 Barcelona, Spain

* Correspondence: mireia.mallandrich@ub.edu

Abstract: Atopic dermatitis (AD) is a chronic autoimmune inflammatory skin disorder which causes a significant clinical problem due to its prevalence. The ongoing treatment for AD is aimed at improving the patient's quality of life. Additionally, glucocorticoids or immunosuppressants are being used in systemic therapy. Baricitinib (BNB) is a reversible Janus-associated kinase (JAK)-inhibitor; JAK is an important kinase involved in different immune responses. We aimed at developing and evaluating new topical liposomal formulations loaded with BNB for the treatment of flare ups. Three liposomal formulations were elaborated using POPC (1-palmitoyl-2-oleoyl-glycero-3-phosphocholine), CHOL (Cholesterol) and CER (Ceramide) in different proportions: (i) POPC, (ii) POPC:CHOL (8:2, mol/mol) and (iii) POPC:CHOL:CER (3.6:2.4:4.0 mol/mol/mol). They were physiochemically characterized over time. In addition, an in vitro release study, ex vivo permeation and retention studies in altered human skin (AHS) were also performed. Histological analysis was used to study the tolerance of the formulations on the skin. Lastly, the HET-CAM test was also performed to evaluate the irritancy capacity of the formulations, and the modified Draize test was performed to evaluate the erythema and edema capacity of the formulations on the altered skin. All liposomes showed good physicochemical properties and were stable for at least one month. POPC:CHOL:CER had the highest flux and permeation, and the retention in the skin was equal to that of POPC:CHOL. The formulations exhibited no harmful or irritating effects, and the histological examination revealed no changes in structure. The three liposomes have shown promising results for the aim of the study.

Keywords: liposomes; baricitinib; JAK-inhibitor; transepidermal delivery; skin permeation

Citation: Garrós, N.; Bustos-Salgados, P.; Domènech, Ò.; Rodríguez-Lagunas, M.J.; Beirampour, N.; Mohammadi-Meyabadi, R.; Mallandrich, M.; Calpena, A.C.; Colom, H. Baricitinib Lipid-Based Nanosystems as a Topical Alternative for Atopic Dermatitis Treatment. *Pharmaceuticals* **2023**, *16*, 894. https://doi.org/10.3390/ph16060894

Academic Editors: Ana Catarina Silva, João Nuno Moreira and José Manuel Sousa Lobo

Received: 3 April 2023
Revised: 15 June 2023
Accepted: 15 June 2023
Published: 18 June 2023

1. Introduction

Lipid-based nanosystems (LBN) are formed through a lipid phase and surfactants [1]. They have demonstrated that they improve the delivery of various active principles to specific skin layers, with stated localization in the upper layers of the skin [2]. There are different kinds of LBN: liposomes, ethosomes, transferosomes, solid lipid nanoparticles, nanostructured lipid carriers, cubosomes, and monoolein aqueous dispersions [3].

The study of liposomes for drug delivery or targeting on specific sites of the body has been going on since 1970. Liposomes possess structural flexibility in terms of their size, composition, surface charge, bilayer fluidity, and their capacity to incorporate virtually any drug irrespective of its solubility, or to display cell-specific ligands on their surface. Consequently, liposomes can be customized in numerous ways so as to create formulations that are ideal for clinical use [4].

The structural similarity between the lipids composing the nano systems and those composing the skin represents one of the main advantages of LBN, allowing the interaction between the nanosystem matrix and the *stratum corneum* [3]. CHOL, CER and free fatty acids are present in the stratum corneum, the superficial layer of the skin. All of them are involved in different cellular processes at some level, such as transport functions and immune activity [5,6]. Different subclasses of CER exist in the skin, all interacting with the lipids [6]. Patients with AD have a different composition of lipids in their skin, and, in particular, this arises from them having a lower proportion of CER and increased proportions of unsaturated free fatty acids. These differences with normal skin lead to a different organization of the lipids in the skin and thus a different skin structure [7–9]. AD affects populations of all ages, particularly children. It is a worldwide chronic autoimmune inflammatory skin disorder highly prevalent in developed countries and it has been increasing over the most recent decades. This disease implies a deterioration of quality of life, worn down by the symptoms and secondary infections [10]. The treatment of the disease will depend on the degree to which these manifestations are present in the patients. It is also very important to be aware of the individual trigger factors so as to avoid them and reduce flare-ups (Figure 1) [11]. The European Academy of Dermatology and Venereology classifies the different treatments, grading them into six signs: erythema, exudation, excoriation, dryness, cracking and lichenification [12]. Additional therapeutic options should be considered in every treatment phase if established therapy is insufficient or in cases of major infections.

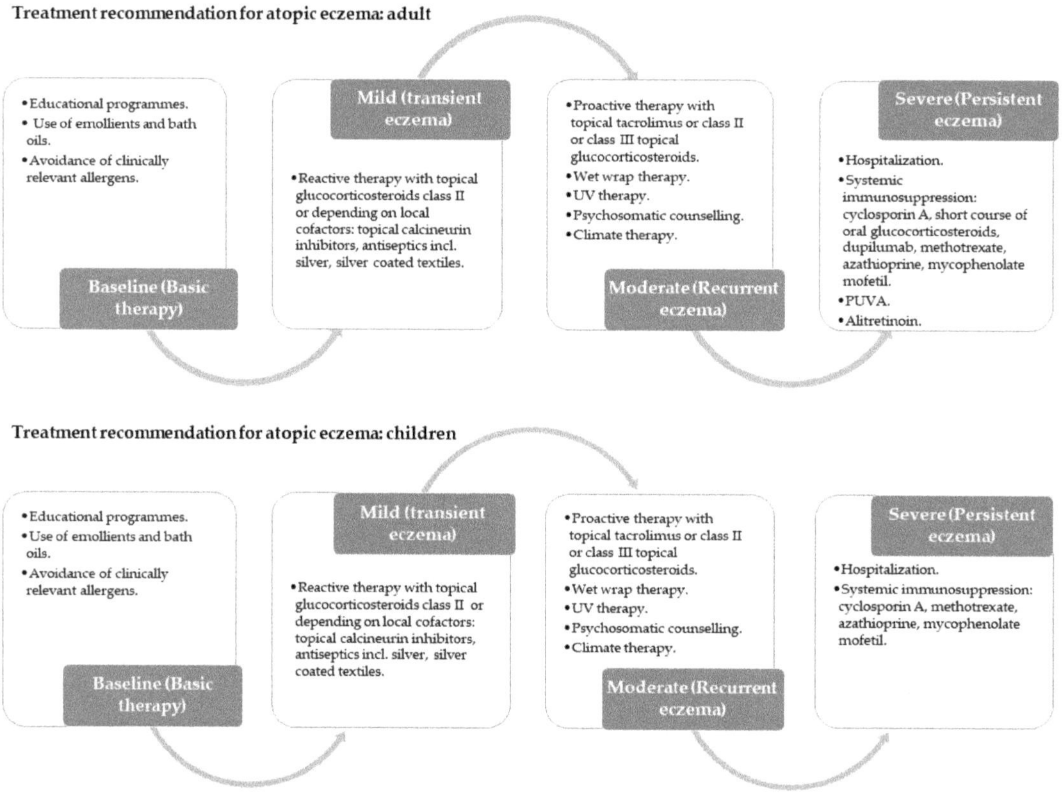

Treatment recommendation for atopic eczema: adult

Treatment recommendation for atopic eczema: children

Figure 1. Treatment recommendations for adults and children with atopic eczema according to European guidelines. PUVA = Psoralen and ultraviolet light therapy.

Baricitinib (BNB) is a reversible Janus-associated kinase (JAK)-inhibitor. JAK is important because it stimulates the signal transducers and activators of transcription (STAT) that cause different immune responses. These include monocyte activation, antibody secretion, erythropoiesis and acute phase reactant production [13]. Furthermore, BNB has recently been introduced orally in cases of moderate-to-severe AD, showing good results in reducing clinical symptoms and improving the quality of life. The most frequent oral doses used are 2 and 4 mg, resulting in a therapeutic plasma concentration of 0.055 μg/mL [14]. However, it has some side effects such as infectious diseases, cardiovascular events and deep venous thrombosis [15]. Topical drug administration is an alternative to avoid systemic effects. To our knowledge, there are no published studies of BNB for the topical route of administration. The main aim of this work was to develop liposomes loaded with BNB for topical administration using natural lipids as a possible topical alternative to the oral route currently available for patients with AD. To achieve this, the following specific objectives were set: (i) to study the physicochemical characteristics of each liposome differentiated by the formulations of three natural lipids: POPC (1-palmitoyl-2-oleoyl-glycero-3-phosphocholine), CHOL (Cholesterol) and CER (Ceramide) in different proportions; (ii) to investigate their drug release profile, as well as the permeation of BNB through physically altered human skin (AHS), the skin being a model of a compromised permeability barrier, which is a particular feature in AD; and (iii) to study the drug retention capacity on AHS, and the tolerability of the formulations by a modified Draize rabbit test and hen's egg chorioallantoic membrane test (HET-CAM test). It is worth mentioning that POPC is a natural lipid found in different microorganisms but not in human skin [16], while CHOL and CER are found in the stratum corneum, as previously mentioned.

2. Results

2.1. Liposomes Physicochemical Characterization

Three liposome formulations were prepared: POPC liposomes, POPC:CHOL liposomes and POPC:CHOL:CER liposomes. The formulations were characterized for pH, particle size and size distribution, encapsulation efficiency and surface charge. This was carried out when the formulations were freshly prepared and when they had been stored at 4 °C.

The pH value for all the liposomes prepared was the same (7.4 ± 0.1), which is adequate for atopic skin treatments [17]. Likewise, the liposomal formulations exhibited comparable efficiency of encapsulation (EE): EE (%) of $6.21 \pm 0.55\%$ for POPC; $5.57 \pm 0.50\%$ for POPC:CHOL; and $6.21 \pm 0.63\%$ for POPC:CHOL:CER.

The results of vesicle size, polydispersity index (PDI) and Zeta potential (ZP) for each liposome are presented in Table 1. All liposomes share similar characteristics, except for liposome POPC:CHOL:CER, which has a higher ZP.

Table 1. Liposomes composition: hydrodynamic diameter, PDI and ZP; and physical stability for 1 month. The results are presented as mean $\pm$ SD ($n = 3$).

Composition	Hydrodynamic Diameter (nm)		PDI		Zeta Potential (mV)	
	1 Day	1 Month	1 Day	1 Month	1 Day	1 Month
POPC	86.0 ± 1.4	86.9 ± 1.1	0.120	0.119	-14.2 ± 0.3	-13.9 ± 0.8
POPC:CHOL (8:2, mol/mol)	53.5 ± 0.9	55.4 ± 1.3	0.174	0.172	-13.2 ± 1.3	-13.5 ± 0.9
POPC:CHOL:CER (3.6:2.4:4.0 mol/mol/mol)	64.1 ± 0.3	65.0 ± 0.7	0.120	0.117	-18.3 ± 1.9	-18.1 ± 1.3

A one-way ANOVA test was carried out and then followed by Tukey's multiple comparison test. All three liposome sizes are statistically different from each other ($p < 0.0001$). Similarly, the ZP of POPC:CHOL:CER is different from the other two liposomes ($p < 0.05$). Liposome POPC and POPC:CHOL do not have a significantly different ZP compared to each other.

These values were also calculated one month after their elaboration and no-significant change was observed, the maximum being 4%.

2.2. In Vitro Drug Release Study

The drug release from the liposomes was evaluated by Franz diffusion cells using a dialysis membrane at the cutaneous temperature, 32 °C, yielding the cumulative amount of BNB released as a function of time. The data were then fitted to different kinetic models. The BNB release profiles from the three liposomes varied; Table 2 indicates the corresponding equations. The liposomes POPC:CHOL:CER and POPC:CHOL fitted a hyperbola model, while liposome POPC was in accordance with a polynomial (second order) model. The modeling of the release profile is shown in Figure 2.

Table 2. Liposome formulations' best-fit values in the kinetic release modeling.

Liposome	Equation	Best-Fit Values According to the Equation				
		A	B	C	B_{max} (µg)	K_d (h)
POPC	Polynominal: Second Order $y = A + Bx + Cx^2$	0.21	0.08	0.002	-	-
POPC:CHOL	One site binding (hyperbola) $y = B_{max}x/(K_d + x)$	-	-	-	18.37	38.34
POPC:CHOL:CER	One site binding (hyperbola) $y = B_{max}x/(K_d + x)$	-	-	-	5.55	1.45

A, B and C = parabola coefficients. Hyperbola parameters B_{max} = maximum amount of BNB that can be released; and Kd = drug release constant.

The liposome POPC:CHOL:CER releases the drug faster than the other two liposomes; after 8 h, the release of BNB had already reached a plateau, indicating that the maximum amount of the drug that could be released had been reached. Nevertheless, the total amount of drug released is lower than with the other liposomes. In contrast, the liposomes, POPC and POPC:CHOL, have a sustained release of up to 53 h. At this time, those liposomes exhibited a 2-fold drug release compared to liposome POPC:CHOL:CER, as demonstrated in Figure 2.

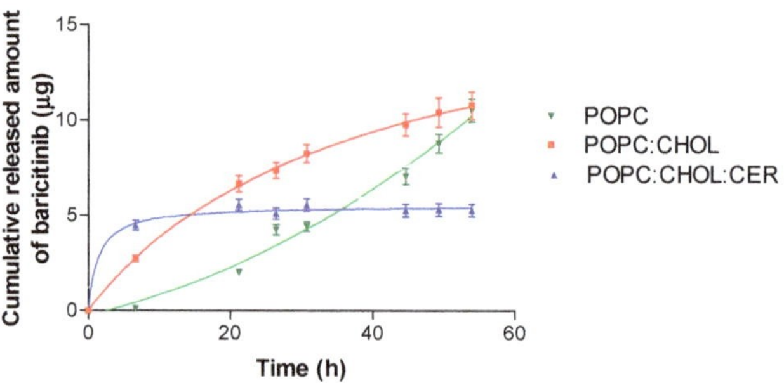

Figure 2. The BNB release profiles from liposomes POPC, POPC:CHOL and POPC:CHOL:CER. BNB cumulative released amount (µg) vs. time (h). The results are presented as mean ± SD ($n = 5$).

To compare different drug release profiles, non-modelistic parameters such as area under the curve (AUC), release efficiency and mean release time (MRT) were calculated. Figure 3 shows the non-modelistic parameters as well as the statistical parameters test, which confirmed there were differences between the three liposomes. Liposome POPC:CHOL displayed the highest values of AUC and the greatest efficiency percentage, but, in contrast, it has the lowest MRT value.

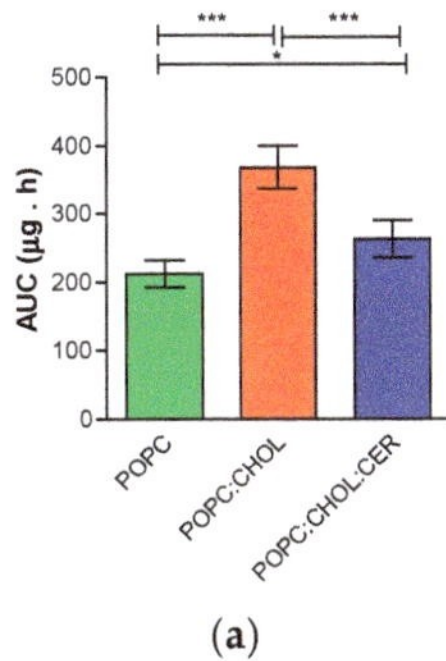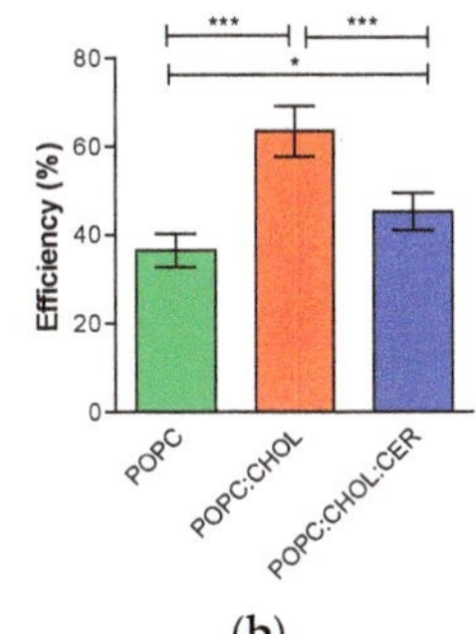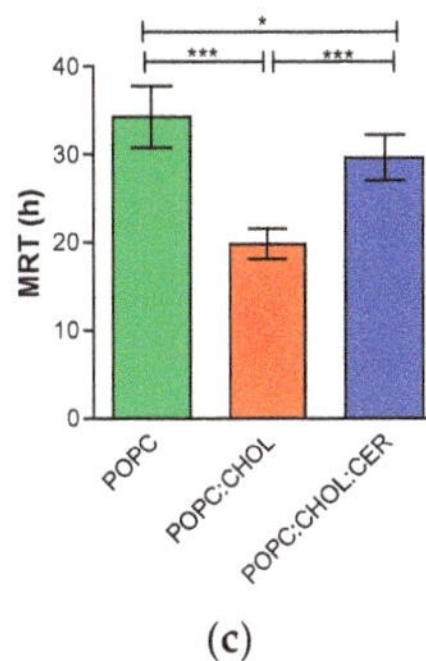

(a)   (b)   (c)

Figure 3. Non-modelistic parameters of: (**a**) area under the curve (AUC: μg/h); (**b**) efficiency (E:%); (**c**) mean release time (MRT: h). A one-way ANOVA test was carried out, followed by Tukey's multiple comparison test (* $p < 0.05$, *** $p < 0.0001$). The results are presented as the mean $\pm$ SD ($n = 5$).

2.3. Ex Vivo Permeation Study

As with the in vitro drug release study, the amount of BNB that was capable of permeating through the human skin was evaluated by Franz cells. Since dermatitis atopic skins present increased permeability relative to healthy skin, the skin was subjected to microneedles to obtain a more permeable skin (hereinafter AHS) and was then mounted on the Franz cells.

The permeation profile, as the cumulative amount permeated through AHS over 25 h, is outlined in Figure 4. It shows that the liposome POPC:CHOL exhibited the highest permeation, with liposome POPC:CHOL:CER following behind, and liposome POPC showing the lowest permeation of the three liposomes tested. The permeation parameters calculated are presented in Table 3.

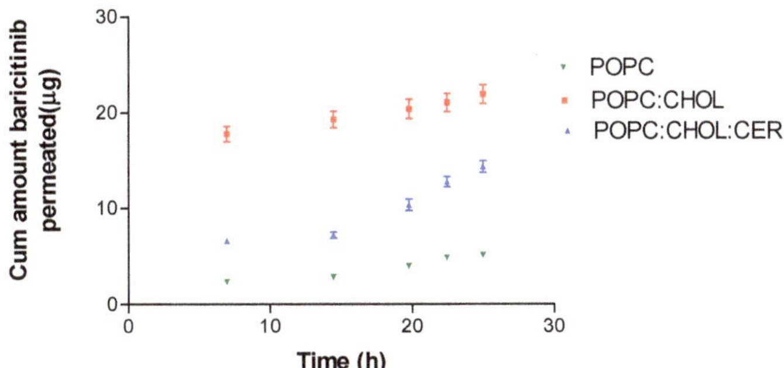

Figure 4. BNB permeation profile: cumulative amount of BNB permeated (μg) vs. time (h). The results are presented as mean $\pm$ SD ($n = 5$).

Table 3. Permeation parameters of three liposomes: cumulative amount of BNB permeated at 25 h (AP_{25h}, μg), flux (Jss, μg/h), permeability coefficient (Kp, cm/h) and predicted steady-state plasma concentration in human steady state on a 10 cm² surface application (Css, ng/mL).

	AP_{25h} (μg)	Jss (μg/h)	Kp (10^{-4} cm/h)	Css (ng/mL)
POPC	5.13 $\pm$ 0.52	0.22 $\pm$ 0.03	1.14 $\pm$ 0.16	0.36 $\pm$ 0.05
POPC:CHOL	21.93 $\pm$ 2.20	0.29 $\pm$ 0.03	1.52 $\pm$ 0.16	0.48 $\pm$ 0.05
POPC:CHOL:CER	14.36 $\pm$ 1.40	0.77 $\pm$ 0.07	4.01 $\pm$ 0.37	1.28 $\pm$ 0.12

ANOVA test analysis of variance, followed by Tukey's multiple comparison test, were performed, and all were statistically different from each other ($p < 0.001$). Results are expressed by mean $\pm$ SD ($n = 5$).

Figure 5 illustrates the quantity of BNB retained in the tissues and the corresponding statistical outcomes. Liposome POPC demonstrated significant statistical differences when compared to liposome POPC:CHOL and liposome POPC:CHOL:CER. However, no significant differences were observed between liposome POPC:CHOL and liposome POPC:CHOL:CER.

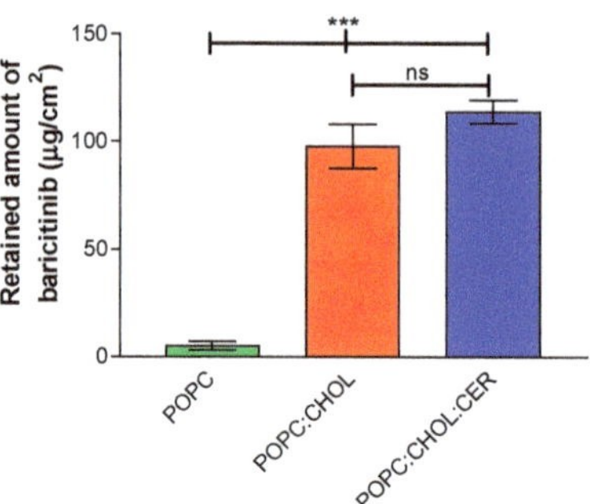

Figure 5. Retained amount (μg/cm^2) of BNB at 25 h in the AHS. Results are expressed as mean $\pm$ SD (n = 5). *ANOVA* test analysis of variance, followed by Tukey's multiple comparison test, were performed. Statistically significant difference: *** = $p < 0.0001$; ns = no statistically significant difference.

2.4. Tolerance Study and Histological Analysis

2.4.1. In Vivo Tolerance Study

The tolerability of the liposomal formulations on altered skin (previously subjected to microneedle punches) was evaluated on New Zealand rabbits. Figure 6 shows the progression of altered rabbit's skin (ARS) monitored for 3 h 30 min after applying xylol so as to induce erythema and edema. This was intended to stimulate AD flare-ups. All three liposomes appear to delay the onset of edema and erythema caused by xylol. The use of POPC liposomes was found to reduce the damage caused by xylol. The negative control of ARS was not treated with any substance or formulation.

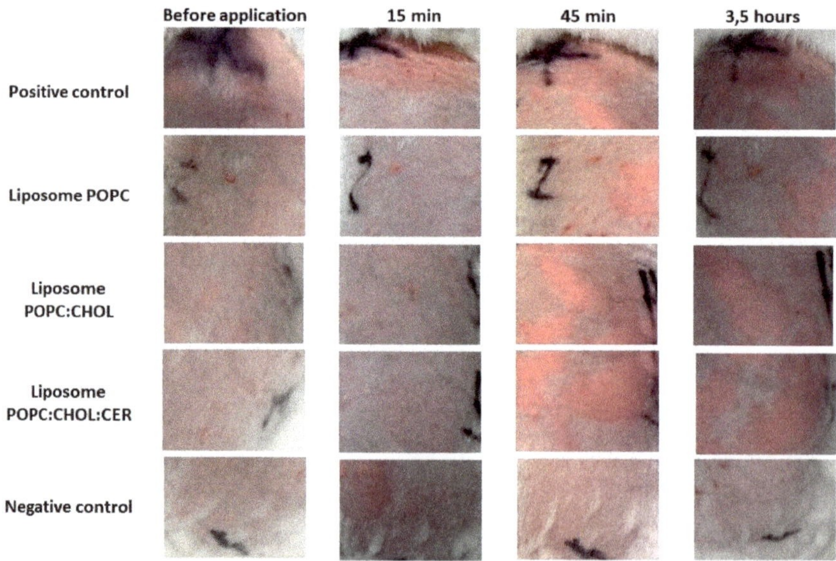

Figure 6. Pictures of 5 groups of rabbits used for the modified Draize test: before the application of xylol and liposomes, at 15 min, 45 min and 3 and a half hours after the respective applications.

The erythema and edema presented on the rabbits' backs are classified by the view scoring system (see Table 4).

Table 4. A modified Draize score was employed to evaluate erythema and edema resulting from xylol exposure, both with and without subsequent application of the liposomes (mean $\pm$ SD, $n = 5$).

Chemicals	Before Induced Er and Ed		15 min		45 min		3 h	
	Erythema	Edema	Erythema	Edema	Erythema	Edema	Erythema	Edema
Negative control	0.00 ± 0.00	0.00 ± 0.00	0.00 ± 0.00	0.00 ± 0.00	0.00 ± 0.00	0.00 ± 0.00	0.00 ± 0.00	0.00 ± 0.00
Liposome POPC	0.00 ± 0.00	0.00 ± 0.00	0.00 ± 0.00	0.00 ± 0.00	0.00 ± 0.00	0.00 ± 0.00	0.00 ± 0.00	0.00 ± 0.00
Liposome POPC:CHOL	0.00 ± 0.00	0.00 ± 0.00	0.00 ± 0.00	0.00 ± 0.00	1.00 ± 0.53	0.00 ± 0.00	0.65 ± 0.40	0.00 ± 0.00
Liposome POPC:CHOL:CER	0.00 ± 0.00	0.00 ± 0.00	0.00 ± 0.00	0.00 ± 0.00	1.45 ± 0.42	0.00 ± 0.00	0.37 ± 0.03	0.00 ± 0.00
Positive control (xylol)	0.00 ± 0.00	0.00 ± 0.00	3.54 ± 0.20	1.62 ± 0.41	3.50 ± 0.40	1.84 ± 0.13	2.40 ± 0.30	0.50 ± 0.02

Er = erythema; Ed = Edema.

The pictures of Figure 6 are supported by the graphs shown in Figure 7, which show the evolution of the transepidermal water loss (TEWL), and the evolution of the skin hydration, of rabbits with altered skin.

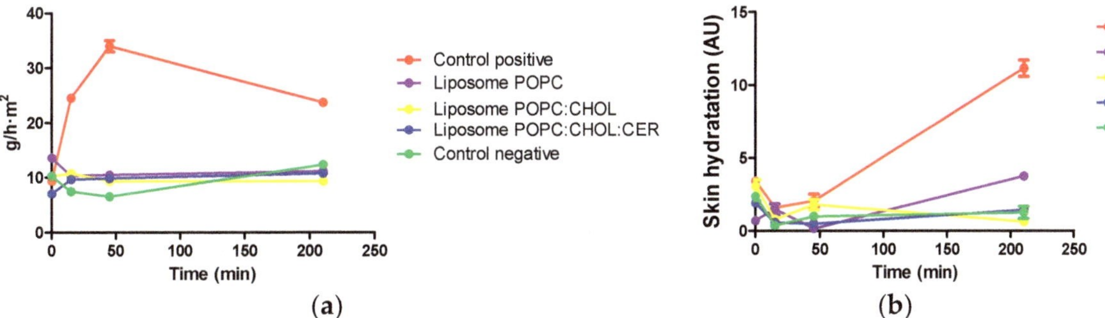

Figure 7. Results of TEWL and skin hydration during 210 min before and after formulations application on rabbits with induced dermatitis by xylol, except for the negative control. (**a**) TEWL; (**b**) Skin hydronation (AU). Results are expressed as mean $\pm$ SD ($n = 5$).

2.4.2. Histological Analysis

Once the modified Draize test had been finished, a histological study was conducted to evaluate whether any structural change had occurred to the altered skin due to the application of the formulations. The histology results of the different liposomes, as well as the positive and negative controls, are set out in Figure 8. The skin treated with liposome POPC:CHOL:CER presented stratum corneum loss (Figure 8e) indicating some disruptive effect. This is in contrast to the skins treated with either liposomes POPC or POPC:CHOL, which do not demonstrate any alteration to the skin.

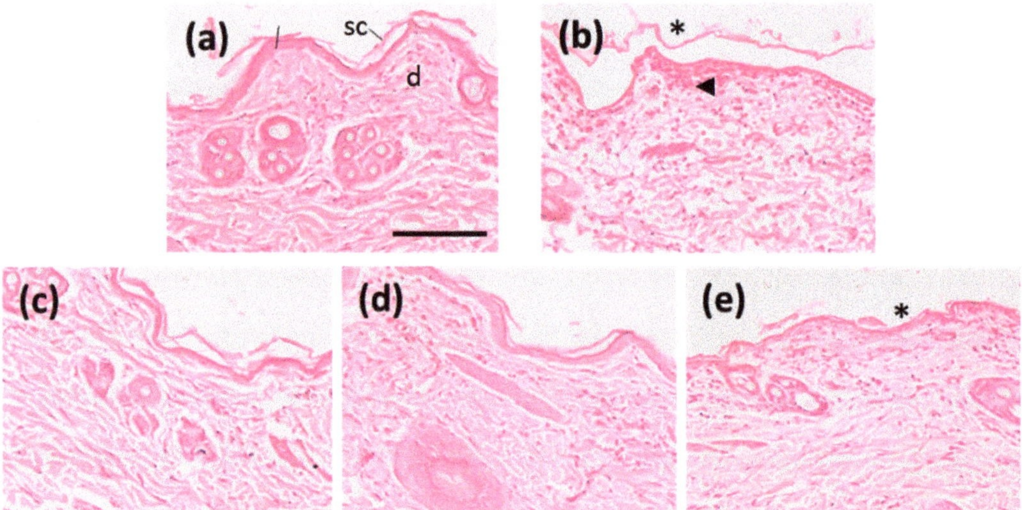

Figure 8. Skin sections colored with eosin and hematoxylin. (**a**) Control negative skin; (**b**) positive control; (**c**) treated with POPC; (**d**) treated with POPC:CHOL; and (**e**) treated with POPC:CHOL:CER. sc = stratum corneum, d = dermis, * shows loss of stratum corneum, Δ arrowhead indicates leukocyte infiltrate. Magnification = 200×, scale bar = 100 μm.

2.4.3. In Vitro Tolerance of the Liposomal Formulations for Periocular Application

AD can also be present on facial skin, with symptoms such as dryness, redness, sensitivity and itching, and facial skin might need the application of soothing formulations. This is why the potential tolerance of the liposomal formulations on the eye, after a periocular application on the eye, was assessed by the in vitro technique HET-CAM of fertilized chicken eggs. Table 5 shows the irritation score (IS) estimated for the liposomal formulations. The three liposomes resulted in non-irritant formulations exhibiting IS values similar to the negative control, whereas the positive control resulted in higher IS values corresponding to a severely irritant substance.

Table 5. Irritation score calculated for the liposomal formulations (mean $\pm$ SD of $n = 3$). The scores obtained for the positive and negative controls are also reported.

	Formulation				
	Negative control	Positive control (0.1 N NaOH)	POPC	POPC:CHOL	POPC:CHOL:CER
Irritation score (IS)	0.07 ± 0.00	16.10 ± 0.08	0.07 ± 0.00	0.07 ± 0.00	0.07 ± 0.00

IS $\leq$ 0.9, non-irritating/slightly irritating; 0.9 < IS $\leq$ 4.9, moderately irritating; 4.9 < IS $\leq$ 8.9, irritating; and 8.9 < IS $\leq$ 21, severely irritating [18].

Figure 9 shows the results from the HET-CAM test. They revealed no irritant effect of any kind; no hemorrhage, coagulation or lysis vessel were observed 5 min after 300 μL of the respective formulations had been applied. This is opposite to the positive control, in which lysis vessel and coagulation appeared (Figure 9b).

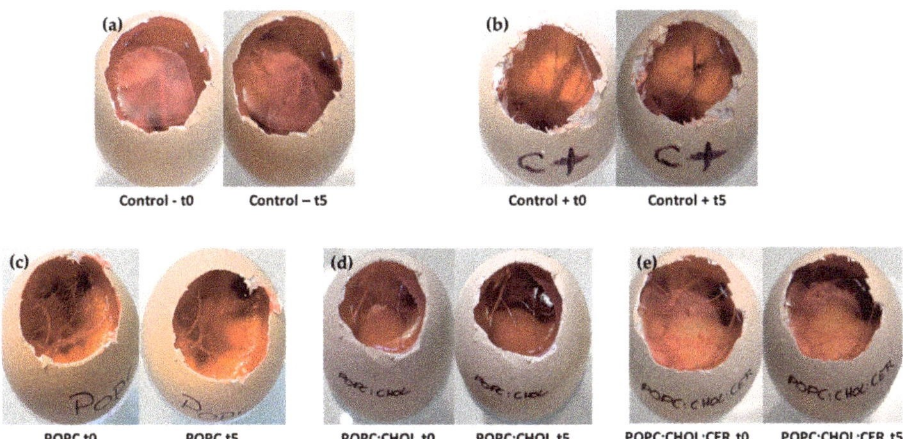

Figure 9. The irritant effect of the formulations was evaluated using the HET-CAM method, with (**a**) a negative control using saline solution, and (**b**) a positive control using 0.1 N sodium hydroxide solution. The other three images show the evolution of the liposomal formulations: (**c**) POPC liposome, (**d**) POPC:CHOL liposome and (**e**) POPC:CHOL:CER liposome.

3. Discussion

All physicochemical characteristics, such as pH, vesicle size and ZP, influence the liposome interaction with the skin [19]. Liposome POPC was the largest vesicle, followed by POPC:CHOL, and the smallest was POPC:CHOL:CER. All of them had a PDI below 0.2, which is indicative of the uniformity of the particle size, and their small size and the low PDI mean the formulations tend to pass more easily through the sterilizing filters, which, in turn, renders them suitable for skins that are grazed or scratched and could become infected. Instead, the ZP helps to predict the stability of particles. A high ZP indicates a stable formulation, so the liposome POPC:CHOL:CER is the most stable of the tested liposomes [20]. Differences in the lipid used for each liposome elaboration may lead to different release profiles described by different kinetic models [21]. In our work, the two liposomes containing CHOL displayed the same kinetic model suggesting that the presence of CHOL in the liposome strongly impacts on their drug release characteristics. The fastest BNB release over a short period of time was presented only by liposome POPC:CHOL:CER but not by liposome POPC:CHOL (Figure 2). Although liposomes POPC and POPC:CHOL exhibited similar BNB released at 54 h, POPC:CHOL showed a higher AUC than POPC:CHOL:CER, indicating a superior performance by POPC:CHOL. The mathematical modelling in the release studies is an excellent tool to evaluate differences between formulations [22–24]. Furthermore, the non-modelistic parameters are useful to compare formulations which exhibit different kinetic models. In this work, the non-modelistic parameters showed a relation between the amount of BNB that is released from the formulation and the release efficiency, with the cumulative permeated amount throughout the 25 h period being the liposome POPC:CHOL, the formulation with the highest values. Baricitnib is a molecule with poor water solubility under physiological conditions, as observed from its structure. It does not present charged structures at pH 7.40, suggesting that it could be found deep within the lipid bilayer. Moreover, it presents several groups capable of stabilizing the molecule in hydrophobic regions through hydrogen bonds. These facts point to baricitinib incorporating into the liposome lipid membrane, remaining there and not being released to permeate through the skin. To overcome this problem, liposomes containing baricitinib were supplemented with 5% Transcutol. The structure of Transcutol allows it to be incorporated in parallel to hydrocarbon chains with its OH group near the headgroup of the phospholipids, distorting the phospholipid bilayer. Then, when liposomes containing baricitinib interact with the skin surface, baricitinib can easily be released from the liposome, and Transcutol molecules can increase the water solubility of baricitinib and facilitate its distribution towards the surface of the skin.

Different authors have demonstrated that, if the lipids are like those in the stratum corneum, more drugs will penetrate the skin [19]. It is worth mentioning that human skin contains CHOL and CER and disturbances in their levels cause disruption of the skin barrier function. Yet, harmonizing the CHOL and CER levels in the skin restores its barrier function [25]. Sinico and Fadda explained that a greater permeation and release could be produced when the liposomes are composed of lipids that are more similar to those of the skin [26]. This would explain the higher permeation of POPC:CHOL and POPC:CHOL:CER compared with liposome POPC without CHOL. The liposome POPC:CHOL:CER triplicated the results values of flux, permeability coefficient and theoretical plasma concentration in human steady state compared with the other studied liposomes (POPC and POPC:CHOL, see Table 3). Therefore, CER could be acting like a permeation enhancer. CERs have been considered the principal factor in the control of the skin barrier as the enhancer effect of CER analogues has been demonstrated in diverse studies [27]. Since the predicted plasma concentration at steady state did not reach therapeutic levels, it is likely that BNB only exerts a local effect on the skin [14].

Retention of BNB in the skin was not statistically different between POPC:CHOL and POPC:CHOL:CER, so both liposomes would be a good option in order to achieve a local effect of BNB because both liposomes reached values a hundred times higher than liposome POPC (Figure 5). Liposomes with CHOL and CER—which are the lipids found in the skin—were able to diffuse through the skin, thus creating a reservoir effect in the BNB. This achieved concentrations inside the skin higher than those obtained in the blood in oral therapy for AD treatment [28], considering the human skin density to be 1 g/mL [29].

The HET-CAM test showed no irritation effect caused by any of the three liposomes and, in reference to the modified Draize test, we observed a good Draize score for erythema and edema (Table 4). Liposome POPC effectively counteracted the impact of xylol on the skin and neither erythema nor edema were observed over the 3 h of the study. Xylol caused both reactions, erythema and edema, which were observed from the first assessment (after 15 min) and up to the end of the tolerance study, which was after 3 h. Liposomes POPC:CHOL and POP:CHOL:CER also effectively counteracted the edema caused by xylol. However, after 45 min of application, a slight erythema appeared in the areas where liposomes POPC:CHOL and POPC:CHOL:CER were tested. Nevertheless, this effect was more than 2-fold and 3-fold lower than the erythema caused by xylol. TEWL values were constant for all the liposomes with similar values to the negative control (within the range of 8–15 g/h·m^2, which means a healthy value for rabbits), whereas the positive control showed a significant increase. The results are in accordance with those obtained in control rabbits, as observed by Babu M. Medi and Angela Anigbogu [30,31]. The skin hydration values were constant and followed the trend of the negative control, while the positive control showed a steady increase during the tolerance study. Finally, the histological study demonstrated that liposome POPC and POPC:CHOL avoided any damage to the tissue structures. Based on these promising results, further biochemical studies should be carried out to test the efficacy of these liposomal formulations on animal models of the disease, including mutant animals, before proceeding to clinical trials.

4. Materials and Methods

4.1. Materials

BNB, Ammonium Formate and POPC were purchased from Sigma–Aldrich (Madrid, Spain). Transcutol® P [Diethylene glycol monoethyl ether] was bought at Gattefossé (Barcelona, Spain). Fisher Chemical (Loughborough, UK) supplied the Acetonitrile. Finally, CHOL (ovine wool > 98%) and CER (bovine spinal cord ≥ 98%) were acquired at Avanti Polar Lipid Inc. (Alabaster, AL, USA). A microneedle roller (Currentbody, Barcelona, Spain) contains 540 titanium needles that are 0.25 mm long, corresponding to 72.3 microneedles/cm^2.

BNB (C16H17N7O2S) is a pyrrolopyrimidine, the chemical structure of which is shown in the figure below, Figure 10, which has been obtained from PubChem, an open chemistry database at the National Institute of Health (NIH).

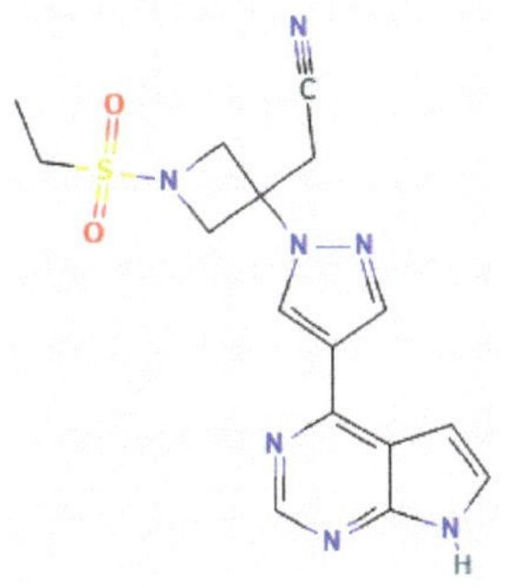

Figure 10. Chemical structure of BNB.

4.2. Biological Materials

The abdominal human skin (protocol code 93-01162 02/18 approved on 17 January 2020 by the 99 Bioethics Committee of SCIAS Hospital de Barcelona), was dermatomed to 400 μm thickness (Aesculap GA 630, Aesculap, Tuttligen, Germany). All the skin was subjected to a physical alteration with microneedles in order to simulate an AD skin by piercing the epidermis. Since the needles do not come into contact with the nerves or blood vessels, this technique is painless when performed on live animals.

4.3. Methods

4.3.1. Preparation of the Liposomes

Three different liposome formulations were prepared: (i) pure POPC liposomes, (ii) POPC:CHOL (0.8:0.2, mol/mol) liposomes and (iii) POPC:CHOL:CER (0.36:0.24:0.40, mol/mol/mol) liposomes.

All liposomes samples were elaborated in accordance with the methods published in other articles [32]. In short, to elaborate each liposome sample, we added 500 mg of BNB in a round bottom flask to the corresponding chloroform–methanol (2:1, v/v) lipid solutions to achieve the desired molar lipid concentration for each composition. Then, the mixture was sonicated for 10–15 s to make sure all BNB was dissolved. Following the removal of the solvent using a rotary evaporator, the thin lipid film was kept in a high vacuum overnight in the absence of light to ensure the absence of organic solvent traces. The thin films were rehydrated using a solution containing 10 mM TRIS·HCl ([tris(hydroxymethyl)aminomethane] 150 mM NaCl), and 5% (v/v) of Transcutol® P pH 7.40. Vigorous vortexing was performed for 5 cycles, at a temperature above that of the lipid mixture's transition, so as to obtain large multilamellar vesicles. The liposome size was homogenized using an ultrasound bath with temperature control for 15 min. Finally, the liposomes were passed through a Sephadex® G50 column mounted in a 5 mL syringe and centrifuged at 1000 rpm for 10 s using a Rotanta 460R centrifuge (Andreas Hettich GmbH & Co. KG, DE, Tuttlingen, Germany) to eliminate non-encapsulated BNB.

4.3.2. Liposomes' Physicochemical Characterization

The physicochemical properties of the liposomes were analyzed using various parameters, including pH, vesicle size, polydispersity index, ZP and encapsulation efficiency. pH measurement was carried out, using a pH-meter micro pH 2001 (Crison Instruments SA, Alella, Spain), in triplicate. The Zetasizer Nano S (Malvern Instrument, Malvern, UK) was used to determine the liposomes size, PDI and ZP. All the physicochemical characteristics were determined in triplicate [33]. All the measures were analyzed by one-way ANOVA test followed by a Tukey's multiple comparison test. These measurements were repeated on samples stored for up to 1 month at 4 °C to assess the stability of the liposomes.

To study the EE percentage (EE%), the liposomes were broken down with Transcutol® P: Triton at 10% (8:1), so that they released the BNB, and quantified using HPLC (see Section 4.3.6). The comparison between the initial amount and the extracted amount gave the *EE%* (Equation (1)) [32]:

$$EE\% = \frac{Q_f}{Q_0} \times 100 \tag{1}$$

where Q_f is the total mass of BNB retained inside the liposomes and Q_0 is the total mass of BNB initially used to prepare the liposomes. Both quantities are expressed in mg.

4.3.3. In Vitro Drug Release Study

In order to investigate the release of the drug, we employed a dialysis membrane that had a molecular cut-off weight of 14,000 Da (Sigma–Aldrich, Madrid, Spain) in Franz-type diffusion cells. These cells had a diffusion area of 0.64 cm^2 and a receptor chamber of 4.9 mL (Crown Glass Company, Inc., Jersey City, NJ, USA) [34,35]. Prior to use, the membrane was hydrated in methanol:water (1:1) for 24 h and then washed before being set in the Franz diffusion cells. The receptor medium used was Transcutol® P which was stirred at 500 r.p.m. to keep sink conditions. The experiment was conducted at 32 °C by means of a thermostatic water bath. An amount of 500 μL of formulation was added to the donor compartment; five replicates per each liposome were included. During the experiment, samples of 200 μL were collected at specific time intervals and, in order to maintain a constant volume in the cells, Transcutol® P was added after each sample collection. The collected samples were analyzed by a validated HPLC-fluorescence method, as described in Section 4.3.6. The cumulative amounts of BNB released from each liposomal formulation were plotted over time, and the data were analyzed by different kinetic models to describe the drug release profile. The determination coefficient (r^2) was used to assess the goodness of fit [36].

Moreover, some non-modelestic parameters were calculated to compare different release profiles. These estimated parameters were the MRT of BNB from the formulation, the AUC representing the amount of BNB that was released from the formulation [37] and the efficiency (E) as the percentage of BNB released from the initial formulation.

4.3.4. Ex Vivo Permeation Study

The permeation studies were conducted using Franz diffusion cells with a surface area measuring 0.64 cm^2 and a receptor chamber of 4.9 mL. The altered abdominal human skin was placed between the donor and the receptor compartments [34,35]. The receptor medium was Transcutol® P. Amounts of 500 μL of each liposome was put on the donor compartment. Samples of 200 μL were taken over 25 h and replaced by Transctuol® P after every sampling time. We analyzed the samples using the validated HPLC-fluorescence method (see Section 4.3.6).

Three permeation parameters of each liposome were calculated: flux (*Jss*, μg/h), permeability coefficient (*Kp*, cm/h) and theoretical predicted plasma concentration in human steady state applied to a 10 cm^2 surface (*Css*, ng/mL). Flux is the slope calculated with the aligned points in the permeation profile [35]. The permeability coefficient was obtained by the following equation:

$$Kp = \frac{Jss}{C_0 \cdot A} \tag{2}$$

where C_0 (μg/mL) is the initial concentration of BNB in the liposome and A is the surface of the diffusion area (cm^2) [34].

Css was calculated by the equation detailed below:

$$C_{ss} = \frac{Jss \cdot TSA}{Clp \cdot A} \tag{3}$$

where *Jss* (µg/h) is the flux, *TSA* (cm^2) is the theoretical surface area of application, *Clp* (ml/min) is the human plasma clearance of BNB and *A* (cm^2) is the diffusion area of the Franz cells [34]. The area of application considered was 10 cm^2.

After completing the permeation study, we removed all tissues from the diffusion cells and washed away any liposomes remaining on the surface with distilled water. Then, we extracted the BNB that was retained in the permeation area of the tissue, cutting it, weighing it and immersing it in 1 mL of Transcutol® P. The sample was then sonicated for 10 min using an ultrasonic water bath [33]. The final step was to analyze the Transcutol® P with the extracted BNB using HPLC. We calculated the retained BNB in the tissues (Q_{ret}) using Equation (4) and the results were stated, normalized by the weight of the tissue and the diffusion area (0.64 cm^2) and multiplied by the recuperation of the drug:

$$Q_{ret} = \frac{Q_{ext}}{W \times A} \times \frac{100}{R} \tag{4}$$

In this equation, Q_{ext} represents the quantity of drug extracted from the tissue and is measured in µg, *W* denotes the weight of the tissue in grams, while *A* is the diffusion area in cm^2. Finally, *R* represents the proportion of BNB that is recovered in each tissue [35].

4.3.5. Baricitinib Determination by HPLC

The measurement of BNB in each sample was carried out using high-performance liquid chromatography (HPLC) equipped with a fluorescence detector. The HPLC system consisted of a Chromatograph Waters Alliance 2695 and a Fluorescence Jasco FP-1520 detector that operated at an excitation wavelength of 310 nm and an emission wavelength of 390 nm. The chromatographic column was a Symmetry C18 (4.6 × 75 mm, 3.5 µm) and the mobile phase was Ammonium Formate 10 mM pH 7.4 (75:25 *v/v*); the flux was 1 mL/min and the volume of injection was 10 µL. The validated range for the quantification of BNB was from 0.03 to 1 µg/mL.

4.3.6. Tolerance Study and Histological Analysis

Liposomes were also evaluated by a modified Draize skin test to study the effect on induced erythema and edema with xylol to simulate atopic skin. We used non-anesthetized New Zealand healthy rabbits (Harlan, Barcelona, Spain). They were cared for in accordance with the standard conditions, receiving food and water ad libitum. The objective was to detect the possible signs of damage on altered skin as indicated by the level of erythema and edema [38,39]. The studies were conducted under a protocol in accordance with the Mexican Official Norm for Animal Care and Handling (NOM-062-ZOO-1999).

To obtain an ARS, we used microneedles so as to compromise the skin barrier function on the rabbits' backs. This was carried out one day after having measured their basal values and having shaved them. The animals were divided into different groups: the negative control group which only underwent microneedles; the positive control group which, in addition to the microneedles, received xylol to induce skin irritation; 3 other groups which received microneedles, plus xylol, plus one of the liposomes. Next, we applied 0.5 mL of xylol to all the rabbits minus the negative control (which also did not have liposomes). The positive control received microneedles plus xylol.

The responses were recorded at 15 min, 45 min and 3 h 30 min. At the same points in time, the transepidermal water loss (TEWL) and skin hydration were measured. For the positive control, 0.5 mL of xylol was applied and evaluated at the same times as the liposomes. A visual scoring system was used to evaluate inflammation; this system classifies from 1 to 4 according to whether the erythema and edema were practically imperceptible or had reached a large area of exposure [40]: 0 denotes no erythema and no edema, 1 denotes a little sign of erythema or edema, 2 denotes explicit erythema or slight edema, 3 denotes a moderate to severe erythema or edema and 4 refers to serious erythema (beet redness) through to the first signs of depth injuries or severe edema [41].

Xylol was used as an irritant component to induce allergic contact dermatitis (ACD), characterized by manifestations such as skin redness, swelling, warmth and itching and accompanied by dryness and flaking. Other articles, like those of Patricia L Nadworny et al. [42] or Liu Tang et al. [43], used dinitrochlorobenzene, or Paul L. Stanley et al. [44], who used 12-O-tetradecanoylphorbol-13-acetate (TPA).

TEWL is the amount of water that can diffuse through the skin stratum corneum per unit of time. The appropriate structure of intracellular lipids in the stratum corneum is one of the key factors in retaining transdermal water [45,46]. TEWL was measured by Tewameter (TEWL-Dermalab, Agaram Industries, India). An increment of this value means there is damage on the skin barrier [47]. The skin hydration was measured by a Corneometer (EnviroDerm, Ireland), which can quantify the amount of water within the corneum.

After monitoring the mentioned parameters for 3 h, the treated animal parts were histologically evaluated to assess the effect of the liposomes. To ensure this, the animals were euthanized with xylazine (Rompun® 20 mg/mL, Bayer Hispania, Sant Joan Despí, Spain) and ketamine (Imalgene® 100 mg/mL, Boehringer Ingelheim Animal Health España, Sant Cugat del Vallès, Spain). The mixture was injected via the right ear vein at 4 mg/kg [48]. After clinical death, the back skin was immediately excised, rinsed with PBS pH 7.4, and set overnight at room temperature in 4% buffered formaldehyde and subsequently embedded in paraffin wax. Transverse sections measuring 5 μm were stained with hematoxylin and eosin and then examined using a light microscope (Olympus BX41 and camera Olympus XC50) on blinded-coded samples to assess the histological structure [49].

Finally, a HET-CAM test was conducted to evaluate the potential risk of causing irritation to the eye after a periocular application. The HET-CAM test assesses the potential toxicity of formulations when applied to the CAM of a 10-day embryonated hen's egg (supplied by the G.A.L.L.S.A. farm, Tarragona, Spain). The CAM was observed for five minutes following application, with any reactions, such as bleeding (hemorrhage), blood vessel disintegration (coagulation) and protein denaturation (intra- and extra-vascular vessel lysis coagulation), being noted [18]. To this end, we applied 300 μL of liposomes to the CAM and we waited 5 min to see if there had been any reaction working with the INVITTOX protocol [50]. The positive control used was a 0.1 N solution of NaOH, while the negative control was a solution containing 0.9% NaCl [50]. The IS was calculated, as described by Garrós et al., including 3 replicates per formulation [49].

5. Conclusions

Three liposomal formulations containing BNB, a Janus kinase inhibitor, were developed for the topical treatment of complement flare-ups in AD. The liposomes were prepared using three different lipids: POPC, CHOL and CER. The POPC:CHOL:CER formulation showed higher flux and permeation compared to the other formulations. However, there were no statistically significant differences in the retention concentration in the skin between POPC:CHOL and POPC:CHOL:CER. These formulations also showed that they retained higher amounts of BNB than liposome POPC; this may be due to them having a longer effect. However, further biomedical investigations should be carried out. The formulations did not demonstrate any irritant effect in the HET-CAM test, and the liposomes POPC and POPC:CHOL did not cause any structural alteration according to the histological analysis.

Author Contributions: Conceptualization, Ò.D., M.M. and A.C.C.; methodology, Ò.D., M.M. and H.C.; validation, M.M. and H.C.; formal analysis, N.G.; investigation, N.G., M.J.R.-L., N.B. and R.M.-M.; resources, Ò.D., M.M., A.C.C. and M.J.R.-L.; data curation, P.B.-S., Ò.D. and M.M.; writing—original draft preparation, N.G. and P.B.-S.; writing—review and editing, P.B.-S. and M.M.; visualization, M.M.; supervision, A.C.C., M.M. and H.C.; project administration, M.M., A.C.C. and H.C.;

funding acquisition, A.C.C., M.M. and H.C. All authors have read and agreed to the published version of the manuscript.

Funding: This research received no external funding.

Institutional Review Board Statement: The protocol used to carry out the studies was in accordance with the Mexican Official Norm for Animal Care and Handing (NOM-062-ZOO-1999) and with the approval of the Academic Committee of Ethics of the Vivarium of the Autonomous University of the Morelos State of Mexico, number 0122013. Moreover, the experiments were carried out in agreement with the guidelines stated in the protocol "Principles of Laboratory Animal Care" (publication 214/97 of 30 July).

Informed Consent Statement: Not applicable.

Data Availability Statement: The data presented in this study are available on request from the corresponding author.

Acknowledgments: The authors would like to thank Pol Alegret and Alexander Parra-Coca for their excellent technical support. We also thank Harry Paul for revising the English language.

Conflicts of Interest: The authors declare no conflict of interest. The funders had no role in the design of the study; in the collection, analyses, or interpretation of data; in the writing of the manuscript, or in the decision to publish the results.

References

1. Naseri, N.; Valizadeh, H.; Zakeri-Milani, P. Solid Lipid Nanoparticles and Nanostructured Lipid Carriers: Structure, Preparation and Application. *Tabriz Univ. Med. Sci.* **2015**, *5*, 305–313. [CrossRef]
2. Bose, S.; Michniak-Kohn, B. Preparation and Characterization of Lipid Based Nanosystems for Topical Delivery of Quercetin. *Eur. J. Pharm. Sci.* **2013**, *48*, 442–452. [CrossRef]
3. Sguizzato, M.; Esposito, E.; Cortesi, R.; Terrinoni, A. Molecular Sciences Lipid-Based Nanosystems as a Tool to Overcome Skin Barrier. *Int. J. Mol. Sci.* **2021**, *22*, 8319. [CrossRef]
4. Gregoriadis, G.; Florence, A.T. Liposomes in Drug Delivery. *Drugs* **1993**, *45*, 15–28. [CrossRef]
5. Coderch, L.; López, O.; De La Maza, A.; Parra, J.L. Ceramides and Skin Function. *Am. J. Clin. Derm.* **2003**, *4*, 107–129. [CrossRef] [PubMed]
6. Boncheva, M. The Physical Chemistry of the Stratum Corneum Lipids. *Int. J. Cosmet. Sci.* **2014**, *36*, 505–515. [CrossRef]
7. Danso, M.; Boiten, W.; van Drongelen, V.; Gmelig Meijling, K.; Gooris, G.; El Ghalbzouri, A.; Absalah, S.; Vreeken, R.; Kezic, S.; van Smeden, J.; et al. Altered Expression of Epidermal Lipid Bio-Synthesis Enzymes in Atopic Dermatitis Skin Is Accompanied by Changes in Stratum Corneum Lipid Composition. *J. Derm. Sci.* **2017**, *88*, 57–66. [CrossRef] [PubMed]
8. Elias, P.M. Lipid Abnormalities and Lipid-Based Repair Strategies in Atopic Dermatitis. *Biochim. Et Biophys. Acta.-Mol. Cell Biol. Lipids* **2014**, *1841*, 323–330. [CrossRef]
9. van Smeden, J.; Janssens, M.; Gooris, G.S.; Bouwstra, J.A. The Important Role of Stratum Corneum Lipids for the Cutaneous Barrier Function. *Biochim. Et Biophys. Acta.-Mol. Cell Biol. Lipids* **2014**, *1841*, 295–313. [CrossRef] [PubMed]
10. Dharmage, S.C.; Lowe, A.J.; Matheson, M.C.; Burgess, J.A.; Allen, K.J.; Abramson, M.J. Atopic Dermatitis and the Atopic March Revisited. *Allergy* **2014**, *69*, 17–27. [CrossRef]
11. Wollenberg, A.; Barbarot, S.; Bieber, T.; Christen-Zaech, S.; Deleuran, M.; Fink-Wagner, A.; Gieler, U.; Girolomoni, G.; Lau, S.; Muraro, A.; et al. Consensus-Based European Guidelines for Treatment of Atopic Eczema (Atopic Dermatitis) in Adults and Children: Part I. *J. Eur. Acad. Dermatol. Venereol.* **2018**, *32*, 657–682. [CrossRef] [PubMed]
12. Oranje, A.P. Practical Issues on Interpretation of Scoring Atopic Dermatitis: SCORAD Index, Objective SCORAD, Patient-Oriented SCORAD and Three-Item Severity Score. *Curr. Probl. Dermatol.* **2011**, *41*, 149–155. [PubMed]
13. Jorgensen, S.C.J.; Tse, C.L.Y.; Burry, L.; Dresser, L.D. Baricitinib: A Review of Pharmacology, Safety, and Emerging Clinical Experience in COVID-19. *Pharmacother. J. Hum. Pharmacol. Drug. Ther.* **2020**, *40*, 843–856. [CrossRef]
14. Committee for Medicinal Products for Human Use (CHMP). *Olumiant-Assessment Report*; Committee for Medicinal Products for Human Use (CHMP): London, UK, 2020.
15. Saeki, H.; Ohya, Y.; Furuta, J.; Arakawa, H.; Ichiyama, S.; Katsunuma, T.; Katoh, N.; Tanaka, A.; Tsunemi, Y.; Nakahara, T.; et al. Executive Summary: Japanese Guidelines for Atopic Dermatitis (ADGL) 2021. *Allergol. Int.* **2022**, *71*, 448–458. [CrossRef]
16. National Library of Medicine (US); National Center for Biotechnology Information PubChem Compound Summary for CID 5497103, 1-Palmitoyl-2-Oleoyl-Sn-Glycero-3-Phosphocholine. Available online: https://pubchem.ncbi.nlm.nih.gov/compound/1-Palmitoyl-2-oleoyl-sn-glycero-3-phosphocholine (accessed on 27 September 2022).
17. Jurecek, L.; Rajcigelova, T.; Kozarova, A.; Werner, T.; Vormann, J.; Kolisek, M. Beneficial Effects of an Alkaline Topical Treatment in Patients with Mild Atopic Dermatitis. *J. Cosmet. Derm.* **2021**, *20*, 2824–2831. [CrossRef]
18. Mallandrich, M.; Calpena, A.C.; Clares, B.; Parra, A.; García, M.L.; Soriano, J.L.; Fernández-Campos, F. Nano-Engineering of Ketorolac Tromethamine Platforms for Ocular Treatment of Inflammatory Disorders. *Nanomedicine* **2021**, *16*, 401–414. [CrossRef]

19. González-Rodríguez, M.; Rabasco, A. Charged Liposomes as Carriers to Enhance the Permeation through the Skin. *Expert Opin. Drug. Deliv.* **2011**, *8*, 857–871. [CrossRef]
20. Paranjpe, M.; Müller-Goymann, C.C. Nanoparticle-Mediated Pulmonary Drug Delivery: A Review. *Int. J. Mol. Sci.* **2014**, *15*, 5852–5873. [CrossRef]
21. Schroeder, A.; Kost, J.; Barenholz, Y. Ultrasound, Liposomes, and Drug Delivery: Principles for Using Ultrasound to Control the Release of Drugs from Liposomes. *Chem. Phys. Lipids* **2009**, *162*, 1–16. [CrossRef] [PubMed]
22. Campos, F.F.; Calpena Campmany, A.C.; Delgado, G.R.; Serrano, O.L.; Naveros, B.C. Development and Characterization of a Novel Nystatin-Loaded Nanoemulsion for the Buccal Treatment of Candidosis: Ultrastructural Effects and Release Studies. *J. Pharm. Sci.* **2012**, *101*, 3739–3752. [CrossRef] [PubMed]
23. Domínguez-Villegas, V.; Clares-Naveros, B.; García-López, M.L.; Calpena-Campmany, A.C.; Bustos-Zagal, P.; Garduño-Ramírez, M.L. Development and Characterization of Two Nano-Structured Systems for Topical Application of Flavanones Isolated from Eysenhardtia Platycarpa. *Colloids Surf. B Biointerfaces* **2014**, *116*, 183–192. [CrossRef]
24. D'Souza, S. A Review of In Vitro Drug Release Test Methods for Nano-Sized Dosage Forms. *Adv. Pharm.* **2014**, *2014*, 1–12. [CrossRef]
25. Pappas, A. Epidermal Surface Lipids. *Dermatoendocrinol* **2009**, *1*, 72–76. [CrossRef] [PubMed]
26. Sinico, C.; Fadda, A.M. Vesicular Carriers for Dermal Drug Delivery. *Expert Opin. Drug. Deliv.* **2009**, *6*, 813–825. [CrossRef] [PubMed]
27. Chen, Y.; Quan, P.; Liu, X.; Wang, M.; Fang, L. Novel Chemical Permeation Enhancers for Transdermal Drug Delivery. *Asian J. Pharm. Sci.* **2014**, *9*, 51–64. [CrossRef]
28. Shi, J.G.; Chen, X.; Lee, F.; Emm, T.; Scherle, P.A.; Lo, Y.; Punwani, N.; Williams, W.V.; Yeleswaram, S. The Pharmacokinetics, Pharmacodynamics, and Safety of Baricitinib, an Oral JAK 1/2 Inhibitor, in Healthy Volunteers. *J. Clin. Pharm.* **2014**, *54*, 1354–1361. [CrossRef]
29. Rins, M.; Diez, I.; Calpena, A.C.; Obach, R. Skin Density in the Hairless Rat. Evidence of Regional Differences. *Eur. J. Drug. Metab. Pharm.* **1991**, *Spec No 3*, 456–457.
30. Medi, B.M.; Singh, J. Skin Targeted DNA Vaccine Delivery Using Electroporation in Rabbits: II. Safety. *Int. J. Pharm.* **2006**, *308*, 61–68. [CrossRef]
31. Anigbogu, A.; Patil, S.; Singh, P.; Liu, P.; Dinh, S.; Maibach, H. An in Vivo Investigation of the Rabbit Skin Responses to Transdermal Iontophoresis. *Int. J. Pharm.* **2000**, *200*, 195–206. [CrossRef]
32. Vázquez-González, M.L.; Botet-Carreras, A.; Domènech, Ò.; Teresa Montero, M.; Borrell, J.H. Planar Lipid Bilayers Formed from Thermodynamically-Optimized Liposomes as New Featured Carriers for Drug Delivery Systems through Human Skin. *Int. J. Pharm.* **2019**, *563*, 1–8. [CrossRef]
33. Moussaoui, S.E.; Abo-horan, I.; Halbaut, L.; Alonso, C.; Coderch, L.; Garduño-ramírez, M.L.; Clares, B.; Soriano, J.L.; Calpena, A.C.; Fernández-campos, F.; et al. Polymeric Nanoparticles and Chitosan Gel Loading Ketorolac Tromethamine to Alleviate Pain Associated with Condyloma Acuminata during the Pre- and Post-ablation. *Pharmaceutics* **2021**, *13*, 1784. [CrossRef]
34. Moussaoui, S.E.; Fernández-Campos, F.; Alonso, C.; Limón, D.; Halbaut, L.; Garduño-Ramirez, M.L.; Calpena, A.C.; Mallandrich, M. Topical Mucoadhesive Alginate-Based Hydrogel Loading Ketorolac for Pain Management after Pharmacotherapy, Ablation, or Surgical Removal in Condyloma Acuminata. *Gels* **2021**, *7*, 8. [CrossRef]
35. Mallandrich, M.; Fernández-Campos, F.; Clares, B.; Halbaut, L.; Alonso, C.; Coderch, L.; Garduño-Ramírez, M.L.; Andrade, B.; del Pozo, A.; Lane, M.E.; et al. Developing Transdermal Applications of Ketorolac Tromethamine Entrapped in Stimuli Sensitive Block Copolymer Hydrogels. *Pharm. Res.* **2017**, *34*, 1728–1740. [CrossRef] [PubMed]
36. Kurakula, M.; Srinivas, C.; Kasturi, N.; Diwan, P. V Formulation and Evaluation of Prednisolone Proliposomal Gel for Effective Topical Pharmacotherapy. *Int. J. Pharm. Sci. Drug. Res.* **2012**, *4*, 35–43.
37. Pérez-González, N.; Bozal-De Febrer, N.; Calpena-Campmany, A.C.; Nardi-Ricart, A.; Rodríguez-Lagunas, M.J.; Morales-Molina, J.A.; Soriano-Ruiz, J.L.; Fernández-Campos, F.; Clares-Naveros, B.; Dinu, V. New Formulations Loading Caspofungin for Topical Therapy of Vulvovaginal Candidiasis. *Gel* **2021**, *7*, 259. [CrossRef]
38. Lee, M.; Hwang, J.-H.; Lim, K.-M. Alternatives to In Vivo Draize Rabbit Eye and Skin Irritation Tests with a Focus on 3D Reconstructed Human Cornea—Like Epithelium and Epidermis Models. *Toxicol. Res.* **2017**, *33*, 191–203. [CrossRef] [PubMed]
39. Gupta, P.K. Chapter 12-Toxicological Testing: In Vivo Systems. In *Fundamentals of Toxicology*; Academic Press: Cambridge , MA, USA, 2016; pp. 131–150. [CrossRef]
40. Singh, S.; Singh, J. Dermal Toxicity and Microscopic Alterations by JP-8 Jet Fuel Components in vivo in Rabbit. *Env. Toxicol. Pharm.* **2004**, *16*, 153–161. [CrossRef]
41. Mehanna, M.M.; Abla, K.K.; Elmaradny, H.A. Tailored Limonene-Based Nanosized Microemulsion: Formulation, Physicochemical Characterization and In Vivo Skin Irritation Assessment. *Adv. Pharm. Bull.* **2020**, *11*, 274–285. [CrossRef]
42. Nadworny, P.L.; Wang, J.; Tredget, E.E.; Burrell, R.E. Anti-Inflammatory Activity of Nanocrystalline Silver-Derived Solutions in Porcine Contact Dermatitis. *J. Inflamm.* **2010**, *7*, 13. [CrossRef]
43. Tang, L.; Cao, X.; Li, X.; Ding, H. Topical Application with Conjugated Linoleic Acid Ameliorates 2, 4-dinitrofluorobenzene-induced Atopic Dermatitis-like Lesions in BALB/c Mice. *Exp. Derm.* **2021**, *30*, 237–248. [CrossRef] [PubMed]
44. Stanley, P.L.; Steiner, S.; Havens, M.; Tramposch, K.M. Mouse Skin Inflammation Induced by Multiple Topical Applications of 12-O-Tetradecanoylphorbol-13-Acetate. *Ski. Pharm. Physiol.* **1991**, *4*, 262–271. [CrossRef] [PubMed]

45. Verdier-Sévrain, S.; Bonté, F. Skin Hydration: A Review on Its Molecular Mechanisms. *J. Cosmet. Derm.* **2007**, *6*, 75–82. [CrossRef] [PubMed]
46. Alexander, H.; Brown, S.; Danby, S.; Flohr, C. Research Techniques Made Simple: Transepidermal Water Loss Measurement as a Research Tool. *J. Investig. Dermatol.* **2018**, *138*, 2295–2300.e1. [CrossRef] [PubMed]
47. Netzlaff, F.; Kostka, K.H.; Lehr, C.M.; Schaefer, U.F. TEWL Measurements as a Routine Method for Evaluating the Integrity of Epidermis Sheets in Static Franz Type Diffusion Cells in Vitro. Limitations Shown by Transport Data Testing. *Eur. J. Pharm. Biopharm.* **2006**, *63*, 44–50. [CrossRef]
48. Parra-Coca, A.; Boix-Montañés, A.; Calpena-Campmany, A.C.; Colom, H. In Vivo Pharmacokinetic Evaluation of Carprofen Delivery from Intra-Articular Nanoparticles in Rabbits: A Population Modelling Approach. *Res. Vet. Sci.* **2021**, *137*, 235–242. [CrossRef] [PubMed]
49. Garrós, N.; Mallandrich, M.; Beirampour, N.; Mohammadi, R.; Domènech, Ò.; Rodríguez-Lagunas, M.J.; Clares, B.; Colom, H. Baricitinib Liposomes as a New Approach for the Treatment of Sjögren's Syndrome. *Pharmaceutics* **2022**, *14*, 1895. [CrossRef]
50. Interagency Coordinating Committee on the Validation of Alternative Methods (ICCVAM). *Test Method Protocol: Hen's Egg Test-Chorioallantoic Membrane (HET-CAM) Test Method*; Interagency Coordinating Committee on the Validation of Alternative Methods (ICCVAM): Bethesda, MD, USA, 2010.

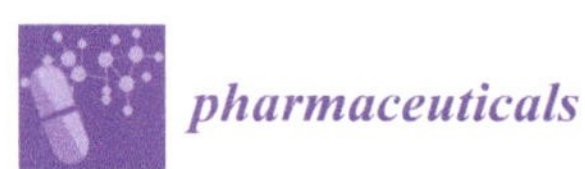
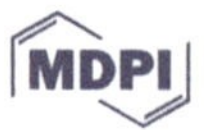

Article

Preparation, Characterization, and In Vivo Evaluation of Gentiopicroside-Phospholipid Complex (GTP-PC) and Its Self-Nanoemulsion Drug Delivery System (GTP-PC-SNEDDS)

Yingpeng Tong [1,2,†], Wen Shi [2,†], Qin Zhang [2] and Jianxin Wang [1,2,3,*]

[1] Institute of Natural Medicine and Health Product, School of Advanced Study, Taizhou University, Taizhou 318000, China
[2] Department of Pharmaceutics, School of Pharmacy, Fudan University, Key Laboratory of Smart Drug Delivery, Ministry of Education, Shanghai 201203, China
[3] Institute of Integrative Medicine, Fudan University, Shanghai 201203, China
[*] Correspondence: jxwang@fudan.edu.cn
[†] These authors contributed equally to this work.

Abstract: The objective of the present study was to develop a gentiopicroside-phospholipid complex (GTP-PC) and its self-nanoemulsion drug delivery system (GTP-PC-SNEDDS) to increase the oral bioavailability of gentiopicroside (GTP). The factors affecting the formation of GTP-PC were studied with the complexation efficiency and dissociation rate. The properties of the complex were investigated by means of differential scanning calorimetry (DSC), X-ray diffraction (XRD), Fourier transform infrared spectra (FT-IR), dissolution, etc. Then, GTP-PC was loaded into SNEDDS by investigating the effects of weight ratios of GTP-PC to blank SNEDDS, preparation technology, dilution media, and dilution multi, based on the screening results of oils, surfactants, and cosurfactants. In rats, GTP, GTP-PC, and GTP-PC-SNEDDS were orally administered at different times, and GTP concentrations were determined using RP-HPLC. The optimal GTP-PC was prepared with tetrahydrofuran as the reaction solvent, GTP:phospholipid = 1:2, and stirring for 4 h. The optimal prescription for GTP-PC-SNEDDS was as follows: Maisin 35-1:Miglycol = 30%, Labrasol:Cremophor EL = 1:4 = 40%, Transcutol P = 30%; Maisin 35-1:Miglycol = 12, and the ratio of GTP-PC to blank was 1:10—then the mixture was stirred at 37 °C for 1 d and then placed for 2 d to form stable GTP-PC-SNEDDS. After oral administration of GTP, GTP-PC and GTP-PC-SNEDDS, and mean plasma GTP concentration–time curves were all in accordance with the single-compartment model. The C_{max}, $AUC_{0-\infty}$, and Fr of the three formulations were significantly higher than that of GTP, demonstrating that GTP was metabolized rapidly, and its higher bioavailability could be achieved by the formation of GTP-PC and GTP-PC-SNEDDS. Among the three formations, the bioavailability of GTP-PC-SNEDDS was highest, with approximately 2.6-fold and 1.3-fold of Fr value, compared with GTP-PC (suspension) and GTP-PC (oil solution), respectively. Compared with GTP, GTP-PC and GTP-PC-SNEDDS enhanced the bioavailability of GTP significantly. In the future, this study could serve as a reference for clinical trials using GTP-PC and GTP-PC-SNEDDS.

Keywords: gentiopicroside; phospholipid complex; self-nanoemulsion drug delivery system; oral bioavailability; pharmacokinetics

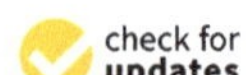
check for updates

Citation: Tong, Y.; Shi, W.; Zhang, Q.; Wang, J. Preparation, Characterization, and In Vivo Evaluation of Gentiopicroside-Phospholipid Complex (GTP-PC) and Its Self-Nanoemulsion Drug Delivery System (GTP-PC-SNEDDS). *Pharmaceuticals* **2023**, *16*, 99. https://doi.org/10.3390/ph16010099

Academic Editors: Ana Catarina Silva, João Nuno Moreira and José Manuel Sousa Lobo

Received: 9 October 2022
Revised: 1 January 2023
Accepted: 5 January 2023
Published: 9 January 2023

1. Introduction

Gentiopicroside (GTP, Figure 1A), a kind of iridoid glycoside, is one of the key active components from Gentiana species [1–3]. It exhibits many activities, including anti-inflammatory, analgesic, antioxidant, and anti-hepatotoxic activities, which imply its benefit in the treatment of rheumatoid arthritis, liver illness (hepatitis), fever, digestive, intestinal disorders, and so on [4–9].

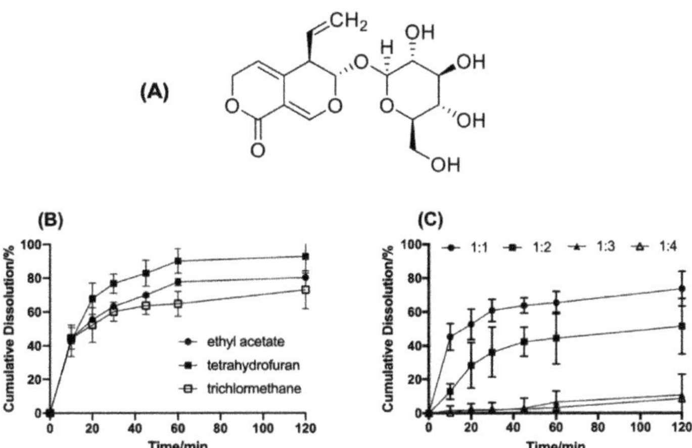

Figure 1. The structure of GTP and its influencing factors on the formation of phospholipid complexes. (**A**): The structure of GTP. (**B**): Cumulative Dissolution of phytosome of different type of solvent in phosphate buffer saline (pH 6.8). (**C**): Cumulative Dissolution of phytosome of different molar ratios of GTP and phospholipids.

Unfortunately, the clinical efficacy was limited by the low bioavailability of oral GTP. Several studies attributed the low bioavailability of oral GTP to the first-pass metabolism, bacterial metabolic processes, or decomposition in the intestine, as well as to poor absorption from the gastrointestinal tract [10–16]. To overcome the problem of the slight clinical efficacy of GTP, it is important to improve its bioavailability. Some reports had exposed that the bioavailability of GTP could be significantly improved by the interaction of the compound–compound in an herb extract [11] or the herb–herb in a formulae decoction [12,16]. Additionally, no data about pharmaceutical approaches have been published, in relation to improving the bioavailability of GTP after oral administration.

The formation of a drug–phospholipid complex is an important, and the most common, way to improve bioavailability. Up until now, several drug–phospholipid complexes have been approved to use in clinical treatment, such as Meriva® (curcumin-PC) [17], Siliphos® (Silybin-PC) [17]. SNEDDS, which consists of a drug, oil, surfactant, and co-surfactant, can produce an oil-in-water (O/W) nanoemulsion with a droplet size of less than 100 nm by gently mixing with water [18–21]. It is another pharmaceutical means to enhance the drug's bioavailability. More importantly, the combination of PC and SNEDDS can overcome the same limitations of drugs with low oral bioavailability. It has been proposed that combining PC with SNEDDS can enhance the oral bioavailability of bioactive compounds or biomacromolecules, such as morin [22–25], akebia saponin D [26,27], rosuvastatin calcium [28], paclitaxel [29], curcumin [30], ellagic acid [31], baicalin [32], and matrine [33].

In the above experiments, the tested compounds are water insoluble and belong to classes 2 or classes 4 of the biopharmaceutical classification system. However, there are no related studies on class 3 compounds. Classified as class 3 drugs, they are highly soluble in gastrointestinal fluids, but possess low absorption membrane permeability, often resulting in low bioavailability [34]. GTP was a typical class 3 compound with high water solubility (7.65 g/100 g at 23 °C) and low membrane permeability [35]. So, GTP was adopted in this study, and then GTP-PC and GTP-PC-SNEDDS were optimized to test their advantages on enhancing GTP's oral bioavailability.

2. Results and Discussion

2.1. Factors Affecting the Formation of GTP-Phospholipid Complex

2.1.1. Different Type of Phospholipids

The complexation efficiency and dissociation rate of GTP-PC of different type of phospholipids, including hydrogenated phospholipids, soybean phospholipids, and egg yolk phospholipids, are shown in Table 1. The results display that the complexation efficiency of the GTP-PC prepared by the soybean phospholipid and egg yolk phospholipid exceeded 95%. The dissociation rate of GTP-PC in pH 6.8 PBS was hydrogenated phospholipid > egg yolk phospholipid > soybean phospholipid, indicating that the stability of hydrogenated phospholipids prepared by hydrogenated phospholipid was poor, and it was easy to dissociate in aqueous environment. The cost of egg yolk phospholipid is higher than that of soybean phospholipid. Considering the complexation efficiency, dissociation rate, and cost factors, soybean phospholipid was selected for preparing GTP-PC.

Table 1. Complexation efficiency and dissociation rate of GTP-PC of different types of phospholipids.

Type of Phospholipids	Complexation Efficiency (%)	K (h^{-1})
soybean phospholipid	97.15 ± 3.27	1.60
egg yolk phospholipid	100 ± 4.92	2.49
hydrogenated phospholipid	88.20 ± 4.74	8.52

2.1.2. Dissolving Solvents

The solubility of GTP and GTP-PC is shown in Table 2. The results show that GTP is insoluble in dichloromethane, ethyl acetate, and tetrahydrofuran, but GTP-PC and soybean phospholipid are easily soluble. In this case, the formation of GTP-PC could be judged according to the change of solubility. Then, the most suitable solvent was chosen further by complexation efficiency and dissociation. The results are shown in Table 3 and Figure 1B, indicating that the phospholipid complex prepared in tetrahydrofuran had the highest complexation efficiency and slowest dissociation. Therefore, tetrahydrofuran was identified as the dissolving solvent.

Table 2. Dissolubility of GTP, GTP-PC, and phospholipids in different solvents (mg/mL).

Solvents	Soybean Phospholipid	GTP	GTP-PC
Water	※	++	※
Methanol	+	++	+
Ethanol	−	−	※
Acetone	++	−	−
Dichloromethane	++	−	++
Tetrahydrofuran	++	−	++
Ethyl Acetate	++	−	++
Trichloromethane	++	+	++
Ethyl Ether	−	−	−
n-hexane	++	−	−

− indicates substance is not soluble in the solvent within 48 h; + indicates substance is soluble in the solvent within 24 h; ++ indicates substance is easily dissoluble in the solvent within 8~12 h; ※ indicates substance is dispersed in the solvent within 48 h.

Table 3. Complexation efficiency and dissociation rate of GTP-PC of different types of solvent.

Type of Solvent	Complexation Efficiency (%)	K (h^{-1})
trichloromethane	61.71 ± 5.38	3.17
tetrahydrofuran	97.15 ± 3.31	1.99
ethyl acetate	86.77 ± 4.24	2.53

2.1.3. Molar Ratio of GTP to Phospholipid

Complexation efficiency and dissociation of the GTP-PC of different molar ratios of GTP and phospholipid are shown in Table 4 and Figure 1C. The data indicated that the complexation efficiency of phospholipid complex was close to 100% for the GTP of GTP:phospholipid $\leq$ 1:1. The dissociation rate increased with the ratio of GTP-to-phospholipid increase, suggesting that the greater the amount of phospholipid, the higher the stability of GTP-PC. However, the content of phospholipid could not be too much, due to the poor dispersion and fluidity of the GTP-PC of the drug-to-lipid ratio $\geq$ 1:3. Additionally, according to the results of the bioavailability, the molar ratio of GTP and phospholipid was identified as 1:2 [36].

Table 4. Complexation efficiency and dissociation rate of phytosome of different molar ratios of GTP and phospholipid.

Molar Ratio of GTP and Phospholipids	Complexation Efficiency (%)	K (h^{-1})
2:1	86.82 ± 6.53	5.21
1:1	97.15 ± 3.31	3.72
1:2	99.87 ± 3.21	2.39
1:3	99.66 ± 1.14	0.72
1:4	99.79 ± 2.23	0.55

2.1.4. Stirring Time

It was found that, with the stirring time increasing from 0.5 to 4 h, the complexation efficiency increased from 83.57% to 99.50%, and at 4 h reached the peak. When stirring for 5 h and 6 h, the complexation efficiency declined to 92.63% and 88.63%. This may be due to the instability of GTP. Therefore, the optimal stirring time was 4 h.

2.2. Characterization of GTP-PC

2.2.1. Differential Scanning Calorimetry (DSC)

In DSC, an interaction can be detected by eliminating endothermic peaks, showing new peaks, changing peak shape, and changing the peak temperature and relative peak area or enthalpy [37]. The DSC curves of the GTP, phospholipids, physical mixture, and GTP-PC are shown in Figure 2A. The GTP displayed an abroad endothermal peak at 260.5 °C (Figure 2Aα). The phospholipid had a peak at 100.6 °C (Figure 2Aβ). The DSC of the phospholipid complex showed that the phospholipid peak vanished, and the onset temperature was lower than GTP's, which was at 245.08 °C (Figure 2Aδ). The GTP and phospholipids were thought to interact through hydrogen bonds or van der Waals forces. As the GTP and phospholipid polarity parts were combined, the carbon–hydrogen chain of phospholipids was free to turn and enclose the polarity parts and GTP of the phospholipids. After that, the sequence between the aliphatic hydrocarbon chains of phospholipids decreased and the peak of phospholipids disappeared, lowering the onset temperature of GTP [38]. The physical mixture of the GTP and phospholipid showed two peaks. The former was 60.5 °C, lower than the onset temperature of phospholipid; the other was 245.8 °C, the same with the onset temperature of GTP-PC (Figure 2Aχ). It was thought that, as the temperature increased, the phospholipid melted, and the drugs dissolved into it, partially forming phospholipid complexes.

2.2.2. X-ray Diffractometry (XRD)

The powder X-ray diffraction patterns of the GTP, phospholipids, physical mixture, and complex are shown in Figure 2B. The GTP displayed sharp crystalline peaks. In contrast, phospholipids were amorphous and lacking crystalline peaks. Despite the physical mixtures of the GTP and phospholipid, some drug signals could still be detected. However, the crystalline peaks had disappeared in the GTP-PC. The combination of the polar ends of phospholipid with GTP led to their being highly dispersed, thus inhibiting their crystalline characteristics.

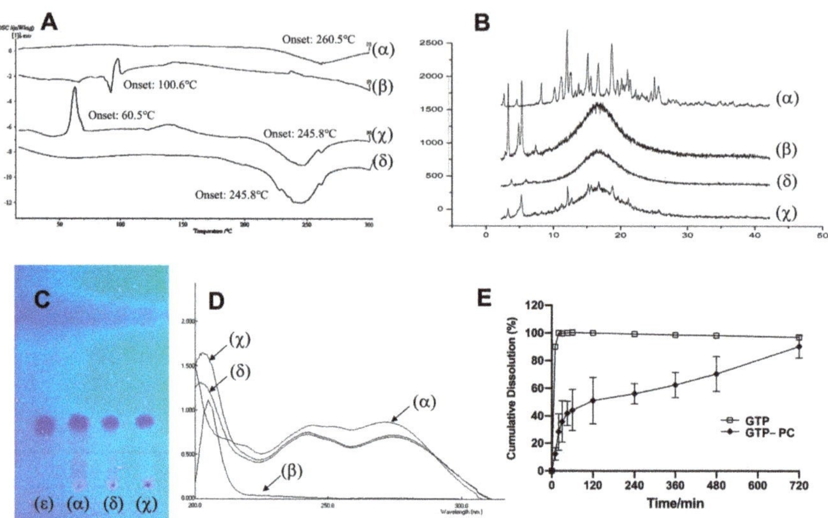

Figure 2. Characterization of GTP-PC. (**A**): Differential scanning calorimetry (DSC). (**B**): X-ray diffractometry (XRD). (**C**): Thin-layer chromatography (TLC). (**D**): Ultraviolet (UV) spectra. (**E**): Degradation of GTP-PC in phosphate buffer solutions and diluted hydrochloric acid at different pH (n = 3). GTP (α), phospholipids (β), physical mixture (χ), GTP-PC (δ), and standard GTP (ε).

2.2.3. Fourier Transform Infrared Spectra (FT-IR)

The FT-IR of the GTP, phospholipids, physical mixture, and GTP-PC are shown in Figure 3A–D, respectively. The FT-IR spectrum of GTP was shown in Figure 3A, disclosing a broad band of 3600–3000 cm^{-1} for hydrogen-bonded O-H stretching vibrations. The absorption bands at 1713.35, 1609.84 cm^{-1} related to the C=O and C=C stretching. The signal at 1273.48 and 1007.06 cm^{-1} were assigned to C–O–C vibration. This FT-IR spectrum was consistent with the previously published reports. The stretching vibration of hydroxyl in GTP (υOH, 3420.86) and phospholipids (υOH, 3389.75) were superimposed in the physical mixture, forming a large, wide peak. The vibration of the hydrocarbon of saturated long-chain fatty (υCH, 2924.56, 2853.51), carbonyl of fatty acid ester (υC=O, 1737.68), phosphorus oxygen double bond (υP=O, 1241.04), and phosphorus oxygen single bond (υP-O-C, 1089.90) in phospholipid can be found, indicating little interaction between the GTP and phospholipid in the physical mixture (Figure 3C). In the phospholipid (Figure 3B), there were strong hydrogen bonds, so the vibration of hydroxyl was very strong and had a relatively low wavenumber (3389.75). This was due to the fact that the phospholipid phosphate and quaternary ammonium in the phospholipids had a strong ability to ionize, and hydrogen bonds formed by positive and negative ions were significantly strong, possibly with ionic character. However, the combination of phospholipid and GTP made new hydrogen bonds, formed between the two, and also destroyed part of the hydrogen bonds between the phospholipids (Figure 3D), resulting in the vibration of the hydroxyl moving to a higher wavenumber (υOH, 3396.32). Moreover, the υC=O and υP-O-C in phospholipids moved to a lower wavenumber (υC=O, 1737.68 to 1735.78; υP-O-C, 1089.90 to 1085.39), indicating that new hydrogen bonds may have been formed.

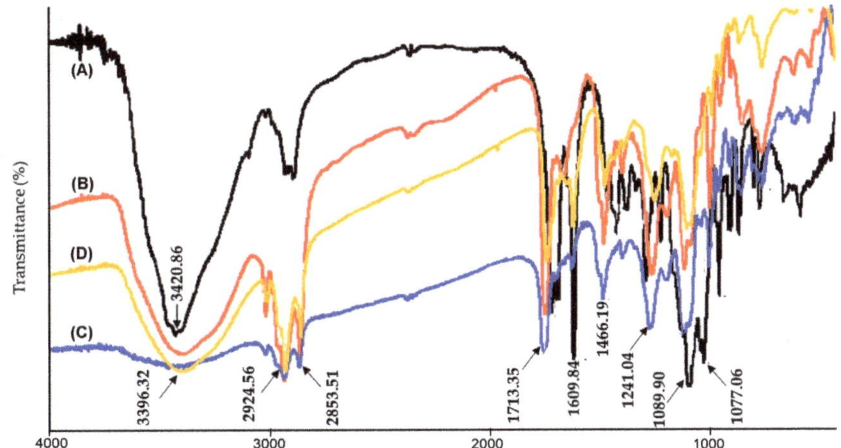

Figure 3. Fourier Transform Infrared spectra (FT-IR) of GTP-PC. GTP (**A**), phospholipids (**B**), physical mixture (**C**), GTP-PC (**D**).

The FT-IR of the GTP, phospholipids, physical mixture, and GTP-PC is shown in Figure 3A–D, respectively. The GTP spectrum (Figure 3A) disclosed the characteristic hydrogen-bonded O-H stretching vibration at 3600–3000 cm^{-1}, C=O stretching vibration at 1713.35 cm^{-1}, C=C stretching vibration at 1609.84 cm^{-1}, and C–O stretching vibrations at 1273.48, 1083.96, and 1007.06 cm^{-1}. The characteristic C-H stretching and bending vibrations of the long fatty acid chain of PC shown in Figure 3B were at 2924.56, 2853.51, and 1466.19 cm^{-1}. Carbonyl of fatty acid ester (υC=O) at 1737.68 cm^{-1}, phosphorus oxygen double bond (υP=O) at 1241.04 cm^{-1}, and phosphorus oxygen single bond (υP-O-C) at 1089.90 cm^{-1} in phospholipid can also be found. In the spectrum of the physical mixture of GTP and PC, the peaks of O-H stretching vibrations of GTP and PC were superposed to form a wide peak at 3409.70 cm^{-1}, with the other main peaks from GTP and PC still existing in the physical mixture of GTP and PC, but the intensity of some peaks from GTP were significantly weakened, such as the C=C stretching vibration at 1609.84 cm^{-1} and C–O stretching vibration at 1007.06 cm^{-1}. However, the combination of the phospholipid and GTP may form new hydrogen bonds between them and destroy part of the hydrogen bonds between the phospho-lipids (Figure 3D), resulting in the hydroxyl vibration of PC moving to higher wavenumber at 3396.32 cm^{-1}. The intensity of the peaks from GTP at 1609.84 cm^{-1} and 1007.06 cm^{-1} were also weakened, but they were relatively stronger than those from the physical mixture of GTP and PC.

2.2.4. Thin-Layer Chromatography (TLC)

Only one spot with the same Rf as GTP was observed in the chromatogram of GTP-PC, similar to that of the physical mixture (Figure 2C). As the GTP and phospholipid have no chemical groups that can react with each other under our preparation conditions, they were unable to form new compounds. Therefore, the TLC did not reveal any new spots, and the UV confirmed the result.

2.2.5. Ultraviolet (UV) Spectra

As can be seen in Figure 2D, the phospholipid exhibited only end absorptions close to 200 nm, while GTP, the physical mixture, and GTP-PC showed nearly identical absorption curves. All of them exhibited two characteristic absorption bands at 240 and 270 nm. Therefore, the UV spectra of GTP was not changed during the combination with the phospholipid, indicating that no chemical groups could react between the GTP and the phospholipid.

2.2.6. Dissolution Studies in Phosphate Buffer Saline (pH 6.8)

Figure 2E shows the dissolution profile of GTP from the GTP-PC and GTP in phosphate buffer saline (pH 6.8). The dissolution of GTP was complete in 30 min, while the GTP from GTP-PC had a fast dissolution in the 0–2 h (about 50%); then, the dissolution tended to increase slowly in 2–12 h, and eventually, the phospholipid complex almost completely dissolved in 12 h. Therefore, the GTP and GTP-PC had significantly different dissolution characteristics, in that the dissolution of GTP in GTP-PC was delayed, compared with the GTP material.

2.3. Preparation Process of GTP-PC-SNEDDS

2.3.1. Screening of Oils, Surfactants and Cosurfactant

Among the oils surfactants and cosurfactants that have been experimentally investigated and shown in Table 5, imwitor 742, labrasol, and transcutol P had the highest solubility, which were 0.146 ± 0.028, 0.107 ± 0.011, and 0.315 ± 0.012 g/g, respectively. Additionally, the mixtures of Maisin 35-1/Miglycol 812N, Imwitor742/Miglycol 812N, and Labrasol/Cremophor EL with different ratios also had a relatively high solubility.

Table 5. The solubility of GTP-PC in various vehicles at 37 °C (n = 3, g/g).

Vehicle	Solubility of GTP-PC (g/g)
Oils	
Imwitor742	0.146 ± 0.028
Maisin 35-1	0.037 ± 0.016
Miglycol 812N	-
Maisin 35-1:Miglycol 812N = 1:2	0.095 ± 0.016
Maisin 35-1:Miglycol 812N = 1:1	0.105 ± 0.013
Maisin 35-1:Miglycol 812N = 2:1	0.065 ± 0.009
Labrafill M 1994 CS	0.074 ± 0.019
Imwitor742:Miglycol 812N = 2:1	0.127 ± 0.013
Imwitor742:Miglycol 812N = 1:2	0.132 ± 0.011
Imwitor742:Miglycol 812N = 1:1	0.138 ± 0.038
Plurol Qleique CC 497	0.016 ± 0.006
Surfactant	
Labrasol	0.107 ± 0.011
Cremophor EL	0.025 ± 0.005
Labrasol:Cremophor EL = 1:1	0.058 ± 0.005
Labrasol:Cremophor EL = 1:2	0.070 ± 0.009
Labrasol:Cremophor EL = 1:3	0.069 ± 0.014
Labrasol:Cremophor EL = 1:4	0.060 ± 0.009
Tween 80	0.012 ± 0.004
Co-surfactant	
Transcutol P	0.315 ± 0.012
PEG400	-
Absolute ethanol	-
95% ethanol	-

In previous preliminary studies on the blank formulation of SNEDDS, the SNEDDS could not have been formed by choosing Imwitor 742 or maisin 35-1 as the oil, Labrasol as the surfactant, or Transcutol P as the cosurfactant. Only when the oil loading was less than 10% could the microemulsion be infinitely diluted, but layered after 30 min, which might be related to the weak emulsifying ability of Labrasol. It was reported that the combination of Labrasol and Cremophor EL in the formulation could easily form self-microemulsion because of the high emulsifying ability of Cremophor EL and the excellent dissolving capacity of Labrasol. When the ratio of Labrasol:Cremophor EL = 1:4, the microemulsion area was larger. When the surfactant was changed to Labrasol:Cremophor EL = 1:4, the formed SNEDDS would not layer after 24 h, while the oil loading was still less than 10%, which might have been related with the weak polarity of Imwitor 742. However, the mixture of Maisin 35-1:Miglyol 812N and Imwitor742:Miglyol 812N would significantly improve the oil loading of SNEDDS, which is consistent with the previous reports. After the Maisin 35-1 was mixed with Miglyol 812N, the mixture would change the polarity of the oil phase, improve the ability of oil phase molecule penetrating into surfactant, and reduce the interfacial tension between oil and water, which would result in the formulation of stable microemulsion droplets. In the mixture, the combination of the long-chain oils solubilizing in microemulsions and short-chain oils acting as cosurfactants would help the hydrophilic groups of oil molecules to disperse in polar cephalic groups of surfactants form chelating effect, which would increase the formation area of microemulsions.

Based on previous results shown above, the pseudo-ternary phase diagrams were constructed by selecting Imwitor742:Miglyol 812N = 1:1 or Maisin 35-1:Miglyol 812N = 1:1 as the oil phase, Labrasol:Cremophor EL = 1:4 as the surfactant, and Transcutol P as the cosurfactant. It can be seen that the self-microemulsifying region of Maisin 35-1:Miglyol 812N = 1:1 was bigger than that of Imwitor742: Miglyol = 1:1 (Figure 4A,B). The effects of different weight ratios of Maisin 35-1 and Miglyol 812N on the self-microemulsifying region was shown in Figure 4B,C, and Maisin 35-1:Miglyol 812N = 1:2 was chosen as oil phase because of its lager self-microemulsifying region and higher oil loading. Labrasol:Cremophor EL = 1:4 would also been selected by comparing the effects of different weight ratios on the self-microemulsifying region and oil loading, which are presented in Figure 4C–F.

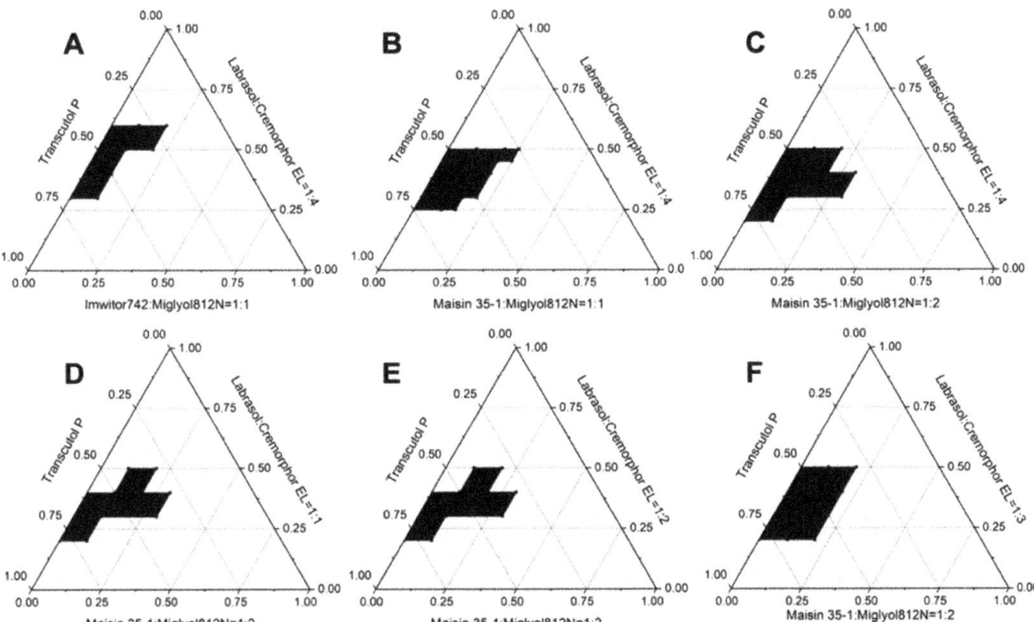

Figure 4. Pseudo-ternary phase diagrams of different compositions of oil, surfactant, and cosurfactant. The region of self-microemulsifaction is in black. (**A,B**) indicates effects of different oil on the efficient self-microemulsifacation. The oil phase was as follows: (**A**) as Imwitor742:Miglyol 812N = 1:1; (**B**) as Maisin 35-1:Miglyol 812N = 1:1. (**C–F**) indicates effects of different ratios between Labrasol and Cremophor EL from 1:1 to 1:4 on the efficient self-microemulsifacation, respectively.

2.3.2. Factors Affecting the Formation of GTP-PC-SNEDDS

In the present work, the effect factors for preparation of GTP-PC-SNEDDS, including the weight ratios of GTP-PC to blank SNEDDS, preparation technology, dilution media, and dilution multi, were further optimized, and the results are presented in Tables 6–9.

Table 6. The particle size of GTP-PC-SNEDDS with different ratios of drug/blank formula (*w/w*) in 0.1 M HCl, pH 6.8 PBS, and water (nm).

GTP-PC/Blank Formula (*w/w*)	0.1 M HCl Particle Size (nm)	pH 6.8 PBS Particle Size (nm)	Water Particle Size (nm)
1:5	190.0 ± 23.5	527.5 ± 34.7	205.6 ± 38.1
1:7	47.5 ± 15.2	150.1 ± 21.1	44.6 ± 12.8
1:10	27.8 ± 3.9	52.7 ± 8.4	24.6 ± 3.4

Table 7. The effect of preparation technology on the efficiency of self-microemulsifacation of GTP-PC-SNEDDS.

Preparation Technology	Particle Size (nm)	Time (s)	Appearance	Appearance after Dilution
Ultrasonic	31.2 ± 0.6	69 ± 15	Clear liquid	Turbid, clear after 30 min
Stirring (at room temperature, 25 °C)	27.8 ± 3.9	21 ± 6	Clear liquid	Clear liquid
Volution	32.6 ± 3.0	47 ± 12	Clear liquid	Turbid, clear after 30 min
Placed at 4 °C	26.2 ± 2.0	32 ± 9	Layering	Clear liquid
Placed at 25 °C	31.7 ± 2.4	26 ± 5	Layering	Clear liquid
Placed at 30 °C	31.3 ± 0.4	23 ± 7	Layering	Clear liquid
Placed at 40 °C	27.7 ± 0.1	29 ± 3	Layering	Clear liquid

Table 8. The effects of different dilution media on the efficiency of self-microemulsifacation of GTP-PC-SNEDDS.

Different Media	Particle Size (nm)
0.1 M HCl	27.8 ± 3.9
pH 6.8 PBS	46.7 ± 2.1
Distilled Water	24.6 ± 3.4

Table 9. The effects of different dilution multi on the efficiency of self-microemulsifacation of GTP-PC-SNEDDS.

Diluted Multi	Particle Size (nm)
100	29.7 ± 4.4
250	27.8 ± 3.9
500	27.5 ± 4.5
1000	3.2 ± 0.6

As described in Table 6, the formulation with the weight ratio of 1:10 (GTP-PC:blank SNEDDS) could form a stable self-microemulsion in both the PBS and HCl. This might be related to the solubility of GTP-PC. When the weight ratio was 1:10, the most stable self-microemulsion with the smallest particle size could be formed. With the increase of drug concentration, resulting in the increase of phospholipids, the particle size of self-microemulsion became bigger, which would affect the efficiency of the self-microemulsification. In addition, the undissolved drugs also had some influence on the particle size and stability of the system. Therefore, the ratio of drug-to-blank medium was 1:10 (*w/w*).

As shown in Table 7, the GTP-PC-SNEDDS prepared by ultrasonic method and volution would become turbid after dilution, and then be clear after standing for 30 min. Therefore, the excessively vigorous preparation process had a certain influence on the self-microemulsifying drug delivery system. Prepared by placing at different temperature, the self-microemulsifying drug delivery system would become layered, implying that it was an unstable system. The GTP-PC-SNEDDS, prepared by stirring at room temperature, was the most stable system with the smallest particle size and the shortest self-microemulsification time.

The effects of different dilution media on the efficiency of self-microemulsifacation is shown in Table 8. After being diluted 250 times by different media, the particle diameters of GTP-PC-SNEDDS, from large to small, were: pH 6.8 PBS > 0.1 M HCl ≈ distilled water. It might be due to the NaCl in the PBS, which can cause salting out to lower the surfactant content and reduce the solubility of the surfactant, resulting in an increase in particle size. After repeated verification, the particle size in PBS was about two times larger than that in HCl, and the system was relatively stable. Considering the cost and ease of operation, the 0.1 M HCl was used to replace pH 6.8 PBS for the following investigation.

As described in Table 9, there was not a significant effect on the particle size of GTP-PC-SNEDDS when it was diluted 100–500 times by 0.1 M HCl. However, the particle size was remarkably reduced when it was diluted 1000 times, which might be due to the fact that SNEDDS was in a solution state after being infinitely diluted. In keeping with the previous investigations, the dilution factor was chosen to be 250 times.

In summary, the preparation process with the following parameters had the highest efficiency of self-microemulsifacation of GTP-PC-SNEDDS: the ratio of GTP-PC to blank was 1:10, and then the mixture was stirred at room temperature to form GTP-PC-SNEDDS, which was diluted 250 times by 0.1 M HCl, subsequently.

After many validation tests, the formulation with the most stable system was determined, and it had the highest solubility, a suitable particle size (<100 nm), and a shorter emulsion time (<2 min). Therefore, the optimal prescription was as follows: Maisin 35-1:Miglycol = 30%, Labrasol: Cremophor EL = 14 = 40%, Transcutol P = 30%, and Maisin 35-1:Miglycol = 12, and the ratio of GTP-PC to blank was 1:10; then, the mixture was stirred at 37 °C for 1 d and placed for 2 d to form stable GTP-PC-SNEDDS.

2.4. Characterization of GTP-PC-SNEDDS

2.4.1. Transmittance Electron Microscope

The diluted GTP-PC-SNEDDS was examined by a transmission electron microscope. Because the particle size of GTP-PC-SNEDDS was only about 20 nm, which could easily form a relatively uniform spherical emulsion, the emulsion droplets were small and evenly dispersed under transmission electron microscope after negative staining with 1% phosphotungstic acid.

2.4.2. Droplet Size and Zeta Potential

As presented in Figure 5A,B, the average droplet sizes of GTP-PC-SNEDDS diluted by pH 1.0 HCl or pH 6.8 PBS were (25.2 ± 5.3) nm and (46.7 ± 8.2) nm, respectively, showing Gaussian distribution. The Zeta potentials of the GTP-PC-SNEDDS diluted by pH 1.0 HCl or pH 6.8 PBS were (−19.23 ± 5.84) mV and (−23.43 ± 3.93) mV, respectively, showing no significant difference ($p > 0.05$).

2.4.3. Stability of Microemulsion Particle Size after Microemulsification

As described in Table 10, the particle size of the self-microemulsifying solution was not significantly changed within 8 h after dilution with 0.1 M HCl and distilled water ($p > 0.05$), and there was no drug for crystallization. However, the particle size of GTP-PC-SNEDDS diluted in pH 6.8 PBS significantly increased with time, and this might be due to the present of salt in PBS, which can reduce the surfactant content by salting out. The decrease of the surfactant content will reduce the surfactant solubilizing ability and weaken the self-microemulsifying ability, resulting in an increase in particle size. The larger particle size may be also due to the easily aggregation of the particles when dispersed in pH 6.8 PBS, with time increasing [39].

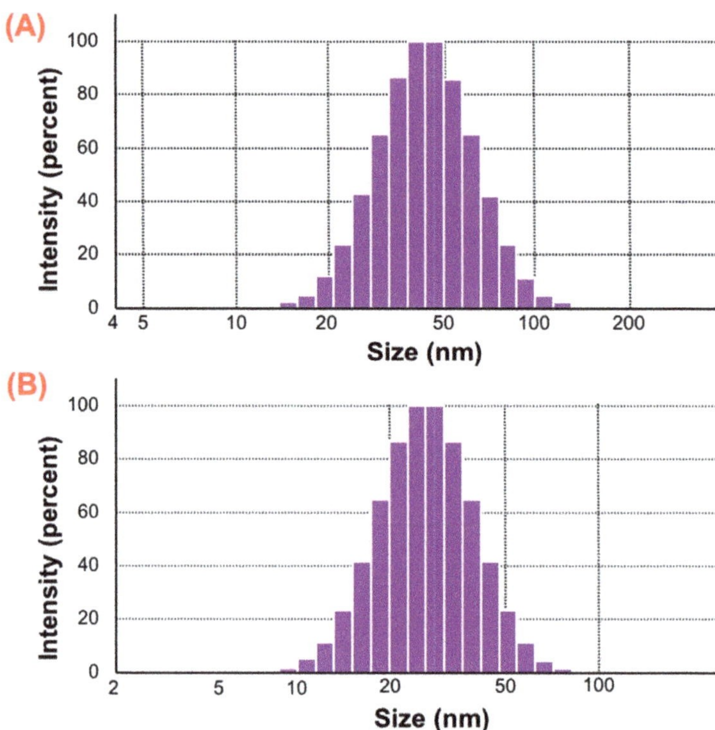

Figure 5. Characterization of GTP-PC-SNEDDS. (**A**): Particle Size distribution in dynamic light scattering (DLS) of SNEDDS at the dilution of 1:250 by pH 6.8 PBS. (**B**): Particle Size distribution DLS of SNEDDS at the dilution of 1:250 by pH 1.0 HCl.

Table 10. Stability of particle size after self-microemulsifying in 0.1 M HCl, pH 6.8 PBS, and distilled water at 37 °C.

Time (h)	HCl Particle Size (nm)	pH 6.8 PBS Particle Size (nm)	Distilled Water Particle Size (nm)
0	27.8 ± 3.9	46.7 ± 2.1	24.6 ± 3.4
1	30.5 ± 5.0	56.7 ± 8.5	28.2 ± 4.1
2	31.5 ± 4.4	62.7 ± 8.4	30.8 ± 4.8
4	32.7 ± 4.3	61.6 ± 5.7	31.4 ± 3.9
8	35.4 ± 5.7	65.3 ± 6.2	34.6 ± 2.5

Therefore, since various salts are present in the intestinal tract, the particle size of the self-microemulsifying liquid in the intestinal tract easily became larger.

2.5. Bioavailability Experiments in Rats

Figure 6 shows the complete separation of the GTP in plasma under analytical conditions (A = 0.0133 C + 0.004, r = 0.9996), where C is the concentration ratio of GTP to theophylline, and A is the corresponding peak-area ratio of GTP/theophylline. The results attained from the RSD inter-days of low, middle, and high concentrations were 8.45%, 2.39%, and 3.78%, respectively. The corresponding RSD intra-days were 7.99%, 2.59%, and 5.42%, and the recoveries were (96.67 $\pm$ 6.22)%, (102.24 $\pm$ 2.71)%, and (102.40 $\pm$ 5.58)%, which indicated recoveries and RSD inter-days, and the RSD intra-days were satisfying, with the lowest detection limit at 50 ng·mL^{-1}.

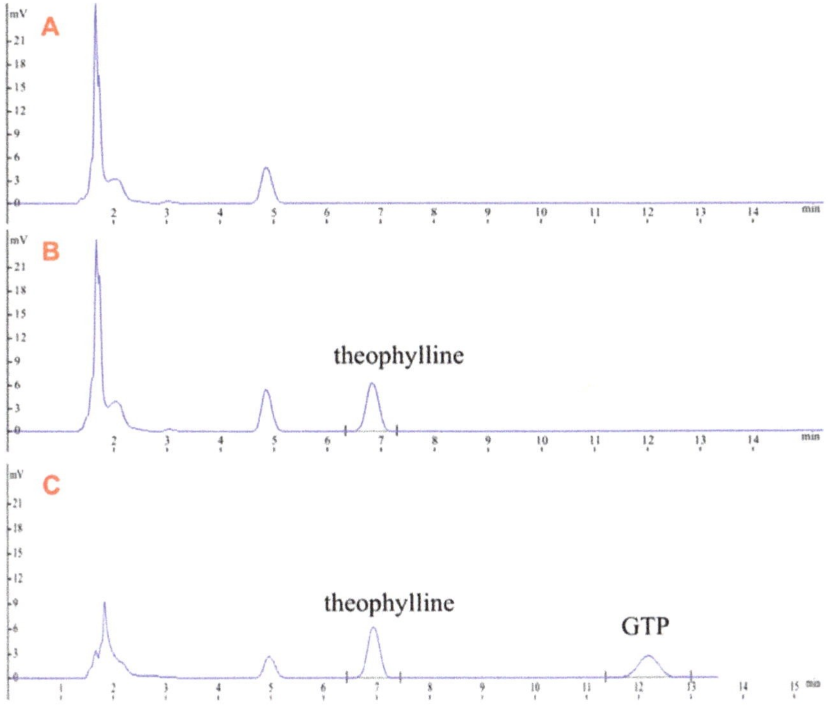

Figure 6. Typical chromatograms of (**A**) blank rat plasma; (**B**) blank rat plasma with theophylline; (**C**) blank rat plasma with theophylline and GTP.

Figure 7 and Table 11 illustrate the mean plasma concentration–time curve of GTP in rats after oral administration of GTP, GTP-PC, and GTP-PC-SNEDDS (equivalent to 80 mg/kg of GTP). All of them followed a single-compartment absorption model with first order. The main pharmacokinetic parameters of GTP and the other three formulations are presented in Table 11. As shown in Table 11, the C_{max}, $AUC_{0-\infty}$, and Fr of three formulations were significantly higher than that of GTP, demonstrating that GTP was metabolized rapidly, and its higher bioavailability could be achieved by the formation of GTP-PC and GTP-PC-SNEDDS. Among the three formations, the bioavailability of GTP-PC-SNEDDS was highest, with approximately 2.6-fold and 1.3-fold of Fr value, compared with GTP-PC (suspension) and GTP-PC (oil solution), respectively. The improved bioavailability by GTP-PC and GTP-PC-SNEDDS might be attributed to the following reasons: (1) phospholipids are an important component of cell membrane, having the effects of keeping the cell membrane fluidity. Moreover, phosphatidylcholine and its digestion product lysophosphatidylcholine could promote lymphatic transport efficiently [40–42]. (2) Compared with that of GTP, the lipophilicity of GTP-PC was effectively increased, and the dissolution rate of GTP in GTP-PC was reduced. Therefore, improved bioavailability could be achieved by the use of delivery systems, which could enhance the rate and/or the extent of drug absorbing into intestinal mucosa [43]. (3) The instability of GTP in GI tract might decrease the bioavailability and activity of the GTP; however, the GTP-PC and GTP-PC-SNEDDS might protect it from metabolization by gastric secretions and gut bacteria [44–46] and improve the absorption of GTP. (4) By enhancing the solubility of bile to GTP, liver targeting may be facilitated, and phosphatidylcholine also acts as a hepatoprotective, hence giving the synergistic effect. Additionally, compared with GTP-PC, these fine droplets, with nano-size, produced by GTP-PC-SNEDDS could further enhance the dispersion of drug dissolved inside the oil phase into gastrointestinal fluid, resulting in the significant improvement of absorption in gastrointestinal (GI) tract.

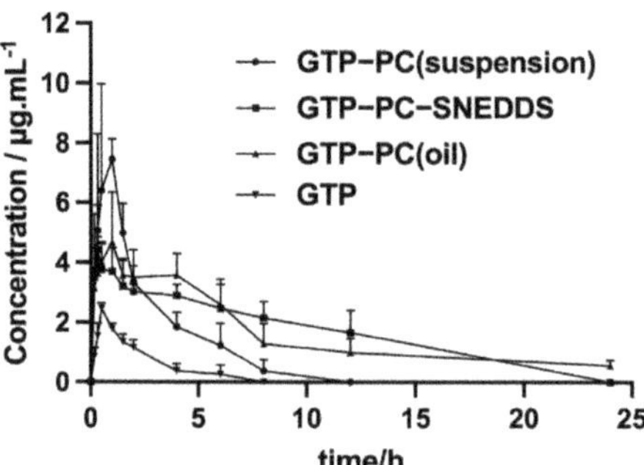

Figure 7. Mean plasma concentration–time curve of GTP, GTP-PC (suspension), GTP-PC (oil) solution, and GTP-PC-SNEDDS after single po dose of 80 mg/kg GTP in SD rats, n = 6.

Table 11. Pharmacokinetic parameters and bioavailability of GTP, GTP-PC (suspension), and GTP-PC (oil solution) to SD rats (n = 6).

Parameter	GTP	GTP: Phospholipids = 1:2 (Suspension)	GTP: Phospholipids = 1:2 (Oil Solution)	GTP-PCSMEDDS
A	3.486 ± 1.391	8.961 ± 2.677	4.666 ± 0.904	3.954 ± 0.554
K_a/h^{-1}	5.362 ± 3.319	2.275 ± 0.411	6.303 ± 3.873	18.123 ± 15.921
K_e/h^{-1}	0.550 ± 0.295	0.338 ± 0.059	0.115 ± 0.038	0.086 ± 0.045
$T_{1/2Ka}/h$	0.160 ± 0.099	0.310 ± 0.056	0.110 ± 0.061	0.061 ± 0.042
$T_{1/2Ke}/h$	1.473 ± 0.790	2.085 ± 0.364	6.049 ± 1.351	10.233 ± 6.400
T_{max}/h	0.604 ± 0.138	1.001 ± 0.070 *	0.665 ± 0.388	0.452 ± 0.306 *
$C_{max}/\mu g \cdot mL^{-1}$	2.417 ± 0.227	7.365 ± 0.760 **	4.682 ± 1.645 *	4.369 ± 1.503 *
$AUC_{0-\infty}/\mu g \cdot mL^{-1} \cdot h$	6.273 ± 2.123	23.375 ± 10.665 **	47.009 ± 20.532 **	60.749 ± 33.759 **
Fr (%)	-	372.65	749.45	968.49

* $p < 0.05$ and ** $p < 0.01$ indicate a statistically significant difference, when compared with GTP concentration used Student's *t* test; K_a: rate constant of absorption; K_e: rate constant of elimination; $T_{1/2Ka}$: absorption half-life; $T_{1/2Ke}$: elimination half-life; T_{max}: time to reach peak concentration; C_{max}: the maximum concentration; $AUC_{0-\infty}$: the area under the plasma concentration–time curve; Fr: relative bioavailability.

3. Materials and Methods

3.1. Material and Animals

National Institute for Control of Pharmaceuticals supplied the reference substances of GTP with purity of 98%. GTP extract with a purity of 85% (*w/w*) was isolated in our laboratory and used for preparation of GTP-PC and GTP-PC-SNEDDS. Soybean phospholipids were obtained from Shanghai Tai-Wei pharmaceutical Co. Ltd. (Shanghai, China), and the phosphatidylcholine content was about 98% (*w/w*). Egg yolk phospholipid and hydrogenated phospholipid were presented by Lipoid Company (Ludwigshafen, LS, Germany). Imwitor 742 and Migyol 812N were presented by SASOL Company (Johannesburg, JB, South Africa). Maisin 35-1, Labrasol, Plurol Qleique CC 497, and Transcutol P were presented by GATTEFOSSE SAS Company (SAINT-PRIEST, SP, France). Cremophor EL was purchased from Shanghai Licheng Food Industry Co., Ltd (Shanghai, China). HPLC-grade methanol was purchased from TEDIA company, Inc. (Fairfield, CA, USA). A Milli-Q water purification system (Millipore, Bedford, MA, USA) was used to purify the water. All other chemicals were of analytical grade.

Male SD rats (180 ± 20 g) were supplied by Experimental Animal Center of Chinese Academy of Sciences. The rats were housed in an environmentally controlled room. Unless otherwise indicated, standard laboratory food and water were given. The Animal Experimentation Ethics Committee of Fudan University recommended all animal experimentation procedures (2019-03-YJ-WJX-01).

3.2. Chromatography

The GTP in GTP-PC was analyzed by LC-20AB HPLC system with SPD-20A UV detector (SHIMADZU, Kyoto, Japan) at 270 nm. The chromatography was performed on a Venusil MP C_{18} column 300A (150 mm × 4.6 mm, 5 μm) by using a mixture of methanol–water (30:70, *v/v*) as mobile phase at 1 mL/min and 30 °C. The GTP concentration in plasma samples were also detected following this method, except for the mobile phase, which was changed to a mixture of methanol–water (24:76, *v/v*).

The GTP content in GTP-PC was determined according to the external standard method. The peak area of GTP had a good linear relationship, with a concentration ranging from 19.84 to 744 μg/mL. The standard curve equation between peak area of GTP (A) and its concentration (C, μg/mL) was A = 6808.5C + (r = 0.9999). While the GTP was quantitatively determined by internal standard method, theophylline was used as internal standard. The linear regression curve between GTP concentration (C, μg/mL) and peak radio between GTP and theophylline (A) was calculated. The r value was 0.9996, indicating this curve had a good linear relationship (A = 0.033 C + 0.004).

3.3. Preparation of GTP-PC

3.3.1. Complexation Efficiency of GTP-PC

The complexation efficiency of GTP-PC was measured as previously reported [36]. Briefly, methanol and dichloromethane were used to dissolve two samples of GTP-PC with approximately the same amount. After the dichloromethane solution was filtered, the GTP contents in both the methanol and dichloromethane solutions were determined by HPLC, as described in Section 3.2. The GTP in dichloromethane and methnol was regarded as complexed GTP and total GTP in GTP-PC (complexed and uncomplexed), respectively, because methanol can easily dissolve complexed and uncomplexed GTP in GTP-PC, while only complexed GTP in GTP-PC is dissolvable in dichloromethane. Therefore, the complexation efficiency was calculated as follows:

$$\text{Complexation efficiency } \% = \text{Wc/Wt} \times 100\%$$

where Wc is the GTP content dissolved in dichloromethane, and Wt is the GTP content in methanol.

3.3.2. Measurement of Dissociation Rate of GTP-PC

GTP was easily dissolved in water, but GTP-PC was practically insoluble. GTP dissolved in water was considered to be from the dissociation of GTP-PC. The dissolution studies could be carried out using the paddle method to assess the dissociation of GTP-PC [47]. At 37 °C, 200 mL of pH 6.8 phosphate buffer saline (PBS) was continually stirred at 50 rpm in dissolution flasks. The stirred medium was first containing GTP-PC (0.2 g). At 10, 20, 30, 45, 60, and 120 min, 5 mL samples were withdrawn and filtrated with 0.45 μm cellulose nitrate membranes, and then 5 mL fresh mediums were added into flask. The GTP concentration in the resulting solution was determined by HPLC by mixing 0.4 mL filtrate with 4 mL PBS. The dissociation rate was calculated according to the following equation [48]:

$$\text{Log C} = \text{Log C}_0 - \text{Kt}/2.303$$

where C_0 is the initial concentration of GTP, K is the first order rate constant, and t is the time in hours.

3.3.3. Investigations of GTP-PC

GTP and phospholipid were placed in a round-bottom flask and suspended in different solvents (trichloromethane, ethyl acetate, and tetrahydrofuran) with a certain molar ratio (GTP: phospholipids = 2:1, 1:1, 1:2, 1:3, and 1:4). Then, the mixture was stirred at 40 °C for different times (0.5 h, 1 h, 2 h, 3 h, 4 h, 5 h, and 6 h). The dried residues were collected as GTP-PC after the solvent was evaporated off under vacuum at 40 °C. By measuring complexation efficiency and dissociation, the optimal preparation process for GTP-PC was determined.

3.4. Characterization of GTP-PC

3.4.1. Differential Scanning Calorimetry (DSC)

In a nitrogen atmosphere, samples sealed in aluminum crimp cells were heated at 10 °C/min from 0 °C to 300 °C (PERKIN-ELMER 7, Waltham, MA, USA). The peak transition onset temperatures of four types of samples were compared, including phospholipid, GTP, the mixture of phospholipid and GTP, and the GTP-PC.

3.4.2. X-ray Diffractometry (XRD)

Using a graphite monochromator with Cu/Ka radiation with a voltage window of 40 kV and current density of 60 mA with a scanning rate of 4 °C/min ranging from 5 °C to 45 °C, the X-ray diffraction (D/MAXX Rigaku, Tokyo, Japan) was performed.

3.4.3. Fourier Transform Infrared Spectra (FT-IR)

Samples were compressed into a KBr pellet, and their FT-IR spectra were recorded by FT-IR spectrometer (Avatar TM 360E.S.P.TM, Avatar).

3.4.4. Thin-Layer Chromatography (TLC)

Sample was prepared by dissolving standard GTP, GTP-PC, the physical mixture, and GTP-PC in methanol. The experiment was carried out according to a TLC test of China pharmacopoeia. A total of 5 µL solution was spotted onto a silica gel GF254 plate with ethyl acetate-menthol-water (20:2:1, *v/v/v*) as developing solvent. The resulting plate had a picture taken under ultraviolet lamp (254 nm).

3.4.5. Ultraviolet (UV) Spectra

Sample methanol solutions were scanned by a UV spectrometer over the wavenumber range of 200–400 nm.

3.4.6. Dissolution Studies in Phosphate Buffer Saline (pH 6.8)

The dissolution studies were carried out according to paddle method demonstrated in Section 3.3.2. Additionally, samples were withdrawn at 10 min, 20 min, 30 min, 1 h, 2 h, 4 h, 6 h, 8 h, and 12 h.

3.5. Preparation of GTP-PC-SNEDDS

3.5.1. Solubility Studies

Suitable excipients for preparation of GTP-PC were screened by solubility studies. Briefly, excess GTP-PC was added into about 1 g of various oils, surfactants, or co-surfactants, respectively. Then, the mixture was shaken at 37 °C for 48 h; after centrifuging at rpm for 10 min, the content of GTP was assayed by HPLC, and the GTP solubility of GTP-PC in each oily medium was calculated.

3.5.2. Construction of Pseudo-Ternary Phase Diagrams

Pseudo-ternary phase diagrams can be used for preliminary screening of self-microemulsifying systems. The points in the triangle represent the different composition ratios of ternary systems, such as oil phase, surfactant, and cosurfactant. In this work, about 1 g of blank formulation (only including different ratios of oil phase, surfactant, and cosurfactant) was first weighed accurately, and then about 10% (*w/w*) of GTP-PC was added. The mixture was stirred at 37 °C for 24 h and followed to keep for 48 h to observe whether all the drugs were dissolved and formed a uniform and transparent solution. If so, part of formulation (equivalent to 4 mg of GTP) was diluted 250 times with 0.1 M HCl and then stirred at 37 °C and 50 rpm. If a clear and transparent solution could be formed, it is believed that the formulation, including this ratio of oil phase, surfactant, and cosurfactant, could been used to form microemulsion and draw pseudo-ternary phase diagrams, in turn.

3.5.3. Investigations of GTP-PC-SNEDDS

In order to optimize the preparation process of GTP-PC-SNEDDS, the effects of weight ratios of GTP-PC to blank SNEDDS, preparation technology, dilution media, and dilution multi were further investigated.

3.5.4. Characterization of GTP-PC-SNEDDS
Morphological Characterization

Transmission electron microscope (TEM) (PHILIPS CM-120, Eindhoven, EIN, Netherlands) was used to observe the morphology of SMEDDS. SMEDDS was diluted with distilled water 1:25 and gently shaken to mix. Afterwards, a drop of the diluted sample was placed on copper grids, and the excess was rubbed off with filter paper. The grids were then stained with 1% phosphor-tungstic acid solution for 30 s.

Droplet Size and Zeta Potential

Droplet size distribution and zeta potential of GTP-PC-SNEDDS were determined using NICOMP 380 ZLS Zeta Potential/Particle Sizer (PSS-380, NICOMP, Santa Barbara, CA, USA).

Solubility

Excess GTP-PC was added into about 0.5 g of blank formulation, which was shaken at 37 °C for 48 h and then centrifuged at 15,000 rpm for 10 min. The solubility of GTP in blank formulation was evaluated by the content measurement of GTP in supernatant by HPLC.

Self-Microemulsifying Time

The self-microemulsifying time of GTP-PC-SNEDDS was analyzed according to Chinese pharmacopoeia (2015 edition). Certain amount of formulation (equivalent to 4 mg of GTP) was diluted 250 times with 0.1 M HCl, and then stirred at 37 °C and 50 rpm. Self-microemulsifying time was recorded, since the droplets contacted with the liquid level to a clear and transparent solution was formed. According to the literature, the time of self-microemulsification should not exceed 2 min.

3.6. Bioavailability Experiments in Rats
3.6.1. Plasma Sample Preparation and Validity

A total of 250 µL internal standard solution (4.031 µg/mL theophylline in methanol solution) was added to 100 µL plasma and agitated for 30 s. Then, the solution was centrifuged (15 min). Aliquots (20 µL) of the supernatant were injected for HPLC analysis.

Rat plasma blanks were supplemented with different amounts of GTP for validation of the method. The resulting concentrations of GTP were 0.13, 0.53, 5.3, 21.2, and 42.4 µg/mL. For testing the method's precision, accuracy, and detection limit, the calibrations were subjected to the above analytical procedure.

3.6.2. Pharmacokinetic Study

Twelve four male rats (150–200 g) were divided randomly into four groups, and each group had six animals. They were fasted for 24 h, but allowed to take water freely. They were orally administered GTP solution in water (equivalent to 80 mg/kg of GTP), GTP-PC suspension in oil (equivalent to 80 mg/kg of GTP), GTP-PC suspension in water (equivalent to 80 mg/kg of GTP), and GTP-PC–SNEDDS (equivalent to 80 mg/kg of GTP), respectively. About 0.4 mL blood samples were collected from the tail vein into tubes containing heparin at 0.17, 0.33, 0.5, 1, 1.5, 2, 4, 6, 8, 12, and 24 h. Plasma was separated by centrifugation (5000 rpm, 10 min) and stored at −20 °C until analysis.

Peak concentration (C_{max}) and peak times (t_{max}) were derived directly from the experiment points, and $AUC_{0-\infty}$ was calculated by trapezoidal method. A computer program called 3p87 was used to compute the rest of the pharmacokinetic parameters.

4. Conclusions

In this study, we firstly prepared GTP-PC by studying the factors affecting the formation of GTP-PC with complexation efficiency and a dissociation experiment. DSC, XRD, FT-IR, TLC, and UV measurements confirmed that GTP is bonded to phospholipids only through hydrogen bonds and/or van der Waals forces. Then, GTP-PC was loaded into SNEDDS by investigating the effects of the weight ratios of GTP-PC to blank SNEDDS, preparation technology, dilution media, and dilution multi based on the screening results of the oils, surfactants, and cosurfactants. As a result, the dissolution of the GTP in GTP-PC was delayed, compared with GTP material. In rats, GTP-PC and GTP-SNEDDS could significantly enhance GTP bioavailability, compared with GTP. Our study may serve as a basis for the clinical applications of GTP-PC and GTP-PC-SNEDDS.

There are also the same limits for this work, for example, the morphology and sizes of aggregates of GTP-PC were not characterized. The characterization of SNEDDS without GTP-PC, including size, Z-potential, and PDI, was not clarified. Furthermore, several studies need to be further executed, such as regarding the absorbed mechanism of GTP-PC and GTP-PC-SNEDDS, an experiment with the delivery of GTP to show that the GTP-PC and GTP-PC-SNEDDS are really able to work in vivo.

Author Contributions: Conceptualization, J.W.; data curation, W.S. and Y.T.; writing—original draft preparation, Y.T. and W.S.; writing—review and editing, Y.T., J.W. and Q.Z.; methodology, W.S. and Q.Z., formal analysis, Y.T., J.W. and Q.Z.; supervision, J.W. All authors have read and agreed to the published version of the manuscript.

Funding: This research was funded by National Natural Science Foundation of China (No. 81573616 and No. 81773911) and the Development Project of Shanghai Peak Disciplines-Integrative Medicine (20180101).

Institutional Review Board Statement: The animal study protocol was approved by The Animal Experimentation Ethics Committee of Fudan University (2019-03-YJ-WJX-01).

Informed Consent Statement: Not applicable.

Data Availability Statement: Data is contained within the article.

Conflicts of Interest: The authors declare no conflict of interest.

References

1. Zhang, X.; Zhan, G.; Jin, M.; Zhang, H.; Dang, J.; Zhang, Y.; Guo, Z.; Ito, Y. Botany, traditional use, phytochemistry, pharmacology, quality control, and authentication of Radix Gentianae Macrophyllae-A traditional medicine: A review. *Phytomedicine* **2018**, *46*, 142–163. [CrossRef] [PubMed]
2. Li, X.H.; Yang, C.L.; Shen, H. Gentiopicroside exerts convincing antitumor effects in human ovarian carcinoma cells (SKOV3) by inducing cell cycle arrest, mitochondrial mediated apoptosis and inhibition of cell migration. *J. Buon.* **2019**, *24*, 280–284. [PubMed]
3. Mudrić, J.; Janković, T.; Šavikin, K.; Bigović, D.; Đukić-Ćosić, D.; Ibrić, S.; Đuriš, J. Optimization and modelling of gentiopicroside, isogentisin and total phenolics extraction from *Gentiana lutea* L. roots. *Ind. Crops Prod.* **2020**, *155*, 112767. [CrossRef]
4. Zhang, Q.-L.; Zhang, J.; Xia, P.-F.; Peng, X.-J.; Li, H.-L.; Jin, H.; Li, Y.; Yang, J.; Zhao, L. Anti-inflammatory activities of gentiopicroside against iNOS and COX-2 targets. *Chin. Herb. Med.* **2019**, *11*, 108–112. [CrossRef]
5. Chang, Y.; Tian, Y.; Zhou, D.; Yang, L.; Liu, T.-M.; Liu, Z.-G.; Wang, S.-W. Gentiopicroside ameliorates ethanol-induced gastritis via regulating MMP-10 and pERK1/2 signaling. *Int. Immunopharmacol.* **2021**, *90*, 107213. [CrossRef]
6. Zhang, Y.; Yang, X.; Wang, S.; Song, S.; Yang, X. Gentiopicroside prevents alcoholic liver damage by improving mitochondrial dysfunction in the rat model. *Phytotherapy Res.* **2021**, *35*, 2230–2251. [CrossRef]
7. Xu, Z.; Zhang, M.; Wang, Y.; Chen, R.; Xu, S.; Sun, X.; Yang, Y.; Lin, Z.; Wang, S.; Huang, H. Gentiopicroside Ameliorates Diabetic Renal Tubulointerstitial Fibrosis via Inhibiting the AT1R/CK2/NF-κB Pathway. *Front. Pharmacol.* **2022**, *13*, 848915. [CrossRef]

8. Xiao, H.; Sun, X.; Lin, Z.; Yang, Y.; Zhang, M.; Xu, Z.; Liu, P.; Liu, Z.; Huang, H. Gentiopicroside targets PAQR3 to activate the PI3K/AKT signaling pathway and ameliorate disordered glucose and lipid metabolism. *Acta Pharm. Sin. B* **2022**, *12*, 2887–2904. [CrossRef]

9. Jia, N.; Ma, H.; Zhang, T.; Wang, L.; Cui, J.; Zha, Y.; Ding, Y.; Wang, J. Gentiopicroside attenuates collagen-induced arthritis in mice via modulating the CD147/p38/NF-κB pathway. *Int. Immunopharmacol.* **2022**, *108*, 108854. [CrossRef]

10. Wang, C.-H.; Wang, Z.-T.; Bligh, S.W.A.; White, K.N.; White, C.J.B. Pharmacokinetics and tissue distribution of Gentiopicroside following oral and intravenous administration in mice. *Eur. J. Drug Metab. Pharmacokinet.* **2004**, *29*, 199–203. [CrossRef]

11. Wang, C.H.; Cheng, X.M.; He, Y.-Q.; White, K.N.; Bligh, S.W.A.; Branford-White, C.J.; Wang, Z.-T. Pharmacokinetic behavior of gentiopicroside from decoction of Radix Gentianae, Gentiana macrophylla after oral administration in rats: A pharmacokinetic comaprison with gentiopicroside after oral and intravenous administration alone. *Arch. Pharmacal Res.* **2007**, *30*, 1149–1154. [CrossRef] [PubMed]

12. Wang, C.-H.; Cheng, X.-M.; Bligh, S.W.A.; White, K.N.; Branford-White, C.J.; Wang, Z.-T. Pharmacokinetics and bioavailability of gentiopicroside from decoctions of Gentianae and Longdan Xiegan Tang after oral administration in rats—Comparison with gentiopicroside alone. *J. Pharm. Biomed. Anal.* **2007**, *44*, 1113–1117. [CrossRef] [PubMed]

13. Xiong, K.; Gao, T.; Zhang, T.; Wang, Z.; Han, H. Simultaneous determination of gentiopicroside and its two active metabolites in rat plasma by LC–MS/MS and its application in pharmacokinetic studies. *J. Chromatogr. B-Anal. Technol. Biomed. Life Sci.* **2017**, *1065*, 1–7. [CrossRef] [PubMed]

14. Zeng, W.; Han, H.; Tao, Y.; Yang, L.; Wang, Z.; Chen, K. Identification of bio-active metabolites of gentiopicroside by UPLC/Q-TOF MS and NMR. *Biomed. Chromatogr.* **2013**, *27*, 1129–1136. [CrossRef] [PubMed]

15. Chang-Liao, W.-L.; Chien, C.-F.; Lin, L.-C.; Tsai, T.-H. Isolation of gentiopicroside from Gentianae Radix and its pharmacokinetics on liver ischemia/reperfusion rats. *J. Ethnopharmacol.* **2012**, *141*, 668–673. [CrossRef] [PubMed]

16. Lu, C.-M.; Lin, L.-C.; Tsai, T.-H. Determination and Pharmacokinetic Study of Gentiopicroside, Geniposide, Baicalin, and Swertiamarin in Chinese Herbal Formulae after Oral Administration in Rats by LC-MS/MS. *Molecules* **2014**, *19*, 21560–21578. [CrossRef]

17. Babazadeh, A.; Zeinali, M.; Hamishehkar, H. Nano-Phytosome: A Developing Platform for Herbal Anti-Cancer Agents in Cancer Therapy. *Curr. Drug Targets* **2018**, *19*, 170–180. [CrossRef]

18. Salem, H.F.; Kharshoum, R.M.; Sayed, O.M.; Hakim, L.F.A. Formulation development of self-nanoemulsifying drug delivery system of celecoxib for the management of oral cavity inflammation. *J. Liposome Res.* **2019**, *29*, 195–205. [CrossRef]

19. Patel, P.; Pailla, S.R.; Rangaraj, N.; Cheruvu, H.S.; Dodoala, S.; Sampathi, S. Quality by Design Approach for Developing Lipid-Based Nanoformulations of Gliclazide to Improve Oral Bioavailability and Anti-Diabetic Activity. *AAPS PharmSciTech* **2019**, *20*, 45. [CrossRef]

20. Ashfaq, M.; Shah, S.; Rasul, A.; Hanif, M.; Khan, H.U.; Khames, A.; Abdelgawad, M.A.; Ghoneim, M.M.; Ali, M.Y.; Abourehab, M.A.S.; et al. Enhancement of the Solubility and Bioavailability of Pitavastatin through a Self-Nanoemulsifying Drug Delivery System (SNEDDS). *Pharmaceutics* **2022**, *14*, 482. [CrossRef]

21. Kuche, K.; Bhargavi, N.; Dora, C.P.; Jain, S. Drug-Phospholipid Complex—A Go Through Strategy for Enhanced Oral Bioavailability. *AAPS PharmSciTech* **2019**, *20*, 43. [CrossRef] [PubMed]

22. Zhang, J.; Peng, Q.; Shi, S.; Zhang, Q.; Sun, X.; Gong, T.; Zhang, Z. Preparation, characterization, and in vivo evaluation of a self-nanoemulsifying drug delivery system (SNEDDS) loaded with morin-phospholipid complex. *Int. J. Nanomed.* **2011**, *6*, 3405–3414. [CrossRef]

23. Zhang, J.; Li, J.; Ju, Y.; Fu, Y.; Gong, T.; Zhang, Z. Mechanism of Enhanced Oral Absorption of Morin by Phospholipid Complex Based Self-Nanoemulsifying Drug Delivery System. *Mol. Pharm.* **2015**, *12*, 504–513. [CrossRef] [PubMed]

24. Zhang, J.; Shuai, X.; Li, J.; Xiang, N.; Gong, T.; Zhang, Z. Biodistribution, hypouricemic efficacy and therapeutic mechanism of morin phospholipid complex loaded self-nanoemulsifying drug delivery systems in an experimental hyperuricemic model in rats. *J. Pharm. Pharmacol.* **2016**, *68*, 14–25. [CrossRef]

25. Li, J.; Yang, Y.; Ning, E.; Peng, Y.; Zhang, J. Mechanisms of poor oral bioavailability of flavonoid Morin in rats: From physico-chemical to biopharmaceutical evaluations. *Eur. J. Pharm. Sci.* **2019**, *128*, 290–298. [CrossRef]

26. Li, F.; Shen, J.; Bi, J.; Tian, H.; Jin, Y.; Wang, Y.; Yang, X.; Yang, Z.; Kou, J. Preparation and evaluation of a self-nanoemulsifying drug delivery system loaded with Akebia saponin D–phospholipid complex. *Int. J. Nanomed.* **2016**, *11*, 4919–4929. [CrossRef]

27. Wang, Y.; Shen, J.; Yang, X.; Jin, Y.; Yang, Z.; Wang, R.; Zhang, F.; Linhardt, R.J. Mechanism of enhanced oral absorption of akebia saponin D by a self-nanoemulsifying drug delivery system loaded with phospholipid complex. *Drug Dev. Ind. Pharm.* **2019**, *45*, 124–129. [CrossRef]

28. Beg, S.; Alam, M.N.; Ahmad, F.J.; Singh, B. Chylomicron mimicking nanocolloidal carriers of rosuvastatin calcium for lymphatic drug targeting and management of hyperlipidemia. *Colloids Surf. B Biointerfaces* **2019**, *177*, 541–549. [CrossRef]

29. Ding, D.; Sun, B.; Cui, W.; Chen, Q.; Zhang, X.; Zhang, H.; He, Z.; Sun, J.; Luo, C. Integration of phospholipid-drug complex into self-nanoemulsifying drug delivery system to facilitate oral delivery of paclitaxel. *Asian J. Pharm. Sci.* **2019**, *14*, 552–558. [CrossRef]

30. Shukla, M.; Jaiswal, S.; Sharma, A.; Srivastava, P.K.; Arya, A.; Dwivedi, A.K.; Lal, J. A combination of complexation and self-nanoemulsifying drug delivery system for enhancing oral bioavailability and anticancer efficacy of curcumin. *Drug Dev. Ind. Pharm.* **2017**, *43*, 847–861. [CrossRef]

31. Avachat, A.M.; Patel, V.G. Self nanoemulsifying drug delivery system of stabilized ellagic acid–phospholipid complex with improved dissolution and permeability. *Saudi Pharm. J.* **2015**, *23*, 276–289. [CrossRef]

32. Wu, H.; Long, X.; Yuan, F.; Chen, L.; Pan, S.; Liu, Y.; Stowell, Y.; Li, X. Combined use of phospholipid complexes and self-emulsifying microemulsions for improving the oral absorption of a BCS class IV compound, baicalin. *Acta Pharm. Sin. B* **2014**, *4*, 217–226. [CrossRef] [PubMed]

33. Ruan, J.; Liu, J.; Zhu, D.; Gong, T.; Yang, F.; Hao, X.; Zhang, Z. Preparation and evaluation of self-nanoemulsified drug delivery systems (SNEDDSs) of matrine based on drug–phospholipid complex technique. *Int. J. Pharm.* **2010**, *386*, 282–290. [CrossRef] [PubMed]

34. Phan, T.N.Q.; Shahzadi, I.; Bernkop-Schnürch, A. Hydrophobic ion-pairs and lipid-based nanocarrier systems: The perfect match for delivery of BCS class 3 drugs. *J. Control. Release* **2019**, *304*, 146–155. [CrossRef] [PubMed]

35. Zhao, W.-N.; Shang, P.-P.; Sun, W.-J. HPLC determination of apparent n-octanol/water partition coefficient of gentiopicroside. *Chin. J. Pharm. Anal.* **2009**, *7*, 1093–1095.

36. Shi, W.; Gao, D.-Y.; Wang, J.-X.; Han, L.-M. Analysis method of gentiopicroside in rat plasma and its application in investigation of preparation technology of phytosome. *Fudan Univ. J. Med. Sci.* **2009**, *3*, 342–345.

37. Maiti, K.; Mukherjee, K.; Gantait, A.; Saha, B.P.; Mukherjee, P.K. Curcumin–phospholipid complex: Preparation, therapeutic evaluation and pharmacokinetic study in rats. *Int. J. Pharm.* **2007**, *330*, 155–163. [CrossRef]

38. Yanyu, X.; Yunmei, S.; Zhipeng, C.; Qineng, P. The preparation of silybin–phospholipid complex and the study on its pharmacokinetics in rats. *Int. J. Pharm.* **2006**, *307*, 77–82. [CrossRef]

39. Azadbakht, M.; Nayebi, E.; Fard, R.E.; Khaleghi, F. Standardization and formulation of an herbal appetite-stimulating drug from Gentiana olivieri. *J. Herb. Med.* **2020**, *19*, 100306. [CrossRef]

40. Koo, S.I.; Noh, S.K. Phosphatidylcholine Inhibits and Lysophosphatidylcholine Enhances the Lymphatic Absorption of α-Tocopherol in Adult Rats. *J. Nutr.* **2001**, *131*, 717–722. [CrossRef]

41. Tso, P.; Lam, J.; Simmonds, W.J. The importance of the lysophosphatidylcholine and choline moiety of bile phosphatidylcholine in lymphatic transport of fat. *Biochim. Biophys. Acta Mol. Cell Biol. Lipids.* **1978**, *528*, 364–372. [CrossRef] [PubMed]

42. Trevaskis, N.L.; Porter, C.J.H.; Charman, W.N. The Lymph Lipid Precursor Pool Is a Key Determinant of Intestinal Lymphatic Drug Transport. *J. Pharmacol. Exp. Ther.* **2006**, *316*, 881–891. [CrossRef] [PubMed]

43. Yue, P.-F.; Yuan, H.-L.; Li, X.-Y.; Yang, M.; Zhu, W.-F. Process optimization, characterization and evaluation in vivo of oxymatrine–phospholipid complex. *Int. J. Pharm.* **2010**, *387*, 139–146. [CrossRef]

44. Kidd, P.; Head, K. A review of the bioavailability and clinical efficacy of milk thistle phytosome: A silybin-phosphatidylcholine complex (Siliphos). *Altern. Med. Rev.* **2005**, *10*, 193–203.

45. Bombardelli, E.; Della Loggia, R.; Sosa, S.; Spelta, M.; Tubaro, A. Aging skin: Protective effect of Silymarin-Phytosome (R). *Fitoterapia* **1991**, *62*, 115–122.

46. Kumar, P.; Yadav, S.; Agarwal, A.; Kumar, N. Phytosomes: A novel phyto-phospholipid carriers: An overview. *Int. J. Pharm. Res. Dev.* **2010**, *2*, 1–7.

47. Committee of the Chinese Pharmacopoeia. *Pharmacopoeia of the People's Republic of China*; China Medical Science Press: Beijing, China, 2020; Volume 4.

48. Telange, D.R.; Nirgulkar, S.B.; Umekar, M.J.; Patil, A.T.; Pethe, A.M.; Bali, N.R. Enhanced transdermal permeation and anti-inflammatory potential of phospholipids complex-loaded matrix film of umbelliferone: Formulation development, physico-chemical and functional characterization. *Eur. J. Pharm. Sci.* **2019**, *131*, 23–38. [CrossRef]

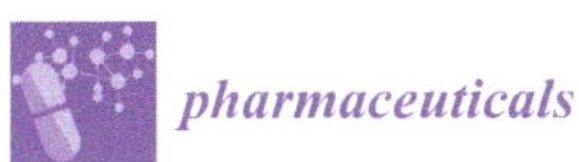

pharmaceuticals

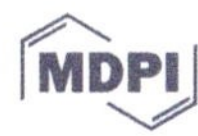

Article

Quality by Design of Pranoprofen Loaded Nanostructured Lipid Carriers and Their Ex Vivo Evaluation in Different Mucosae and Ocular Tissues

María Rincón [1], Lupe Carolina Espinoza [2], Marcelle Silva-Abreu [3,4,*], Lilian Sosa [5], Jessica Pesantez-Narvaez [6], Guadalupe Abrego [7], Ana Cristina Calpena [3,4] and Mireia Mallandrich [3,4]

[1] Department of Materials Science and Physical Chemistry, Faculty of Chemistry, University of Barcelona, C. Martí i Franquès 1-11, 08028 Barcelona, Spain
[2] Departamento de Química, Universidad Técnica Particular de Loja, Loja 1101608, Ecuador
[3] Department of Pharmacy, Pharmaceutical Technology and Physical Chemistry, Faculty of Pharmacy and Food Sciences, University of Barcelona, Av. Joan XXIII 27-31, 08028 Barcelona, Spain
[4] Institut de Nanociència i Nanotecnologia IN2UB, University of Barcelona, 08028 Barcelona, Spain
[5] Pharmaceutical Technology Research Group, Faculty of Chemical Sciences and Pharmacy, National Autonomous University of Honduras (UNAH), Tegucigalpa 11101, Honduras
[6] Departamento de Estadística, Facultad de Ciencias Sociales, Universidad Carlos III, C. Madrid, 126, 28903 Madrid, Spain
[7] Department of Chemical and Instrumental Analysis, Faculty of Chemistry and Pharmacy, University of El Salvador, Ciudad Universitaria, 28040 Madrid, Spain
* Correspondence: silvadeabreu@ub.edu

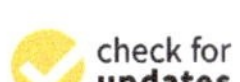

Citation: Rincón, M.; Espinoza, L.C.; Silva-Abreu, M.; Sosa, L.; Pesantez-Narvaez, J.; Abrego, G.; Calpena, A.C.; Mallandrich, M. Quality by Design of Pranoprofen Loaded Nanostructured Lipid Carriers and Their Ex Vivo Evaluation in Different Mucosae and Ocular Tissues. *Pharmaceuticals* **2022**, *15*, 1185. https://doi.org/10.3390/ph15101185

Academic Editors: Ana Catarina Silva, João Nuno Moreira and José Manuel Sousa Lobo

Received: 20 August 2022
Accepted: 19 September 2022
Published: 24 September 2022

Publisher's Note: MDPI stays neutral with regard to jurisdictional claims in published maps and institutional affiliations.

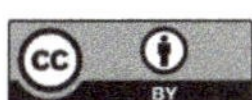

Abstract: Transmucosal delivery is commonly used to prevent or treat local diseases. Pranoprofen is an anti-inflammatory drug prescribed in postoperative cataract surgery, intraocular lens implantation, chorioretinopathy, uveitis, age-related macular degeneration or cystoid macular edema. Pranoprofen can also be used for acute and chronic management of osteoarthritis and rheumatoid arthritis. Quality by Design (QbD) provides a systematic approach to drug development and maps the influence of the formulation components. The aim of this work was to develop and optimize a nanostructured lipid carrier by means of the QbD and factorial design suitable for the topical management of inflammatory processes on mucosal tissues. To this end, the nanoparticles loading pranoprofen were prepared by a high-pressure homogenization technique with Tween 80 as stabilizer and Lanette® 18 as the solid lipid. From, the factorial design results, the PF-NLCs-N6 formulation showed the most suitable characteristics, which was selected for further studies. The permeability capacity of pranoprofen loaded in the lipid-based nanoparticles was evaluated by ex vivo transmucosal permeation tests, including buccal, sublingual, nasal, vaginal, corneal and scleral mucosae. The results revealed high permeation and retention of pranoprofen in all the tissues tested. According to the predicted plasma concentration at the steady-state, no systemic effects would be expected, any neither were any signs of ocular irritancy observed from the optimized formulation when tested by the HET-CAM technique. Hence, the optimized formulation (PF-NLCs-N6) may offer a safe and attractive nanotechnological tool in topical treatment of local inflammation on mucosal diseases.

Keywords: design of experiment; porcine mucous membrane; ophthalmic tissues; permeation; nanostructured lipid carriers

1. Introduction

Pranoprofen (PF) or 2-(5H-chromeno[2,3-b]pyridin-7-yl)propanoic acid is a non-steroidal anti-inflammatory drug (NSAID), which can be used as an effective and safe anti-inflammatory treatment option in ocular therapy [1–3]. It is usually indicated in chronic but non-bacterial inflammatory processes affecting the anterior segment of the eye and in the treatment of postoperative pain of cataract or strabismus surgery [4]. PF may also be used to control the inflammation and pain in the posterior segment, such as in the case of posterior chamber intraocular lens implantation, acute central serous chorioretinopathy, uveitis age-related macular degeneration or cystoid macular edema [5]. PF can also be used for acute and chronic management of osteoarthritis and rheumatoid arthritis [6,7]. PF inhibit COX-1 and COX-2 enzymes, and thus it blocks arachidonic acid being converted to eicosanoids and reduces prostaglandins synthesis. Although this drug has shown high anti-inflammatory and analgesic efficiency, and its side effects on the gastrointestinal tract are minimal, the pharmaceutical use of PF is limited due to its inadequate biopharmaceutical profile. PF has a short plasmatic half-life, low water solubility and is unstable in aqueous solution, particularly when exposed to light [6,8].

The application of NSAIDs through the mucosal tissues offers a set of advantages, e.g., it avoids the first pass metabolism, averts the risk of gastrointestinal disturbance, targeting only the areas of disease. The use of ophthalmic NSAIDs is the usual treatment to prevent and treat common ocular disorders inflammatory [9]. However, this conventional dosage form cannot be considered optimal in the treatment of ocular diseases due to the fact that most of the drugs is removed from the surface of the eye, following the instillation, by various mechanisms (tear dilution and tear turn over). Moreover, the relatively impermeable corneal barrier restricts the entry of foreign substances. As a result, less than 5% of the administered drug penetrates the cornea and reaches intraocular tissues [10].

Intranasal drug application is currently most used for the treatment of local inflammations such as common rhinitis, allergic rhinitis or for easing nasal congestion. The main advantage of nasal administration is the rapid drug absorption through this membrane due to the prevailing physical conditions of the nose, such as good blood circulation of the nasal mucosa, resulting in a quick local effect, and the rapid onset of action. Due to the fast local absorption, an unintentional systemic distribution of the active ingredient is prevented, eliminating the first pass metabolism and its side effects are avoided [11,12]. Other advantages are the high permeability of some drugs in the nasal epithelium and better compliance with the recommended treatment, improved comfort for the patient, and a sustained and prolonged effect compared to other delivery systems such as oral drug delivery systems [11].

The administration of drugs through the oral mucosa, particularly the buccal and sublingual mucosa, has been attracting great interest. The main advantage of using the buccal route is the direct access of drugs to the systemic circulation by the internal jugular vein, eliminating the hepatic first-pass metabolism and mitigating possible side effects [13,14]. Nevertheless, buccal drug delivery suffers from some disadvantages such as low permeability and a smaller absorptive surface area, in contrast to the high absorptive surface area of the small intestine [15,16].

Vaginal drug delivery treats or prevents diseases and allows a controlled or enhanced drug absorption with the advantage of a systemic circulation delivery of drugs avoiding the hepatic first-pass effect and gastrointestinal interferences while assuring, in accordance with the selected formulation, stable and/or high local concentrations and reduced, enhanced and/or controlled systemic absorption [17].

In an attempt to overcome, the biopharmaceutical profile and improve the permeability of drugs through the tissues, nanostructured Lipid Carriers (NLCs) are one of the colloidal systems that have been most widely studied due to their characteristics such as small particle size, biocompatibility, prolonged release, drug protection, and incorporation of both hydrophilic and lipophilic drugs [18]. In ocular delivery, conventional ophthalmic formulations are effortlessly drained through the nasolacrimal pathway, while nanoparticles are cleared more slowly and therefore can release the drug upon interaction with the cornea over a longer time period [10].

Taking into account all these considerations, the main purpose of the work in question here was to target PF-loaded NLCs (PF-NLCs) in mucosal tissues (buccal, sublingual nasal, vaginal, cornea and sclera) with controlled release effect, enhancing the contact of the PF and improving its mucosal tissues retention, thus to increase the anti-inflammatory and analgesic. For this purpose, a factorial design and detailed statistical studies shed light on the most adequate lipid and led to the optimized formulation with physicochemical properties to permeate the mucosae in a competent way. Taking into consideration that factorial designs provide the maximum information from the least number of experiments [19], a 2^3 +star central composite factorial design was applied to study the main effects and interactions of three factors: PF concentration (cPF), the concentration of the solid lipid in relation to the liquid lipid (cSL/cLL) and the concentration of Tween® 80 (cTW), on dependent variables: average particle size (Z-Ave), zeta potential (ZP) and polydispersity index (PI), and encapsulation efficacy (EE). From a total of 16 formulations obtained by factorial design, an optimized formulation was selected to carry out additional studies. These formulations were characterized for their morphology rheological and extensibility. The physical stability of the optimized formulation was also evaluated, as well as the ex vivo permeation profile through porcine mucosal tissues (buccal, sublingual nasal, vaginal, cornea and sclera) and the in vitro tolerance study were assessed.

Design of Experiments is extensively used for the implementation of Quality by Design (QbD) in research and industrial settings. In QbD, formula (product) and process understanding are the key enablers of assuring quality in the final product [20]. QbD is not only a guide, but it also provides a systematic approach to drug development, focusing on quality through the application of analytical and risk management methodologies for the design, development and manufacture of new drugs. Likewise, it maps the influence and interaction of various formulations and operating parameters on process performance [21].

2. Results

2.1. Lipid Screening

The PF was dissolved in different solid lipids (SL) and liquid lipids (LL) in order to determine the components of the lipid phase before producing the NLCs containing PF. Therefore, components of the lipid phase were determined by evaluating the solubility of PF in 14 different lipids as shown in Table 1. Selected liquid lipids included LAS (PEG-8 Caprylic/Capric Glycerides), Castor oil, rose mosqueta oil, plantacare oil, Jojoba oil and Miglyol® 812, and isopropyl myristate. The solubility of PF was also evaluated in solid lipids such as stearic acid, Precifac® ATO, Compritol® ATO 888, Precirol® ATO 5, Lanette® 18, Geleol® and Gelucire®. Following on from this, PF (0.1 to 1% of PF was dissolved in different SL and LL or physical mixtures of them (PF, 1.5 to 3%, with regard to total lipid). PF in either physical mixtures or lipids was heated at about 10 °C above the melting point of the SL. The samples obtained were then observed to verify the presence/absence of insoluble drug crystals. The next step was that the mixtures were cooled down to room temperature (RT) for solidification, and this was followed by the analysis of the lipids and PF by Differential Scanning Calorimetry (DSC) to evaluate non-solubilized PF. The analysis was carried out under the conditions described below in the assessment of the lipid matrix crystallinity. Another condition that we imposed is that any resulting solid lipids that were "soft" or "semi-solid" at room temperature were not considered for the design of the NPs (Tables 1 and 2).

Table 1. Solubility of pranoprofen in different solid lipids and liquid lipids.

Lipid Raw Materials	0.1% PF		0.5% PF		1.0% PF	
	Solubility	Appearance	Solubility	Appearance	Solubility	Appearance
SOLID LIPIDS						
Stearic acid	−	Semi-solid	−	Semi-solid	−	Semi-solid
Precifac® ATO	−	Hard	−	Hard	−	Hard
Compritol® 888 ATO	−	Soft	−	Soft	−	Soft
Lanette®18	+	Hard	+	Hard	−	Hard
Precirol® ATO 5	+	Hard	+	Hard	−	Hard
Gelucire® 44	+	Semi-solid	−	Semi-solid	−	Semi-solid
Geleol®	−	Soft	−	Soft	−	Soft
LIQUID LIPIDS						
Isopropyl myristate	+	Clear solution	−	Precipitation	−	Precipitation
Plantacare oil	+	Clear solution	+	Clear solution	−	Precipitation
Miglyol® 812	+	Clear solution	−	Precipitation	−	Precipitation
Rose mosqueta oil	+	Clear solution	−	Precipitation	−	Precipitation
Jojoba oil	+	Clear solution	−	Precipitation	−	Precipitation
Castor oil	+	Clear solution	+	Clear solution	−	Precipitation
LAS (PEG-8 Caprylic/Capric Glycerides)	+	Clear solution	+	Clear solution	+	Clear solution

+ pranoprofen is soluble; − pronoprofen is insoluble.

Table 2. Solubility of pranoprofen in mixtures of lipids.

Physical Mixtures of Lipids	1.5% PF		2.0% PF		3.0% PF	
	Solubility	Appearance	Solubility	Appearance	Solubility	Appearance
LAS:Castor oil (50:50)	+	Clear solution	−	Precipitation	−	Precipitation
LAS:Castor oil (60:40)	+	Clear solution	−	Precipitation	−	Precipitation
LAS:Castor oil (75:25)	+	Clear solution	+	Clear solution	−	Precipitation
Precirol® ATO 5:(LAS-Castor oil (75:25)) 40:60	+	Semi-solid	+	Semi-solid	−	Semi-solid
Precirol® ATO 5:(LAS-Castor oil (75:25)) 50:50	+	Hard	+	Hard	−	Hard
Precirol® ATO 5:(LAS-Castor oil (75:25)) 60:40	+	Hard	−	Hard	−	Hard

+ pranoprofen is soluble; − pronoprofen is insoluble.

Based on the results from the lipid screening, the selected lipids for the preparation of the PF-NLC formulations were Castor oil, LAS and Lanette® 18. In previous studies, we formulated the NLCs with Castor oil, LAS and Precirol® ATO 5, which were chosen and studied [8,18].

2.2. Design of Experiments

The PF-NLC formulations were optimized by means of a 2^3 + star central composite rotatable design (Tables 3 and 4). The main effects and interactions of the independent variables, such as concentration of solid lipid with regard to liquid lipid (cSL/LL), concentration of PF, and concentration of Tween 80® (cTW) were investigated on the mean particle size (Z-Ave), polydispersity index (PI), zeta potential (ZP) and encapsulation efficiency (%EE). A total of 16 experiments are summarized in Table 4.

Table 3. Factors and their corresponding coded levels of experimental design.

Factors	−1.68	−1	0	1	1.68
cSL/LL (%)	43.2	50	60	70	76.8
cPF (%)	0.16	0.5	1	1.5	1.84
cTW (%)	2.16	2.5	3	3.5	3.84

cSL/LL: concentration of solid lipid concerning liquid lipid; cPF: concentration of PF, cTW: concentration of TW 80.

Table 4. Independent and dependent variables of the 2^3 start central composite rotatable factorial design factors.

Formulations	Independent Variables						Dependent Variables			
	cSL/LL		cPF		cTW		Z-Ave (nm)	PI	ZP (mV)	EE (%)
PF-NLCs-N1	1	70	1	1.5	1	3.5	219.3	0.305	−10.70	98.30
PF-NLCs-N2	0	60	0	1	−1.68	2.16	329.5	0.373	−10.56	98.50
PF-NLCs-N3	−1	50	−1	0.5	−1	2.5	449.1	0.452	−12.48	96.90
PF-NLCs-N4	−1.68	43.2	0	1	0	3	345.1	0.365	−8.60	98.54
PF-NLCs-N5	0	60	0	1	0	3	283.5	0.287	−10.20	97.21
PF-NLCs-N6	**−1**	**50**	**1**	**1.5**	**−1**	**2.5**	**214.2**	**0.266**	**−10.81**	**98.33**
PF-NLCs-N7	1	70	−1	0.5	−1	2.5	267.4	0.478	−8.56	94.30
PF-NLCs-N8	0	60	−1.68	0.16	0	3	345.8	0.499	−9.60	93.36
PF-NLCs-N9	−1	50	−1	0.5	1	3.5	321.5	0.419	−10.00	98.15
PF-NLCs-N10	1.68	76.8	0	1	0	3	290.9	0.363	−9.99	98.49
PF-NLCs-N11	0	60	1.68	1.84	0	3	327.9	0.267	−8.96	91.54
PF-NLCs-N12	0	60	0	1	1.68	3.84	359.7	0.486	−8.34	93.58
PF-NLCs-N13	0	60	0	1	0	3	272.8	0.294	−10.50	97.86
PF-NLCs-N14	−1	50	1	1.5	1	3.5	252.4	0.286	−10.34	97.22
PF-NLCs-N15	1	70	1	1.5	−1	2.5	257.1	0.295	−9.84	97.15
PF-NLCs-N16	1	70	−1	0.5	1	3.5	387.8	0.34	−10.3	90.1

cSL/LL: concentration of solid lipid concerning liquid lipid; cPF: concentration of PF; cTW: concentration of TW 80; Z-Ave: mean particle size; PI: poly dispersity index; ZP: zeta potential and EE: encapsulation efficiency.

Four statistical techniques are presented to reveal and visualize the relationship between the aforementioned trials, the independent variables (cLS/L), (cPF), (cTW) and the dependent variables (ZP (mv), Z-Ave (nm), PI and EE (%)).

2.2.1. Principal Component Analysis (PCA)

PCA is a classic multivariate analysis technique used to represent n trials in a synthetic variables space known as *principal components*. This method permits the better visualization of the most representative variables and trials' behavioural patterns of each component. For further details, see the work of Peña [22].

The stages of PCA consist of: (i) plotting and measuring the percentage of explained variability of each principal component, (ii) deciding the number of components, (iii) representing and interpreting results through biplots.

Figure 1 shows a scree plot of the variance of each principal component, and Table 5 shows a descriptive summary of the importance of all the components. The decomposition into 3 first principal components explain 74% of the information. Under the elbow criterion, this threshold might be considered high enough to draw conclusions from it.

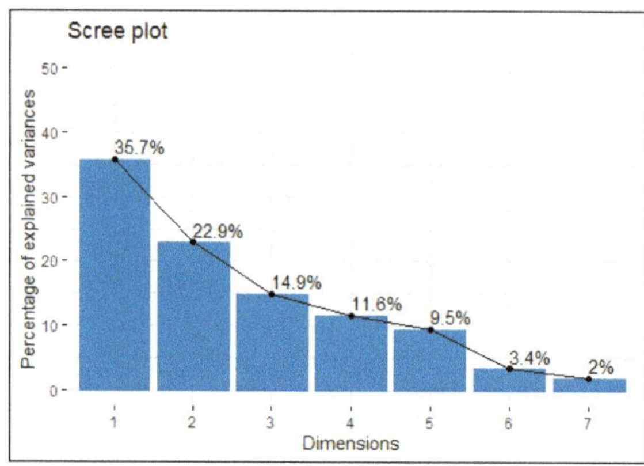

Figure 1. Scree plot of the variance of the components.

Table 5. Summary of importance of principal components.

	PC1	PC2	PC3	PC4	PC5	PC6	PC7
				Importance of Components			
SD	1.5804	1.2667	1.0206	0.9006	0.8158	0.4872	0.3770
Prop V	0.3568	0.2292	0.1488	0.1159	0.0951	0.0339	0.0203
Cum P	0.3568	0.5860	0.7348	0.8507	0.9458	0.9797	1.0000

SD: standard deviation; Prop V: proportion of variance, and Cum P: cumulative proportion.

Table 6 presents a correlation matrix between variables and principal components. We consider a high representation of variables whose correlation with the component is higher than 70%.

Table 6. Correlation matrix of variables and principal components.

	PC1	PC2	PC3	PC4	PC5	PC6	PC7
				Importance of Components			
cLS/LL	−0.01	0.51	−0.79	0.15	−0.25	0.16	0.04
cPF	0.83	0.31	0.18	0.12	0.26	0.25	−0.19
cTW	−0.20	0.56	0.57	0.18	−0.53	0.04	0.00
Z-Ave (nm)	−0.79	−0.29	0.16	0.34	0.21	0.30	0.11
PI	−0.86	−0.14	−0.10	−0.37	−0.12	0.09	−0.25
ZP (mV)	−0.23	0.72	0.13	−0.56	0.28	0.06	0.13
EE(%)	0.58	−0.56	0.06	−0.42	−0.34	0.22	0.10

cLS/LL: concentration of solid lipid concerning liquid lipid; cPF: concentration of pranoprofen; cTW: concentration of Tween 80; Z-Ave: mean particle size; PI: polydispersity index; ZP: zeta potential and EE: encapsulation efficiency.

Figure 2a is a biplot for the first and second principal components (PC1–PC2). The *x*-axis (PC1) is represented mainly by cPF, Z-Ave (nm) and PI. The latter has a negative strong correlation with variables cPF and Z-Ave (nm), specifically the greater the values of cPF, the lower the values cPF and Z-Ave (nm) and vice versa. In particular, trial 8 has the highest levels of PI and Z-Ave (nm), the very opposite of trials 1, 14 and 15.

The most represented variables on the y-axis (PC2) are ZP (mv) and EE, both are inversely related. Trials 12, 16, 7 and 11 have the largest concentrations of ZP (mv); and thus, the lowest EE, in contrast to trial 2 which has the maximum EE (%).

Trials 4, 5 and 10 showed mean concentrations of both types of variables, dependent and independent.

Figure 2b is a biplot for the first and third principal components (PC1-PC3). The *x*-axis (PC1) is weakly represented by cLS/LL and cTW, both variables are inversely correlated. Trials 2 and 10 have the largest levels of cLS/LL and the lowest of TW. In contrast, trials 4 and 9 have the highest TW and cLS/LL. In addition, the *y*-axis (PC3) has no correlations larger than 70%.

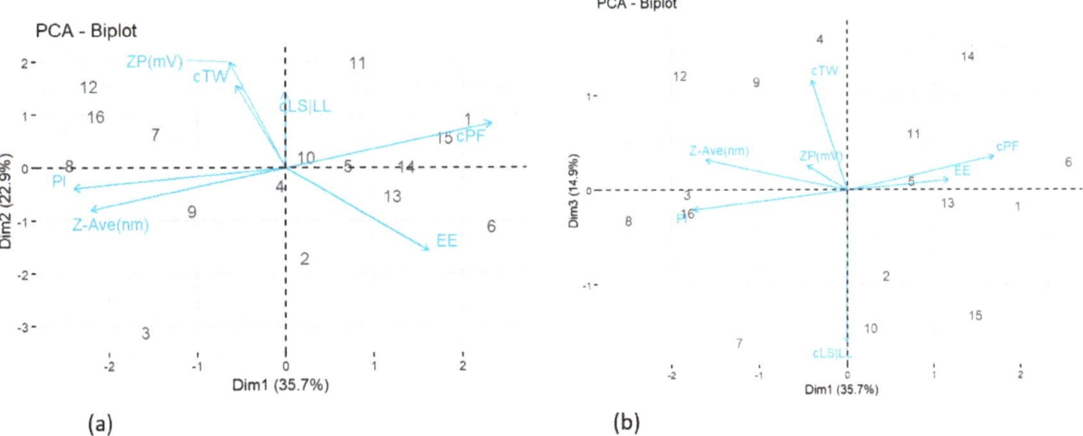

Figure 2. Biplots of (**a**) the First and Second Principal Component; (**b**) the First and Third Principal Component.

2.2.2. Boxplots

Figure 3 shows three boxplots with cLS/LL, cPF and cTW represented on each *x*-axis and compared to their corresponding Z-Ave (nm), Pl, ZP (mV) and EE (%).

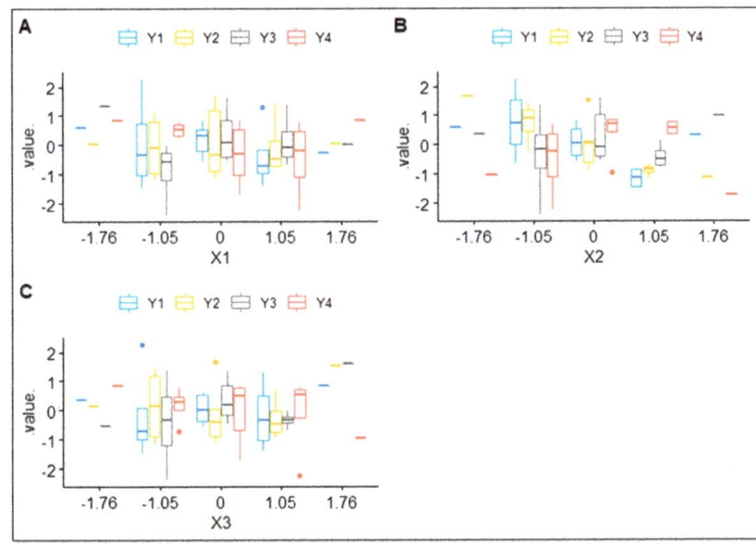

Figure 3. Boxplots of independent variables (cLS/LL, cPF and cTW) according to their corresponding dependent variables (Z-Ave (nm), Pl, ZP (mV) and EE (%)), represented in subfigures (**A–C**) respectively. X1, X2 and X3 denote cLS/LL, cPF and cTW, respectively, and Y1, Y2, Y3 and Y4 denote Z − Ave (nm), Pl, ZP (mV) and EE (%), respectively.

When independent variables take extreme values (-1.76 or 1.76), the interquartile range is extremely small, in fact, dependent variables are barely influenced. However, when independent variables take more intermediate values, the dependent ones present a much higher dispersion; thus, they become more sensitive to changes in cLS/LL, cPF and cTW.

2.2.3. Multivariate Analysis of Variance

The multivariate analysis of variance (MANOVA) is an extension of the ANOVA which includes two or more dependent variables instead of only one. It is used to examine the effects of factor independent variables cLS/LL, cPF, cTW on continuous dependent variables Z-Ave (nm), ZP (mV), Pl and EE (%).

Table 7 shows the results of Manova. cPF is the only statistically significant variable at the 5% level. Therefore, the means of the levels of the factor cPF are significantly different from each other in all the responses (dependent variables).

Table 7. Correlation matrix of variables and principal components.

	Degrees of Freedom	Pillai	Approx F Statistic	Degrees of Freedom (Numerator)	Degrees of Freedom (Denominator)	Pr (>F)
cLS/LL	1	0.26843	0.8256	4	9	0.54092
cPF	1	0.69140	5.0409	4	9	0.02071 *
cTW	1	0.12866	0.3322	4	9	0.84961
Residuals	12	-	-	-	-	0.54092

Significance codes: * = 0.01.

2.2.4. Four-Dimensional Graphics

Figure 4 shows four (A, B, C and D) four-dimensional (4D) plots that reveal the relationship of the independent variables (cLS/LL, cPF and cTW) with the dependent variable (ZP (mV). In this case, cLS/LL is represented on the x-axis and cPF on the y-axis, both variables plotted by each one of the 5 levels of cTW, and coloured by the intensity of ZP (mV), Z-Ave (nm), Pl and EE (%), respectively.

Case A of Figure 4 shows that intermediate values of cLS/LL, cPF and cTW stimulate a medium concentration of ZP (mV), but low values of cLS/LL and cPF with intermediate values of cTW decrease substantially the concentration of ZP (mV).

Case B of Figure 4 shows that intermediate values of cLS/LL, cPF and cTW generate a medium concentration of Z-Ave (nm), in contrast to intermediate levels of cLS/LL and cPF with high levels of cTW that influence Z-Ave (nm) to range from 300 to 400 approximately. Low levels of cLS/LL and cPF with intermediate levels of cTW substantially increase the concentration of Z-Ave (nm). Moreover, high levels of cPF with intermediate levels of cTW tend to decrease the concentration of Z-Ave (nm).

Case C of Figure 4 shows that intermediate levels of cLS/LL, cPF and cTW cause a low concentration of Pl. However, intermediate values of cLL/LL and cPF with high levels of cTW decrease the concentration of Pl. Low levels of cLS/LL and cPF with intermediate levels of cTW cause a medium concentration (0.36–0.45 approximately) of Pl. Moreover, high levels of cPF with intermediate values of cTW decrease the concentration of Pl, while low values of cPF with intermediate values of cLS/LL and TW increase the concentration of Pl.

Case D of Figure 4 shows that intermediate values of cLS/LL and TW generate a medium-high concentration (69–98) of EE (%). However, intermediate values of cLS/LL and cPF with high values of cTW decrease the concentration of EE (%). Low levels of cLS/LL and cPF with intermediate values of cTW cause a medium concentration of EE (%). Intermediate values of cLS/LL and cPF with low values of cTW increase the concentration of EE (%) whilst with high values of cTW, the concentration of EE (%) decreases.

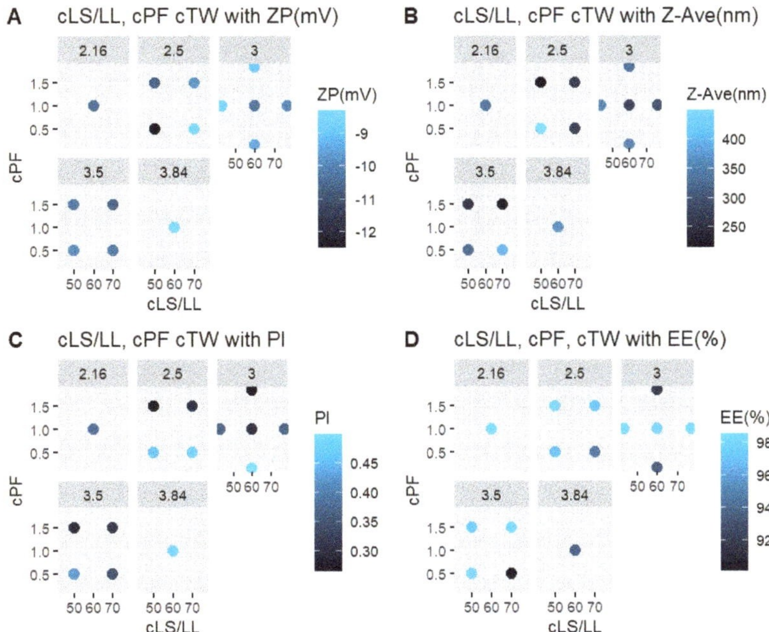

Figure 4. Four-dimensional plots of dependent and independent variables: (**A**) relationship between the independent variables with the zeta potential; (**B**) relationship between the independent variables with the mean particle size; (**C**) relationship between the independent variables with the polydisopersity index; and (**D**) relationship between the independent variables with the encapsulation efficiency.

2.3. Physicochemical Characterization

2.3.1. Particle Size, Zeta Potential and Encapsulation Efficiency

The developed PF-NLCs formulation selected was the number 6 (see Table 4), which exhibited a Z-Ave around 214.20 nm, a negative surface charge with ZP values around −10.81 mV, and PI values of 0.266 that indicate a monomodal distribution (lower than 0.3). The percentage of EE shows values around 98% indicating that PF is inside of the NLCs. To evaluate the presence of large particles, the Z-Ave for PF-NLCs was measured by Laser Diffraction (LD) using a Mastersizer Hydro 2000 (Malvern Instrument Ltd., Malvern UK). After one day of production, PF-NLCs-N6 showed values of 0.087 d (0.1), 0592 d (0.9) and 0.199 d (0.5), which indicated that more than 50% (V) of the particles were smaller than 199 nm in all cases.

2.3.2. Morphological Characterization

The morphology of the optimized PF-NLCs was determined by SEM. The results showed spherical and no aggregated particles (Figure 5); the mean particle size of the sample was 192.37 nm ± 48.56 nm, confirming the results obtained by Photon correlation spectroscopy.

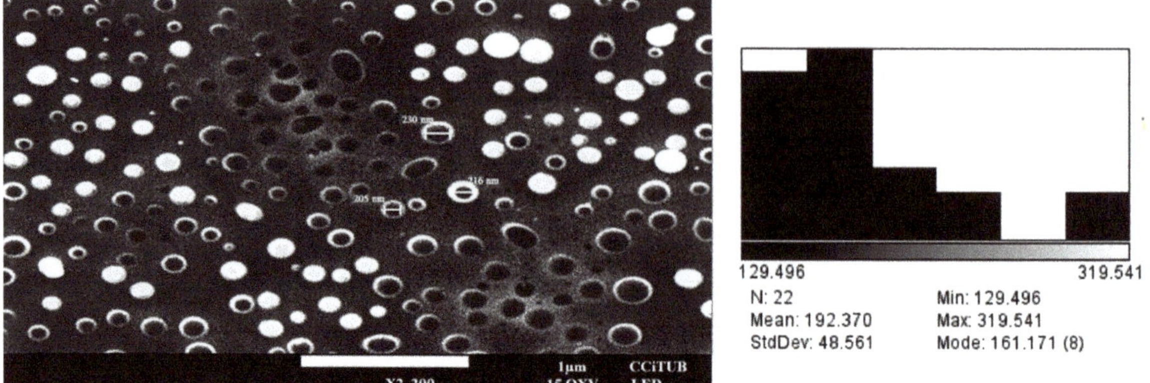

Figure 5. Scanning Electron Microscopy image of PF-NLCs-N6 and the related histogram.

2.4. Rheological Studies

The mathematical Cross best fitted the data. Figure 6 shows the rheological behaviour of PF-NLCs-N6. In addition, the viscosity at 25 °C from the constant velocity period of 50 s^{-1} was $0.77 \times 10^2 \pm 0.76$ mPa·s, demonstrating repeatability between samples ($n = 3$) in the rheological results.

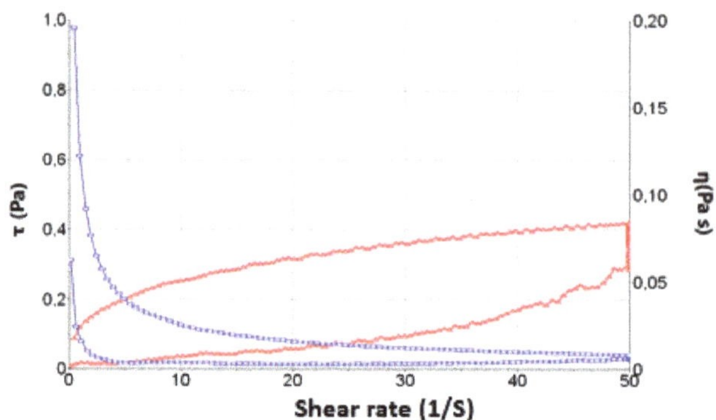

Figure 6. Rheological behaviour of PF-NLCs-N6.

2.5. Extensibility (Spreadability)

PF-NLCs showed a first-order model (Figure 7). The maximum extensibility (Ymax) obtained by the mathematical modelling was 2.023 ± 0.088 cm^2 and the constant (K) was 0.138 ± 0.022 g^{-1}. The data are expressed as mean $\pm$ standard deviation of three replicates ($n = 3$).

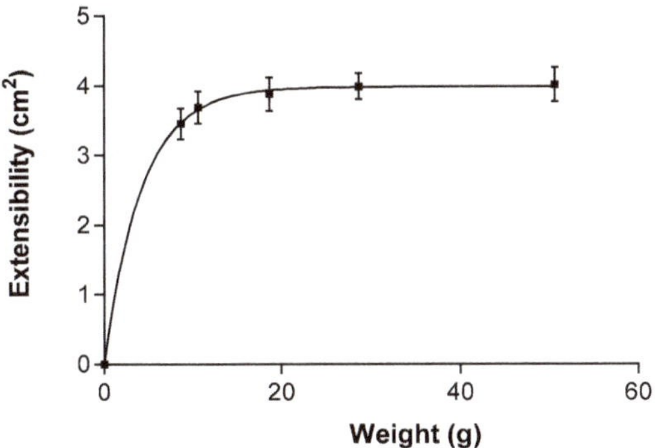

Figure 7. Fitting of PF-NLCs-N6 for the extensibility at 25 ± 2 °C; $60\% \pm 5\%$ RH ($n = 3$). The extensibility followed a first-order model.

2.6. Stability Studies

The prediction of the accelerated stability of the PF-NLCs-N6 was evaluated for 60 days and measured to assess their short-term stability. It was studied after 1, 30 and 60 days of storage at 25 °C. Turbiscan® Lab was used to observe the destabilization processes such as the alteration in the migration speed of the particles (vertical sections of the graph) and the variation in size (horizontal section of the graph) (Figure 8).

The migration of the particles to the top part of the cell leads to a drop in the concentration in the bottom part. This is shown as a drop in the backscatter signal (negative peak) and in reverse for the phenomena that happen in the top part of the vial. It is considered that the backscatter profile with a deviation of $\pm 5\%$ does not present significant variations in particle size. Variations of $\pm 10\%$ indicate that the formulation is unstable. It was observed that the back-scattered light profile did not show fluctuations greater than 5%, which indicates that our formula remained stable stored at 25 °C.

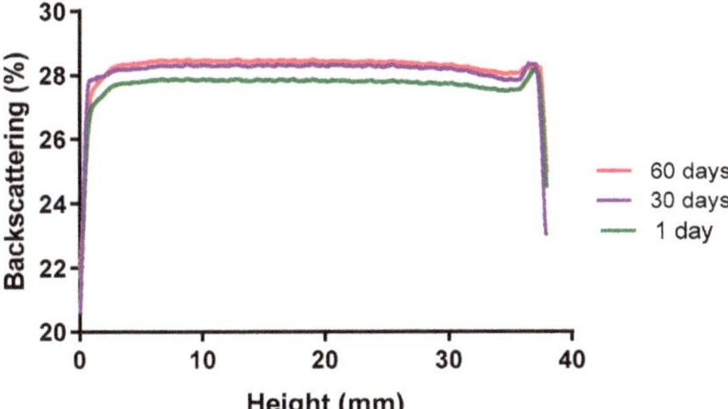

Figure 8. Backscattering of the PF-NLCs-N6 at different stability time points stored at 25 °C ($n = 3$). The left side of the curve represents the bottom of the vial, and the right side is the behaviour in the upper part of the vial.

In addition, physical-chemical properties were measured over 90 days of storage at 25 °C and 4 °C, and the results are shown in Tables 8 and 9.

The graphics of Figure 9a,b show the evolution of Z-Ave (nm), ZP (mV), EE (%) and PI over 90 days when the temperature is 25 °C and 4 °C, respectively. Z-Ave (nm) and ZP (mV) do not show relevant changes across time. However, the behaviour of EE (%) in the first and last days of the trial at 25 °C is in contrast to the trial of 4 °C. PI has a sudden rise, in comparison to the other trial, on the fourteenth day, when the temperature is 4 °C.

Table 8. Physicochemical stability of PF-NLCs-N6 at 25 °C ($n = 3$), monitored by the evaluation of any change in the following parameters: mean particle size, polydispersity index, zeta potential and encapsulation efficiency.

Time (days)	Z-Ave (nm) ± SD	PI ± SD	ZP (mV) ± SD	EE (%)
1	218.09 ± 3.97	0.297 ± 0.03	−10.13 ± 0.11	98.02
7	232.07 ± 5.43	0.299 ± 0.06	−10.01 ± 0.09	97.46
14	267.97 ± 3.93	0.304 ± 0.03	−10.00 ± 0.07	97.54
30	300.72 ± 8.76	0.312 ± 0.05	−9.89 ± 0.16	96.68
60	318.21 ± 5.12	0.329 ± 0.06	−9.53 ± 0.20	96.03
90	326.07 ± 4.88	0.344 ± 0.05	−9.48 ± 0.09	96.52

Table 9. Physicochemical stability of PF-NLCs-N6 at 4 °C ($n = 3$), monitored by the evaluation of any change in the following parameters: mean particle size, polydispersity index, zeta potential and encapsulation efficiency.

Time (days)	Z-Ave (nm) ± SD	PI ± SD	ZP (mV) ± SD	EE (%)
1	220.14 ± 4.92	0.288 ± 0.04	−10.25± 0.10	97.99
7	242.10 ± 3.63	0.301 ± 0.04	−10.16± 0.07	98.45
14	256.24 ± 4.09	0.299 ± 0.05	−9.90 ± 0.09	97.73
30	284.15 ± 5.09	0.309 ± 0.04	−9.76 ± 0.12	97.12
60	303.16 ± 5.94	0.316 ± 0.04	−9.66 ± 0.15	97.23
90	315.02 ± 4.83	0.327 ± 0.06	−9.52 ± 0.08	96.81

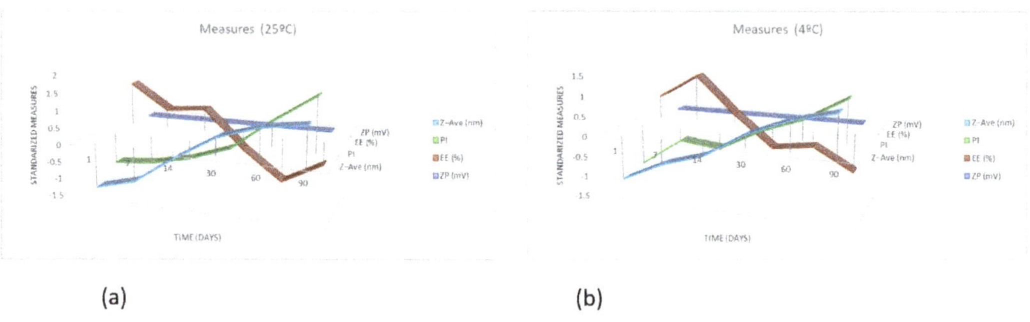

(a)　　　　(b)

Figure 9. Graphics of the evolution of Z − Ave (nm), ZP (mV), EE (%) and PI over 90 days of PF-NLCs-N6 at 25 °C (**a**) ± and 4 °C (**b**) ($n = 3$).

2.7. Ex Vivo Permeation Studies in Porcine Mucosal Tissues

We estimated the permeation parameters starting from the ex vivo permeation studies on different mucosal tissues, including six replicates per tissue. Table 10 reports the results obtained for flux, lag-time, partition and diffusion coefficients as well as the permeability coefficient. Cornea showed the greater flux, whereas similar values were observed for the rest of the mucosae (buccal, sublingual, nasal, vaginal and scleral tissue).

Regarding the lag time Tl (h), which is the time for the drug to reach the steady state, very quick absorption took place in the cornea. Nasal and vaginal mucosae showed intermediate lag-times, and buccal, sublingual and scleral tissue took a long time to reach the steady-state. This is probably correlated to the diffusion coefficient, which apparently is the major mechanism involved in the permeation (versus the partition coefficient), which in turn, may be due to the structural differences of the tissues tested [23,24]. The permeability coefficients were also similar for the four mucous membranes and about twice for the cornea.

Table 10. The results of the permeation parameters of PF at 6 h from the selected formula in the different mucosal tissues tested, $n = 6$ each. The results are reported as the median (maximum and minimum): Flux (Jss), lag time (Tl), partition coefficient P1, diffusion coefficient P2, permeability coefficient (Kp).

	Buccal	Sublingual	Nasal	Vaginal	Sclera	Cornea
Jss (μg/h)	2.46 (2.14–2.96)	2.34 (2.14–2.63)	3.26 (2.45–5.11)	2.59 (1.96–2.84)	2.57 (2.15–2.83)	5.02 (4.15–6.32)
Tl (h)	4.10 (3.92–4.37)	3.67 (3.14–4.99)	1.18 (0.83–1.94)	0.94 (0.51–1.31)	3.66 (2.41–4.93)	0.09 (0.04–0.11)
P2 (10^{-1} h^{-1})	0.41 (0.38–0.42)	0.45 (0.33–0.53)	1.41 (0.86–2.01)	3.26 (1.27–1.77)	0.45 (0.33–0.69)	18.52 (15.15–41.67)
P1 (10^{-3} cm)	0.16 (1.30–2.00)	0.13 (1.00–2.10)	0.06 (0.30–1.60)	0.03 (0.10–0.60)	0.15 (0.80–2.20)	0.007 (0.03–0.11)
Kp (10^{-4} cm/h)	0.65 (0.56–0.78)	0.61 (0.56–0.69)	0.85 (0.64–1.34)	0.68 (0.51–0.74)	0.67 (0.56–0.74)	1.32 (1.09–1.66)

Table 11 shows the recovery of PF from each tissue studied after the application of PF-NLCs-N6. In addition, Table 12 reports the amount of PF remaining in the tissues, expressed per surface area of mucosa exposed and per gram of tissue.

Table 11. The results of the pranoprofen recovery with phosphate-buffered saline (PBS), expressed as a percentage of the recovery, and its relative standard derivation (%RSD); $n = 3$ each.

Membrane	Recovery (%)	RSD (%)
Buccal	17.03	1.60
Sublingual	8.72	0.70
Nasal	16.03	1.36
Vaginal	12.65	0.71
Sclera	12.97	1.15
Cornea	15.01	1.34

Table 12. The results of the retained amount (Qr) of pranoprofen at 6 h from the selected formula (PF-NLCs-N6) in the tissues (buccal, sublingual nasal and vaginal, cornea and sclera), $n = 6$ each. Values are reported as median (maximum and minimum).

Membrane	Qr ($\mu g/cm^2/g$)
Buccal	1488.52 (1227.62–1563.24)
Sublingual	3198.92 (3005.43–3321.72)
Nasal	1879.92 (1765.70–1990.44)
Vaginal	591.01 (437.20–625.30)
Sclera	1842.73 (1711.32–1897.90)
Cornea	745.09 (623.72–804.57)

Table 13 shows the plasma concentration that would be achieved in the steady-state after the application of PF-NLCs-N6 on 1 cm^2 of porcine mucous membrane (buccal, sublingual, nasal and vaginal) and ophthalmic tissues (sclera and cornea). The predicted Css values were below the therapeutic concentrations in plasma 4.89 ± 1.29 µg/mL for young subjects and 10.19 ± 2.43 µg/mL for elderly subjects [25].

Table 13. Predicted plasma levels of PF at the steady-state (Css) for the young and elderly populations, obtained from the selected formulation applied on 1 cm^2 of porcine mucous membrane (buccal, sublingual, nasal and vaginal) and ophthalmic tissues (sclera and cornea). Data are reported as median (min-max).

Membrane	Young Subject Css (ng/mL)	Elderly Subject Css (ng/mL)
Buccal	2.14 (1.87–2.58)	4.04 (3.51–4.87)
Sublingual	2.04 (1.87–2.29)	3.84 (3.51–4.32)
Nasal	2.84 (2.14–4.46)	5.35 (4.02–8.39)
Vaginal	2.26 (1.71–2.48)	4.25 (3.22–4.67)
Sclera	2.24 (1.87–2.47)	4.22 (3.53–4.65)
Cornea	4.38 (3.62–5.51)	8.24 (6.81–10.38)

2.8. Hen's Egg Test on the Chorioallantoic Membrane (HET-CAM)

To establish ocular tolerance, an HET-CAM in vitro test was applied. PF-NLCs-N6 and free PF-NLCs were tested in the CAM of 3 eggs per formulation, to determine the possible rapid irritation reaction. The addition of 0.1 N NaOH (positive control) produced intense vasoconstriction and haemorrhage. In contrast, 0.9% NaCl (negative control) produced no reaction over the time tested. Similarly, the application of PF-NLCs-N6 onto the CAM did not expose any sign of intolerance or vascular alteration. Considering Figure 10, it is possible to confirm the suitability for ocular administration.

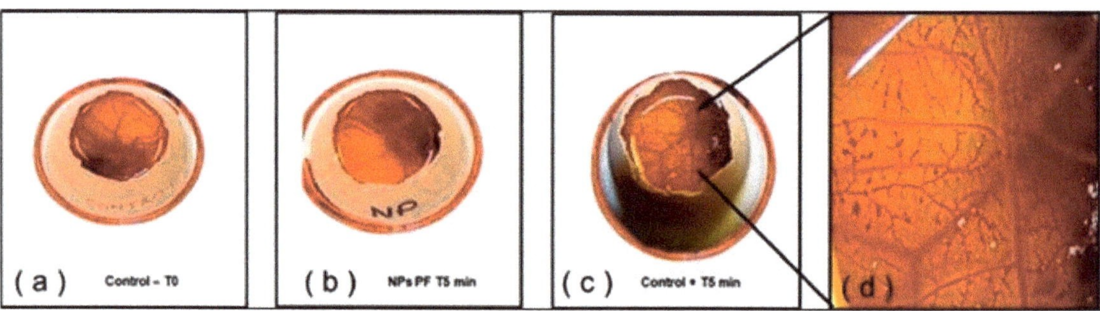

Figure 10. HET-CAM test: (**a**) Saline solution (Negative control-free PF-NPLCs); (**b**) PF-NPLCs-N6; (**c**) 0.1 N sodium hydroxide (Positive control); and (**d**) lesions caused by the positive control.

3. Discussion

AINEs in pig mucous and ocular tissues can be studied to learn a lot about veterinary and human medicine. Pig eyes are useful in comparative studies due to their many parallels to human eyes, including possessing a holangiotic retinal vasculature, cone photoreceptors in the outer retina, no tapetum, and they have a similar scleral thickness, making them very useful in comparative research [26]. When compared to other animal models, porcine buccal mucosa has been employed most frequently as a representative model for human buccal mucosa historically by multiple prestigious research groups worldwide [27,28].

The mouth can be affected by significant inflammatory processes because of localized or systemic diseases manifest in various types of buccal sores, such as lichen planus or canker sores, conditions that commonly present with inflammation and pain. In addition, although the oral cavity has its own bacterial flora, a qualitative and quantitative imbalance of this ecosystem leads to infections that produce inflammatory processes [29]. Regarding porcine vaginal mucosa, comparative studies with human vaginal mucosa reveal similarities in the morphology between species, both possess a nonkeratinized, stratified, squamous surface epithelium. The lipid composition of vaginal epithelium from pigs and humans shows similar concentrations of lipids, including ceramides, glucosyl ceramides, and cholesterol, which are the key permeability barrier components. This similarity in barrier lipids is reflected functionally in the data from permeability studies [30]. Concerning the nasal mucosa, morphological similarities between porcine and human mucosa, combined with ethical considerations when using pig model for studies, are reasons to continue with in vivo nasal absorption studies in various animal models that are correlated with human data and that have recently been presented [31].

A drug's capacity to pass through mucous membrane and ocular tissues, such as PF, depends on both its physicochemical characteristics and the pharmaceutical formulation [32,33]. To reduce inflammation, it is essential to make sure the medicine is delivered to the site of action at therapeutic concentrations, and that these concentrations remain there for a long time. In this regard, using NLCs is a judicious substitute for using traditional medications. PF-NLCs-N6 was selected as the optimized formulation based on the qualities observed in the factorial design (Table 4). It is common knowledge that smaller particles adhere more strongly to surfaces such as tissues. SEM pictures attest to the effectiveness of the preparation strategy. The ZP is a measure of the particle charge which can influence both the stability of the particle and its mucoadhesion. Aggregation is prevented by electrostatic repulsion between particles with the same polarity of electrical charge. There was a net negative charge in every formulation. Although values of about $\pm$ 10 mV in zeta potential value may be considered too low to ensure stability, the results of the stability study demonstrated the PF-NLCs-N6 was a stable system. The stability is probably maintained by the addition of Tween® 80 in the formulation, since non-ionic surfactants stabilize the colloidal systems by the steric effect instead of electrical repulsion between particles [34]. Concerning the relationship between mucoadhesion and the surface particle charge, it is accepted that the presence of a cationic surface charge in the lipidic nanocarrier may increase the residence time compared to negatively charged nanocarriers, because the positively charged systems interact with the corneal epithelium and the mucins from tears fluid and the conjunctiva, which they are all negatively charged [35,36].

The rheological and viscosity results suggest that the formulation can be easily and gently applied, resulting in low values of viscosity. The formulation was evaluated for extensibility or spreadability, which fitted first-order kinetics. The results suggest that the formulation is suitable for use as eyedrops (Figure 7).

The PF-NLCs-N6 showed no signs of destabilisation after 60 days at 25 °C as was shown by the backscattering profile having variations of less than 10%, indicating that the formulation was stable; contrarily variations greater than 10% would have signified an unstable formulation. Additionally, no signals of creaming, sedimentation, flocculation or coalescence were found. This system allows the predicting of the instability processes of NPs sooner than with other techniques [37]. These results are in line with previous studies with PF-NLCs with Precirol® ATO 5 as solid lipid [8,18]. The high physicochemical stability of the formulation was also confirmed by no changes in the physical and chemical parameters Z-ave PI, ZP and EE, and the stability is also supported by negligible changes in the drug content (EE). Based on these results, we concluded that the nanoparticles are stable for at least 90 days at the different storage conditions studied since no apparent agglomeration occurred. In addition to this, the drug seems to have high compatibility with the formulation's components.

An ex vivo permeation assay was carried out using the selected formulation, ex vivo permeation studies provide useful information to predict in vivo behaviour of the formulation [38,39]. It is known that the permeation of NSAIDs through the cornea is higher than through the scleral tissue and other ocular structures [23,40]. We observed the same trend for the flux and permeation coefficient in the permeation tests. The flux is the diffusion rate of pranoprofen into the eye and as, already mentioned, these differences may have their origin in different anatomical structures. This is the opposite of other studies that suggest that despite the fact that both tissues have a similar thickness (900µm), the sclera is ten times more permeable than the cornea [41]. The same pattern was observed for the permeability coefficient, the greatest value of Kp was found in the cornea. In addition, the Tl in corneal tissue is lower compared to the buccal mucous (minutes versus several hours). Taking into account that the Tl is representative of the time required for the drug to reach a steady state, the results suggest that PF-NLCs-N6 is rapidly absorbed in the cornea with a high diffusion. This is a desirable situation in anti-inflammatory drugs, which are aimed at achieving rapid action. Moreover, Tween® 80 as a surfactant could expand the cornea membrane by potentially increasing its permeability, which could be key in the drug delivery of PF into the eye and even to the posterior segment of the eye [39]. The higher amount of PF retained in the cornea than the sclera (about 2.5-fold) favours a deposit of PF that could act over a longer time. Other researchers also investigated the amount of PF retained in ophthalmic tissues from nanostructured formulations and observed a lower amount of drug retained in the membranes. A similar study with human skin and PF-NLC with Precirol® ATO 5 as solid lipid showed a Qr of about 24.29 $\mu g/cm^2/g$ [18]. Other studies carried out with nanoparticles loading an NSAID drug with similar results in the physicochemical characterization also resulted in lower drug retention [2,23]. However, in both cases, the nanoparticles consisted of poly D, L-lactic-co-glycolic acid (PLGA), which suggests that the formulation strongly impacts the permeation capacity of PF through the ophthalmic tissues.

Among the studied tissues, sublingual mucosa exhibited the highest amount of PF retained in the membrane, and the vaginal mucosa the lowest. Finally, the nasal and buccal mucosae showed intermediate values. The high amount of PF deposited in the sublingual mucosa suggests the PF-NLCs-N6 as a promising vehicle for the local delivery of PF in the sublingual mucosa.

From all the mucosae studied, the predicted plasma levels that were obtained at the steady state would be below the therapeutic concentration in plasma, considering when PF-NLCs-N6 is applied on 1 cm^2 of tissue, meaning that no systemic effect would be observed and hence confirming the safety of formulation topically applied, while having a local analgesic and anti-inflammatory effect.

By observing negative changes that take place in the chorioallantoic membrane of the egg after being exposed to test substances, it is possible to identify compounds that may cause irritation (Figure 10). PF-NLCs-N6 is classified as a non-irritating drug at the ocular level, as shown in investigation. These findings are consistent with information obtained by other authors who also developed nanoparticles for ocular administration [42].

These results, which are in accordance with our earlier research, offer enormous opportunities for the local treatment of numerous inflammatory illnesses in humans or pigs, while pranoprofen side effects will be reduced. Despite this, additional research is needed to develop a pharmaceutical dosage form that makes its administration more convenient and effective.

4. Materials and Methods

4.1. Materials

Pranoprofen (2-(5H-chromeno[2,3-b]pyridin-7-yl)propanoic acid) (CAS 52549-17-4) was gratefully provided by Alcon Cusi (Barcelona, Spain). Tween® 80 (Polyethylene glycol sorbitan monooleate) and Castor oil (Ricinus communis L.) (CAS 8001-79-4) were acquired from Sigma-Aldrich Química (Barcelona, Spain). Lanette® 18 (stearyl alcohol) was acquired from Cognis (Dusseldorf, Germany). LAS (PEG-8 Caprylic/Capric Glycerides), Precifac® ATO (cetyl palmitate), Compritol® ATO 888 (glyceryl behenate), Precirol® ATO 5 (glycerol mono, di and tripalmitostearate), Geleol® (Glyceryl Monostearate) and Gelucire® 44/14 (Polyoxylglycerides) were supplied by Gattefosse (Saint-Priest, France). Rose mosqueta oil, Plantacare oil, Jojoba oil and Miglyol® 812 were provided by Roig Farma-Fagron (Tarrasa, Spain), isopropyl myristate was supplied by Merck (Darmstadt, Germany), and stearic acid (a saturated fatty acid (of C18) was provided by Croda Industrial Specialities (Nettetal, Germany). MilliQ water (resistivity > 18 MOhm.cm) was obtained by a MilliQ® Plus System lab supplied. Phosphate buffer saline (PBS) pH 7.4 (tablets) was purchased from Sigma (Germany) and prepared as indicated by the manufacturer. All the other reagents and chemicals used in this research were of analytical grade.

4.2. Lipid Screening

Based on a list of suitable lipids (solid and liquid), the solubility of PF in different solid lipids (SL) and liquid lipids (LL) was performed to determine the components of the lipid phase before producing the NLCs containing PF.

4.3. Development of NLCs

A high-pressure homogenization technique was used to produce the NLCs, as described beforehand [18]. The lipid phase, which was 5% w/w of the total amount of formulation, consisted of Castor oil, the liquid lipid (LL) and Lanette® 18 (75:25), the solid lipid (SL). The lipid phase in conjunction with PF was melted at 85 °C in a water bath resulting in a homogeneous lipid solution. An aqueous solution of Tween® 80 as surfactant was heated in parallel at the same temperature and then added to the lipid phase, obtaining a primary emulsion by an Ultra-Turrax T25 (IKA, Staufen, Germany) at 8000 rpm for 45 s. Next, the emulsion was homogenized by a high-pressure homogenizer (Homogeniser FPG 12800, Stansted, UK) at 800 bar and 85 °C in three homogenization cycles. The NLCs were formed once the lipid recrystallized during the cool-down to room temperature. The NLCs were characterized for Z-Ave, PI, ZP and %EE, as described before [8].

4.4. Design of Experiments

A design of experiments (DoE) was performed to optimize formulation parameters. A central composite factorial design 2^3 (containing 2 replicated centre points, 8 factorial points and 6 axial points) was developed using the statistical program Statgraphics Centurion XVI.II® v. 16.2.04 (Warrenton, VA, USA).

In this section, we present some statistical techniques to reveal and visualize the relationship between the aforementioned trials with the independent variables (cLS/L), (cPF), (cTW) and the dependent variables (ZP (mv), Z-Ave (nm), PI and EE (%)). The selected techniques for this analysis are principal component analysis (PCA), MANOVA, boxplots and four-dimensional plots performed with R, statistical software, version (4.0.0).

Considering the fact that trials are measured by different experimental units, the first two techniques are applied based on standardized input data (by subtracting the mean and dividing by the standard deviation) so that variables are treated equally, and the outcomes are not influenced by the units of measurement.

4.5. Physicochemical Characterization

4.5.1. Particle Size and Zeta Potential

Photon correlation spectroscopy (PCS) technique by a Zetasizer Nano ZS (Malvern Instruments, Malvern, UK) [8,18], was used to determine the Z-Ave and PI of PF-NLCs. Samples were diluted (1:20 v/v) with Milli-Q water and measurements were carried out in triplicate at 25 °C in disposable quartz cells. In addition, the ZP was determined by electrophoresis laser-Doppler using the same instrument, with prior dilution in Milli-Q water (1:10 v/v) [19].

Furthermore, the particle size of PF-NLCs-N6 was measured by Laser Diffraction (LD) using a Mastersizer Hydro 2000 (Malvern Instrument Ltd., Malvern, UK) to evaluate the presence of large particles [18,34]. The volume distribution method served to determine the diameter values by Mie analysis including d (0.1), d (0.5), and d (0.9). The diameter values indicate the percentage of particles showing a diameter equal to or lower than the given value. Prior to all the measurements, the samples were dispersed in Milli-Q water using an Elma Transsonic Digital S T490 DH ultrasonic bath (Elma, Singen, Germany).

4.5.2. Entrapment Efficiency

The encapsulation efficiency (EE) of PF was measured indirectly by quantification of the unloaded amount of PF in the dispersing agent by a reverse-phase high-performance liquid chromatography (RP-HPLC) [43]. Nanoparticles were isolated using a filtration/centrifugation procedure with Ultracel YM-100 filter (Amicon® Millipore Corporation, Bedford, MA, USA) at 6000 rpm for 30 min (Sigma 301K 8 centrifuge, Osterode am Harz, Germany), with prior dilution in PBS pH 7.4 (1:20). Validation of the methodology was performed beforehand in accordance with international guidelines (EMEA, 2011) [8,44]. The EE was determined by Equation (1):

$$EE(\%) = \frac{Total\ amount\ of\ PF - Free\ PF}{Total\ amount\ of\ PF} \times 100\,, \tag{1}$$

Samples were analysed in a Waters 1525 pump System (Waters, Milford, CT, USA) with a UV-Vis 2487 detector (Waters, Milford, CT, USA) at the wavelength $\lambda = 235$ nm using a Kromasil® column (C-18, 150 $\times$ 4.6 mm, 5 μm) and methanol/glacial acetic acid 5% (70:30; $v:v$) as the mobile phase at the flow rate of 1 mL/min.

4.5.3. Morphological Characterization

Scanning Electron Microscopy (SEM) was used to examine the morphology of the selected formulation. Samples were centrifuged at 14,000 rpm at 4 °C for 30 min. The supernatant content was discarded and the precipitate (corresponding to the PF-NLCs) was collected very carefully, and dried under vacuum for 8 days [45–48] using a vacuum desiccator. The samples were adhered to a metal tube which contained an adhesive tape where part of the dry sample was placed, and finally it was covered with carbon to generate conductivity. Images were collected using a JEOL J-7100F (Peabody, MA, USA). The SEM image was processed by Image J (1.53 t) to measure the particle size taking 22 measurements.

4.6. Rheological Behavior

The rheological characterization of the formulations was performed in triplicate at 25 °C using a Thermo Scientific Haake RheoStress 1 rheometer (Thermo Fisher Scientific, Karlsruhe, Germany) with a cone rotor geometry C60/2-Ti (60 mm diameter, 2° angle, 0.105 mm gap between cone-plate), coupled to a thermostatic circulator (Thermo Haake Phoenix II + Haake C25P) and operated by the software the Haake Rheowin® Job Manager v 3.3 software (Thermo Electron Corporation, Karlsruhe, Germany). Haake Rheowin® Data manager v. 3.3 software (Thermo Electron Corporation, Karlsruhe, Germany) was used to perform the data analyses. The viscosity and flow curves were obtained under rotational runs at 25 °C for 3 min during the ramp-up period from $0\ s^{-1}$ to $50\ s^{-1}$, a subsequent 1-min period at $50\ s^{-1}$ (constant share rate period), and followed by a ramp-down period of 3 min from $50\ s^{-1}$ to $0\ s^{-1}$. The viscosity was determined at $50\ s^{-1}$ after 3 days of production. The data was fitted to different mathematical models: Newton, Casson, Ostwald, Bingham Herschel-Bulkley and Cross [29].

4.7. Extensibility (Spreadability)

The extensibility or spreadability was determined at room temperature by placing a weight of 0.05 g of the formulation selected inside a 10 cm diameter cavity, a glass plate was positioned on top of it and pieces of increasing standard weight (5, 10, 15, 25, and 50 g) were added successively and allowed to stand on top of the glass plate for 1 min forcing the formulation to spread. The expansion in diameter was recorded as a function of the weight applied. The experiment was carried out in triplicate and fitted to a mathematical model using Graph Pad Prism® software version 6.0 (GraphPad Software Inc., San Diego, CA, USA) [49].

4.8. Ex Vivo Permeation Study in Porcine Mucosal Tissues

To evaluate the capacity of PF to penetrate and diffuse through the mucous membranes and ophthalmic tissues, ex vivo permeation tests were conducted using different mucosal membranes from female pigs (cross Landrace × Large White, 25–30 kg), under the approval of the Ethics Committee of Animals Experimentation of the University of Barcelona. The tissues included in the study were: buccal, sublingual, nasal, vaginal mucosa, and two ophthalmic structures (sclera and cornea). The tissues were frozen to $-20\,°C$ after excision. Buccal and nasal mucosae were dermatomed (dermatome GA 630 Aesculap, Tuttlingen, Germany), at 500 μm thick slabs, the sublingual mucosa at 300 μm, and vaginal mucosa at 400 μm.

The tissues were clamped in vertical Franz cells (FDC 400, Crown Glass, Somerville, NY, USA) with a surface available diffusion area of 0.64 cm^2 and 4.5 mL of capacity. The receptor medium was PBS pH 7.4, which was continuously in contact with the inner part of the tissue while the external side faced the donor compartment, where 500 μL of PF-NLCs-N6 was added and sealed with Parafilm® to prevent evaporation. Six replicates for each tissue were included in the study. The receptor fluid was kept at $37 \pm 0.5\,°C$ under continuous magnetic stirring, except for cornea cells which were kept at $32 \pm 0.5\,°C$. The experiments lasted 6 h during which 300 μL of the receptor compartment were collected at selected times. The same volume was replaced with fresh receptor medium after each sample collection to keep constant the volume of the receptor compartment. Samples were analysed by HPLC [8,18].

The quantification of PF retained inside the membranes and recovery required an extraction before analysis. Regarding the amount of PF retained in the tissues, we proceeded as follows: the mucous membranes and ophthalmic tissues were disassembled from the Franz cell, cleaned with a 0.05% dodecyl sulphate solution, rinsed with distilled water and weighed accurately. The tissues were pierced several times using a small needle, minced carefully, and weighed accurately. The PF was extracted with PBS pH 7.4 under sonication for 30 min in an ultrasonic water bath. The samples from drug extraction were analysed by HPLC, rendering the amount of PF extracted from the skin. The recovery was performed by incubating weighed tissues in a known concentration of PF solution in PBS pH 7.4 (Co). The incubation took place at the same temperature and with the same duration as the ex vivo experiments. After the incubation, the solution was collected, and the tissues were gently blotted and weighed again. Afterwards, the drug that had penetrated the skin was extracted by PBS as described for the retained amount. After the sonication process, the resulting solution was collected (Ex) [50]. All samples were analysed by HPLC.

We calculated the permeation parameters resulting from the permeation assays: the flux values per unit area (J_{ss} in mg/h cm^2), the permeability coefficients (Kp in cm/h) and the lag times (Tl) were calculated at the steady state by linear regression analysis using the Graph Pad Prism® software version 6.0 (GraphPad Software Inc., San Diego, CA, USA). Stationary flux values across membranes were obtained by applying Equation (2):

$$J_{ss} = \frac{Q_t}{A \times t}, \tag{2}$$

where Q_t is the amount of PF which diffuses to the receptor medium (μg), A is the active diffusional area (cm^2), and t is the time (h) of exposure per unit area. Deriving our results from the foregoing, we determined the permeability coefficient Kp, (cm/h) based on Equation (3):

$$Kp = \frac{J_{ss}}{Co} \, , \qquad (3)$$

where J_{ss} is the flux at the steady state normalized by unit area, and Co is the initial drug concentration of the formulation tested and applied to the donor compartment. Partition ($P1$) and diffusion ($P2$) parameters were computed from Equations (4) and (5):

$$Tl = \frac{1}{6} \times P2 \, , \qquad (4)$$

where Tl is the lag time and $P2$ the diffusion coefficient.

$$Kp = P1 \times P2 \, , \qquad (5)$$

To predict if systemic levels of PF would be achieved after the topical application of PF-NLC-N6 to a specific surface area, we calculated the predicted plasma concentration at the steady state (Css) using the Equation (6):

$$Css = \frac{J_{ss} \times A}{Clp} \, , \qquad (6)$$

where Css is the concentration in plasma at the steady-state, J_{ss} is the flux computed in this study, A is the hypothetical application area of 1 cm^2, and Clp is the plasma clearance obtained from the literature; we considered two populations, the young subjects (Clp = 1146.60 cm^3/h) and the elderly subjects (Clp = 609.00 cm^3/h) [1,51].

Equation (7) was used to calculate the amount of PF retained in the tissue (Qr, μg/g/cm^2):

$$Qr = \frac{\frac{Ex}{Px}}{A} \times \frac{100}{R} \, , \qquad (7)$$

where Ex (μg) is the amount of PF extracted from the tissue, Px (g) is the weight of the tissues exposed to the permeation, A (cm^2) is the active area for diffusion and R is the recovery of the PF from the tissue, expressed as a percentage.

4.9. Stability Studies

Short-term physical stability was assessed after 1, 30, and 60 days analysing light backscattering (BS) profiles by using the Turbiscan®Lab (Formulaction Co., L'Union, France). For this purpose, a cylindrical glass measurement cell was filled with 20 mL of PF-NLCs-N6 stored at 25 °C for two months. The radiation source was a pulse near infrared light (λ = 880 nm) and it was received by backscattering detectors at an angle of 45° from the incident beam due to the opacity of the formulation.

Additionally, morphometric parameters (Z-Ave, PI and ZP) and EE were also measured at 25 °C and 4 °C, monitored for 24 h and after 7, 14, 30, 60 and 90 days to evaluate any potential changes.

4.10. In Vitro Ocular Tolerance Study: Hen's Egg Test on the Chorioallantoic Membrane (HET-CAM)

In vitro ocular tolerance was assessed using the HET-CAM test to ensure that the formulation of PF-NLC-N6 was non-irritating when administered as eye drops. 300 μL of the formulation studied was applied on the chorioallantoic membrane of a fertilized chicken egg and monitored for 5 min after the application of the formulation. The following phenomena were considered: irritation, coagulation, and haemorrhaging.

The development of the test was carried out using 3 eggs for each group (formula PF-NLCs-N6, negative control (0.9% NaCl), positive control (NaOH 0.1 N)). The ocular irritation index (*OII*) was calculated by the sum of the scores of each injury or discomfort according to the following expression (Equation (8)):

$$OII = \frac{(301 - H) \times 5}{300} + \frac{(301 - V) \times 7}{300} + \frac{(301 - C) \times 9}{300},\tag{8}$$

where H, V and C are times (in seconds) until the start of haemorrhaging (H), vasoconstriction (V) and coagulation (C), respectively. The formulations were classified according to the following scores: OII $\leq$ 0.9 non-irritating; 0.9 < OII $\leq$ 4.9 weakly irritating; 4.9 < OII $\leq$ 8.9 moderately irritating; 8.9 < OII $\leq$ 21 irritating [52,53].

5. Conclusions

A nanostructured lipid carrier has been developed by means of QbD, which allowed the influence of the components in the formulation to be understood. It was seen that the factorial design played a key role in optimizing the formulation. Finally, the optimized nanoparticles were tested on ex vivo porcine mucosal tissues (buccal, sublingual nasal, vaginal, cornea and sclera) to evaluate their capacity to diffuse the tissues and, in turn, their potential to treat different inflammatory conditions in mucosal tissues with a topical approach. High permeation and high retention were observed in all the tissues tested. In particular, the highest permeation was found on the cornea; and PF was mostly retained in the sublingual mucosa. The optimized nanoparticles exhibit suitable characteristics for the topical delivery on the tested mucosae, and they were shown to be safe for the ocular route since no irritant effects were observed in the HET-CAM test. Furthermore, the predicted concentration at the steady-state was below the therapeutic concentration of PF in plasma, and this may result in a local anti-inflammatory and analgesic effect on damaged mucosae.

Author Contributions: Conceptualization, G.A., M.S.-A. and A.C.C.; methodology, G.A. and A.C.C.; software, J.P.-N. and A.C.C.; validation, M.R., J.P.-N. and L.S.; formal analysis, A.C.C.; investigation, M.R., G.A. and J.P.-N.; resources, L.C.E., A.C.C. and M.M.; data curation, A.C.C.; writing—original draft preparation, M.R.; writing—review and editing, M.S.-A., L.S. and M.M.; visualization, M.R. and M.M.; supervision, G.A. and A.C.C.; project administration, G.A. and A.C.C.; funding acquisition, L.C.E., A.C.C. and M.M. All authors have read and agreed to the published version of the manuscript.

Funding: This research received no external funding.

Institutional Review Board Statement: The animal study protocol was approved by the Animal Experimentation Ethics Committee of the University of Barcelona (protocol code 10619 and date of approval 30 May 2019).

Informed Consent Statement: Not applicable.

Data Availability Statement: The data presented in this study are available on request from the corresponding author.

Acknowledgments: The authors want to thank Harry Paul for the English language editing. We also acknowledge the support received from Universidad Técnica Particular de Loja—Ecuador. Moreover, thanks to Maria Luisa García for her technical support, Elena Sanchez for helping with HPLC analysis, and Lyda Halbaut for her support with rheological studies.

Conflicts of Interest: The authors declare no conflict of interest.

References

1. Abrego, G.; Alvarado, H.; Souto, E.B.; Guevara, B.; Bellowa, L.H.; Garduño, M.L.; Garcia, M.L.; Calpena, A.C. Biopharmaceutical profile of hydrogels containing pranoprofen-loaded PLGA nanoparticles for skin administration: In vitro, ex vivo and in vivo characterization. *Int. J. Pharm.* **2016**, *501*, 350–361. [CrossRef]
2. Cañadas-Enrich, C.; Abrego, G.; Alvarado, H.L.; Calpena-Campmany, A.C.; Boix-Montañes, A. Pranoprofen quantification in ex vivo corneal and scleral permeation samples: Analytical validation. *J. Pharm. Biomed. Anal.* **2018**, *160*, 109–118. [CrossRef]

3.	Aronson, J.K. Pranoprofen. In *Meyler's Side Effects of Drugs. The International Encyclopedia of Adverse Drug Reactions and Interactions*, 16th ed.; Elsevier: Amsterdam, The Netherlands, 2016; Volume 7, p. 893.

4.	Akyol-Salman, I.; Leçe-Sertöz, D.; Baykal, O. Topical Pranoprofen 0.1% Is As Effective Anti-Inflammatory and Analgesic Agent as Diclofenac Sodium 0.1% After Strabismus Surgery. *J. Ocul. Pharmacol. Ther.* **2007**, *23*, 280–283. [CrossRef]

5.	Yao, B.; Wang, F.; Zhao, X.; Wang, B.; Yue, X.; Ding, Y.; Liu, G. Effect of a Topical Nonsteroidal Anti-Inflammatory Drug (0.1% Pranoprofen) on VEGF and COX-2 Expression in Primary Pterygium. *Front. Pharmacol.* **2021**, *12*, 709251. [CrossRef] [PubMed]

6.	Abrego, G.; Alvarado, H.; Souto, E.B.; Guevara, B.; Bellowa, L.H.; Parra, A.; Calpena, A.; Garcia, M.L. Biopharmaceutical profile of pranoprofen-loaded PLGA nanoparticles containing hydrogels for ocular administration. *Eur. J. Pharm. Biopharm.* **2015**, *95*, 261–270. [CrossRef] [PubMed]

7.	Gong, Y.; Zhang, W.; Yan, P.; Mu, Y. Pranoprofen inhibits endoplasmic reticulum stress-mediated apoptosis of chondrocytes. *Panminerva Med.* **2020**. *ahead of print*. [CrossRef]

8.	Rincón, M.; Calpena, A.C.; Clares, B.; Espina, M.; Garduño-Ramírez, M.L.; Rodríguez-Lagunas, M.J.; García, M.L.; Abrego, G. Skin-controlled release lipid nanosystems of pranoprofen for the treatment of local inflammation and pain. *Nanomedicine* **2018**, *13*, 2397–2413. [CrossRef] [PubMed]

9.	Mallandrich, M.; Calpena, A.C.; Clares, B.; Parra, A.; García, M.L.; Soriano, J.L.; Fernández-Campos, F. Nano-engineering of ketorolac tromethamine platforms for ocular treatment of inflammatory disorders. *Nanomedicine* **2021**, *16*, 401–414. [CrossRef]

10.	Battaglia, L.; Serpe, L.; Foglietta, F.; Muntoni, E.; Gallarate, M.; del Pozo-Rodriguez, A.; Solinis, M.A. Application of lipid nanoparticles to ocular drug delivery. *Expert Opin. Drug Deliv.* **2016**, *13*, 1743–1757. [CrossRef] [PubMed]

11.	Laffleur, F.; Bauer, B. Progress in nasal drug delivery systems. *Int. J. Pharm.* **2021**, *607*, 20994. [CrossRef]

12.	Akel, H.; Ismail, R.; Csóka, I. Progress and perspectives of brain-targeting lipid-based nanosystems via the nasal route in Alzheimer's disease. *Eur. J. Pharm. Biopharm.* **2020**, *148*, 38–53. [CrossRef]

13.	Hua, S. Advances in Nanoparticulate Drug Delivery Approaches for Sublingual and Buccal Administration. *Front. Pharmacol.* **2019**, *10*, 1328. [CrossRef] [PubMed]

14.	Shirvan, A.R.; Hemmatinejad, N.; Bahrami, S.H.; Bashari, A. Fabrication of multifunctional mucoadhesive buccal patch for drug delivery applications. *J. Biomed. Mater. Res. A* **2021**, *109*, 2640–2656. [CrossRef]

15.	Macedo, A.S.; Castro, P.M.; Roque, L.; Thomé, N.G.; Reis, C.P.; Pintado, M.E.; Fonte, P. Novel and revisited approaches in nanoparticle systems for buccal drug delivery. *J. Control. Release* **2020**, *320*, 125–141. [CrossRef] [PubMed]

16.	Langoth, N.; Kalbe, J.; Bernkop-Schnürch, A. Development of buccal drug delivery systems based on a thiolated polymer. *Int. J. Pharm.* **2003**, *252*, 141–148. [CrossRef]

17.	de Oliveira, R.P.; de Oliveira, J.M.; Caramella, C. Special issue on vaginal drug delivery. *Adv. Drug Deliv. Rev.* **2015**, *92*, 1. [CrossRef]

18.	Rincón, M.; Calpena, A.C.; Fabrega, M.-J.; Garduño-Ramírez, M.L.; Espina, M.; Rodríguez-Lagunas, M.J.; García, M.L.; Abrego, G. Development of Pranoprofen Loaded Nanostructured Lipid Carriers to Improve Its Release and Therapeutic Efficacy in Skin Inflammatory Disorders. *Nanomaterials* **2018**, *8*, 1022. [CrossRef]

19.	Fangueiro, J.; Andreani, T.; Egea, M.A.; Garcia, M.L.; Souto, S.B.; Souto, E.B. Experimental factorial design applied to mucoadhesive lipid nanoparticles via multiple emulsion process. *Colloids Surf. B Biointerfaces* **2012**, *100*, 84–89. [CrossRef] [PubMed]

20.	Politis, S.N.; Colombo, P.; Colombo, G.; Rekkas, D.M. Design of experiments (DoE) in pharmaceutical development. *Drug Dev. Ind. Pharm.* **2017**, *43*, 889–901. [CrossRef]

21.	Buttini, F.; Rozou, S.; Rossi, A.; Zoumpliou, V.; Rekkas, D.M. The application of Quality by Design framework in the pharmaceutical development of dry powder inhalers. *Eur. J. Pharm. Sci.* **2018**, *113*, 64–76. [CrossRef] [PubMed]

22.	Peña, D. *Análisis de Datos Multivariantes*; McGraw-Hill/Interamericana: Madrid, Spain, 2002; pp. 137–171.

23.	Gómez-Segura, L.; Parra, A.; Calpena, A.C.; Gimeno, Á.; Boix-Montañes, A. Carprofen Permeation Test through Porcine Ex Vivo Mucous Membranes and Ophthalmic Tissues for Tolerability Assessments: Validation and Histological Study. *Vet. Sci.* **2020**, *7*, 152. [CrossRef] [PubMed]

24.	Domínguez-Villegas, V.; Clares-Naveros, B.; García-López, M.L.; Calpena-Campmany, A.C.; Bustos-Zagal, P.; Garduño-Ramírez, M.L. Development and characterization of two nano-structured systems for topical application of flavanones isolated from Eysenhardtia platycarpa. *Colloids Surf. B Biointerfaces* **2014**, *116*, 183–192. [CrossRef] [PubMed]

25.	Rincón, M.; Silva-Abreu, M.; Espinoza, L.C.; Sosa, L.; Calpena, A.C.; Rodríguez-Lagunas, M.J.; Colom, H. Enhanced Transdermal Delivery of Pranoprofen Using a Thermo-Reversible Hydrogel Loaded with Lipid Nanocarriers for the Treatment of Local Inflammation. *Pharmaceuticals* **2021**, *15*, 22. [CrossRef] [PubMed]

26.	Middleton, S. Porcine ophthalmology. *Vet. Clin. N. Am. Food Anim. Pract.* **2010**, *26*, 557–572. [CrossRef]

27.	Van Eyk, A.D.; van der Bijl, P. Comparative permeability of various chemical markers through human vaginal and buccal mucosa as well as porcine buccal and mouth floor mucosa. *Arch. Oral Biol.* **2004**, *49*, 387–392. [CrossRef]

28.	Liu, C.; Xu, H.N.; Li, X.L. In vitro permeation of tetramethylpyr-azine across porcine buccal mucosa. *Acta Pharmacol. Sin.* **2002**, *23*, 792–796.

29.	Valls, M.M.; Labrador, A.M.; Bellowa, L.H.; Torres, D.B.; Granda, P.; Carmona, M.M.; Limón, D.; Campmany, A.C. Biopharmaceutical Study of Triamcinolone Acetonide Semisolid Formulations for Sublingual and Buccal Administration. *Pharmaceutics* **2021**, *13*, 1080. [CrossRef]

30. Squier, C.A.; Mantz, M.J.; Schlievert, P.M.; Davis, C.C. Porcine Vagina Ex Vivo as a Model for Studying Permeability and Pathogenesis in Mucosa. *J. Pharm. Sci.* **2008**, *97*, 9–21. [CrossRef]

31. Wadell, C.; Björk, E.; Camber, O. Permeability of porcine nasal mucosa correlated with human nasal absorption. *Eur. J. Pharm. Sci.* **2002**, *18*, 47–53. [CrossRef]

32. Gómez-Segura, L.; Parra, A.; Calpena-Campmany, A.C.; Gimeno, Á.; de Aranda, I.G.; Boix-Montañes, A. Ex Vivo Permeation of Carprofen Vehiculated by PLGA Nanoparticles through Porcine Mucous Membranes and Ophthalmic Tissues. *Nanomaterials* **2020**, *10*, 355. [CrossRef]

33. Patel, A.; Bell, M.; O'Connor, C.; Inchley, A.; Wibawa, J.; Lane, M.E. Delivery of ibuprofen to the skin. *Int. J. Pharm.* **2013**, *457*, 9–13. [CrossRef] [PubMed]

34. González-Mira, E.; Egea, M.A.; García, M.L.; Souto, E.B. Design and ocular tolerance of flurbiprofen loaded ultrasound-engineered NLC. *Colloids Surf. B Biointerfaces* **2010**, *81*, 412–421. [CrossRef] [PubMed]

35. López-Machado, A.; Díaz-Garrido, N.; Cano, A.; Espina, M.; Badia, J.; Baldomà, L.; Calpena, A.C.; Souto, E.B.; García, M.L.; Sánchez-López, E. Development of Lactoferrin-Loaded Liposomes for the Management of Dry Eye Disease and Ocular Inflammation. *Pharmaceutics* **2021**, *13*, 1698. [CrossRef] [PubMed]

36. González-Fernández, F.; Bianchera, A.; Gasco, P.; Nicoli, S.; Pescina, S. Lipid-Based Nanocarriers for Ophthalmic Administration: Towards Experimental Design Implementation. *Pharmaceutics* **2021**, *13*, 447. [CrossRef] [PubMed]

37. Celia, C.; Trapasso, E.; Cosco, D.; Paolino, D.; Fresta, M. Turbiscan Lab® Expert analysis of the stability of ethosomes® and ultradeformable liposomes containing a bilayer fluidizing agent. *Colloids Surf. B Biointerfaces* **2009**, *72*, 155–160. [CrossRef]

38. Espinoza, L.C.; Silva-Abreu, M.; Clares, B.; Rodríguez-Lagunas, M.J.; Halbaut, L.; Cañas, M.-A.; Calpena, A.C. Formulation Strategies to Improve Nose-to-Brain Delivery of Donepezil. *Pharmaceutics* **2019**, *11*, 64. [CrossRef]

39. Sánchez-López, E.; Esteruelas, G.; Ortiz, A.; Espina, M.; Prat, J.; Muñoz, M.; Cano, A.; Calpena, A.C.; Ettcheto, M.; Camins, A.; et al. Dexibuprofen Biodegradable Nanoparticles: One Step Closer towards a Better Ocular Interaction Study. *Nanomaterials* **2020**, *10*, 720. [CrossRef]

40. Lindstrom, R.; Kim, T. Ocular permeation and inhibition of retinal inflammation: An examination of data and expert opinion on the clinical utility of nepafenac. *Curr. Med. Res. Opin.* **2006**, *22*, 397–404. [CrossRef]

41. Menduni, F.; Davies, L.N.; Madrid-Costa, D.; Fratini, A.; Wolffsohn, J. Characterisation of the porcine eyeball as an in-vitro model for dry eye. *Contact Lens Anterior Eye* **2018**, *41*, 13–17. [CrossRef]

42. Varela-Fernández, R.; García-Otero, X.; Díaz-Tomé, V.; Regueiro, U.; López-López, M.; González-Barcia, M.; Lema, M.I.; Otero-Espinar, F.J. Design, Optimization, and Characterization of Lactoferrin-Loaded Chitosan/TPP and Chitosan/Sulfobutylether-β-cyclodextrin Nanoparticles as a Pharmacological Alternative for Keratoconus Treatment. *ACS Appl. Mater. Interfaces* **2021**, *13*, 3559–3575. [CrossRef]

43. Folle, C.; Marqués, A.M.; Díaz-Garrido, N.; Espina, M.; Sánchez-López, E.; Badia, J.; Baldoma, L.; Calpena, A.C.; García, M.L. Thymol-loaded PLGA nanoparticles: An efficient approach for acne treatment. *J. Nanobiotechnol.* **2021**, *19*, 359. [CrossRef] [PubMed]

44. International Conference on Harmonization (ICH). *Validation of Analytical Procedures: Text and Methodology, Q2(R1)*; ICH: Geneva, Switzerland, 2005.

45. Prasertpol, T.; Tiyaboonchai, W. Nanostructured lipid carriers: A novel hair protective product preventing hair damage and discoloration from UV radiation and thermal treatment. *J. Photochem. Photobiol. B Biol.* **2020**, *204*, 111769. [CrossRef]

46. Riangjanapatee, P.; Khongkow, M.; Treetong, A.; Unger, O.; Phungbun, C.; Jaemsai, S.; Bootsiri, C.; Okonogi, S. Development of Tea Seed Oil Nanostructured Lipid Carriers and In Vitro Studies on Their Applications in Inducing Human Hair Growth. *Pharmaceutics* **2022**, *14*, 984. [CrossRef] [PubMed]

47. Velmurugan, R.; Selvamuthukumar, S. Development and optimization of ifosfamide nanostructured lipid carriers for oral delivery using response surface methodology. *Appl. Nanosci.* **2016**, *6*, 159–173. [CrossRef]

48. Angelo, T.; El-Sayed, N.; Jurisic, M.; Koenneke, A.; Gelfuso, G.M.; Filho, M.C.; Taveira, S.F.; Lemor, R.; Schneider, M.; Gratieri, T. Effect of physical stimuli on hair follicle deposition of clobetasol-loaded Lipid Nanocarriers. *Sci. Rep.* **2020**, *10*, 176. [CrossRef]

49. Sosa, L.; Calpena, A.C.; Silva-Abreu, M.; Espinoza, L.C.; Rincón, M.; Bozal, N.; Domenech, O.; Rodríguez-Lagunas, M.J.; Clares, B. Thermoreversible Gel-Loaded Amphotericin B for the Treatment of Dermal and Vaginal Candidiasis. *Pharmaceutics* **2019**, *11*, 312. [CrossRef] [PubMed]

50. El Moussaoui, S.; Abo-Horan, I.; Halbaut, L.; Alonso, C.; Coderch, L.; Garduño-Ramírez, M.L.; Clares, B.; Soriano, J.L.; Calpena, A.C.; Fernández-Campos, F.; et al. Polymeric Nanoparticles and Chitosan Gel Loading Ketorolac Tromethamine to Alleviate Pain Associated with Condyloma Acuminata during the Pre- and Post-Ablation. *Pharmaceutics* **2021**, *13*, 1784. [CrossRef] [PubMed]

51. Yoshio, I.; Iwata, A.; Isobe, M.; Takamatsu, R.; Higashi, M. The pharmacokinetics of pranoprofen in humans. *Yakugaku Zasshi.* **1990**, *110*, 509–515. [CrossRef]

52. López-Machado, A.; Díaz, N.; Cano, A.; Espina, M.; Badía, J.; Baldomà, L.; Calpena, A.C.; Biancardi, M.; Souto, E.B.; García, M.L.; et al. Development of topical eye-drops of lactoferrin-loaded biodegradable nanoparticles for the treatment of anterior segment inflammatory processes. *Int. J. Pharm.* **2021**, *609*, 121188. [CrossRef] [PubMed]

53. Derouiche, M.T.T.; Abdennour, S. HET-CAM test. Application to shampoos in developing countries. *Toxicol. Vitr.* **2017**, *45*, 393–396. [CrossRef] [PubMed]

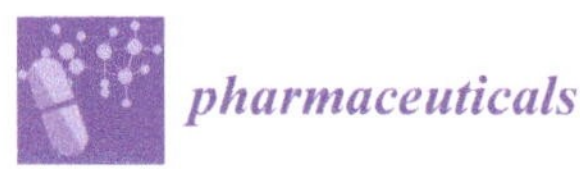 *pharmaceuticals*

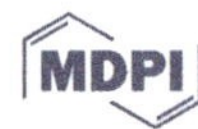

Review

Use of Nanocarriers Containing Antitrypanosomal Drugs for the Treatment of Chagas Disease

Diogo de Freitas Paiva [1], Ana Paula dos Santos Matos [1], Denise de Abreu Garófalo [1], Tatielle do Nascimento [1], Mariana Sato de Souza de Bustamante Monteiro [1], Ralph Santos-Oliveira [2] and Eduardo Ricci-Junior [1,*]

[1] Laboratory of Pharmaceutical Nanotechnology, Department of Drugs and Medications, Faculty of Pharmacy, Universidade Federal do Rio de Janeiro (UFRJ), Rio de Janeiro 21941-902, Brazil; di0g0fp2@gmail.com (D.d.F.P.); anapaulasmatos@gmail.com (A.P.d.S.M.); denise_gar@hotmail.com (D.d.A.G.); tatiellenascimento@hotmail.com (T.d.N.); mari-sato@hotmail.com (M.S.d.S.d.B.M.)

[2] Nuclear Engineering Institute (IEN), University Campus of the Federal University of Rio de Janeiro, Rio de Janeiro 21941-906, Brazil; roliveira@ien.gov.br

* Correspondence: ricci@pharma.ufrj.br

Abstract: Chagas disease, caused by the *Trypanosoma cruzi* parasitic protozoan, is a neglected tropical disease (NTD) of significant incidence in Latin America. Transmission to humans and other mammals is mainly via the vector insect from the Reduviidae family, popularly known as the kissing bug. There are other transmission means, such as through congenital transmission, blood transfusions, organ transplantations, and the consumption of contaminated food. For more than 50 years, the disease has been treated with benznidazole and nifurtimox, which are only effective during the acute phase of the disease. In addition to their low efficacy in the chronic phase, they cause many adverse effects and are somewhat selective. The use of nanocarriers has received significant attention due to their ability to encapsulate and release therapeutic agents in a controlled manner. Generally, their diameter ranges from 100 to 300 nanometers. The objective of this scoping review was to perform a search of the literature for the use of nanocarriers as an alternative for improving the treatment of Chagas disease and to suggest future research. Bibliographic searches were carried out in the Web of Science and PubMed scientific databases from January 2012 to May 2023, using the "Chagas disease and *Trypanosoma cruzi* and nanoparticles" keywords, seeking to gather the largest number of articles, which were evaluated using the inclusion and exclusion criteria. After analyzing the papers, the results showed that nanocarriers offer physiological stability and safety for the transport and controlled release of drugs. They can increase solubility and selectivity against the parasite. The in vitro assays showed that the trypanocidal activity of the drug was not impaired after encapsulation. In the in vivo assays, parasitemia reduction and high survival and cure rates in animals were obtained during both phases of the disease using lower doses when compared to the standard treatment. The scoping review showed that nanocarriers are a promising alternative for the treatment of Chagas disease.

Keywords: nanocarriers; Chagas disease; *Trypanosoma cruzi*; in vivo assays

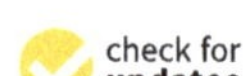 check for **updates**

Citation: Paiva, D.d.F.; Matos, A.P.d.S.; Garófalo, D.d.A.; do Nascimento, T.; Monteiro, M.S.d.S.d.B.; Santos-Oliveira, R.; Ricci-Junior, E. Use of Nanocarriers Containing Antitrypanosomal Drugs for the Treatment of Chagas Disease. *Pharmaceuticals* **2023**, *16*, 1163. https://doi.org/10.3390/ph16081163

Academic Editors: Ana Catarina Silva, João Nuno Moreira and José Manuel Sousa Lobo

Received: 12 July 2023
Revised: 9 August 2023
Accepted: 11 August 2023
Published: 15 August 2023

1. Introduction

Chagas disease, or American trypanosomiasis, was discovered by the Brazilian Carlos Chagas in 1909 [1]. It is an infection caused by the *Trypanosoma cruzi* parasitic protozoan. The World Health Organization (WHO) estimates that there are from 6 to 8 million people infected with the parasite in the world, with a higher incidence in endemic areas of South American countries [2,3]. Approximately 10,000 people die every year because of the disease [4,5]. It is considered a neglected tropical disease (NTD) due to the pharmaceutical companies lacking interest in investing in the search for new treatments and increasing professional specialization for faster and more efficient diagnoses. Despite that, the disease is no longer exclusive to developing countries [1]. Due to the increase in immigration to other countries, many cases are diagnosed in European countries, Canada, Australia, Japan, and the United States [2,4,6].

The main transmission means is vectorial by blood-sucking insects of the Reduviidae family, popularly known as the kissing bug [7]. When the insect bites, it defecates in the region close to the bite, generating itching. This makes the person scratch the area, taking feces and urine containing the infective form of *T. cruzi* inside the wound [4,6]. Other transmission means are already known, through blood transfusions in banks that do not carry out screening, organ transplants, congenital transmission, and oral transmission by the consumption of food or beverages contaminated with the infected vector [1,6].

Trypanosoma cruzi presents in three different forms in its development cycle and needs two different types of hosts: invertebrate ones (hematophagous insects) and vertebrate ones (mammals) [6,8]. The epimastigote form is found in the vector, replicative but non-infectious. The circulating trypomastigote form is found in the hosts; it is infectious and not replicative. The intracellular amastigote form is only replicative and is present in vertebrate hosts [9]. When the vector bites a contaminated host, it ingests blood in the metacyclic trypomastigote form, which in the invertebrate organism will differentiate into epimastigotes that multiply by binary fission [6,9]. Subsequently, these epimastigote forms are differentiated into trypomastigotes that will be released in triatomine excretions. Upon entering the wound of the human host, the trypomastigote form penetrates the cells and transforms into amastigotes, which will multiply and differentiate into trypomastigotes through several binary division cycles until causing the cell to break, which releases amastigotes and trypomastigotes, infecting neighboring cells and spreading [9]. The infective forms of the parasite can penetrate any type of nucleated cell, including defense cells such as macrophages [1,4]. They present tropism via myocytes, which explains their presence in cardiac muscle cells causing heart dysfunction [1].

Chagas disease is divided into two clinical phases: acute and chronic. The acute phase can manifest early in time or progress to being undetermined, silent, and asymptomatic. In the early acute stage, the disease can disappear spontaneously without causing complications in most infected individuals due to adaptive immunity control or present with nonspecific symptoms [1,2]. It can be characterized by the onset of inflammation in the parasite entry region and present with more ease of parasitemia detection [2,6]. In the undetermined silent and asymptomatic phase, the parasites hide in different tissues, hindering diagnosis [2]. When progressing to the chronic phase of the disease, the patient has a 30% to 40% chance, after years or decades, of developing megaesophagus, megacolon, and chronic chagasic cardiomyopathy, which is the most severe form of the disease and, without treatment that can revert the clinical picture, possibly presenting with thromboembolism, cardiac arrhythmias, and cardiac arrest [1,2,6,8].

Since the 1960s, the only treatments known for Chagas disease have been two nitro-heterocyclic compounds: nifurtimox and benznidazole (Figure 1) [3,9]. Despite a therapeutic efficacy of up to 80% presented during treatment in the acute phase, the drugs have low efficacy in the chronic phase [1,3]. In addition, they have high toxicity, low solubility in aqueous media, difficulty crossing biological barriers, low selectivity, and serious adverse effects, leading many patients to abandon drug treatment [3,8,9]. Such high toxicity can be related to the high doses required for the drugs to achieve the effective concentration to cause intracellular death [1].

The treatment with nifurtimox causes stronger adverse effects than using benznidazole, even when administered in low doses. The most frequent adverse effects are gastrointestinal symptoms, anorexia, sleepiness, and paresthesia [9].

Benznidazole is the first-choice drug for treating the infection, despite the low cure rate in the chronic phase of the disease [3]. Its main adverse effects are peripheral neuropathy, cutaneous manifestations, paresthesia, anorexia, gastrointestinal symptoms, and more severe ones such as decrease in bone marrow and agranulocytosis [9,10]. Other factors can influence the outcome of the treatment with benznidazole, such as the different parasite strains, emergence of drug-resistant strains, the patient's age, the progression of the disease, the long period required for the treatment, and the lack of appropriate infant formulations [6,9,10].

Nifurtimox

Benznidazole

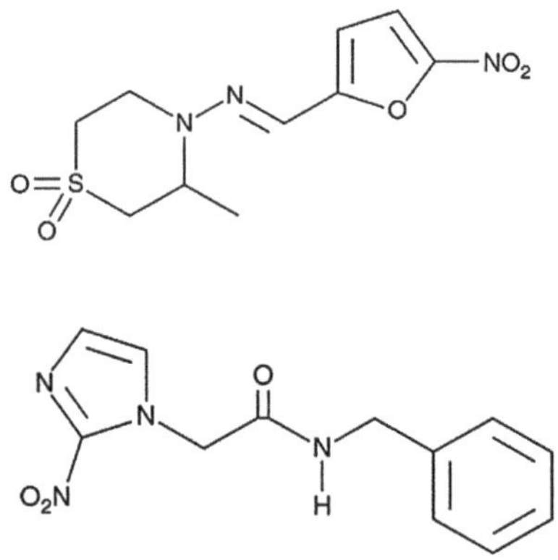

Figure 1. Chemical structures of nifurtimox and benznidazole.

The WHO has determined that the ideal drug for treatment should present a parasitological cure and show dose efficacy during the acute and chronic phases, not present adverse effects, or cause resistance, or induce teratogenic effects. The problem is that no currently known drug manages to cover all these needs [9].

Due to the limitations presented by the only treatments currently known to combat the Chagas disease infection, it has become necessary to search for and learn about new therapeutic options that can improve the desired parameters.

In recent years, nanotechnology has been a promising option for studies aimed at finding ways to improve the treatments of various diseases. It is a type of technology that uses nanoscience practically with multiple functions performed by structures at a nanometric scale, from 1 to 100 nm [11,12]. Nanoparticles can improve bioavailability, promote sustained release, and decrease toxicity. Nanoparticles can stimulate immune system cells, such as macrophages, promoting the elimination of intracellular parasites [13]. Nanoparticles can bind to receptors located on the surface of cells, resulting in cellular uptake [14].

Drugs and nanocarriers can cross the cell membrane by endocytosis or direct permeation. In direct permeation, molecules and particles cross the cell membrane by a mechanism controlled by diffusion or pore formation. However, nanocarriers with polar surfaces and hydrophilic drugs do not cross the plasma membrane easily with a lipophilic nature. To cross the cell membrane, hydrophilic drugs and nanocarriers of polar nature need active transport that involves energy expenditure, such as endocytosis, in which the cell captures extracellular materials through invaginations of the membrane to form endosomes. There are two forms of endocytosis: phagocytosis and macropinocytosis. In phagocytosis, nanomaterials are captured by activated phagocytes through the process of opsonization, in which opsonins, such as immunoglobulins and complement system proteins, coat the target particle. In macropinocytosis, the cell captures liquids and solids (nanoparticles and nanocarriers) with the formation of vesicles called pinosomes. Endocytosis can occur by clathrin-mediated endocytosis, caveolin-mediated endocytosis, and clathrin–caveolin independent endocytosis. Thus, the cellular internalization of nanocarriers depends not only on physicochemical properties, such as the size, shape, surface charge and polarity, but also on the presence of ligands on the surface [15].

Nanoparticles can be classified into polymeric, lipid, metallic, and mesoporous silica (Figure 2) [13]. Lipid nanoparticles are divided into two types: solid lipid nanoparticles (SLNs), and nanostructured lipid carriers (NLCs). Due to the presence of lipids, SLNs are biocompatible and biodegradable and present high bioavailability. They are composed of the same mixture of liquid and solid lipids. Their rigidity confers better protection to the incorporated drug. They are fairly stable, produced on a large scale, and can encapsulate drugs to provide controlled release [6,13,14]. NLCs are like SLNs but can incorporate various types of drugs and liquid lipids in their internal parts [14].

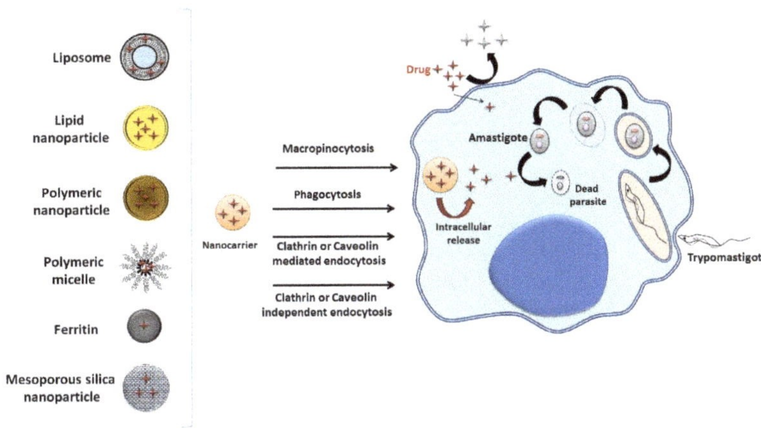

Figure 2. Nanocarriers used for the treatment of Chagas disease and cell uptake routes.

Polymeric nanoparticles are solid colloidal particles generally composed of biodegradable and biocompatible polymers approved by the US regulating agency, the Food and Drug Administration (FDA). They can be dissolved, encapsulated, or absorbed in the constituent polymeric matrix in systems for the release of therapeutic agents and be used as adjuvants in vaccines. They can be produced using countless types of natural or synthetic polymers, such as poly (lactic co-glycolic acid) (PLGA); polylactic acid (PLA); polyglycolide acid (PGA); polycaprolactone (PCL); chitosan; and polyethylene glycol (PEG) [6,13].

Mesoporous silica nanoparticles are potent drug releasers formed by a complex organized network of pores with homogeneous sizes and can assist in the functionalization of drugs. The metallic nanoparticles are formed by clusters of metal atoms [6,13].

In addition to nanoparticles, other nanocarriers are also widely used for the controlled release of drugs, such as liposomes and polymeric micelles. Liposomes are vesicular systems composed of one or more lipid bilayers of a spherical format with sizes ranging from 50 to 500 nm. They are employed extensively due to their ability to encapsulate drugs, thanks to their hydrophobic and hydrophilic characteristics, high bioavailability, and biocompatibility [16].

Polymeric micelles are amphiphilic polymer structures that have a hydrophobic part and a hydrophilic component. They can have different formats and are prepared in various ways. Among their advantages as drug vehicles, they have a nanoscale size, selective targeting, storage stability, and reduction in adverse effects [17].

Also, cage-like proteins such as Ferritin can be used as drug carriers [18]. Ferritins can be particularly important in delivering drugs to cure leishmaniasis since ferritins are phagocytized by the macrophages where the parasites live and multiply [19].

The objective of this scoping review is to identify and analyze knowledge gaps and examine how research is conducted in relation to the use of nanocarriers containing trypanocidal drugs to treat Chagas disease, highlighting articles with in vivo studies. This scoping review differs from the others because it will search scientific databases for articles focusing on in vivo studies containing robust in vitro studies published in the last ten years, using nanocarriers as an alternative for the treatment of infection caused by the *Trypanosoma cruzi* parasite.

2. Results

2.1. Bibliographic Research of Articles in the Databases

The number of articles found during the research in the databases chosen to prepare this paper is presented in Table 1.

Table 1. Keyword research and number of articles found.

Keywords	PubMed	Web of Science	Total
Chagas disease and nanoparticles	69	63	123
Trypanosoma cruzi and nanoparticles	49	71	120
Chagas disease and *Trypanosoma cruzi* and nanoparticles	43	44	87

Added to the results of the searches carried out in the PubMed and Web of Science databases covering the period from January 2012 to May 2023, 123 articles were found with the "Chagas disease and nanoparticles" keyword, 120 for "*Trypanosoma cruzi* and nanoparticles", and 87 using "Chagas disease and *Trypanosoma cruzi* and nanoparticles". All 87 articles found in the research using the "Chagas Disease and *Trypanosoma cruzi* and nanoparticles" keywords were selected to proceed to the following stage.

All 87 articles were analyzed according to the exclusion criteria, removing 23 duplicates and 17 review articles. No congress abstracts, patents, or book chapters were found. Only one article was excluded for having been published in a journal with an impact factor below 1.0. The remaining 46 papers had their content assessed by reading, excluding those that did not deal with the topic of interest. A total of 28 articles were removed; among them: one article on vaccines, eight articles on new diagnostic techniques for detecting the disease, nine articles that did not use nanocarriers, two studies on cell migration, three studies that addressed other diseases such as leishmaniasis and toxoplasmosis, and five studies on extracellular vesicles (Evs). In the end, 18 articles were selected for review. The process to select the articles is shown in the flowchart in Figure 3.

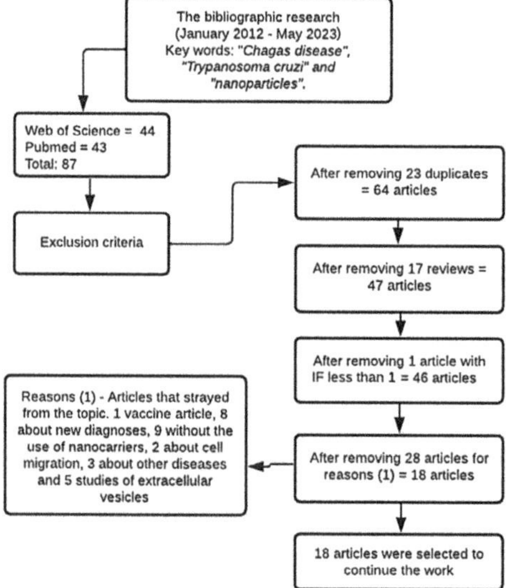

Figure 3. Flowchart corresponding to selection of the articles for the bibliographic review, as PAGE et al. [20].

The assessment of the remaining 18 articles is presented in Table 2.

Table 2. Evaluation of the articles selected, according to the binary code 0/1, where 0 = not present and 1 = present. The value 0 indicates not present and value 1 indicates present. Table adapted from Cruz [21].

Reference	[22]	[23]	[24]	[2]	[25]	[4]	[3]	[10]	[1]	[26]	[5]	[27]	[28]	[29]	[8]	[30]	[31]	[7]
Title	1	1	1	1	1	1	1	1	1	1	1	1	1	0	1	1	1	1
Abstract	1	1	1	1	1	1	1	1	1	1	1	1	1	1	1	1	1	1
Introduction																		
Contextualization	1	1	1	1	1	1	1	1	1	1	1	1	1	1	1	1	1	1
Objective	1	1	1	1	1	1	1	1	1	1	1	1	1	1	1	1	1	1
Methods																		
Ethics statement	0	0	0	0	1	0	0	1	1	1	0	1	1	1	1	1	1	1
Study design	0	0	0	0	1	0	0	1	1	1	0	1	1	1	1	1	1	1
Complete physicochemical characterization	0	0	1	1	0	0	0	1	1	0	1	0	0	1	0	0	1	0
Nanometric size	1	1	1	1	1	1	0	1	1	1	1	1	1	1	1	1	1	1
Animals	0	0	0	0	1	0	0	1	1	1	0	1	1	1	1	1	1	1
Sample size	0	0	0	0	1	0	0	1	1	1	0	1	1	1	1	1	1	1
In vitro study	1	1	1	1	0	1	1	1	1	0	1	1	1	1	0	0	0	1
In vivo study	0	0	0	0	1	0	0	1	1	1	0	1	1	1	1	1	1	1
Trypanocidal effect	1	1	1	0	1	1	1	1	1	1	1	1	1	1	1	1	1	1
Statistics	1	1	1	1	1	1	0	1	1	1	1	1	1	1	1	1	1	1
Results and discussion																		
Interpretation	1	1	1	1	1	1	1	1	1	1	1	1	1	1	1	1	1	1
Limitations	1	0	1	0	1	1	1	1	1	1	1	1	1	1	0	1	1	1
Conclusion	1	1	1	1	1	1	1	1	1	1	1	1	1	1	1	1	1	1
Score	**11**	**10**	**12**	**10**	**14**	**12**	**9**	**17**	**17**	**15**	**12**	**16**	**16**	**16**	**14**	**15**	**16**	**16**

As shown in Table 2, two articles [1,10] obtained the maximum score, as they presented all the topics selected for the assessment. The article that obtained the lowest score was [3], as it only conducted in vitro assays, obtaining a null score in all the topics related to in vivo assays, in addition to not presenting other issues such as physicochemical characterization and the nanometric size of the nanocarrier. The articles [2,3,5,22–24] received a zero for the topics of ethics statement, study design, animals, sample size, and in vivo studies, as they did not present in vivo studies, only in vitro ones.

The articles that presented in vivo tests were [1,7,8,10,25,27–31].

All the articles were scored for presenting full abstracts, contextualization, and objectives in their introduction and interpretation of the results with a conclusion [1–5,7,8,10,22–31].

The article of Abriata [29] had the topic of the title scored as zero, as it did not specify the content of in vitro assays, even if present in the paper. Nhavene [3] was the only article that did not report the nanometric scale size of the nanoparticle. In the article of Branquinho [31], the complete physicochemical characterization had been previously performed by Branquinho [32]. Some articles did not present the characterization of the morphology [4,7,8,22,26–28,30] and the polydispersity index [3,22,23,25] of the nanoparticles; therefore, they obtained a zero in physicochemical characterization.

Only the article [2] did not present an efficient trypanocidal effect in the tests with the nanoparticles and, along with articles [8,23], obtained zero points on the topic of limitations. The only article that did not present any statistics was [3].

2.2. Nanocarriers

The composition and characterization of the structures of the nanocarriers used are shown in Table 3.

Most of the research used polymeric nanoparticles as drug nanocarriers [4,7,8,24,25,29–31], followed by polymeric micelles [26–28], and by solid lipid nanoparticles [2,10]. In addition to solid lipid nanoparticles (SLN), the article by Vinuesa [2] evaluated nanostructured lipid carriers (NLCs) and liposomes in the tests. Of the selected articles, only one employed silver nanoparticles [5], and another resorted to mesoporous silica nanoparticles [3]. One of the articles applied the organic nanoparticle system called MOF (Metal–Organic Framework), composed of hybrid polymers [23]. The article by Tessarolo [22] presented an inorganic $CaCO_3$ particle containing encapsulated BZN. Li [1] worked with vesicular nanocarriers known as polymerosomes. The types of nanostructures used in the papers are represented in Figure 4.

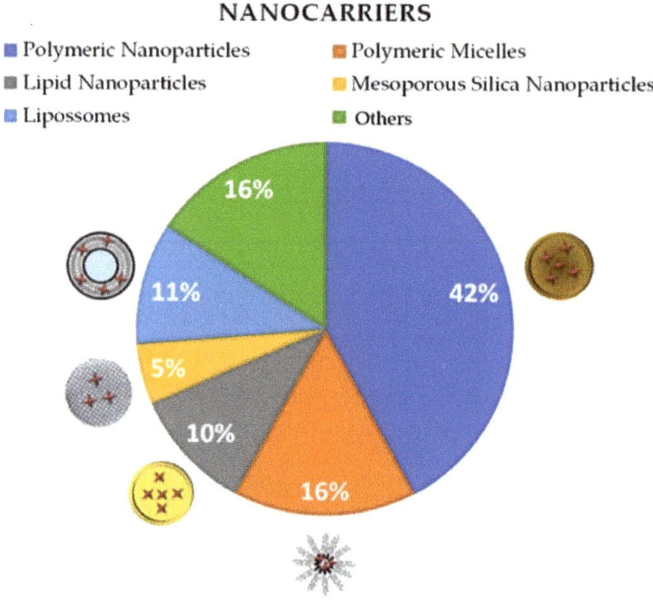

Figure 4. Types of nanocarriers used for delivery of anti-*T. cruzi* drugs. Others: metallic nanoparticles, composite nanoparticles, and polymerosomes.

Table 3. Composition and physicochemical characterization of the Nanocarriers.

			Polymeric Nanoparticle				
Reference	System	Composition	Drug	Drug Concentration	Preparation Method	Characterization	Size (nm)/PDI
[4]	Chitosan polymeric nanoparticles (CS-NPs) and S-nitroso-MSA-CS NPs (NO-releasing nanoparticles)	CS, TPP, MSA, NaNO$_2$, DTNB, EDTA, PBS, [3-(4,5-dimethylthiazol-2-yl)-2,5-diphenyl-2H-tetrazolium bromide] and acetic acid	Mercaptosuccinic acid (MSA) and NO for NaNO$_2$	400 mmol/L of MSA and equimolar amount of NaNO$_2$	Ionotropic gelation, stirring and suspension	Mean hydrodynamic diameter, PDI, and zeta potential by DLS. MSA EE in CS-NPs and nitrosation of MSA-CS NPs by UV-Vis spectrophotometry. Kinetics of decomposition through linear regression.	101.0 ± 2.535 nm/ PDI = 0.280 ± 0.006
[7]	Biodegradable polymeric nanoparticles (NPs) with encapsulated LYC	LYC, monomethoxy-polyethylene glycol-block-poly(lactide) polymer, n-dimethylacetamide: polyethylene glycol 300 (DMA-PEG), isotonic glucose solution	LYC	10 mg of LYC with 60 mg of PLA.	Interfacial polymer deposition followed by solvent displacement method.	Mean hydrodynamic diameter and PDI determined by DLS	105.1 ± 4.4 nm/ PDI = Below 0.3
[8]	LYC-loaded polymeric nanoparticles	LYC, DMA-PEG 300, Glucose, Acetone, Poloxamer 188, PLA-PEG Polymer, Resomer 203, Epikuron 170, Miglyol 810 N	LYC	10 mg de LYC with 80 mg PCL Drug loading 95% to LYC-loaded in PCL-NP 10 mg de LYC with 80 mg (40 mg of PLA-Peg + 40 mg Resomer 203) Drug loading 100% to LYC-loaded in (PLA-Peg/PLA)-NP	Interfacial polymer deposition followed by solvent displacement method.	Mean size and PDI	182.5 ± 3.2 nm/ PDI = Below 0.3

Table 3. *Cont.*

	Polymeric Nanoparticle						
Reference	System	Composition	Drug	Drug Concentration	Preparation Method	Characterization	Size (nm)/PDI
[24]	Polymeric PLA nanoparticles containing DETC	DETC, acetone, ethanol, and PLA at 0.5% (w/v)	Diethyldithio-carbamate	1:12 DETC/polymer ratios, which corresponds to 8.2% (w/w) of the drug in the system	Nanoprecipitation with solvent evaporation methodology	Physical characterization by DLS, SEM, and AFM. Particle diameter by DLS, zeta potential by electrophoretic mobility. EE, DL, UV-Vis spectrophotometry, and FTIR-ATR	168 nm/ PDI below 0.3
[25]	Polymeric nanoparticle	PLGA, curcumin, ethyl acetate, polyvinyl alcohol, 5% sucrose solution. (coating), miltefosine (co-release vehicle)	BZN and Curcumin	500 mg of PLGA with 75 mg of Cur	Emulsification followed by evaporation	DLS size, zeta potential, and AFM morphology	250–300 nm
[29]	Polymeric PCL nanoparticles	UA, PCL, acetone, and surfactant (Poloxamer™ 407).	Ursolic acid	125 mg of PCL with 12.5 mg of ursolic acid	Nanoprecipitation	Size, zeta potential, PDI, EE, morphology by SEM, and thermal behavior by DSC	1:1 = 197.6 $\pm$ 0.85 nm 1:2 = 173.2 $\pm$ 7.28 nm/ PDI = 0.09 $\pm$ 0.03
[30]	Polymeric PEG nanoparticles containing LYC (LYC-NPs)	LYC, PCL, Miglyol 810 N, Epikuron, Acetone, Poloxamer 188, PLA-PEG and PLA	LYC	20 mg of LYC with 80 mg of PCL. 20 mg of LYC with 60 mg of PLA-PEG diblock polymer blended with 60 mg of PLA homopolymer.	Interfacial polymer deposition followed by solvent displacement method.	Mean hydrodynamic diameter and PDI by DLS. Zeta potentials by laser Doppler anemometry associated with microelectrophoresis	LYC-PCL-NP 190.2 $\pm$ 5.7 nm LYC-PLA-PEG-NP 106.1 $\pm$ 6.3 nm/ PDI below 0.3
[31]	Lychnopholide Polymeric Nanoparticles (LYC-PLA-PEG-NP)	LYC, PLA-PEG. Acetone, Epikuron, Miglyol, Poloxamer	LYC	20 to 40 mg de LYC with 120 mg (60 mg of PLA-Peg + 60 mg Resomer 203) LYC loading in PLA-PEG-NP of 9 wt%	Interfacial polymer deposition followed by solvent displacement method.	Mean hydrodynamic diameter, PDI, zeta potential, HPLC-UV, AFM, and LYC loading.	107 $\pm$ 8 nm PDI = Below 0.3

Table 3. *Cont.*

Reference	System	Composition	Drug	Drug Concentration	Preparation Method	Characterization	Size (nm)/PDI
				Polymeric Nanoparticle			
				Lipid Nanoparticles			
[2]	SLNs, NLCs and liposomes.	BNZ, Precirol® dichloromethane solution, Poloxamer 188 at 1% and Polysorbate 80 for SLNs. Precirol® ATO 5, Miglyol® 812, Polysorbate 80 and Poloxamer 188 for NLCs. Cholesterol with PEG1000 for Liposomes.	BZN	-	Emulsification techniques for SLNs. Hot homogenization technique using high pressure homogenizer for NLCs. Fluid compression technique called DELOS-SUSP for liposomes.	Size, PDI, Zeta potential, EE, and cumulative release	SLNs (166 nm) NLCs (202 nm) Liposomes (118 nm) PDI SLNs (0.219 $\pm$ 0.02–0.263 $\pm$ 0.02) NLCs = 0.371 $\pm$ 0.03–0.447 $\pm$ 0.00) Liposomes (0.190 $\pm$ 0.005)
[10]	H2bdtc-loaded SLNs (H2bdtc-SLNs)	Sodium taurodeoxycholate, melted stearic acid, soy lecithin and H2bdtc	H2bdtc	0.02% w/v of H2bdtc with 0.12% w/v of sodium taurodeoxycholate and 0.95% w/v of stearic acid	Microemulsion	D-stroke size by PCS. Zeta potential by mobility electrophoresis of the nanoparticles. Morphology by AFM. DL by UV-Vis spectroscopy. EE%	127.4 $\pm$ 10.2 nm/ PDI = 0.229 $\pm$ 0.130
				Mesoporous Silica Nanoparticles			
[3]	Mesoporous Silica Nanoparticles (MSNs)	BZN, CS, EtOH, GPTMS, NaOH, HCl, C$_4$H$_4$O$_3$, TEOS, CTAB.	BZN	-	Positively charged CTAB model and NaOH catalyst in diluted aqueous conditions, through hydrolysis and condensation of tetraethoxysilane	Zeta potential, TEM, EFTEM, CHN, XPS, SS NMR and DFT	Not reported

Table 3. *Cont.*

					Polymeric Nanoparticle		
Reference	System	Composition	Drug	Drug Concentration	Preparation Method	Characterization	Size (nm)/PDI
				Silver Nanoparticles			
[5]	Silver nanoparticles	*Iresine. herbstii* leaves, corn cob xylan, silver nitrate	Xylan (bioactive polysaccharide)	10 mg/mL (1:9 w/v) solution of xylan with a solution of 1.0 mM silver nitrate.	Green Synthesis process, continuous agitation, centrifugation and lyophilization	Ultraviolet-visible spectroscopy, FTIR, Raman spectroscopy, EDS, SEM, AFM, ICP-OES, DLS, PDI, and zeta potential	55 nm mean size by SEM and AFM DLS showed 102 ± 1.7 nm PDI = 0.178
				Polymeric Micelles			
[26]	Polymeric micelles (BZN-PMs)	BZN, ethanol and Lutrol F-68 (P188)	BZN	200 mg of BZN dissolved in 10 mL of EtOH and 300 mg of P188	Solvent diffusion method	Size, zeta potential, and PDI	61–65 nm/ PDI = 3.35 ±0.1
[27]	BNZ polymeric micelles (BZN-PMs)	BZN, EtOH (solvent), water (antisolvent), Lutrol F-68 (P188)	BZN	200 mg of BZN dissolved in 10 mL of EtOH and 300 mg of P188	Solvent diffusion method and nanoprecipitation technique with P188 as stabilizer	Size by DLS, PDI, ID, z mean diameter, and zeta potential (ζ). Saturation solubility studies	63.30 ± 2.82 nm/ PDI = 3.35 ± 0.10
[28]	Polymeric micelles (BZN-PMs)	BNZ, EtOH and Lutrol F-68 (P188)	BZN	200 mg of BZN dissolved in 10 mL of EtOH and 300 mg of P188	Solvent diffusion method and nanoprecipitation technique with P188 as stabilizer	Size (PCS), zeta potential measurement (electrophoretic mobility) and PDI	63.3 ± 2.82 nm/ PDI = 3.35 ± 0.1
				Liposomes			
[1]	BNZ-loaded polymerosomes	PEG thioacetate, PEG mesylate, propylene sulfide, BZN and tetrahydrofuran	BZN	1.5 mg of BNZ with 30 mg of the copolymer (PEG_{17}-PPS_{60}-PEG_{17})	Anionic polymerization, methanol precipitation, and thin film rehydration.	NMR spectroscopy and gel permeation chromatography, TEM, DLS, LC-MS, liquid chromatography–coupled mass spectrometry, SEM. Loading efficiency, EE, size, zeta potential, and morphology	115 nm/ PDI = 0.11 ± 0.02.

Table 3. *Cont.*

				Polymeric Nanoparticle			
Reference	System	Composition	Drug	Drug Concentration	Preparation Method	Characterization	Size (nm)/PDI
				Others Nanocarriers			
[22]	CaCO$_3$ nanoparticles containing BZN (BZN@CaCO$_3$)	Calcium chloride, Pluronic F-68, Sodium carbonate and BNZ.	BZN	1 mg of BZN in a solution A containing 50 mL of calcium chloride which has been mixed with a solution B containing 50 mL of sodium carbonate and 50 mL of sodium citrate	Emulsification	Zeta potential, AFM, IR, and UV-Vis spectrophotometry.	27.83–64.01 nm
[23]	MOF nanoparticles coupled to EP (MOFs-EP)	Zn (NO$_3$)$_2$·6H$_2$O, L1, L2 and	EP	50 mg of EP with 100 mg of Zn-MOFs	Heating and cooling for crystal formation (synthesis of MOF nanoparticles). Sensitized photo-oxygenation in methanol with eosin (synthesis of EP). Mechanochemistry for coupling.	IR, XRD, TEM, and SEM	28.67–80.44 nm

Key: AFM = Atomic Force Microscopy; BZN = Benznidazole; C$_4$H$_4$O$_3$ = Succinic anhydride; CHN = Elemental Analysis; CS = Chitosan; CTAB = Hexadecyl trimethylammonium bromide; DETC = Sodium diethyldithiocarbamate, DFT = Density Functional Theory Techniques; DL = Content; DLS = Dynamic Light Scattering (or Dispersion); DSC = Differential Scanning Calorimetry; D-Stroke = Dispersion Index; DTNB = 5,5$'$-dithiobis(2-nitrobenzoic acid); EDS = Energy Dispersive X-ray Spectroscopy; EDTA = Ethylenediamine Tetra-acetic Acid; EE = Encapsulation Efficiency; EFTEM = Energy-Filtered Transmission Electron Microscopy; EP = Ergosterol peroxide; EtOH = Pure ethyl alcohol; FTIR = Fourier Transform Infrared Spectroscopy; FTIR-ATR = Infrared Absorption Spectroscopy; GPTMS = 3-glycidyloxypropyl trimethoxysilane; HCl = Hydrochloric acid; HPLC = High Performance Liquid Chromatography; HPLC-UV = High-efficiency Liquid Chromatography with Ultraviolet Detection; ICP-OES = Inductively Coupled Plasma—Optical Emission Spectroscopy; ID = Size distribution; IR = Infrared Spectrometry; LYC = Lychnopholide; MSA = Mercaptosuccinic Acid; MOF = Metal-Organic Frameworks; NaNO$_2$ = Sodium nitrate; NaOH = Sodium hydroxide; NLC = Nanostructured Lipid Carriers; PBS = Phosphate Buffered Saline; PCL = Poly-ε-caprolactone; PCS = Photon Correlation Spectrometry; PDI = Polydispersity Index; PEG = Polyethylene glycol; PLA = Polylactic Acid; PLGA = Poly (Lactic Co-Glycolic Acid); PLA-PEG = Polylactic Acid/Polyethylene glycol; SEM = Scan Electron Microscopy; SLN = Solid Lipid Nanoparticles; SS NMR = Solid-State Nuclear Magnetic Resonance; TEM = Transmission Electron Microscopy; TEOS = Tetraethyl orthosilicate; TPP = Sodium Triphosphate; UA = Ursolic acid; UPLC = Ultra-Performance Liquid Chromatography; XPS = X-ray Photoelectron Spectroscopy; XRD = X-ray Diffraction; Zn(NO$_3$)$_2$·6H$_2$O = Zinc nitrate hexahydrate.

2.3. Components

To produce polymeric nanoparticles, among the components used in the studies there are PLGA [25], different types of polyethylene glycol (PEG) [7,8,30,31], PCL [29–31], and poloxamer [7,29–31]. In the papers that produced lipid nanoparticles or lipid carriers, among the components used are poloxamer 188, polysorbate 80, sodium taurodeoxycholate, Precirol®, and Miglyol® [2,10]. For the silver nanoparticles, silver nitrate and *Iresine herbstii* leaves were used to extract the natural active substance [5]. Chitosan was used in the paper that employed the chitosan polymeric nanoparticle [4] and in the one that produced the mesoporous silica nanoparticle [3]. To produce the hybrid polymer nanoparticles, metal–organic frameworks (MOFs) were used [23]. Poloxamer 188 (Lutrol F-68) was also used as a stabilizer in the synthesis of polymeric micelles [26–28]. PEG thioacetate and mesylate were used in the production of the polymersome [1].

Metal–organic frameworks (MOFs) are hybrid polymers belonging to a new class of nanocarriers of drugs. They can be produced at a nanoscale and their use presents benefits such as a greater surface area at the nanoscale, porosity, and crystallization, which improves the interaction potential with other molecules [23].

The use of chitosan in the articles [3,4] is explained by its biodegradability, biocompatibility, structural stability, low toxicity, and cationic nature, which result in good interaction with cell membranes and increased endocytosis. It was quite often used in drug carriers for biomedical systems in the articles [4,33].

PCL was used for the formation of polymeric nanoparticles and is a synthetic polymer used as a carrier for controlled drug release [29–31]. It is widely applied because it is designed to have good biocompatibility and biodegradability [29].

2.4. Anti-T. cruzi Drugs

The drug used by most of the studies was benznidazole [1–3,22,25–28], which is the first-choice medication for the treatment of Chagas disease. One other drug frequently studied was a natural product, lychnopholide (LYC), a sesquiterpene lactone extracted from *Lychnophora trichocarpha* with anti-*T. cruzi* activity previously reported by De Oliveira [34]. It was employed in the papers [7,8,30,31]. In addition to LIC, other natural active molecules were also used, such as corn cob xylan, a bioactive polysaccharide extracted from the *Iresine herbstii* leaves [5]; curcumin, a polyphenolic flavonoid with anti-inflammatory, antioxidant, and immunomodulatory properties [25], which was combined with benznidazole in the study by Hernández [25]; and ursolic acid, a natural pentacyclic triterpene that has already shown efficacy in the treatment against *Trypanosoma cruzi* infection in vivo [29].

In addition to these compounds, ergosterol peroxide was also used, which, according to data previously obtained, has trypanocidal activity in vitro [23] and sodium diethyldithiocarbamate, which has already shown activity against *T. cruzi* in studies, by chelating metals and stimulating reactive oxygen species (ROS), causing damage to the parasites [24]. In addition, 5-hydroxy-3-methyl-5-phenyl-pyrazoline-1-(S-benzyl dithiocarbonate) (H2bdtc) was used, a cyclic compound derived from S-dithiocarbonate and 1,3-diketones, with significant trypanocidal activity [10] and mercaptosuccinic acid with nitrosation to release nitric oxide (NO), which may be able to kill the parasite and control disease progression [4]. Figure 5 presents a scheme of anti-*T. cruzi* drugs encapsulated in nanocarriers.

2.5. Preparation Method

Most of the studies used the interfacial polymer deposition method after solvent displacement. It is a conventional method for preparing nanoparticles and is also called solvent diffusion or nanoprecipitation [7,8,24,26–31]. The articles [8,26,31] reported that the method had been previously described by Scalise et al. [28], Branquinho et al. [35], and Branquinho et al. [32]. The emulsification method was employed in the papers [22,25]. Vinuesa et al. [2] used the hot homogenization technique to produce NLCs, emulsification for SLNs, and the fluid compression technique, called DELOS-SUSP, for liposomes.

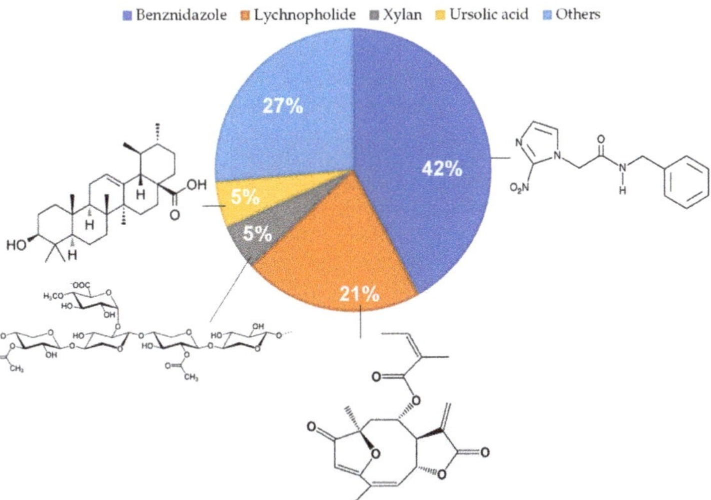

Figure 5. Anti-*T. cruzi* drugs encapsulated in nanocarriers. Others: Curcumin, ergosterol peroxide, sodium diethyldithiocarbamate, 5-hydroxy-3-methyl-5-phenyl-pyrazoline-1-(S-benzyl dithiocarbonate) (H2bdtc), and mercaptosuccinic acid with nitric oxide (NO).

For the synthesis of MOF nanoparticles, the article by Morales-Baez [23] used heating and cooling in crystal formation. For the synthesis of ergosterol peroxide, sensitized photooxygenation in methanol with eosin was used. Finally, mechanochemistry was employed for coupling. In other studies, microemulsion [10], ionotropic gelation with agitation and suspension for chitosan nanoparticles [4], anionic polymerization with precipitation in methanol and thin film rehydration [1], and green synthesis process with continuous agitation for the production of silver nanoparticles [5] were used. In the synthesis of mesoporous silica nanoparticles, the study [3] followed the procedure previously described by Fan et al. [36] in which a model of positively charged N-cetyltrimethylammonium bromide (CTAB) and a NaOH catalyst were used through hydrolysis and condensation. The methods used in the papers are summarized in Figure 6.

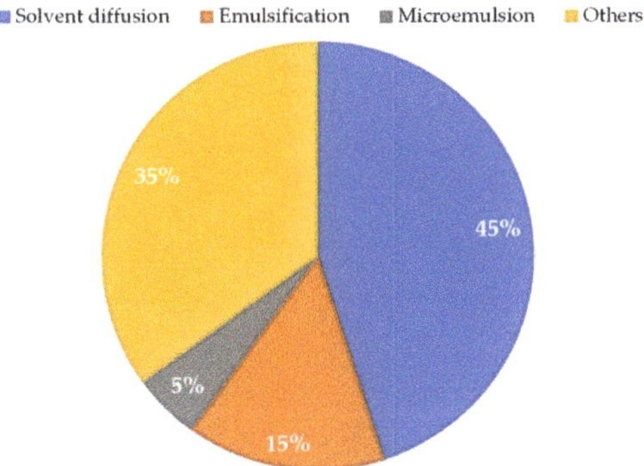

Figure 6. Methods used by the papers in the syntheses of nanocarriers. Others: Hot homogenization technique, emulsion techniques (O/W), heating and cooling in the formation of crystals, sensitized photo-oxygenation in methanol with eosin, mechanochemistry, ionotropic gelation, anionic polymerization with methanol precipitation and thin film rehydration, green synthesis, condensation hydrolysis and the fluid compression technique called DELOS-SUSP.

2.6. Physicochemical Characterization

All the papers reported the nanometric size achieved [1,2,4,5,7,8,10,22–31], except [3]. The techniques used for size characterization were atomic force microscopy (AFM) [5,22, 24,31], dynamic light scattering (DLS) [1,2,4,5,7,8,24,25,27,29–31], scanning electron microscopy (SEM) [5,23], and photon correlation spectroscopy (PCS) [10,26,28].

For the morphology of the nanocarriers, the papers used transmission electron microscopy (TEM) [1,3,23], SEM [2,29], and AFM [10,24,25,31] techniques. The other articles did not present the morphology of the nanocarriers [4,7,8,22,26–28,30].

Zeta potential was obtained by DLS [1–5,27,31], AFM [25], electrophoretic mobility [10,24,26,28], electrophoretic light scattering (ELS) [29], and laser Doppler anemometry associated with microelectrophoresis [30]. The articles [7,8,23] did not present the zeta potential of the nanocarriers. Tessarolo et al. [22] did present the zeta potential value, although without specifying the technique used.

For the polydispersity index (PDI), most articles used the DLS technique [1,2,4,5,7,8, 24,27,29–31]. The PCS technique was used by Carneiro et al. [10] to determine the PDI. Rial et al. [26] and Scalise et al. [28] presented the PDI values without specifying the technique used. The articles [3,22,23,25] did not present the PDI in their studies. Some articles also showed results of the encapsulation efficiency (EE) characterization [1,2,4,10,24,29] and loading efficiency [1,24] of the nanostructures using UV-Vis spectrophotometry and high-efficiency liquid chromatography (HPLC) techniques.

For the quantification of the drug and analysis of coupling with the nanocarrier, infrared (IR) spectroscopy [22,23] and X-ray diffraction (XRD) [23] were used. Vinuesa et al. [2] evaluated the cumulative release for SLNs and NLCs and Abriata et al. [29] obtained the thermal behavior by differential scanning calorimetry (DSC). For the surface characterization of nanocarriers and copolymers, solid-state nuclear magnetic resonance (SS NMR) was used in the studies [1,3]. Nhavene et al. [3] also characterized the elemental composition by energy-filtered transmission electron microscopy (EFTEM), the quantification of organic molecules by elemental analysis (CHN), and the chemical composition and binding state of the elements on the surface of the nanoparticles by X-ray photoelectron spectroscopy (XPS). Other techniques used in the characterization studies were Fourier transform infrared spectroscopy (FTIR) [5], infrared absorption spectroscopy (FTIR-ATR) [24], high-performance liquid chromatography with ultraviolet detection (HPLC-UV) [31], and content (DL) [10,24]. Brito et al. [5] also used Raman spectroscopy, energy dispersion X-ray spectroscopy (EDS), and inductively coupled plasma optical emission spectroscopy (ICP-OES) for the characterization.

2.7. In Vitro Assays

Table 4 presents the in vitro assays and their respective results found by the studies analyzed in this review. The papers selected for the bibliographic research that are not included in the table did not conduct in vitro assays [8,25,26,30,31].

Table 4. In vitro assays.

Reference	Cells	Anti-Epimastigotes	Anti-Trypomastigotes	Anti-Amastigotes	CC_{50}—Cells	IC_{50}—Epimastigotes	IC_{50}—Trypomastigotes	IC_{50}—Amastigotes
				Polymeric Nanoparticle				
[4]	LLCMK2 cells (kidney epithelial cells from Macaca mulatta, CCL-7). Cytotoxicity (MTT) in peritoneal macrophages.	Antiproliferative effect against epimastigotes by direct count in a hemocytometer. Scanning and transmission electron microscopy of epimastigotes.	Effect on trypomastigotes viability in hemocytometer under a light microscope.	-	400 ± 5.7 µg/mL	75.0 ± 6.5 µg/mL	$IC_{50} = 25.0 \pm 5.0$ µg/mL	-
[7]	Potential toxicity of LIC by calcium homeostasis in isolated cardiomyocytes from healthy mice	-	-	-	-	-	-	-
[24]	MTT against three cell lines: RAW (ATCC number TIB-71), derived from macrophages, 3T3 (ATCC CRL-1658), derived from fibroblasts, and Vero (ATCC CCL-81), derived from renal epithelial cells.	Induction of ROS production by parasites in the epimastigote form exposed to DETC nanoparticles.	Antiparasitic activity against different of *T. cruzi* strains in trypomastigotes determined by resazurin reduction and ROS production.	-	-	-	(Dm28c strain) Nanoparticle IC_{50} = 15.47 ± 2.71 µM. Free BZN = 70.58 ± 6.87 µM. (Y strain) Nanoparticle IC_{50} = 45.15 ± 5.44 µM. Free BZN = 85.24 ± 5.22 µM. (Bolivia Strain) Nanoparticle IC_{50} = 47.89 ± 3.98 µM. Free BZN was 79.78 ± 6.18 µM.	-
[29]	Cytotoxicity by the resazurin method in LLCMK2 fibroblasts and *Trypanosoma cruzi* cells.	-	Cytotoxicity in *Trypanosoma cruzi* cells in the trypomastigote form by the resazurin method.	-	-	-	-	-

Table 4. *Cont.*

Reference	Cells	Anti-Epimastigotes	Anti-Trypomastigotes	Anti-Amastigotes	CC_{50}—Cells	IC_{50}—Epimastigotes	IC_{50}—Trypomastigotes	IC_{50}—Amastigotes
Lipid Nanoparticles								
[2]	WST (water soluble tetrazolium test) cytotoxicity in L-929 murine fibroblasts (NCTC 929 clone, ECACC 88102702) and human hepatocellular Hep G2 cell line (American Type Culture Collection (ATCC))	Biological activity of SLNs, NLCs, and liposomes against epimastigotes. Growth inhibition assays.	Growth inhibition assays.	Growth inhibition assays.	-	SLNs (5, 10, 20): 48.8 ± 14.3 μM–123.9 ± 19.7 μM. NLCs: 41.3 ± 9.9 μM–256.0 ± 19.9 μM. BNZ: 17.7 ± 2.1 μM. Liposomes: It was not viable.	NLCs 20″: 17.6 ± 3.3 μM. BNZ: 0.8 ± 0.4 μM	NLCs 20″: 17.6 ± 3.3 μM BNZ: 0.8 ± 0.4 μM
[10]	Cytotoxicity by flow cytometry in spleen cells isolated from C57BL/6 mice previously cultured in fibroblasts (LLCMK2)	-	Evaluation of the trypanocidal activity of free H2bdtc, H2bdtc-SLNs, and BZN after 24h of incubation with trypomastigotes forms	-	-	-	Free H2bdtc—IC_{50} of 0.50 ± 0.12 μM, H2bdtc-SLNs of 1.8 ± 0.18 μM and BZN of 0.50 ± 0.39 μM.	-
Mesoporous Silica Nanoparticles								
[3]		Biological assays—trypanocides for the epimastigotes forms of the *T. cruzi* CL Brener strain.	-	-	-	-	-	-

Table 4. *Cont.*

Reference	Cells	Anti-Epimastigotes	Anti-Trypomastigotes	Anti-Amastigotes	CC$_{50}$—Cells	IC$_{50}$—Epimastigotes	IC$_{50}$—Trypomastigotes	IC$_{50}$—Amastigotes
				Silver Nanoparticles				
[5]	Cytotoxicity (MTT) on murine macrophages (RAW 264.7 ATCC TIB-71) and mouse fibroblasts (3T3 ATCC CCL-92).	Evaluation of the antiparasitic activity of nano xylan by colorimetric MTT. Flow cytometry.	-	-	-	-	-	-
				Polymeric Micelles				
[27]	Quantification of reactive oxygen species (ROS) and *T. cruzi*-specific antibody production in cardiac tissue inflammation in Vero cells (African green monkey renal epithelial cells) by fluorescence assay.	-	-	-	-	-	-	-
[28]	Toxicity (MTT) in Vero cells.	-	-	Amastigote growth inhibition assay in mouse cardiac myocytes (CMs) and Vero cells.	-	-	-	-
				Liposomes				
[1]	It did not assess cell cytotoxicity. Mouse myoblast H9C2 cells for trypanocidal effect	-	Trypanocidal efficacy against trypomastigotes	Trypanocidal efficacy against amastigotes	-	-	BNZ = 55.87 ± 11.39 μM. BNZ-PSs = 56.06 ± 12.21 μM	IC$_{50}$ de BNZ = 33.07 ± 8.17 μM BNZ-PSs = 3.51 ± 0.79 μM.

Table 4. *Cont.*

Reference	Cells	Anti-Epimastigotes	Anti-Trypomastigotes	Anti-Amastigotes	CC$_{50}$—Cells	IC$_{50}$—Epimastigotes	IC$_{50}$—Trypomastigotes	IC$_{50}$—Amastigotes
				Other Nanocarriers				
[22]	Cytotoxicity (MTT) in LLCMK2 mammalian cells (Rhesus monkey kidney epithelial cells)	Trypanocidal effect against epimastigotes (6.25–50 µg/mL)	Trypanocidal effect against trypomastigotes	Trypanocidal effect against amastigotes—Bz-NP (8.7 and 17.4 µg/mL) and Bz (56.7 and 113.4 µg/mL)	55.35 ± 9.03 µg/mL for encapsulated BZN and 160.4 ± 75.09 µg/mL for free BZN	Encapsulated BZN—24 h of 8.72 µg/mL, 48 h of 8.02 µg/mL and 72 h of 4.8 µg/mL. For free BZN: 24 h of 56.7 µg/mL, 48 h of 15.91 µg/mL and 72 h of 4.3 µg/mL	Free BZN LC$_{50}$: 66.9 ± 20.3 µg/mL. Encapsulated BZN: LC$_{50}$ 1.77 ± 0.58 µg/mL	BZN encapsulated IC50 (8.72 µg/mL). Free BZN IC$_{50}$ (56.7 µg/mL)
[23]	Cytotoxicity (MTT) on NIH-3T3 mammalian cells (isolated mouse fibroblast cell line), J774A.1 (monocyte, mouse macrophage), and Vero (African green monkey renal epithelial cells).	Trypanocidal activity at the following concentrations: 5, 10, 20, 50, 100, and 500 µg/mL of MOFs and MOFs-EP. In addition to MOF suspensions in culture media.	Trypanocidal activity at the following concentrations: 5, 10, 20, 50, 100, and 500 µg/mL of MOFs and MOFs-EP. In addition to MOF suspensions in culture media.	-	(MOFs) CC$_{50}$ of 392.0 µg/mL for NIH3T3 cells. CC$_{50}$ of 593.6 µg/mL for J774A.1 cells. CC$_{50}$ of 1030.0 µg/mL for Vero cells. (MOFs-EP)	Results not shown because they are like those found for trypomastigotes	(MOFs-EP) IC$_{50}$ of 4.81 µg/mL and 3.0 µg/mL for 24 and 48 h	Not performed.

Key: CC$_{50}$ = Cytotoxic drug concentration required to kill 50% of the cells; DETC = Sodium diethyldithiocarbamate; H2bdtc = 5-hydroxy-3-methyl-5-phenyl-pyrazoline-1-(S-benzyl dithiocarbonate); IC$_{50}$ = Inhibitory concentration of the drug capable of killing 50% of the parasites; SI = Selectivity index; LIC = Lychnopholide; MOFs = Metal–Organic Frameworks; NLCs = Nanostructured Lipid Carriers; ROS = Reactive Oxygen Species; SLNs = Solid Lipid Nanoparticles, WST = Water Soluble Tetrazolium Test.

The studies used different cell types to conduct the in vitro assays. The cell lines used were LLCMK2 (Rhesus monkey renal epithelial cell) [4,10,22,29], NIH-3T3 (isolated mouse fibroblast cell line) [5,23,24], J774A.1 (monocyte, mouse macrophage) [23], Vero (African green monkey renal epithelial cells) [23,24,27,28], L-929 (murine fibroblasts) [2], Hep G2 (human hepatocellular cell line) [2], H9C2 from mouse myoblasts [1], and RAW (derived from macrophages) [24]. Peritoneal macrophage cell lines [4], cardiomyocytes from healthy mice [7], and spleen cells isolated from C57BL/6 mice [10] were also used.

The test most employed in the articles was MTT, which measures the cytotoxicity of the nanoparticles conferred to the cells, through extracellular reduction of the tetrazolium salts [4,5,22–24,28]. The study [29] assessed cytotoxicity using the resazurin method. Carneiro et al. [10] resorted to flow cytometry to assess cytotoxicity. Branquinho et al. [7] evaluated the toxicity potential of the drug through calcium homeostasis in healthy mouse cells. Vinuesa et al. [2] used the water-soluble tetrazolium (WST) assay to assess cytotoxicity. The studies [1,3] did not employ any cell cytotoxicity assay. The paper by Rial [27] performed tests to quantify ROS and the production of specific *T. cruzi* antibodies in cardiac tissue inflammation.

The papers described tests to evaluate the trypanocidal effect of drugs in free form and of the nanocarriers against the different forms of the evolutionary cycle of *Trypanosoma cruzi*. For the epimastigote, trypomastigote, and amastigote forms, tests of trypanocidal activity at different concentrations, growth inhibition assays, and effect on viability and efficacy were applied [1–5,10,22–24,28]. Many of the papers selected did not perform tests for the amastigote form [3–5,7,10,23,24,27,29]. The articles [3,5] only carried out tests for the epimastigote form, a non-infective form, present in the invertebrate vector. Scalise et al. [28] only employed the growth inhibition assay in the intracellular amastigote form. For more robust results, all studies should present tests against the three forms of *Trypanosoma cruzi*; mainly against circulating trypomastigotes and intracellular amastigotes, because they are the forms present in vertebrates. The lack of these tests is considered a limitation of the studies.

Few studies presented results for CC_{50}, which assesses the drug and nanoparticle concentrations required to kill 50% of the uninfected cells [4,22,23]. The articles [2,22] obtained results of the drug and nanoparticle concentrations required to kill 50% of the parasites present in the infected cells (IC_{50}) in all three *T. cruzi* forms. Morales-Baez et al. [23] and Contreras Lancheros et al. [4] did not perform tests to obtain IC_{50} in amastigotes, just as Li et al. [1] did not obtain it for the epimastigote form. The articles [10,24] presented the IC_{50} result only for the trypomastigotes forms. The papers [3,5,7,27–29] did not present CC_{50} or IC_{50} data.

Some articles calculated the selectivity index (SI), which evaluates the activity of the compound against infected cells, without causing cellular cytotoxicity in the host [2,4,22]. Understanding the degree of cytotoxicity of free drugs and drugs encapsulated in nanocarriers is important to assess the impact on parasite elimination without harming host cells. Thus, it is essential to calculate the selectivity index (SI), which can be obtained through CC_{50} and IC_{50} studies.

2.8. In Vivo Assays

Table 5 lists the in vivo assays conducted with animals infected and not infected with *Trypanosoma cruzi* by the papers selected in this bibliographic review. The studies that did not conduct in vivo assays are not included in Table 5 [2–4,22–24,27].

Table 5. In vivo assays.

Reference	Animal Model	Infection	Treatment	Control Group	Assays
			Polymeric Nanoparticles		
[7]	Male C57BL/6 mice aged seven weeks old		Daily intravenous injections of free LIC solution (2.0 mg/kg/day; 8 mice), LYC loaded in biodegradable polymeric NP (LYC-NP; 2.0 mg/kg/day, 10 mice), blank NP (10 mice), and vehicle (control group; 10 rats) for 20 consecutive days	Control group (vehicle, 10 mice)	Transthoracic echocardiography. Single-cell and real-time Ca^{2+} contracting—imaging. Studies of the cardio-toxicological effects of LYC on cardiac function. Effect of LYC encapsulation on NP.
[8]	Swiss mice aged between 28 and 30 days old and weighing from 20 to 25 g	Infection by trypomastigotes injection 104—Intraperitoneal route	LYC—2 mg/kg/day for 10 and 20 days in the acute phase of the disease. Multiple doses of BZN, free LYC, LIY-PCL NP, unloaded NP, LYC-PLA-PEG NP, and DMA-PEG 300 (i.v. control solution) according to the strain and days. Route—intravenous	Untreated control (infected but untreated), NC unloaded control (UN-NP), and DMA-PEG 300 control (control solution)	Parasitemia level by the Filardi and Brener method. Evaluation of parasitological cure by parasitological methods (examination of fresh blood, blood culture, and PCR in peripheral blood) and conventional serology. (Quantitative PCR). Atrial natriuretic peptide measurements (ELISA). Serum creatine kinase (CK) activity (NADP-reduction photometric assay).
[25]	C57BL/6 mice (Female and male mice aged eight weeks old)	10,000 Trypomastigotes/mouse—Intraperitoneal route	BZN + PLG-Cur. 0.15 mL by gavage/day. BZN. One quarter of 25 mg/kg/day. Cur nanoparticle—One 200 mg/kg daily dose	Uninfected and infected but untreated	Histopathological analysis of the heart (hematoxylin, eosin, and Masson's trichrome). Myocardial cytokine and chemokine concentrations (ELISA). Enzyme activity by gelatin zymography and transmission densitometry.

Table 5. *Cont.*

Reference	Animal Model	Infection	Treatment	Control Group	Assays
[29]	Male C57BL/6 mice (20–22 g)	1×10^3 trypomastigotes (Y strain)—Intraperitoneal route	BZN 2.5 µg/animal/day; blank polymeric nanoparticles; Polymeric PN-UA-2 (13.15 µg/animal/day)—Intra retro-orbital route of samples diluted in 50 µL of PBS	Control group not treated (negative control)	Trypanocidal activity, parasitemia by counting trypomastigote forms of the parasite per 5 µL. Liver markers.
[30]	Female Swiss mice aged 28–30 days and weighing 20–25 g.	10,000 trypomastigotes (Y strain) for the acute phase—Intraperitoneal route. 500 trypomastigotes (Y strain) for chronic phase—Intraperitoneal route	For acute phase: LYC (free LYC, LYC-PCL-NP, and LYC-PLA-PEG-NP) 5 mg/kg for 20 days. A group with BZN for a murine model (100 mg/kg) orally via gavage (0.2 mL). For chronic phase: LIC (free LYC, LYC-PCL-NP, and LYC-PLA-PEG-NP) with LYC doses of 5 mg/kg/day. LYC at 2 mg/kg/day. Two groups received daily BZN doses of 100 mg/kg/day (0.1 mL) and 50 mg/kg/day (0.2 mL)—Orally (gavage) or intravenously (rear vein)	Untreated animals (infected and untreated), animals treated with solution excipients (DMA-PEG), and animals treated with blank NP	Therapeutic efficacy by fresh blood test, blood culture, PCR, and enzyme-linked immunosorbent assay (ELISA). Parasitemia level by FBE method, survival rates, blood culture (BC).
[31]	Female Swiss mice (age: 28–30 days; body weight: 20–25 g)	*T. cruzi* VL-10 strain. Acute phase model: 10,000 trypomastigotes—Intraperitoneal route. Chronic phase model: 500 blood trypomastigotes—Intraperitoneal route.	Free LYC (12 mg/kg of body weight/day), LYC-PLA-PEG-NP (8 or 12 mg/kg/day) or BZN at 100 mg/kg/day—via oral route	Infected and untreated	Treatment efficacy was evaluated by fresh blood test, blood culture, PCR, and enzyme-linked immunosorbent assay (ELISA). *T. cruzi* VL-10 strain DTU II. Survival rates and heart histopathology.

Table 5. *Cont.*

Reference	Animal Model	Infection	Treatment	Control Group	Assays
			Lipid Nanoparticles		
[10]	Swiss mice (6–8 weeks old), weighing 20–25 g.	*T. cruzi* Y strain (Type II linage). 2.0×10^3 trypomastigotes—Intraperitoneal route	BZN, free H2bdtc and H2bdtc-SLNs administered orally at 4 μmol/kg (BZN 1.0 mg/kg/day; free H2bdtc and H2bdtc-SLNs 1.4 mg kg/day) per day for 10 consecutive days	Group 1 = PBS infected and untreated	Cytotoxicity and trypanocidal activity of free H2bdtc and H2bdtc-SLNs in Swiss mice (6–8 weeks old). Evaluation of parasitemia and mortality. Measurement of creatine kinase-MB (CK-MB) and glutamic–pyruvate transaminase levels. Histological analysis to assess inflammatory infiltration through light microscopy DP71.
			Polymeric Micelles		
[26]	Female C57BL/6J mice aged 1 month old.	Chronic model of the *Trypanosoma cruzi* Nicaragua infection. Route—Intraperitoneal with 3000 trypomastigotes.	30 BZN-MP daily doses at 50 mg/kg/day; 30 BZN-MP daily doses at 25 mg/kg/day; 13 BZN-MP intermittent doses at 75 mg/kg; 13 BZN-MP intermittent doses at 50 mg/kg. Intermittent—One dose every 7 days BZN-MP doses Via—Oral gavage	Infected and untreated (only oil)	Induction of immunosuppression and evaluation of parasitemia by DNA amplification. ECGs performed with electrocardiogram, measurement of IgG antibody response by ELISA, histopathological studies. Monitoring of parasitemia and of the survival rates.
[27]	Female C3H/HeN mice aged 1 month old.	*Trypanosoma cruzi* Nicaragua. 1000 trypomastigotes. Route—Intraperitoneal	BZN 50 mg/kg for 30 days; BZN-MP 50 mg/kg/day for 30 days; BZN-MP 25 mg/kg/day for 30 days; BZN-MP 10 mg/kg/day for 30 days. Route—oral gavage	Infected without treatment	Induction of immunosuppression with cyclophosphamide and estimated number of parasites as described by PCR. Analysis of IgG antibody levels by enzyme-linked immunosorbent assay (ELISA). Histopathological studies by microscopy.

Table 5. *Cont.*

Reference	Animal Model	Infection	Treatment	Control Group	Assays
[28]	Female C3H/HeN mice aged 1 month old.	1000 trypomastigotes—Intraperitoneal route.	R-BZN and BZN-MPs were dispersed in olive oil and administered to mice via oral gavage. R-BZN 50 mg/kg/day for 15 days; BZN-MPs 50 mg/kg/day for 15 days; BZN-MPs 50 mg/kg/day for 30 days; BZN-MPs 25 mg/kg/day for 15 days; BZN-MPs 25 mg/kg/day for 30 days; BZN-MPs 10 mg/kg/day for 15 days; BZN-MPs 10 mg/kg/day for 30 days; BZN-MPs 50 mg/kg/day for 30 days (uninfected)	Infected without treatment	Assay in the acute phase of infected mice, parasitemia, antiparasitic effect of BNZ-MPs, survival curve during the acute phase, Kaplan–Meier test to differentiate the curves.
Liposomes					
[1]	Female BALB/c mice (4–6 weeks old)	Infected with the *T. cruzi* Y strain. 2×10^3—Intraperitoneal route.	PS 0.3 mg/mL by i.v. injection; BZN 100 mg/kg/day orally for 14 days; BZN-PS i.v. at a BZN dose of 1.5 mg/kg (2 doses); BZN-PS i.v. at a BZN dose of 0.15 mg/kg (2 doses), BZN-PS at a BZN dose of 0.03 mg/kg (2 doses)	Infected and untreated	Monitoring of parasitemia, cardiac parasitosis quantified by quantitative PCR, cardiac inflammation, and cardiac histology. Hepatotoxicity. Assessment of toxicity and determination of serum alanine aminotransferase.

Key: BZN = Benznidazole; Cur = Curcumin; ECG = Electrocardiogram; ELISA = Enzyme-Linked Immunosorbent Assay; H2bdtc = 5-hydroxy-3-methyl-5-phenyl-pyrazoline-1-(S-benzyl dithiocarbonate); IgG = Immunoglobulin G; LYC = Lychnopholide; NC = Nanocapsule; PBS = Phosphate Buffer Sodium; PCR = Polymerase Chain Reaction; SLNs = Solid Lipid Nanoparticles.

To carry out the in vivo tests, the researchers used the following animal models: C57BL/6 mice [7,25,26,29], BALB/c mice [1], C3H/HeN mice [27,28], and Swiss mice [8,10,30,31] aged around 1-month-old and of both sexes. The study [29] was the only one that did not report the animals' age. The *T. cruzi* infection in animals was carried out intraperitoneally in all studies [1,8,10,25–31]. Branquinho et al. [7] did not provide information on the route used to infect the animals. All animals were infected by the trypomastigote form of *Trypanosoma cruzi*, which is the circulating and infective form of the parasite.

The studies used the infected and untreated animals as the control group [1,7,8,10,26–31]. Hernández et al. [25] used a group of untreated healthy animals and another group of untreated infected animals as control groups. The studies [1,8,27–29] conducted the animals' treatment during the acute phase of the disease. The studies [25,26] conducted the treatment in the chronic phase. In turn, the papers [7,30,31] applied the treatment during both phases of the infection. Carneiro [10] did not report the phase in which the treatment was conducted. For the administration of drugs and nanoparticles, many studies used the oral route by gavage [1,10,25–28,30,31]. The papers [1,30] were also administered via the intravenous route; in turn, those by Branquinho et al. [7,8] only resorted to the intravenous route.

After the treatment, the main assays applied were to assess the parasitemia level [1,8, 10,25–31] and the survival rate [27,28,30,31]. In addition, assays for the detection of cardiac enzymes [10,25] and histological analysis of the heart [27,28,30,31] were used.

3. Discussion

3.1. In Vitro Data Discussion

The discussion was carried out after analyzing the in vitro results of the articles selected in the Table 4.

3.1.1. Polymeric Nanoparticles

Polymeric nanoparticles were widely used by the articles in this review, although only Contreras Lancheros [4] and De Freitas Oliveira [24] showed better results as compared to the free drug.

Contreras Lancheros et al. [4] synthesized chitosan polymeric nanoparticles containing NO. During the infection by the parasite, macrophages release nitric oxide. It is believed that these molecules are responsible for inhibiting the replication of the parasite. The problem is that NO is short-lived and can be toxic to some tissues [4]. The study coupled mercaptosuccinic acid (MSA), an NO precursor molecule, into polymeric nanoparticles with subsequent nitrosation by adding an equimolar amount of sodium nitrite ($NaNO_2$) to form S-nitroso-MSA-CS NPs (NO-releasing nanoparticles). The paper evaluated cellular cytotoxicity in peritoneal macrophages and the effects of the nanoparticles against the *T. cruzi* forms, finding the following results: in the cellular viability evaluation by the MTT method, the CC_{50} value found was 400 ± 5.7 µg/mL after 72 h of exposure to the MSA polymeric nanoparticle (S-nitroso-MSA-CS NPs). For the different forms of *T. cruzi*, tests of effect against parasite proliferation were performed by direct count in a hemocytometer under a light microscope, finding IC_{50} values of 75.0 ± 6.5 µg/mL for epimastigotes and 25.0 ± 5.0 µg/mL for circulating trypomastigotes. The nanoparticles were also effective in reducing the intracellular amastigote forms. With these results, it was possible to carry out the calculation to obtain the selectivity index (SI), which was 5.3 for epimastigotes and 16 for trypomastigotes. The result was positive because it indicates greater selectivity of the nanoparticles by the parasite and sustained NO release when compared to the free donor [4].

De Freitas Oliveira et al. [24] synthesized polymeric nanoparticles of sodium diethyldithiocarbamate (DETC), a compound from the class of carbamates previously studied by the authors with promising results in combating Chagas disease. Its mechanism of action consists of stimulating ROS and chelating metals, which are harmful to the parasite. However, they can be harmful to the host. To avoid toxic effects and maintain an action against the parasite, the study encapsulated diethyldithiocarbamate in PLA [24]. The authors carried out tests to evaluate cytotoxicity by MTT in three different cell lines and the antiparasitic activity of the DETC nanoparticles against the circulating trypomastigote form. Free BZN was used as a positive control. When tested by different concentrations of the nanoparticles containing diethyldithiocarbamate in the cytotoxicity assays, all three cell lines: RAW, derived from macrophages; 3T3, derived from fibroblasts; and Vero, derived from renal epithelial cells, remained constant in viability. There was a significant reduction in viability only in the Vero cells, by 60%, at the highest concentration tested: 132 μM. When evaluating the antiparasitic activity, the study obtained IC_{50} results of the diethyldithiocarbamate nanoparticles for three different *T. cruzi* strains and compared them to the results found with free BZN [24]. For the Dm28c strain, the IC_{50} of the nanoparticles was 15.47 $\pm$ 2.71 μM, while the one for free BZN was 70.58 $\pm$ 6.87 μM. In the evaluation of the Y strain, IC_{50} was 45.15 $\pm$ 5.44 μM and 85.24 $\pm$ 5.22 μM for the diethyldithiocarbamate nanoparticles and for free BZN, respectively. For the Bolivia strain, the IC_{50} of the nanoparticles was 47.89 $\pm$ 3.98 μM and, for free BZN, it was 79.78 $\pm$ 6.18 μM. As can be seen, for all three strains of *Trypanosoma cruzi*, the IC_{50} was lower when using the diethyldithiocarbamate nanoparticles when compared to free BZN. The study did not present the selectivity index (SI) but concluded that the DETC nanoparticles demonstrated low toxicity when compared to the drug in free form due to its capacity for controlled release, reducing cell damage. The nanoparticles showed an IC_{50} similar to the one already found by the authors with the free drug in previous studies, which shows that there was no reduction in activity against the parasite in the encapsulated form with the controlled release [24].

3.1.2. Lipid Nanoparticle

Several studies compared trypanocidal effects and cytotoxicity using another type of nanostructure: lipid nanoparticles. Vinuesa et al. [2] resorted to assays with different concentrations of SLNs, NLCs, and free BZN against all three forms of the *T. cruzi* cycle. For the circulating trypomastigote and intracellular amastigote forms, the IC_{50} values found were 17.6 $\pm$ 3.3 μM for NLCs, and 0.8 $\pm$ 0.4 μM for free BZN. For the epimastigote forms, the IC_{50} results were between 48.8 $\pm$ 14.3 μM and 123.9 $\pm$ 19.7 μM with SLNs, 41.3 $\pm$ 9.9 μM and 256.0 $\pm$ 19.9 μM for NLCs, and 17.7 $\pm$ 2.1 μM for free BZN. As can be seen, the values found for free BZN were better than with the use of lipid nanoparticles. This is also reflected by the numbers presented for the selectivity index, which were 21 and 69 for epimastigotes and trypomastigotes, respectively, with the use of NLCs, and 54 for epimastigotes and 904 for trypomastigotes with free BZN. In the cytotoxicity evaluation by WST performed in murine fibroblasts (L 929) and human liver cells (Hep G2), the article found mixed results for SLNs, requiring a reassessment of the accuracy of the test, which caused these nanoparticles to be removed from the study [2].

Carneiro et al. [10] compared in vitro the trypanocidal effects of the free compound H2bdtc (5-hydroxy-3-methyl-5-phenyl-pyrazoline-1-(S-benzyl dithiocarbonate)) with its conjugated form in a solid lipid nanoparticle (H2bdtc-SLNs) and with free BZN against the circulating trypomastigote form. With free H2bdtc, the IC_{50} found was 0.50 $\pm$ 0.12 μM, for the solid lipid nanoparticle loaded with H2bdtc it was 1.83 $\pm$ 0.18 μM, and with free BZN, the IC_{50} was 0.50 $\pm$ 0.39 μM. Cytotoxicity was evaluated with cells isolated from C57BL/6 mice. No significant cytotoxicity was found with the free and encapsulated form of H2bdtc. Despite the trypanocidal effect of free and H2bdtc-loaded in SLNs being like that of free BZN, the drug has a positive result, as it was not toxic to the cells [10].

3.1.3. Other Nanoparticles

Tessarolo et al. [22] synthesized inorganic calcium carbonate nanoparticles loaded with 1 mg/mL of benznidazole (BZN encapsulated in $CaCO_3$ nanoparticles) using the emulsification method. The use of calcium carbonate to produce the nanoparticle was due to its use in previous studies in the selective and targeted release of chemotherapy drugs in cancer treatments. The study used in vitro cytotoxicity and effect tests against all three forms of *T. cruzi* with the use of free BZN and calcium carbonate nanoparticles loaded with BZN at different times and concentrations, for comparison purposes. In the MTT cytotoxicity evaluation, the study used LLCMK2 mammalian cells. CC_{50} was 55.35 ± 9.03 µg/mL for BZN-loaded calcium carbonate nanoparticles and 160.4 ± 75.09 µg/mL for free BZN. The results show an increase in the cytotoxicity of BZN encapsulated in nanoparticles concerning the free drug, but that was not reflected in the SI, as the SI of encapsulated BZN was 30.5 and the one for free BZN was 2.38. The higher the SI value, the more selective the compound is for the parasite, without causing toxicity to the host cell. With the use of flow cytometry, the parasites were analyzed, and it was discovered that cell death was caused by interference with mitochondrial metabolism. As for the effect against the evolutionary forms of *Trypanosoma cruzi*, the paper presented the IC_{50} values for the nanoparticles containing BZN and free BZN. For the epimastigote form, the antiparasitic effects were evaluated at 24, 48, and 72 h. With BZN encapsulated in $CaCO_3$ nanoparticles, IC_{50} values of 8.72 µg/mL, 8.02 µg/mL, and 4.8 µg/mL were obtained at 24 h, 48 h, and 72 h, respectively. With the use of free BZN, IC_{50} was 56.7 µg/mL at 24 h, 15.91 µg/mL at 48 h, and 4.3 µg/mL at 72 h. The results show that lower concentrations of the calcium carbonate nanoparticles loaded with BZN were necessary to kill the parasite in a shorter period when compared to free BZN. For the circulating trypomastigotes, the study showed results of the minimum lethal concentration for the parasites (LC_{50}), reaching 1.77 ± 0.58 µg/mL with the calcium carbonate nanoparticles loaded with BZN, a value 37 times lower than the one achieved by free BZN, which was 66.9 ± 20.3 µg/mL at 24 h. Circulating trypomastigotes were killed within 24 h at all concentrations tested (50–0.39 µg/mL). However, free BZN was less effective in eliminating the parasite as higher concentrations in the range of 12.5–50 µg/mL had to be administered to reach LC_{50}. In tests of inhibition of the intracellular amastigote forms, compound BZN encapsulated in $CaCO_3$ nanoparticles was able to reduce by 25% the number of infected cells and by 46% the number of amastigotes per cell with an IC_{50} of 8.72 µg/mL. Free BZN also reduced the number of infected cells by 25% and the number of amastigotes within each cell by 32%, but with a much higher IC_{50} (56.7 µg/mL). Encapsulated BZN showed trypanocidal efficacy against all three forms of *Trypanosoma cruzi* at lower doses when compared to free BZN [22].

Another article that showed significant results in in vitro assays was Morales-Baez et al. [23], who synthesized nanoparticles of hybrid materials called MOFs and coupled them to ergosterol peroxide (MOFs-EP), as they have immunosuppressive, antiparasitic, and anti-inflammatory activity. The study analyzed the trypanocidal activity of free MOFs and MOFs coupled to ergosterol peroxide against epimastigotes and trypomastigotes at different concentrations and the toxicity of free MOF nanoparticles by the MTT assay in three cell types. The IC_{50} value of the MOF nanoparticles coupled to ergosterol peroxide was the same for both forms of the *T. cruzi* cycle: 4.81 µg/mL at 24 h and 3.0 µg/mL at 48 h. The application of free MOF nanoparticles at different concentrations and incubation times showed no effect against parasite growth when compared to nifurtimox (positive control), but it was effective when applied in the form of MOF nanoparticles coupled to ergosterol peroxide (MOFs-EP), causing a decrease in parasite growth at different concentrations and incubation times. The cytotoxicity evaluation test by MTT was performed with different concentrations of free MOF nanoparticles applied to cell monolayers in triplicate in three different cell types. The MTT result showed that the free MOF nanoparticles were not cytotoxic when used at different low concentrations; it only showed cell damage when the cells were incubated with 1% Triton X-100 (positive control). The CC_{50} results found for the free MOF nanoparticles were as follows: 392.0 µg/mL for NIH3T3 cells, 593.6 µg/mL for J774A.1 cells, and 1030.0 µg/mL for Vero cells. It was concluded that the MOF nanoparticles did not induce cytotoxicity in cells and may be a promising alternative for the treatment of the acute phase of Chagas disease, due to their selectivity for the plasma membrane, their inhibitory effect against the circulating trypomastigote forms of *T. cruzi*, and for not presenting adverse effects. The study failed to perform tests against the intracellular amastigote form and required complementary testing to assess adverse effects. The selectivity index

(SI) was not obtained, and it was not possible to calculate it, as the study did not present CC_{50} results for the MOF nanoparticles containing ergosterol peroxide [23].

When comparing both studies, the results obtained by Tessarolo et al. [22] were more complete and had more significant effects. The study managed to obtain 100% of circulating parasites killed within 24 h of treatment with the calcium carbonate nanoparticles loaded with BZN at all administered doses, with an LC_{50} (lethal dose for 50% of the parasites) of 1.77 ± 0.58 µg/mL, lower than the IC_{50} found in the study by Morales-Baez et al. [23]. In addition to that, they carried out tests for all three forms of *T. cruzi*. Although the cytotoxicity of BZN increased when coupled to the nanoparticles, the selectivity index was satisfactory and showed greater selectivity of the calcium carbonate nanoparticles loaded with BZN for the parasite than the free BZN. In the study of Morales-Baez et al. [23], the CC_{50} value was only obtained by the free form of the MOF nanoparticles, and it was not possible to calculate the selectivity index.

3.1.4. Liposomes and Vesicular Nanocarriers

Another study that presented results of in vitro assays was that of Li et al. [1]. The article compared the effects of free BZN with those of the vesicular nanocarrier (poly (ethylene glycol)-block-poly (propylene sulfide) (BZN-PSs)) loaded with BZN. The vesicular nanocarrier (BZN-PSs) was chosen because it had already been used in therapy for effective delivery and reduced toxicity [1]. Trypanocidal efficacy was evaluated in two stages of the *T. cruzi* cycle, against intracellular amastigotes and circulating trypomastigotes. The IC_{50} found for the vesicular nanocarrier loaded with BZN in the effect test against intracellular amastigotes was 3.51 ± 0.79 µM and, for free BZN, it was 33.07 ± 8.17 µM. In assays against circulating trypomastigotes, IC_{50} was 55.87 ± 11.39 µM for the vesicular nanocarrier containing BZN and 56.06 ± 12.21 µM for free BZN. Despite not presenting results on the selectivity index and CC_{50}, the study by Li et al. [1] demonstrates, as well as that of Tessarolo et al. [22], significant efficacy in reducing the concentration of the drug against the intracellular amastigote form of the parasite. The IC_{50} result in circulating trypomastigotes was like that of the free BZN found in this study. The article explains that this occurs because the nanostructure manages to take the same route as *T. cruzi* in cell penetration and disintegrate only inside the cell, slowly releasing BZN, which makes it better against intracellular amastigote forms, in addition to contributing to the decrease in toxicity [1].

Vinuesa et al. [2] also performed tests with free and BZN-loaded liposomes to assess cytotoxicity in two mammalian cells (L-929 and Hep G2) and the antiparasitic effect against *T. cruzi*. The results found in the cytotoxicity assays were 0 to 39.4 ± 2.4 µg/mL in L-929 fibroblasts and 0 to 36.2 ± 4.9 µg/mL in the Hep G2 cell line for free liposomes. For BZN-loaded liposomes, the results were 0 to 14.9 ± 1.9 µg/mL in L-929 fibroblasts and 0 to 1.5 ± 2.6 µg/mL in Hep G2 cells. The results varied according to the concentrations. Liposome toxicity was considered insignificant in the study. The toxicity result for free BZN in L-929 fibroblast cells was 3.9 ± 4.5 µM and the IC_{50} of the effect against epimastigotes was 14.8 ± 4.9 µM. It was not possible to obtain the IC_{50} of the BZN-loaded liposome, as the BZN concentrations achieved by the liposome were very low, less than 12 µM, rendering its effect against the parasite negligible. The study concluded that liposomes were inefficient in transporting and releasing BZN [2].

Among the two articles that used liposomes as BZN carriers in vitro assays, Li et al. [1] managed to achieve better results with the BZN-loaded polymersome vesicular nanocarrier, as it required lower concentrations of encapsulated BZN when compared to its free-form in the effect against intracellular amastigotes.

Because of all the values presented, the articles that obtained the best results in the in vitro tests were those that worked with inorganic [22], organic [23], and polymeric [4,24] nanocarriers. They showed efficiency in reducing the toxicity and dose of the drug when coupled with nanocarriers. The articles that worked with liposomes and lipid nanocarriers did not obtain satisfactory results [1,2,10].

3.2. In Vivo Data Discussion

The discussion was carried out after analyzing the in vivo results of the articles selected in Table 5. Regarding the in vivo tests, the articles were evaluated regarding the results of the tests for reducing animals' parasite load, survival rate, and mortality. Some papers described tests only in the acute phase of the disease [1,8,27–29], and others only did so in the chronic phase [25,26], evaluating the appearance of cardiac and hepatic markers. Other articles obtained results for both phases of the disease [7,30,31]. The nanocarriers used in the in vivo tests were polymeric nanoparticles, lipid nanoparticles, polymersomes, and polymeric micelles.

3.2.1. Polymeric Nanoparticles

Branquinho et al. [8] used polymeric nanoparticles for treating the acute phase of Chagas disease. Polymeric nanoparticles were synthesized with LYC encapsulated based on PCL and PLA-PEG and their in vivo effects were compared to the drug and to free BZN. Mice were separated into groups for four experiments and infected with different *T. cruzi* strains: CL (sensitive to BZN) and Y (partially resistant to BZN). All administrations were performed intravenously into the rear veins. Free BZN and free LYC were administered in a mixture of DMA-PEG 300 solution diluted in 5% glucose. In all experiments of this study, 2 mg/kg/day doses of free and encapsulated LYC in nanoparticles and 50 mg/kg/day doses of free BZN were administered [8]. In the analysis of the parasitemia peak of the groups infected by the CL strain (sensitive to BZN), in experiment I, initiated 24 h after the infection and lasting 10 days, the result was a reduction in parasitemia by 98.6% with free BZN, by 56.3% with free LYC, and by 96.3% for the LYC-loaded nanoparticles (LYC-PCL NC), when compared to the untreated control groups. As for the survival rate of animals infected by the CL strain (sensitive to BZN), those in the untreated control group survived for approximately 20 days. The groups treated with free BZN and with the LYC-loaded PCL nanoparticles had a 100% survival rate for 6 months after treatment and the animals that received only free LYC had a 75% survival rate in the same period. The remaining 25% survived for 24 days. Experiment II carried out with the CL strain, initiated 7 days after the infection and lasting 20 days, obtained a reduction during the parasitemia peak of 99.2% for free BZN, 57.7% for free LIC, 98.2% for the LYC-loaded PCL nanoparticles, and 99.30% for the LYC-loaded PLA nanoparticles. The results show that free LYC had a lower parasitemia reduction rate than the groups treated with free BZN and with LYC-loaded PLA-PEG and PCL nanoparticles. The survival rate was 21 days for the untreated groups. A total of 50% of the animals treated with free LYC survived for 34 days and 100% of the animals treated with free BZN and with both LYC-loaded nanoparticles survived during the entire acute phase for 6 months after the treatment, until they were necropsied [8].

The animals infected by the Y strain (partially resistant to BZN) were treated in experiment III, initiated 24 h after the infection and lasting 10 days. They obtained peak parasitemia reductions of 94.3% with free BZN, 37.8% with free LYC, and 96.9% by the LYC-loaded PCL nanoparticles when compared to the untreated control group. This experiment did not use the PLA-PEG nanoparticles. Once again, the parasitemia of free LYC remained higher when compared to free BZN and LYC encapsulated in the nanoparticles, although it achieved a greater reduction when compared to the untreated control group [8].

The survival rate was 100% for the groups treated with free BZN and with the LYC-loaded PCL nanoparticles. The animals in the untreated control group survived for only 16 days and treatment with free LYC did not improve survival. In experiment IV, the group began to be treated 4 days after the infection, for a total of 20 days, with PLA-PEG and PLC nanoparticles loaded with LYC and with free BZN, obtaining reductions in the parasitemia peak of 99.55% with the LYC-loaded PCL nanoparticles, of 95.76% for the LYC-loaded PLA-PEG nanoparticles, and of 98.20% for free BZN. The survival rate was the same as in the previous group [8].

Treatment efficacy was assessed by parasitological cure. In experiment I, of the animals infected by the CL strain, those treated with free BZN had a 100% cure, while those treated with the LYC-loaded PCL nanoparticles achieved a 50% cure. In experiment II, the animals treated with both nanoparticles and with free BZN had a 100% cure. In both experiments (I and II), none of the animals treated with free LYC or those in the untreated control group were cured. In experiment III, the animals treated with the LYC-loaded PCL nanoparticles achieved a 50% cure, while none of the mice treated with free LYC and free BZN were cured. In experiment IV, a 75% cure was obtained with free BZN, 100% with the LYC-loaded PLA-PEG nanoparticles, and 62.2% with the LYC-loaded PCL nanoparticles. No cure was achieved for the mice in the untreated control group. It is concluded that LYC was able to reduce parasitemia by 56% to 99% and by 37% to 99% in the CL and Y strains, respectively, with intravenous administration of 2 mg/kg/day, depending on the type of formulation and the schedule used [8]. The results could be even better with higher doses. The animals survived without signs of toxicity in the experimental tests with free LYC and with the LYC-loaded PLA-PEG and PCL nanoparticles. Free BZN in a DMA-PEG 300 solution was able to cure 75% of the animals with a 50 mg/kg/day dose, a better result than the one found with the standard dose of 100 mg/kg/day used for treating Chagas disease, which reached a 50% healing rate [8].

Despite the reduction in parasitemia and the survival rate of mice infected with the CL strain, experiment I achieved a cure rate of 50% using the LYC-loaded PCL nanoparticles, not outdoing free BZN, which reached 100%. The study explains that this result could be due to the high sensitivity of the CL strain to BZN and to the short treatment period, which was initiated 24 h after the infection and lasted only 10 days. The results of experiment II were better, achieving total survival and complete cure with the LYC-loaded PLA-PEG nanoparticles, with the LYC-loaded PCL nanoparticles, and with free BZN. The treatment in experiment II was initiated 7 days after the infection and lasted 20 days. It is believed that the results were better than experiment I because, after this period, the intracellular amastigote forms had already multiplied and ruptured the host cells, releasing the circulating trypomastigote form in the bloodstream, encountering the drugs and with the nanoparticles [8]. The same occurred in the experiments with the Y strain, partially resistant to BZN. The action of encapsulated LYC was better than that of free LYC due to the ability of the nanoparticles to carry out a prolonged release of the drug. As was the case in experiment I, experiment III carried out the treatment for 10 days, starting it 24 h after the infection, which resulted in a reduction in parasitemia and cure in 50% of the animals only with the use of the LYC-loaded PCL nanoparticles. Once again, the above shows the importance of longer treatment and waiting times to start after the infection. Experiment IV obtained a 100% parasitological cure with the LYC-loaded PLA-PEG nanoparticles, 75% with free BZN, and 62.5% with the LYC-loaded PCL nanoparticles. Free LYC ceased to be used in this experiment due to its lower results to the nanoparticles. In the entire treatment, 50% of the animals treated with free LYC did not survive and did not present a parasitological cure. The above shows the importance of encapsulation in nanocarriers [8].

De Mello et al. [30] also used PLA-PEG and PCL polymeric nanoparticles containing the LYC-encapsulated natural active ingredient for in vivo assays. The nanoparticles were prepared by the technique of interfacial deposition of the preformed polymer followed by solvent displacement. The paper carried out tests during the acute and chronic phases of the disease in mice infected with the *T. cruzi* Y strain (partially resistant to BZN) and compared the results. The animals were infected intraperitoneally with 10,000 circulating trypomastigotes for the acute phase and 500 circulating trypomastigotes for the chronic phase. In the acute phase, the animals were orally treated with both LYC-loaded nanoparticles and with free LYC at a dose of 5 mg/kg/day for 20 days, starting on the 4th day after the infection, as was performed in experiment IV of the article by Branquinho [8]. In the chronic phase, free LYC and both LYC-loaded nanoparticles were administered orally (5 mg/kg/day) and intravenously (2 mg/kg/day) for 20 days, starting 90 days after the infection. For comparison purposes, two groups of animals were treated with 100 mg/kg/day of free BZN orally and 50 mg/kg/day intravenously [30].

Fresh blood tests, PCR, blood culture, and enzyme-linked immunosorbent assay (ELISA) were performed to assess therapeutic efficacy. The cure rate achieved with the use of the LYC-loaded PLA-PEG nanoparticles was 62.5% in the acute phase by the oral route, 55.6% in the chronic phase by the oral route, and 50% in the intravenous route. With the LYC-loaded PCL nanoparticles, the cure rates were 57.0% in the acute phase by the oral route, 30.0% in the chronic phase by the oral route, and 33.3% by the intravenous route. As in the results obtained by Branquinho et al. [8], no animal was cured with the use of free LYC, despite managing to reduce parasitemia and increase the survival rate when compared to the control group without treatment. The animals treated with free BZN achieved a cure rate like those treated with nanoparticles during the acute phase. In the chronic phase, only the animals treated with the LYC-loaded nanoparticles were cured, both in oral and intravenous administration. Treatment with the LYC-loaded PLA-PEG nanoparticles and free BZN achieved total parasitemia suppression in the acute phase. The survival rate of the animals was 75% with free LYC, 87% with the LYC-loaded PCL nanoparticles, and 100% with the LYC-loaded PLA-PEG nanoparticles up to 6 months after treatment when they were necropsied. In the control groups, the animals survived for approximately 20 days [30].

The survival rate in the chronic phase was 70% (orally) and 40% (i.v.) with free LYC, 80% (orally) and 50% (i.v.) with free BZN, 100% (orally) and 90% (via i.v.) with the LYC-loaded PCL nanoparticles, and 90% (orally) and 100% (via i.v.) with the LYC-loaded PLA-PEG nanoparticles. The survival rate of the untreated groups was 70% by the oral route. The results demonstrated greater efficacy of the LYC-loaded PLA-PEG nanoparticles in the treatment of the disease when compared to free LYC. The higher efficiency of nanoparticles containing LYC against the parasite is due to the controlled release of the active drug, as it has a smaller particle size, the ability to stabilize the drug in the gastrointestinal tract, and to influence tissue diffusion and LYC uptake into the blood [30].

Despite having good permeability, rapid absorption, and distribution in its free form, LYC has poor solubility. In addition to that, it requires the administration of repeated doses due to its rapid elimination. In oral administration, it shows chemical instability in contact with the pH of the gastrointestinal tract [30]. Encapsulation in polymeric nanoparticles controls the drug release in a slow and sustained way, which improves pharmacokinetics and biodistribution; in addition to reducing the need for multiple doses, which consequently reduces toxicity. Polymeric nanoparticles are more stable than other nanocarriers, such as lipid-based ones, liposomes, and micelles. The polymeric wall stabilizes the encapsulated drug and increases circulation time by reducing opsonization and release by the phagocytic system. Degradation of the polymeric wall and the release of LYC to the external environment are reduced by preventing the entry of proteins into the oil core. As they do not have elimination and accelerated metabolism like free LYC, LYC-loaded polymeric nanoparticles manage to accumulate in regions of inflamed tissues, improving their activity and being more effective [30]. Although the results achieved by the nanoparticles are close to those found with free BZN, it is important to emphasize that this shows the significant efficacy of these nanocarriers, as they do not compromise the action of the drugs but achieve excellent results by reducing the dose required for the treatment, which is essential to obtain the lowest possible level of adverse effects. In addition to that, the aqueous suspension of LYC-encapsulated nanoparticles is a physiologically acceptable vehicle for oral administration. Having achieved a cure in the chronic phase by this study is encouraging, as it is a phase of the disease with virtually no effective conventional treatments.

Branquinho et al. [31] also evaluated in vivo assays of the action of the PLA-PEG polymeric nanoparticles loaded with LYC. Treatment was performed by administering higher doses orally to mice infected with a strain (VL-10) resistant to BZN and nifurtimox during the acute and chronic phases of the disease. During the acute phase, treatment was initiated 9 days after the infection and lasted 20 days. In the chronic phase, it was initiated 90 days after the infection, with the same duration. A total of 12 mg/kg/day of free LYC, 8 or 12 mg/kg/day of LYC-loaded PLA-PEG nanoparticles, or 100 mg/kg/day of free BZN were administered. With the tests in the acute phase of the disease, the LYC-loaded PLA-PEG nanoparticles managed to suppress parasitemia by 100% with a 12 mg/kg/day dose and by 50% with the lowest dose: 8 mg/kg/day. At a dose of 12 mg/kg/day of the LYC-loaded PLA-PEG nanoparticles, the results obtained were 75% cure in the acute phase and 88% cure in the chronic phase of the disease. At a dose of 8 mg/kg/day, the cure was 43% both in the acute and chronic phases. The animals treated with free BZN and free LYC were not cured, as was also the case with untreated controls. In all groups, the survival rate was 87.5% in the acute phase and, with the LYC-loaded PLA-PEG nanoparticles, it was 100%. In the chronic phase, the survival rate with the use of 12 mg/kg/day of the nanoparticles or with 100 mg/kg/day of free BZN was 80%, while with the dose of 8 mg/kg/day of the nanoparticles and free LYC, it was 70% [31].

In all three articles discussed, the treatment with polymeric nanoparticles showed better results when compared to those achieved by the drugs in their free form. The result varies according to the *T. cruzi* strain, the dose used in the treatment, the length of the treatment time, and the start date. The article [8] tested a 2 mg/kg/day dose during treatment (10 and 20 days) and different strains in the acute phase. The results after 20 days were better, as well as in the studies by De Mello et al. [30] and Branquinho et al. [31]. The treatment was also more effective when initiated 4 to 9 days after the infection in the acute phase, as shown in experiments II and IV by Branquinho et al. [8] and in the tests by De Mello et al. [30] and Branquinho et al. [31]. Free LYC failed to cure any of the animals, while free BZN did not cure mice infected with the BZN-resistant VL-10 strain [31] but achieved high cure rates against sensitive (CL) [8] and partially resistant strains to BZN (Y) [30]. LYC-loaded polymeric nanoparticles achieved high cure rates against all strains at lower doses than those administered with free BZN.

The results of the tests carried out in the chronic phase of the disease were encouraging. The article [30] obtained a cure rate of approximately 55% with the LYC-loaded PLA-PEG nanoparticles and approximately 33% with the LYC-loaded PCL nanoparticles. There was no significant difference between the results with oral and intravenous administration. The study by Branquinho et al. [31] obtained a higher cure rate (88%) of mice in tests in the chronic phase with the administration of a higher dose: 12 mg/kg/day. In both studies, free BZN and free LYC failed to cure any animals in the chronic phase tests. In conclusion, the studies showed that LYC encapsulated in polymeric nanoparticles was more effective in reducing parasitemia and in achieving a parasitological cure, and increased animal survival, even when administered at low doses (2 mg/kg/day), when compared to free BZN (100 to 50 mg/kg/day). Encapsulated LYC presented no toxicity in any of all three studies, thus representing a promising alternative for the treatment of Chagas disease.

3.2.2. Lipid Nanoparticles

In addition to the aforementioned in vitro assays, the study by Carneiro et al. [10] carried out in vivo assays comparing the action against the circulating trypomastigote form of *T. cruzi* of the solid lipid nanoparticles loaded with compound H2bdtc (5-hydroxy-3-methyl-5- phenyl-pyrazoline-1-(S-benzyl dithiocarbonate) to its free form and to free BZN. The tests were performed on mice infected with the *T. cruzi* Y strain. The treatment was administered orally with 1.0 mg/kg/day of free BZN (100 times less than the standard concentration for the treatment of Chagas disease) and 1.4 mg/kg/day of free H2bdtc and H2bdtc-encapsulated in SLNs, for 10 consecutive days. The treatment was initiated on the fifth day after the infection, which reached its peak 9 days later. The results showed a 70% reduction in parasitemia with the administration of the 2bdtc-loaded solid lipid nanoparticle, 45% with free H2bdtc, and 15% with free BZN (positive control) when compared to the control group. The survival rate of the mice was 100% using the 2bdtc-loaded solid lipid nanoparticles. This rate is comparable to the one obtained with the standard administration of free BZN at 400 µmol/kg/day, 100 times higher than the one used in this study with the nanoparticles. With free BZN and H2bdtc, the survival rate compared to the control group was 57%. The study also evaluated whether there was heart and liver damage in the animals after the treatment [10]. The results showed that the animals treated with the nanoparticles did not show cardiac lesions, only reduced inflammation. The H2bdtc compound in its free form reduced cardiac damage by 50% when compared to free BZN in the standard treatment. The H2bdtc-loaded in SLNs also reduced liver toxicity and liver inflammation caused by the *T. cruzi* infection. Both in the in vitro and in vivo assays, the encapsulation of the H2bdtc compound obtained better results than those found with free BZN when administered at the same concentrations as in the study. The article shows that the nanoparticles were able to increase the oral bioavailability of the drug and improve solubility, which may facilitate access to the parasite. The study concludes that the compound is more efficient than the drugs currently used against the *T. cruzi* infection [10].

3.2.3. Polymeric Micelles

The articles [26–28] studied BZN-loaded polymeric micelles (BZN-PMs). Rial et al. [27] and Scalise et al. [28] performed in vivo assays during the acute phase of the disease.

Rial et al. [27] administered polymeric micelles dispersed in olive oil by oral gavage at doses of 10, 25, and 50 mg/kg/day in different groups of mice, for 30 days, starting two days after infection, and compared the results obtained to free BZN dispersed in olive oil at a dose of 50 mg/kg/day by oral gavage. All mice treated with free BZN and with the BZN-loaded polymeric micelle survived until the end of the treatment. In the control group, only 15% of the animals survived. The saturation solubility of BZN encapsulated in polymeric micelles had a 10-fold increase (3.99 mg/mL) when compared to the solubility of free BZN (0.44 mg/mL) [27]. Improved solubility and absorption of BZN encapsulated in polymeric micelles (BZN-PMs) provided an increase in the animals' survival rate with a 10 mg/kg/day dose, much lower than the conventional 100 mg/kg/day free BZN dose. The decrease in the dose achieved by encapsulating BZN in polymeric micelles with sustained release improves the pharmacological action, can avoid possible adverse effects, and reduces the administration frequency [27].

Scalise et al. [28] carried out tests for 15 and 30 days with mice separated into groups, administering oral doses of 50, 25, and 10 mg/kg/day with BZN-loaded polymeric micelles (BZN-PMs). At doses of 50 and 25 mg/kg/day, all mice survived for at least 50 days. Mice infected and treated with a 10 mg/kg/day dose had a survival rate of 70%. Thus, it can be stated that the efficacy of the treatment is dose dependent. Furthermore, as in the study by Rial [27], BZN-loaded polymeric micelles had a significant antiparasitic effect and prevention of animal death even at lower doses.

Rial et al. [26] used BZN-loaded polymeric micelles (BZN-PMs) in 1-month-old female C57BL/6J model mice of similar weight infected with the Nicaragua strain of *T. cruzi* during the chronic phase of the disease. The treatment was carried out by separating the animals into different groups and comparing the efficacy of administering BZN-MP continuously with intermittently. For the continuous treatment, the animals received BZN-PM doses of 25 and 50 mg/kg/day for 30 days. For the intermittent treatment, they received 13 doses of 50 and 75 mg/kg every 7 days. The administration was via the oral route. The results showed that the intermittent doses were as effective as those administered continuously, which is beneficial because the total intermittent dose is smaller. All animals survived until the end of treatment. The evaluation of the efficacy of the treatment by qPCR showed that 80% of the animals continuously treated with a 50 mg/kg/day dose had negative results. All other groups treated with BZN-PMs had no parasite load detected. The authors compared the results with previous studies and revealed that 80% of the animals treated with continuous doses of 75 mg/kg did not present parasitemia, while for the group treated with intermittent doses of 100 mg/kg, 75% did not present parasitemia [26].

The study also evaluated levels of *T. cruzi*-specific antibodies. The results showed a reduction in the antibody levels in all treatment groups when compared to the untreated ones, as well as a better reduction with the intermittent BZN-PM administration. Cardiac electrical alterations in mice were evaluated by ECG, considering that the conduction alterations caused by the infection were reverted after BZN-PM administration continuously and intermittently. Despite this, free BZN showed the same efficacy as polymeric micelles. The study also provoked immunosuppression of the animals after the treatment to evaluate the reactivation of the parasite, not detecting blood parasitic load [26].

When compared to previous studies carried out by Rial et al. [26], a significant reduction was obtained concerning the standard dose of 100 mg/kg/day, being equally effective with a dose of 75 mg/kg/day. This equated to an approximately 70% reduction in the total dose. This improvement is due to the BZN encapsulation in micelles, which are smaller than standard BZN and increase solubility from 0.4 mg/mL to 3.99 mg/mL [26]. Good results were obtained in the administration of smaller BZN-PM doses, as shown in this study with intermittent doses, as they can be an alternative to long-term treatments with fewer adverse effects on the patient.

3.2.4. Liposomes

In addition to the tests performed in vitro, the article [1] also evaluated the action of the vesicular nanocarrier (polymersome) with encapsulated BZN (poly (ethylene glycol) —block—poly (propylene sulfide) (BZN-PSs)) in in vitro assays in BALB/c mice infected with the *T. cruzi* Y strain, during the chronic phase of Chagas disease. The animals were separated into groups and the treatment was initiated 7 days after the infection with the administration of three different concentrations of the BZN-loaded vesicular nanocarrier (0.03, 0.15, and 1.5 mg/kg), 100 mg/kg for the group treated with free BZN, empty nanocarrier, and an untreated group. The results showed that the BZN-loaded vesicular nanocarrier obtained better reduction rates in cardiac parasitemia and myocarditis at a concentration of 1.5 mg/kg. The lowest dose of 0.03 mg/kg reduced parasitemia by 50%, while the mean dose of 0.15 mg/kg failed to reduce cardiac parasitemia but did reduce myocarditis (heart inflammation). At its standard treatment dose (100 mg/kg/day), free BZN was less effective in reducing parasitemia when compared to doses of the BZN-loaded vesicular nanocarrier. In addition to that, no hepatotoxicity was detected in mice using BZN-PS. The amount of BZN present in both nanocarriers administered during all 14 days of the treatment was 466 times lower than the one normally used with free BZN, achieving similar results in reducing parasitemia. The most important result achieved by the study was the reduction in myocarditis/cardiomyopathy (heart inflammation), the most serious sequel caused by infection with the parasite. Once again, using the encapsulated form of drugs in nanocarriers demonstrates significant efficacy in reducing the necessary doses for the treatment against the *T. cruzi* parasite, without causing undesirable adverse effects to the patients. Despite being promising, nanocarriers still need to be tested in clinical studies to evaluate their action in humans [1].

After analysis of the articles discussed, it is concluded that the best results were obtained with the use of drugs encapsulated in polymeric nanoparticles, as shown in the studies by Branquinho et al. [8], De Mello et al. [30], and Branquinho et al. [31]. The best length of the treatment in time was 20 days, starting 4 to 7 days after the infection. The studies analyzed the oral and intravenous routes, not showing significant differences in the results, with oral administration as the best choice for the patients' adaptation. In addition to BZN, the first-choice drug used against the *T. cruzi* parasite, LYC is a natural product encapsulated in polymeric nanoparticles that proved to be a great alternative for the treatment, obtaining high parasitemia reduction rates, as well as increased survival and cure rates for the animals during the acute and chronic phases of the disease, with doses much lower than those used in standard treatments with free BZN. Their studies can be improved and progress to future clinical trials.

Studies have shown that nanocarriers offer several advantages over traditional drugs for the treatment of Chagas disease. One of these advantages is that nanocarriers can improve the bioavailability of the drug, allowing it to reach specific sites more efficiently, improving the therapeutic index [13]. Nanocarriers administered orally need to be absorbed in the intestine by permeation for drug release into the blood or for cellular uptake. Furthermore, nanocarriers can slowly release the loaded actives which can reduce blood peaks of the drug and consequently adverse effects [1,23,24].

Nanocarriers can stabilize the active in the gastrointestinal tract and can promote the tissue diffusion and drug uptake into the blood [14,22,30]. Nanocarriers can also increase cellular uptake of the drug (Figure 2), which can kill the parasite in a shorter time compared to the free drug. In addition, nanosystems can accumulate in inflamed tissues, improving action and effectiveness. The use of nanocarriers for the treatment of Chagas disease also has some disadvantages, such as the difficulty in large-scale production, since the production of nanocarriers requires complex processes, which can increase the cost of treatment. In addition, toxicological and genotoxic studies must be performed to investigate the risk of human exposure to nanocarriers. The results showed that nanocarriers are also dose dependent and their effect varies according to the sensitivity of the *T. cruzi* strain in relation to the drug [28,30]. The advantages of nanocarriers as drug delivery systems are real, but there are many challenges to be overcome. It is necessary to evaluate the safety and efficacy of treatments using nanocarriers and to develop methods to produce them on an industrial scale to promote clinical studies.

3.2.5. Nanocarriers of Drugs in the Chronic Phase of Chagas Disease

Chagas disease has two phases: acute and chronic. The acute phase exhibits high numbers of trypomastigotes in the blood and is controlled by the immune system with the help of drugs. After the acute phase, the parasite continues the life cycle being present outside and inside host cells. In the chronic phase, parasitemia in the blood is low and detection is difficult. In addition, the symptoms are not felt for years, but 4 out of 10 patients develop the chronic phase of Chagas disease. Intracellular amastigotes promote tissue damage to the heart, esophagus, and colon. Patients die due to heart failure caused by chronic chagasic cardiomyopathy [37,38].

There are two strategies for targeting nanocarriers to the target site: passive and active targeting. Both strategies work well for treating tumors and inflamed tissues. Cancer treatments involving nanocarriers depend on the enhanced permeability and retention effect (EPR effect). Tumor tissue grows quickly and releases a series of substances capable of stimulating neoangiogenesis. The vessels grow rapidly in a defective way and present defects such as holes allowing the passage of nanocarriers from the blood vessel into the tissue. Nanocarriers in the tissue interstitium can be endocytosed into the cytoplasm of cells. In active targeting, nanocarriers decorated with targeting molecules pass through the holes in the vessels and can bind to cells, facilitating the uptake. Inflamed tissues have permeable blood vessels, and this fact can be used in favor of the passive or active targeting of nanocarriers [37,39,40]. The use of nanocarriers to target tissue is a success in the treatment of tumors and inflammation; however, targeting these delivery systems to cardiac muscle in the chronic phase of Chagas disease is a challenge. Nanocarriers are effective in transporting drugs to cardiomyocytes when these systems escape from blood vessels into the interstitium of cardiac tissue. In the interstitium, nanocarriers can be recognized and taken up by cardiomyocytes by the mechanism of endocytosis, which is a route to reach the amastigotes. However, the number of amastigotes in cardiac tissue is small and the tissue lesions are slow. Thus, for every significant piece of damage to the cardiac tissue caused by amastigotes, local inflammation is established. Initially, inflamed tissue can facilitate the passage of the nanocarriers to the interstitium, but at the end of the inflammatory process there is a reduction in local circulation and hypoxia [37]. Thus, there is probability of success for the nanocarriers to reach cardiomyocytes at the beginning of the chronic phase or indeterminate phase where blood flow has not yet been compromised. In the late chronic phase, cardiac tissue has suffered extensive damage, compromising the blood flow and the effectiveness of nanocarriers.

There are articles published with promising results from the use of drugs encapsulated in nanocarriers for the treatment of Chagas disease in the chronic phase [7,25,26,30,31]. The articles use animal models and, probably, drugs encapsulated in nanocarriers are effective at the beginning of the chronic phase or indeterminate phase, where circulation in the cardiac tissue has not been compromised, with the possibility of escape of the nanocarriers from the blood vessels to the cardiac tissue.

4. Materials and Methods

To prepare this paper, a search of the literature was carried out in the PubMed and Web of Science scientific databases from January 2012 to May 2023, using the following combinations of keywords: "Chagas Disease and nanoparticles", "*Trypanosoma cruzi* and nanoparticles" and "Chagas Disease and *Trypanosoma cruzi* and nanoparticles". Subsequently, the articles found were assessed using the inclusion and exclusion criteria defined for this review. For the inclusion criteria, the articles considered were those that used nanocarriers in in vitro and in vivo studies in the search for new ways to improve the treatment of Chagas disease. According to the exclusion criteria established, review articles, patents, duplicates, book chapters, conference abstracts, articles published in journals with an impact factor less than 1.0, articles on vaccines, and articles that deviated from the topic proposed were excluded. The scoping review was conducted by three individuals to ensure the quality of study selection. For a better detailing of the search, specific spreadsheets were prepared using Microsoft Excel (2019) for the in vitro and in vivo assays, for the composition and physicochemical characterization of the nanostructured systems, as well as a final evaluation table for each article, regarding the presence of certain items, such as title appropriate to the content, abstract, contextualization and objective present in the introduction, ethical statement, study design, complete physicochemical characterization, size of the nanocarriers, animals, sample size, in vitro and in vivo studies, trypanocidal effect, statistics, interpretation of the results, limitations, and conclusion.

5. Conclusions

After a detailed analysis, this study showed that using nanocarriers capable of encapsulating drugs achieved efficient results in the treatment of the disease. In in vitro assays, the encapsulated drugs did not lose their trypanocidal activities against the different forms of *T. cruzi*. In the tests employed, they were able to reduce cellular toxicity and increase the selectivity of the drugs against the parasite. With the in vivo studies, carried out with mice, the tests in both phases of the disease (acute and chronic) showed a reduction in parasitemia and a high survival and cure rate in the animals with the administration of much smaller doses when compared to the standard treatment with free BZN. In addition to healing during the chronic phase, some results with drugs encapsulated in nanocarriers have shown a reduction in liver toxicity and heart inflammation, which is encouraging given the lack of treatments available for this clinical condition.

With the increased circulation of drugs provided by the prolonged release and the possible decrease in adverse effects by reducing the necessary doses, the nanocarriers showed physiological stability, efficacy, and safety in transporting and delivering drugs to the target.

The nanotechnological strategies for drug delivery could open a new horizon of clinical practices for the successful treatment of Chagas disease. One of the strategies, nanoparticles containing drugs, has shown promising results in inducing the host's immune response against the pathogen with few side effects; in addition, it showed promising results in reducing toxicity, elevating efficacy, and the bioavailability of the active compound against the pathogen, by prolonging release, thereby increasing the therapeutic index. However, there is a need for more clinical studies to predict whether the nanoparticles will offer improved effective antichagasic treatments since the benefits of the nanotechnology for this disease are excellent in relation to cellular assays which have stimulated the preliminary animal studies [6,13,37]. Moreover, the unique nanocarrier approved for clinical trials is liposomal amphotericin B (LAMB) with reasonable anti-*T. cruzi* activity. From this perspective, the pre-clinical studies of the nanocarriers containing anti-*T. cruzi* drugs should be encountered, and this situation demands an approach from governmental and private agencies in conjunction with the pharmaceutical industry focusing on the efficient implementation of these nanosystems for drug delivery that will elevate the efficacy of anti-chagasic treatment procedures [6,13].

The limitations of nanocarriers are related to their ability to deliver drugs to tissues with low blood flow during the chronic phase of the disease. The targeting of nanocarriers to cardiac muscle in the chronic phase of Chagas disease is a challenge due to tissue fibrosis and low blood flow.

The results of preclinical studies analyzed by this review were important in the search for new alternatives for the treatment of Chagas disease. More studies can be carried out so that the treatment is perfected and can proceed to future clinical studies that may provide better adherence by the patients.

Author Contributions: D.d.F.P.: methodology, writing and editing; A.P.d.S.M.: methodology and review; D.d.A.G.: writing and review; T.d.N.: methodology, review and editing; M.S.d.S.d.B.M.: formal analysis and review; R.S.-O.: conceptualization and methodology; E.R.-J.: conceptualization, methodology and supervision. All authors have read and agreed to the published version of the manuscript.

Funding: This work was supported by the: Carlos Chagas Filho Foundation for Research Support of Rio de Janeiro State (FAPERJ)—Cientista do Nosso Estado (CNE) [grant number: E-26/201.077/2021], Apoio aos Programas e Cursos de Pós-graduação Stricto Sensu do Estado do Rio de Janeiro [grant number: E-26/210.136/2021] and Rede NanoSaúde [grant number: E-26/010.000981/2019]; Conselho Nacional de Desenvolvimento Científico e Tecnológico (CNPq)—Bolsa Produtividade em Pesquisa PQ [grant number: 309522/2020-0]. This paper was also supported with a scholarship granted by Coordenação de Aperfeiçoamento de Pessoal de Nível Superior (CAPES).

Institutional Review Board Statement: Not applicable.

Informed Consent Statement: Not applicable.

Data Availability Statement: Data sharing not applicable.

References

1. Li, X.; Yi, S.; Scariot, D.B.; Martinez, S.J.; Falk, B.A.; Olson, C.L.; Romano, P.S.; Scott, E.A.; Engman, D.M. Nanocarrier-enhanced intracellular delivery of benznidazole for treatment of *Trypanosoma cruzi* infection. *JCI Insight* **2021**, *6*, e145523. [CrossRef]

2. Vinuesa, T.; Herráez, R.; Oliver, L.; Elizondo, E.; Acarregui, A.; Esquisabel, A.; Pedraz, J.L.; Ventosa, N.; Veciana, J.; Viñas, M. Benznidazole Nanoformulates: A Chance to Improve Therapeutics for Chagas Disease. *Am. J. Trop. Med. Hyg.* **2017**, *97*, 1469–1476. [CrossRef]

3. Nhavene, E.P.F.; da Silva, W.M.; Trivelato, R.R., Jr.; Gastelois, P.L.; Venâncio, T.; Nascimento, R.; Batista, R.J.C.; Machado, C.R.; Macedo, W.A.d.A.; de Sousa, E.M.B. Chitosan Grafted into Mesoporous Silica Nanoparticles as Benznidazol Carrier for Chagas Diseases Treatment. *Microporous Mesoporous Mater.* **2018**, *272*, 265–275. [CrossRef]

4. Contreras Lancheros, C.A.; Pelegrino, M.T.; Kian, D.; Tavares, E.R.; Hiraiwa, P.M.; Goldenberg, S.; Nakamura, C.V.; Yamauchi, L.M.; Pinge-Filho, P.; Seabra, A.B.; et al. Selective Antiprotozoal Activity of Nitric Oxide-Releasing Chitosan Nanoparticles Against *Trypanosoma cruzi*: Toxicity and Mechanisms of Action. *Curr. Pharm. Des.* **2018**, *24*, 830–839. [CrossRef]

5. Brito, T.K.; Silva Viana, R.L.; Gonçalves Moreno, C.J.; da Silva Barbosa, J.; Lopes de Sousa, F., Jr.; Campos de Medeiros, M.J.; Melo-Silveira, R.F.; Almeida-Lima, J.; de Lima Pontes, D.; Sousa Silva, M.; et al. Synthesis of Silver Nanoparticle Employing Corn Cob Xylan as a Reducing Agent with Anti-*Trypanosoma cruzi* Activity. *Int. J. Nanomed.* **2020**, *15*, 965–979. [CrossRef]

6. Choudhury, S.D. Nano-Medicines a Hope for Chagas Disease! *Front. Mol. Biosci.* **2021**, *8*, 655435. [CrossRef]

7. Branquinho, R.T.; Roy, J.; Farah, C.; Garcia, G.M.; Aimond, F.; le Guennec, J.Y.; Saude-Guimarães, D.A.; Grabe-Guimaraes, A.; Mosqueira, V.C.F.; de Lana, M.; et al. Biodegradable Polymeric Nanocapsules Prevent Cardiotoxicity of Anti-Trypanosomal Lychnopholide. *Sci. Rep.* **2017**, *7*, 44998. [CrossRef]

8. Branquinho, R.T.; Mosqueira, V.C.F.; de Oliveira-Silva, J.C.V.; Simões-Silva, M.R.; Saúde-Guimarães, D.A.; de Lana, M. Sesquiterpene Lactone in Nanostructured Parenteral Dosage Form Is Efficacious in Experimental Chagas Disease. *Antimicrob. Agents Chemother.* **2014**, *58*, 2067–2075. [CrossRef]

9. Sales, P.A.; Molina, I.; Murta, S.M.F.; Sánchez-Montalvá, A.; Salvador, F.; Corrêa-Oliveira, R.; Carneiro, C.M. Experimental and Clinical Treatment of Chagas Disease: A Review. *Am. J. Trop. Med. Hyg.* **2017**, *97*, 1289–1303. [CrossRef]

10. Carneiro, Z.A.; Pedro, P.I.; Sesti-Costa, R.; Lopes, C.D.; Pereira, T.A.; Milanezi, C.M.; da Silva, M.A.P.; Lopez, R.F.V.; Silva, J.S.; Deflon, V.M. In Vitro and In Vivo Trypanocidal Activity of H2bdtc-Loaded Solid Lipid Nanoparticles. *PLoS. Negl. Trop. Dis.* **2014**, *8*, e2847. [CrossRef]

11. Bayda, S.; Adeel, M.; Tuccinardi, T.; Cordani, M.; Rizzolio, F. The History of Nanoscience and Nanotechnology: From Chemical-Physical Applications to Nanomedicine. *Molecules* **2020**, *25*, 112. [CrossRef]

12. Mora-Huertas, C.E.; Fessi, H.; Elaissari, A. Polymer-Based Nanocapsules for Drug Delivery. *Int. J. Pharm.* **2010**, *385*, 113–142. [CrossRef]

13. Quezada, C.Q.; Azevedo, C.S.; Charneau, S.; Santana, J.M.; Chorilli, M.; Carneiro, M.B.; Bastos, I.M.D. Advances in Nanocarriers as Drug Delivery Systems in Chagas Disease. *Int. J. Nanomed.* **2019**, *14*, 6407–6424. [CrossRef]

14. Volpedo, G.; Costa, L.; Ryan, N.; Halsey, G.; Satoskar, A.; Oghumu, S. Nanoparticulate Drug Delivery Systems for the Treatment of Neglected Tropical Protozoan Diseases. *J. Venom. Anim. Toxins Incl. Trop. Dis.* **2019**, *25*, 1–14. [CrossRef]

15. Foroozandeh, P.; Aziz, A. Insight into Cellular Uptake and Intracellular Trafficking of Nanoparticles. *Nanoscale Res. Lett.* **2018**, *13*, 1–12. [CrossRef]

16. Nsairat, H.; Khater, D.; Sayed, U.; Odeh, F.; al Bawab, A.; Alshaer, W. Liposomes: Structure, Composition, Types, and Clinical Applications. *Heliyon* **2022**, *8*, e09394. [CrossRef]

17. Perumal, S.; Atchudan, R.; Lee, W. A Review of Polymeric Micelles and Their Applications. *Polymers* **2022**, *14*, 2510. [CrossRef]

18. Wang, Z.; Gao, H.; Zhang, Y.; Liu, G.; Niu, G.; Chen, X. Functional ferritin nanoparticles for biomedical applications. *Front. Chem. Sci. Eng.* **2017**, *11*, 633–646. [CrossRef]

19. Baiocco, P.; Ilari, A.; Ceci, P.; Orsini, S.; Gramiccia, M.; Di Muccio, T.; Colotti, G. Inhibitory Effect of Silver Nanoparticles on Trypanothione Reductase Activity and Leishmania infantum Proliferation. *ACS Med. Chem. Lett.* **2010**, *2*, 230–233. [CrossRef]

20. Page, M.J.; McKenzie, J.E.; Bossuyt, P.M.; Boutron, I.; Hoffmann, T.C.; Mulrow, C.D.; Shamseer, L.; Tetzlaff, J.M.; Akl, E.A.; Brennan, S.E.; et al. The PRISMA 2020 Statement: An Updated Guideline for Reporting Systematic Reviews. *BMJ* **2021**, *372*, 105906. [CrossRef]

21. Cruz, R.; Calasans-Maia, J.; Sartoretto, S.; Moraschini, V.; Rossi, A.M.; Louro, R.S.; Granjeiro, J.M.; Calasans-Maia, M.D. Does the Incorporation of Zinc into Calcium Phosphate Improve Bone Repair? A Systematic Review. *Ceram. Int.* **2018**, *44*, 1240–1249. [CrossRef]

22. Tessarolo, L.D.; de Menezes, R.R.P.P.B.; Mello, C.P.; Lima, D.B.; Magalhães, E.P.; Bezerra, E.M.; Sales, F.A.M.; Barroso Neto, I.L.; Oliveira, M.D.F.; dos Santos, R.P.; et al. Nanoencapsulation of Benznidazole in Calcium Carbonate Increases Its Selectivity to *Trypanosoma cruzi*. *Mineral. Mag.* **2018**, *145*, 1191–1198. [CrossRef]

23. Morales-Baez, M.; Rivera-Villanueva, J.M.; López-Monteon, A.; Peña-Rodríguez, R.; Trigos, Á.; Ramos-Ligonio, A. Trypanocidal Effect of Nano MOFs-EP on Circulating Forms of *Trypanosoma cruzi*. *Iran. J. Parasitol.* **2020**, *15*, 115–123. [CrossRef] [PubMed]

24. de Freitas Oliveira, J.W.; da Silva, M.F.A.; Damasceno, I.Z.; Rocha, H.A.O.; da Silva Júnior, A.A.; Silva, M.S. In Vitro Validation of Antiparasitic Activity of PLA-Nanoparticles of Sodium Diethyldithiocarbamate against *Trypanosoma cruzi*. *Pharmaceutics* **2022**, *14*, 497. [CrossRef] [PubMed]

25. Hernández, M.; Wicz, S.; Pérez Caballero, E.; Santamaría, M.H.; Corral, R.S. Dual Chemotherapy with Benznidazole at Suboptimal Dose plus Curcumin Nanoparticles Mitigates *Trypanosoma cruzi*-Elicited Chronic Cardiomyopathy. *Parasitol. Int.* **2021**, *81*, 102248. [CrossRef]

26. Rial, M.S.; Arrúa, E.C.; Natale, M.A.; Bua, J.; Esteva, M.I.; Prado, N.G.; Laucella, S.A.; Salomon, C.J.; Fichera, L.E. Efficacy of Continuous versus Intermittent Administration of Nanoformulated Benznidazole during the Chronic Phase of *Trypanosoma cruzi* Nicaragua Infection in Mice. *J. Antimicrob. Chemother.* **2020**, *75*, 1906–1916. [CrossRef]

27. Rial, M.S.; Scalise, M.L.; Arrúa, E.C.; Esteva, M.I.; Salomon, C.J.; Fichera, L.E. Elucidating the Impact of Low Doses of Nano-Formulated Benznidazole in Acute Experimental Chagas Disease. *PLoS. Negl. Trop. Dis.* **2017**, *11*, e0006119. [CrossRef]

28. Scalise, M.L.; Arrúa, E.C.; Rial, M.S.; Esteva, M.I.; Salomon, C.J.; Fichera, L.E. Promising Efficacy of Benznidazole Nanoparticles in Acute *Trypanosoma cruzi* Murine Model: In-Vitro and in-Vivo Studies. *Am. J. Trop. Med. Hyg.* **2016**, *95*, 388–393. [CrossRef]

29. Abriata, J.P.; Eloy, J.O.; Riul, T.B.; Campos, P.M.; Baruffi, M.D.; Marchetti, J.M. Poly-Epsilon-Caprolactone Nanoparticles Enhance Ursolic Acid in Vivo Efficacy against *Trypanosoma cruzi* Infection. *Mater. Sci. Eng. C* **2017**, *77*, 1196–1203. [CrossRef]

30. de Mello, C.G.C.; Branquinho, R.T.; Oliveira, M.T.; Milagre, M.M.; Saúde-Guimarães, D.A.; Mosqueira, V.C.F.; de Lana, M. Efficacy of Lychnopholide Polymeric Nanocapsules after Oral and Intravenous Administration in Murine Experimental Chagas Disease. *Antimicrob. Agents Chemother.* **2016**, *60*, 5215–5222. [CrossRef]

31. Branquinho, R.T.; de Mello, C.G.C.; Oliveira, M.T.; Soares Reis, L.E.; de Abreu Vieira, P.M.; Saúde-Guimarães, D.A.; Furtado Mosqueira, V.C.; de Lana, M. Lychnopholide in Poly(D,L-Lactide)-Block-Polyethylene Glycol Nanocapsules Cures Infection with a Drug-Resistant *Trypanosoma cruzi* Strain at Acute and Chronic Phases. *Antimicrob. Agents. Chemother.* **2020**, *64*, 10–1128. [CrossRef]

32. Branquinho, R.T.; Pound-Lana, G.; Marques Milagre, M.; Saúde-Guimarães, D.A.; Vilela, J.M.C.; Andrade, M.S.; de Lana, M.; Mosqueira, V.C.F. Increased Body Exposure to New Anti-Trypanosomal Through Nanoencapsulation. *Sci. Rep.* **2017**, *7*, 8429. [CrossRef] [PubMed]

33. Das, S.; Ghosh, S.; De, A.K.; Bera, T. Oral Delivery of Ursolic Acid-Loaded Nanostructured Lipid Carrier Coated with Chitosan Oligosaccharides: Development, Characterization, in Vitro and in Vivo Assessment for the Therapy of Leishmaniasis. *Int. J. Biol. Macromol.* **2017**, *102*, 996–1008. [CrossRef] [PubMed]

34. de Oliveira, A.B.; Saúde, D.A.; Perry, K.S.P.; Duarte, D.S.; Raslan, S.; Amelia, M.; Boaventura, D.; Chiari, E. Trypanocidal Sesquiterpenes from *Lychnophora* Species. *Phytother. Res.* **1996**, *10*, 292–295. [CrossRef]

35. Branquinho, R.T.; Mosqueira, V.C.F.; Kano, E.K.; de Souza, J.; Dorim, D.D.R.; Saúde-Guimarães, D.A.; de Lana, M. HPLC-DAD and UV-Spectrophotometry for the Determination of Lychnopholide in Nanocapsule Dosage Form: Validation and Application to Release Kinetic Study. *J. Chromatogr. Sci.* **2014**, *52*, 19–26. [CrossRef]

36. Fan, J.; Fang, G.; Wang, X.; Zeng, F.; Xiang, Y.; Wu, S. Targeted Anticancer Prodrug with Mesoporous Silica Nanoparticles as Vehicles. *Nanotechnology* **2011**, *22*, 455102. [CrossRef] [PubMed]

37. Romero, L.; Morilla, J. Nanotechnological approaches against Chagas disease. *Adv. Drug. Deliv. Ver.* **2010**, *62*, 576–588. [CrossRef]

38. Bustamante, J.M.; Lo Presti, M.S.; Rivarola, H.W.; Fernández, A.R.; Enders, J.E.; Fretes, R.E.; Paglini-Oliva, P. Treatment with benznidazole or thioridazine in the chronic phase of experimental Chagas disease improves cardiopathy. *Int. J. Antimicrob. Agents* **2007**, *29*, 733–737. [CrossRef]

39. Montelione, N.; Loreni, F.; Nenna, A.; Catanese, V.; Scurto, L.; Ferrisi, C.; Jawabra, M.; Gabellini, T.; Codispoti, F.A.; Spinelli, F.; et al. Tissue Engineering and Targeted Drug Delivery in Cardiovascular Disease: The Role of Polymer Nanocarrier for Statin Therapy. *Biomedicines* **2023**, *11*, 798. [CrossRef]

40. do Nascimento, T.; Todeschini, A.R.; Santos-Oliveira, R.; de Souza de Bustamante Monteiro, M.S.; de Souza, V.T.; Ricci-Junior, E. Trends in Nanomedicines for Cancer Treatment. *Curr. Pharm. Des.* **2020**, *26*, 3579–3600. [CrossRef]

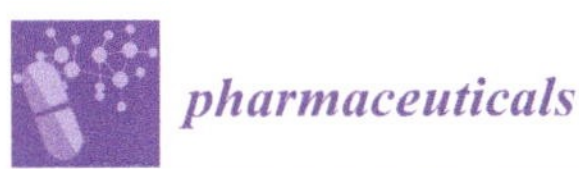

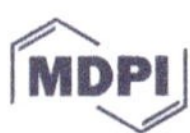

Review

From Bench to Bedside: Implications of Lipid Nanoparticle Carrier Reactogenicity for Advancing Nucleic Acid Therapeutics

Tetiana Korzun [1,2,3,4], Abraham S. Moses [1], Parham Diba [3,4], Ariana L. Sattler [4,5,6], Olena R. Taratula [1], Gaurav Sahay [1], Oleh Taratula [1,2,*] and Daniel L. Marks [4,5,6,*]

1. Department of Pharmaceutical Sciences, College of Pharmacy, Oregon State University, 2730 S Moody Avenue, Portland, OR 97201, USA; korzun@ohsu.edu (T.K.)
2. Department of Biomedical Engineering, Oregon Health & Science University, 3303 SW Bond Avenue, Portland, OR 97239, USA
3. Medical Scientist Training Program, Oregon Health & Science University, 3181 SW Sam Jackson Park Road, Portland, OR 97239, USA
4. Papé Family Pediatric Research Institute, Oregon Health & Science University, 3181 SW Sam Jackson Park Rd, Portland, OR 97239, USA
5. Knight Cancer Institute, Oregon Health & Science University, 2720 S Moody Avenue, Portland, OR 97201, USA
6. Brenden-Colson Center for Pancreatic Care, Oregon Health & Science University, 2730 S Moody Avenue, Portland, OR 97201, USA
* Correspondence: oleh.taratula@oregonstate.edu (O.T.); marksd@ohsu.edu (D.L.M.)

Abstract: In biomedical applications, nanomaterial-based delivery vehicles, such as lipid nanoparticles, have emerged as promising instruments for improving the solubility, stability, and encapsulation of various payloads. This article provides a formal review focusing on the reactogenicity of empty lipid nanoparticles used as delivery vehicles, specifically emphasizing their application in mRNA-based therapies. Reactogenicity refers to the adverse immune responses triggered by xenobiotics, including administered lipid nanoparticles, which can lead to undesirable therapeutic outcomes. The key components of lipid nanoparticles, which include ionizable lipids and PEG-lipids, have been identified as significant contributors to their reactogenicity. Therefore, understanding the relationship between lipid nanoparticles, their structural constituents, cytokine production, and resultant reactogenic outcomes is essential to ensure the safe and effective application of lipid nanoparticles in mRNA-based therapies. Although efforts have been made to minimize these adverse reactions, further research and standardization are imperative. By closely monitoring cytokine profiles and assessing reactogenic manifestations through preclinical and clinical studies, researchers can gain valuable insights into the reactogenic effects of lipid nanoparticles and develop strategies to mitigate undesirable reactions. This comprehensive review underscores the importance of investigating lipid nanoparticle reactogenicity and its implications for the development of mRNA–lipid nanoparticle therapeutics in various applications beyond vaccine development.

Keywords: empty lipid nanoparticles; reactogenicity; xenobiotics; ionizable lipids

Citation: Korzun, T.; Moses, A.S.; Diba, P.; Sattler, A.L.; Taratula, O.R.; Sahay, G.; Taratula, O.; Marks, D.L. From Bench to Bedside: Implications of Lipid Nanoparticle Carrier Reactogenicity for Advancing Nucleic Acid Therapeutics. *Pharmaceuticals* **2023**, *16*, 1088. https://doi.org/10.3390/ph16081088

Academic Editors: Ana Catarina Silva, João Nuno Moreira and José Manuel Sousa Lobo

Received: 7 July 2023
Revised: 24 July 2023
Accepted: 26 July 2023
Published: 31 July 2023

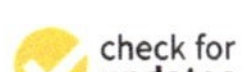

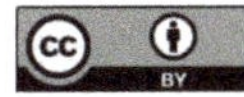

1. Introduction

Nanomaterial-based delivery vehicles are often praised for their ability to encapsulate both hydrophobic and hydrophilic payloads, which include small molecule drugs, imaging agents, and nucleic acids, resulting in their enhanced solubility, extended circulation time, and delayed degradation in the systemic circulation [1]. These properties make nanomedicines an attractive alternative to traditional therapeutic and diagnostic modalities, leading to their extensive use clinically and pre-clinically in various biomedical applications [2]. Extensive research was conducted on the efficacy of lipid nanoparticles (LNPs) for the delivery of messenger RNA (mRNA) as a vaccination tool for the prevention of COVID-19 during the recent pandemic [3–7]. The potential applications of mRNA–LNPs for non-infectious diseases, including those necessitating protein supplementation or replacement therapies, were significantly enhanced by the progress made in this field [8]. These therapeutic interventions apply to a range of disorders, encompassing those linked to chronic inflammation, such as cancer, autoimmune diseases, cardiovascular disorders, diabetes, and other conditions. However, caution must be exercised when considering already reactogenic xenobiotic substances in the presence of pre-existing inflammation. Such a combination is likely to aggravate the underlying inflammation, hamper therapeutic mRNA translation, and interfere with the repeated administration of mRNA therapeutics.

Studies on the reactogenicity of mRNA–LNP formulations were conducted by leveraging the abundance of data derived from clinical trials of COVID-19 vaccines. Systemic and local reactogenic symptoms are known to occur after the administration of COVID-19 mRNA vaccines, including formulations developed by Pfizer-BioNTech and Moderna [4,9]. The observed side effects include fever, muscle aches, headaches, fatigue, chills, and pain at the injection site [3,6,7]. These symptoms are usually mild to moderate in severity and are more common after the second dose of the vaccine [10]. Individuals with underlying chronic inflammation may be at an increased risk of experiencing severe side effects from mRNA–LNP-based therapies and may also have a reduced response to the treatment itself [11]. Furthermore, as shown by COVID-19 vaccine reactogenicity studies, overactivation of immune responses triggered by mRNA–LNP formulations could lead to new-onset autoimmune disorders such as autoimmune liver diseases, Guillain–Barré syndrome, immune thrombotic thrombocytopenia, IgA nephropathy, rheumatoid arthritis, systemic lupus erythematosus, and others [11–13]. Despite the reported unfavorable outcomes, research demonstrates that the manifestation of vaccination side effects is linked to a more robust immune reaction and enhanced protection against COVID-19 [14,15]. However, to guarantee the safety and effectiveness of LNP carrier species for therapeutic applications beyond vaccines and infectious disease prevention, especially when immune activation is unnecessary, a thorough investigation of their toxicity and reactogenicity is indispensable during the formulation development and optimization stages.

The influence of multiple pro-reactogenic elements of mRNA–LNP formulations, such as ionizable lipids, the polyethylene glycol (PEG) coating, and mRNA cargo, should be studied with great caution. Extensive investigation concerning mRNA's reactogenicity, stability, and translatability creates a favorable environment for the current applications of modified mRNA in various therapeutic settings [16–18]. For LNP reactogenicity research, the current focus is now centered on investigating the reactogenic adjuvanticity of LNP formulations to enhance the immunogenicity of mRNA–LNP vaccine formulations [19]. Although a thorough investigation of the LNP carrier's reactogenicity is yet to be accomplished, the current data raise important questions revolving around LNP-associated side effects. For instance, the use of a greater mRNA–LNP dose in the mRNA-1273 vaccine and different ionizable lipids used in the formulation are potential explanations for the increased reactogenicity of mRNA-1273 compared with BNT162b formulations in the Moderna and Pfizer-BioNTech COVID-19 vaccines, respectively [20,21]. Therefore, further research and standardization in the area of reactogenic manifestations and their association with the LNP formulations is necessary to develop effective and safe LNP carrier formulations. By addressing the issue of reactogenicity, mRNA–LNP therapies hold promise for treating a wide range of non-infectious diseases, including those associated with chronic inflammation.

This review summarizes the current understanding of the reactogenicity of LNP carriers, including their potential to exacerbate underlying inflammation, impede the delivered mRNA translation, and potentially interfere with the repeated administration of mRNA therapeutics. Addressing a significant gap in the current literature regarding the reactogenicity of empty LNPs, our review seeks to bridge this critical void by providing a thorough and comprehensive analysis of the reactogenic manifestations associated with LNP carriers.

2. Exploring LNPs as Xenobiotics in Reactogenic Responses

Reactogenicity is a recognized phenomenon that manifests in individuals who are administered xenobiotics, which are defined as any foreign substances introduced into the body. This phenomenon encompasses a range of unfavorable events that may arise due to the immune system's response to such substances, including mRNA–LNP formulations, which are presently employed in COVID-19 vaccines. These reactogenic outcomes in the form of adverse reactions stem from the immune system's response to the LNPs themselves rather than the intended antigen of the vaccine. Although immunogenicity is an anticipated feature of LNP-based vaccines, the reactogenicity of mRNA–LNPs leads to undesirable therapeutic outcomes and unfavorable effects such as pain, fever, chills, and fatigue [4,9,22–24].

Studies are underway to evaluate the reactogenicity of LNPs and their structural components (Table 1) independently of the intended cargo. The typical composition of LNP carriers consists of ionizable lipids, helper lipids, such as distearoylphosphatidylcholine (DSPC), as well as cholesterol and PEG-lipids (Figure 1) [25]. Ionizable lipids are key components of LNPs, as they provide the positive charge that facilitates the encapsulation of negatively charged nucleic acids [26]. Helper lipids, such as DSPC, are often used to optimize the biophysical properties of LNPs. Helper lipids can enhance the stability of the LNP formulation and promote cellular uptake and endosomal escape of nanoparticles [27]. Cholesterol is another essential component of LNPs, as it also influences the biophysical properties of the LNP formulation. The presence of cholesterol within the LNP membrane can enhance its fluidity, thereby promoting the efficient release of nucleic acids from the LNP and facilitating their uptake by cells via enhanced fusogenicity [28]. Lastly, the incorporation of PEG-lipids into LNP formulations serves to augment their stability, decrease the activation of phagocytic immune cells, and enhance their pharmacokinetic properties [26]. In the process of LNP self-assembly, PEG-lipids assume a crucial role by creating a hydrophilic steric barrier through the formation of PEG chains on the LNP surface [29]. Van der Waals forces between the hydrocarbon chains of DSPE, PEG-lipids, and cholesterol molecules are essential for holding the LNPs together and maintaining their structural integrity [30]. The collective result is the formation of a PEG layer around the intact LNP, with the PEG chains protruding from the particle's surface. This arrangement enhances the stability and integrity of the LNP structure, contributing to its overall functionality and effectiveness as a delivery vehicle. Hence, the incorporation of PEG-lipids to create a protective layer around the LNP serves to minimize its recognition by the immune system and enhances its in vivo circulation time. However, it is important to note that PEG-lipid incorporation can also lead to an increase in the immunogenicity of the formulation [31].

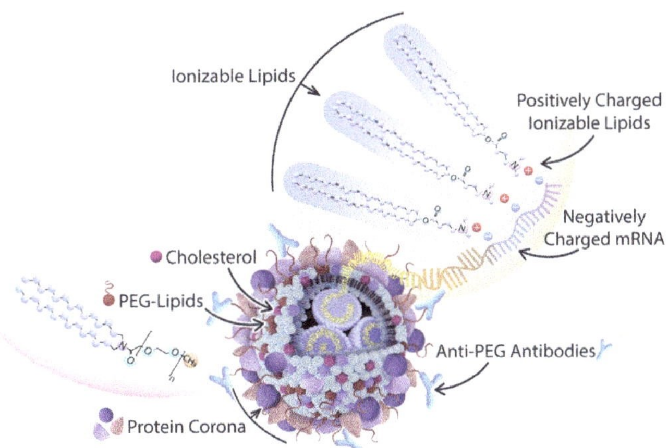

Figure 1. Composition of LNP carriers used in drug delivery: Their composition comprises ionizable lipids, helper lipids such as distearoylphosphatidylcholine (DSPC), cholesterol, and polyethylene glycol

(PEG)-conjugated lipids. Among these components, ionizable lipids and PEG-lipids are the most reactogenic species, posing potential risks for unfavorable immune stimulation and adverse effects. PEG-lipids assume a significant role in LNP self-assembly, creating a hydrophilic steric barrier with protruding PEG chains surrounding the particle, while ionizable lipids bind to the nucleic acid payload through electrostatic interactions.

Table 1. Key building blocks of representative FDA-approved mRNA–LNP formulations.

Category	Common Name	IUPAC Name	Chemical Structure
Ionizable Lipid	Dlin-MC3-DMA [a]	(6Z,9Z,28Z,31Z)-6,9,28,31-Heptatriacontatetraen-19-yl 4-(dimethylamino)butanoate	
Ionizable Lipid	SM-102 [b]	9-Heptadecanyl 8-{(2-hydroxyethyl)[6-oxo-6-(undecyloxy)hexyl]amino}octanoate	
Ionizable Lipid	ALC-0315 [c]	[(4-Hydroxybutyl)imino]di-6,1-hexanediyl bis(2-hexyldecanoate)	
Helper Lipid	DSPC	(2R)-2,3-Bis(stearoyloxy)propyl 2-(trimethylammonio)ethyl phosphate	
Stabilizing component	Cholesterol	(3β)-Cholest-5-en-3-ol	
Shielding component	PEG	poly(oxyethylene)	

Ionizable lipids used in [a] Onpattro therapy, [b] Moderna, and [c] Pfizer-BioNTech COVID-19 vaccines.

Among the components of LNP platforms, ionizable lipids and PEG-lipids are recognized as the most reactogenic elements [32]. Ionizable lipids such as Dlin-MC3-DMA (hereafter referred to as MC3), initially introduced in the therapeutic Onpattro (patirisan); SM-102, employed in the Moderna COVID-19 vaccine; and ALC-0315, utilized in the Pfizer-BioNTech COVID-19 vaccine are frequently evaluated and contrasted based on their reactogenicity and immunogenicity profiles, especially in the context of their implementation in vaccines (Table 1) [33–35]. Ionizable lipids are cationic at low pH and play a crucial role in encapsulating nucleic acids and promoting endosomal escape with the efficient release of cargo into the cytosol [34]. However, their positive charge can also interact with negatively charged endosomal membranes or proteins, resulting in cellular damage and undesired immune activation. Additionally, incorporating PEG-lipids into LNPs to enhance their stability, evade immune cell recognition, and impede opsonization by complement effector molecules can potentially lead to undesirable consequences. These may include the production of anti-PEG antibodies or the accumulation of PEG in various organs and tissues [31]. Importantly, the molecular weight of PEG was shown to play a crucial role in both the production of anti-PEG antibodies and their binding to the PEG moieties. A reduction in anti-PEG IgM formation was observed in mice when treated with LNPs conjugated to a fast-shedding PEG-lipid with short acyl chains, and hence lower molecular weight, in comparison with LNPs conjugated to a slow-shedding PEG-lipid with long acyl chains [36]. Moreover, the pretreatment of mice with slow-shedding PEG-containing LNPs resulted in the suboptimal performance of LNP formulations containing nucleic acids [36]. Interestingly, the administration of high-molecular-weight PEG as a pre-treatment in mice, before introducing PEGylated liposomal formulation, effectively sequestered the existing pool of anti-PEG antibodies [37]. The decrease in available anti-PEG antibodies enabled the prolonged circulation of PEGylated liposomes, avoiding the induction of accelerated clearance and preserving their efficacy. Additionally, PEG with a molecular weight of 2000 Da and larger exhibited the highest affinity for binding anti-PEG antibodies [38].

Therefore, it can be inferred that LNPs themselves, independently of their cargo, possess structural components capable of inducing reactogenic and immunogenic responses. However, evaluating the reactogenicity of individual components of LNP carriers (hereafter referred to as empty LNPs, eLNPs) in isolation is often challenging due to the integral role played by the assembled eLNPs in delivering nucleic acids and the hydrophobicity of separate eLNP components. As such, the comprehensive assessment of the safety and efficacy of the assembled product usually requires an evaluation of the reactogenicity of the intact eLNP platform independently of the intended cargo.

When conducting studies that include reactogenic profiling of mRNA–LNP formulations, researchers use multiple controls beyond the eLNP carriers. These include phosphate-buffered saline, placebo mRNA–LNPs incorporating luciferase or GFP mRNA, diluents, or naked nucleic acids [39–44]. Although LNPs are frequently employed as carriers for mRNA, utilizing eLNPs as a control for comparing their reactogenic effects to mRNA-loaded LNPs and attempting to separate their reactogenic profiles may not always yield optimal results. This is due to the possibility that eLNPs differ from mRNA-loaded LNPs in their size, composition, surface interactions, and fusibility potential. The molar ratio of PEG-lipids, the lipid-to-mRNA mass ratio, and the N/P ratio (representing the positively charged nitrogen of ionizable lipids and the negatively charged phosphates of nucleic acids) are critical factors that influence the ultimate composition of LNPs containing ionizable lipids for mRNA complexation [45]. eLNPs with an altered concentration of helper lipids and interference from ionizable lipids on the surface often display variations in their physicochemical and biological properties compared with mRNA-loaded LNPs, including a positive surface charge, increased splitting dynamics, and a modified protein corona composition [45]. Consequently, eLNPs may display different organ tropism as a result of their differential interaction with homing proteins, such as ApoE, compared with mRNA-loaded LNPs [45]. This, in turn, may augment the local and systemic eLNP reactogenicity.

Considering the major concerns surrounding the reactogenicity of eLNPs and their components, various efforts are underway to develop alternative lipid formulations that can minimize their adverse effects, while still maintaining the desirable properties of LNP platforms. It can be asserted with a high degree of confidence that, at present, the process of constructing LNPs entails adhering to comparable protocols with the primary variance arising from the application of different ionizable lipids (Table 1) but following similar LNP composition ratios (Table 2). For instance, the currently approved mRNA–LNP vaccines demonstrate a commonality in their structural compositions (Table 1). These compositions encompass a diverse range of ionizable lipids, each unique to the specific vaccine formulation, alongside the inclusion of diverse PEGylated lipids. Although the ionizable lipids utilized in each vaccine formulation differ, they all share certain structural features. These structural similarities, such as the amino-alcohol head group and branched hydrocarbon lipid tails characterized by ester linkages, contribute to the stability, mRNA encapsulation efficiency, and facilitation of cellular uptake of mRNA–LNP vaccines.

Despite the development of new formulations, the current Food and Drug Administration (FDA)-approved LNP platforms and their modified versions, which employ similar structural components, continue to serve as the established standard for delivering nucleic acids. Consequently, a comprehensive evaluation of their reactogenicity is imperative to expand the scope of their clinical applications. In light of this, it is essential to note that there are different types of reactogenicity assessments that can be used to evaluate the safety and efficacy of LNP-based therapies.

Table 2. eLNP composition and doses utilized in reactogenicity studies.

Reference	eLNP Composition	Ionizable Lipid	eLNP Dose
[46]	IL: DSPC: cholesterol: PEG-lipid at a molar ratio of 50:10:38.5:1	MC3 and YK009	Not provided; mRNA–LNP dose was equivalent to 10 µg mRNA administered via the IM, SQ, or ID routes
[23]	IL: phosphatidylcholine: cholesterol: PEG-lipid at a molar ratio of 50:10:38.5:1.5 as described in [47]	IL under US10221127B2 patent (Acuitas Therapeutics)	10 µg administered in 4 spots, 2.5 µg/spot, ID, and IV; 10 µg administered IN
[48]	Valera LLC, a Moderna Therapeutics Venture, supplied all vaccines. In-house formulation: IL: DSPC: cholesterol: PEG-lipid: GLA at a molar ratio of 50:9.83:38.5:1.5:0.17	Not discussed	50 µg administered per site, injected ID
[49]	IL: DSPC: cholesterol: PEG-lipid at a molar ratio of 50:10:38.5:1.5	MC3 ionizable lipid	Equivalent to 0.3 mg/kg mRNA–LNP dose, injected IV
[50]	IL: DSPC: cholesterol: PEG-lipid at a molar ratio of 55:10:32.5:2.5 as described in [51]	IL under US10221127B2 patent (Acuitas Therapeutics)	Equivalent to 5 µg/mL total lipids or ~7.5 µg/mL ionizable lipids; eLNP used in in vitro study
[52]	The LNP formulation used in this study is proprietary to Acuitas Therapeutics	IL under US10221127 patent (Acuitas Therapeutics)	Total lipid content: 900 µg; equivalent to the lipid content of 30 µg mRNA-LNP ID and IV
[53]	IL: DSPC: cholesterol: PEG-lipid at a molar ratio of 50:20:28:2 for the MC3 or 50:10:38.5:1.5 for the SM-102 formulations	MC3 and SM-102	eLNP doses are not provided; eLNP injected IV
[54]	IL: phosphatidylcholine: cholesterol: PEG-lipid at a molar ratio of 50:10:38.5:1.5 mol/mol) as described in [47,55]	IL under US10221127 patent (Acuitas Therapeutics)	Equivalent to the lipid content of 2.5 µg mRNA-LNP injected ID
[56]	IL: DSPC: cholesterol: PEG-lipid at a molar ratio of 50:10:38.5:1.5	MC3 and C12-200	2 mg/kg lipids or dose equivalent to 0.32 mg mRNA/kg, injected IV

IL = ionizable lipid; Distearoylphosphatidylcholine = DSPC; ID = intradermally; IV = intravenously; IM = intramuscularly; SQ = subcutaneously; IN = intranasally.

3. Assessment of Reactogenic Manifestations Following LNP Administration

Evaluation of reactogenicity is a crucial component of preclinical safety studies for LNP formulations. Assessing reactogenicity can be carried out in several ways, depending on the administered formulation and the specific adverse events. While the assessment of reactogenicity in human subjects mainly involves evaluating the frequency and severity of local and systemic reactions, as well as monitoring for severe adverse events such as anaphylaxis, preclinical studies involving animal models typically employ a range of approaches. The employed methodologies in animal models encompass behavioral observations, hematological, immunological and biochemical analyses, histopathological examinations, and measurements of specific pro-inflammatory markers through immunohistochemistry and gene expression assays (Figure 2). The comprehensive utilization of these methods facilitates a more thorough understanding of the reactogenic manifestations associated with administered formulations.

Behavioral observation involves monitoring mice for signs of reactogenicity or toxicity, such as changes in food-motivated behavior, activity level, grooming, and respiratory distress. Food intake and body weight are essential parameters often closely examined in preclinical studies. Changes in these parameters provide valuable insights into the overall health of the animals and serve as early indicators of potential reactogenicity to xenobiotics. Therefore, in this review, food intake and body weight will be discussed further as important indicators of reactogenicity in mice.

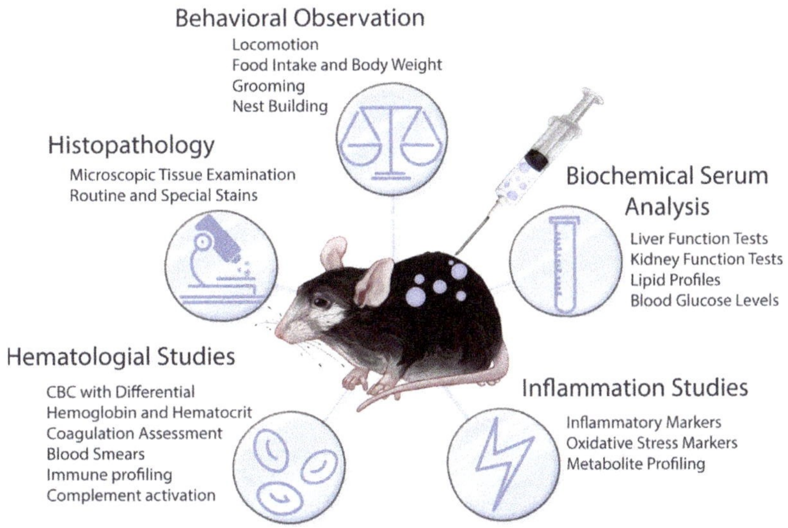

Figure 2. Methodological approaches for investigating reactogenic manifestations in animal models: By integrating different methodologies, such as behavioral observations, histopathological studies, and hematological, biochemical and inflammation analyses, a more comprehensive understanding of the cause-and-effect relationship between treatments and reactogenic manifestations can be achieved, aiding in the development of improved LNP platforms.

The *hematological analysis* focuses on assessing blood samples for parameters such as platelet, white blood cell (WBC), and red blood cell (RBC) counts (i.e., complete blood count (CBC) with differential), hemoglobin concentration, and RBC characteristics. For instance, in rats and monkeys treated with MC3 eLNPs, no change was observed in RBC counts, hemoglobin, hematocrit, and RBC distribution width compared with PBS administration [49]. However, an increase in all these parameters was observed in response to mRNA-loaded LNPs. Additionally, rats exhibited a systemic increase in total WBC count resulting from mRNA-LNP treatment but not from MC3 eLNPs [49]. The systemic increase in WBCs found in that study mirrored the increasing mRNA concentration per administered dose. Interestingly, despite greater WBC counts in the mRNA-LNP treatment group, neutrophils and monocytes were increased in both the mRNA–LNP and MC3 eLNP treatment groups [49]. A transient increase in monocytes and neutrophils in the MC3 eLNP treatment group was observed for a shorter period (specifically, at day 9 post-administration), in comparison with mRNA–LNP treatment groups, where this increase was sustained (up to day 16 post-administration) [49].

In addition to CBC with differential, *immunological investigations*, including immune profiling and complement activation studies, play a crucial role in identifying specific components or characteristics of eLNPs that contribute to their reactogenic properties. Despite the absence of specific studies examining the activation of complement by eLNPs, ample evidence exists regarding complement activation through classical, mannose-binding lectin, and properdin-mediated pathways involving liposomes [57–61]. The activation of the complement cascade can occur through the recognition of structural components of liposomes or antibodies that target these components on the liposomal surface, including cholesterol, PEG, or structural lipids [62–64]. Additionally, the complement cascade can be initiated by the interactions of specific proteins that form the protein corona surrounding nanoparticles [61,65].

In addition to hematological and immunological assessment, blood samples for reactogenic studies can be evaluated for *biochemical parameters*, including liver enzymes, kidney function, and electrolyte balance. The most common biochemical approach utilized to assess systemic reactogenicity in animal models involves the evaluation of hepatic and renal function, as these organs are integral to the metabolism and elimination of foreign substances, including nanoparticles [66]. Exposure to reactogenic substances can result in liver or kidney damage, which is generally reflected by changes in the level of liver enzymes such as alanine and aspartate aminotransferases (AST, ALT) or by changes in markers of renal function, such as increased blood urea nitrogen (BUN) or plasma creatinine levels [67,68]. For instance, AST (but not ALT or alkaline phosphatase) was the only parameter significantly elevated in mice after MC3 eLNPs administration compared with placebo treatment [46]. In rats, the same type of eLNP containing MC3 ionizable lipids increased AST and ALT levels. Moreover, these parameters were increased to the same extent in the rats treated with the highest dose of the mRNA–LNP under investigation [49].

In addition to systemic manifestation, administration of eLNPs also yields local reactogenic reactions. Rodents typically manifest edema, redness, and infiltration of innate immune cells at the injection site. Additionally, innate immune cell infiltration is observed in organs penetrated by LNP-based formulations, such as the lung in studies with intranasal drug administration, mirroring similar responses observed in humans [23,49]. To evaluate the impact of xenobiotics on affected tissues, reactogenicity studies employ an assessment method involving *histopathological examination*, which entails the collection and microscopic analysis of tissue samples from various organs for signs of tissue damage, inflammation, or immune cell infiltration. For instance, histopathological assessment of liver samples showed that MC3 eLNPs induced individual cell necrosis in the livers of rats [49]. Similarly, histopathological approaches are employed to assess the infiltration of immune cells into organs and tissues. In mice, injection-site immune cell infiltrates consist of neutrophils, macrophages, and dendritic cells, and demonstrate the localized release of chemokines in response to eLNPs [23]. The intranasal delivery of labeled LNPs resulted in leukocytic infiltration of lung tissues, with a predominant presence of neutrophils and eosinophils [23]. Additionally, in rhesus macaques, injections with eLNPs and, to a greater extent, mRNA-loaded LNPs led to CD45-positive cell infiltration that denotes non-specific infiltration with hematopoietic cells [48]. Liang et al. also reported that neutrophil and monocyte infiltration in rhesus macaques was similar for mRNA-loaded LNP and eLNP treatments, regardless of administration route, when intramuscular and intradermal routes of injection were compared from immunogenic and reactogenic perspectives [48].

Finally, the assessment of pro-inflammatory effector molecules released in response to eLNP administration encompasses a range of *studies targeting inflammation* that include a wide array of methodologies, including ELISA, flow cytometry, cytokine profiling, quantitative PCR, and microarray analysis. Specifically, chemokine and cytokine expression studies can provide valuable insights into the reactogenicity pathways of eLNPs as a drug delivery system. For instance, the expression of chemokines at the injection site is known to facilitate the trafficking and recruitment of more circulating innate immune cells to the site of active inflammation [69]. Specifically, eLNPs induce the local release of multiple chemokines, including CCL2, CCL3, CCL4, CCL7, CCL12, CXCL1, and CXCL2, that further attract macrophages and monocytes [23]. The potent chemokine CCL2 is also overexpressed by monocytes in response to Acuitas eLNP administration in human peripheral blood mononuclear cells (PBMCs) ex vivo [50]. Collectively, eLNP carriers devoid of payload elicit the recruitment of monocytes and neutrophils, which subsequently amplify this cascade through the local expression of multiple effector molecules. However, eLNP administration elicits a response of shorter duration when contrasted with mRNA-loaded LNP treatments [49]. Our observation further suggests that this disparity may stem from the unique molecular-level responses to mRNA payloads and eLNP carriers, which can be recognized as danger- (DAMPs) or pathogen-associated molecular patterns (PAMPs).

4. Cellular and Molecular Responses to LNP Carriers

Within the intricate landscape of molecular interactions involving LNPs, innate immune cells emerge as the primary first responders to these therapeutics. Among these cellular "arenas", macrophages and neutrophils take center stage as pivotal participants in the dynamic interplay with LNP-based therapies. Employing complex molecular processes, innate immune cells orchestrate a series of reactions that significantly impact the efficacy and safety of LNP formulations. Neutrophils play a critical role in the initiation of acute inflammation and are among the earliest immune cells to be recruited into tissues during such inflammatory processes [70]. Functioning as polymorphonuclear cells, they demonstrate remarkable versatility and contribute significantly to the innate immune response against invading pathogens and tissue damage [71]. Their rapid mobilization to inflamed sites is regulated by a diverse array of signaling molecules, including chemokines and cytokines, which guide their directed migration from the bloodstream to the sites of tissue inflammation [72–74]. Neutrophils interact with different nanoparticles, including LNPs and cationic liposomes [75–78]. Studies reveal that the surface characteristics of lipid-containing nanoparticles, such as PEG density and surface charge, play a pivotal role in modulating the neutrophils' capacity to internalize LNPs [76,78]. Monocytes, the second most abundant cell type responding to LNPs, assume an important role in the context of tissue inflammation. This significance is attributed to their selective recruitment and guided migration into inflamed tissues, which is regulated by an array of inflammatory mediators encompassing cytokines, chemokines, and complement effector molecules [69]. Such an extravasation mechanism enables monocytes to actively participate in immune surveillance and host defense, as they engage with inflamed tissues to facilitate pathogen clearance, tissue repair, and the maintenance of tissue homeostasis [79,80]. Monocytes demonstrate proficient phagocytic capabilities and are equipped with pattern recognition receptors (PRRs), enabling them to actively interact with microbial pathogens, cellular debris, and diverse xenobiotics [81]. Macrophages are also widely recognized to be one of the initial and principal cell types responsible for nanoparticle processing [82]. As nanoparticles interact with the bloodstream, they become coated with opsonins, such as antibodies to PEG or complement effector molecules, which mark them for recognition by the mononuclear phagocytic system [82]. The mononuclear phagocytic system, including monocytes and macrophages, identifies opsonized nanoparticles, facilitating their efficient uptake and clearance from circulation [83–85]. This finely tuned process is essential for the immune surveillance and removal of foreign particles, contributing significantly to the body's defense against potential threats posed by xenobiotics in the bloodstream.

Hematologic studies revealed that the administration of LNP formulations, including eLNPs, leads to a systemic increase in WBC levels. However, a more comprehensive understanding of the biological responses to these formulations can be gained by focusing on the innate immune cells' reactions at the immediate site of administration. For instance, regardless of the eLNP administration mode, be it intravenous (IV), intramuscular (IM), intradermal (ID), or intranasal (IN), the cellular administration sites undergo infiltration by diverse innate immune cells. Among these cellular constituents, neutrophils, monocytes, macrophages, and, to a lesser extent, eosinophils and dendritic cells are identified as the predominant species in areas of infiltration [23,48,50]. This infiltration pattern highlights the robust and multifaceted response of the innate immune system to the presence of administered LNPs and signifies the importance of understanding the specific roles played by these immune cells. Furthermore, a localized approach that defines innate immune cell populations offers a comprehensive view of the early molecular events and interactions that shape the subsequent immune responses, thereby facilitating the development and optimization of LNP-based therapies.

The broad and diverse molecular pathways that underlie eLNP-related reactogenic manifestations as part of DAMP- and PAMP-mediated signaling involve the activation of toll-like receptors (TLRs), primarily TLR4 and TLR2 [50,86]. The interactions between eLNPs and TLRs are studied using downstream effectors and adaptor proteins that facilitate further signal transduction. Signal transduction from TLR4 and TLR2 necessitates the presence of the myeloid differentiation primary response 88 (MyD88) adaptor protein, which is essential for downstream signaling [87]. Additionally, some TLRs, such as TLR4, are known to modify their homophilic interactions with adjacent adaptor proteins based on the acidity of the local environment [87,88]. When TLR4 is internalized along with the forming endosome, the decrease in endosomal pH influences the exchange of the MyD88 adaptor protein for the TIR-domain-containing adaptor-inducing interferon-β (TRIF) adaptor protein [89]. It remains unclear which component of the LNP construct or its protein corona is responsible for TLR ligation, and it is also unknown whether the ligation occurs on the plasma membrane, where TLR4 associates with MyD88, or in the endosome, where TLR4 associates with TRIF for further signal transduction. Furthermore, TLR ligation can be facilitated in the endosome by both LNP surface structures and released LNP components (Figure 3). The acidification of the endosomal environment as endosomes undergo maturation induces the degradation of LNPs, releasing ionizable lipids from the LNP core [90,91]. In the case of LNP-mediated cargo delivery, this conversion occurs during the LNP processing within the endosomal compartment, followed by their escape from the endosomes to facilitate the release of their cargo into the cytosol. It is facilitated by the interactions between the surface of LNPs and the negatively charged membrane of the endosomes in addition to the decrease in ambient pH or by the action of helper lipids or cholesterol or its derivatives [92,93]. Apart from the destabilization of the endosomal membrane caused by LNPs, additional factors, such as the elevation of osmotic pressure or the swelling of particles within the endosome, can contribute to the facilitation of LNP disintegration and subsequent escape from the endosomes [91]. This process allows for the liberation of LNP contents into the cytosol, inevitably compromising the integrity of the intact particles.

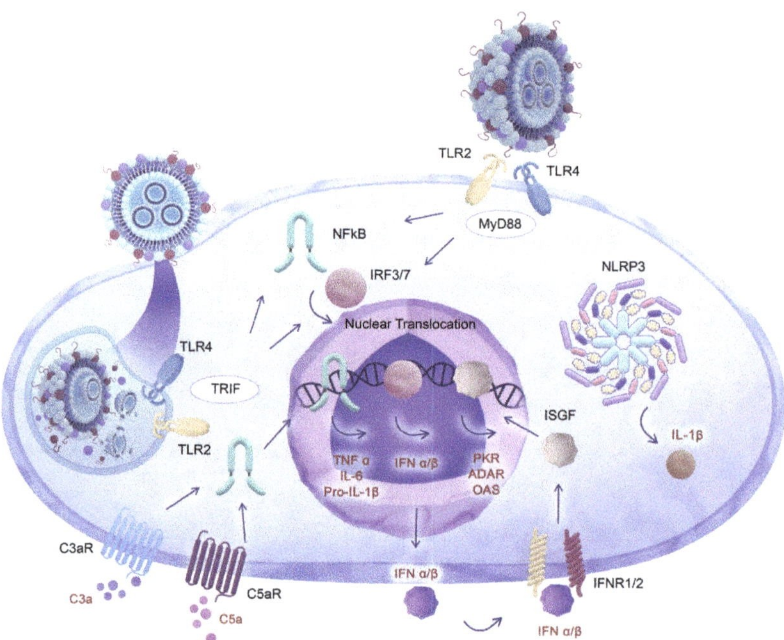

Figure 3. TLR4 signal propagation mediated by MyD88 and TRIF adaptor proteins: Converging pathways involving MyD88 and TRIF adaptors activate the cytokines TNF-α, IL-6, and IL-1β through nuclear translocation of the NF-κB, IRF3, and IRF7 transcription factors. Positive feedback loops and type I interferons enhance cytokine expression, activating additional pro-inflammatory effectors, and inducing cessation of mRNA expression. Complement cascade activation exacerbates cytokine-dependent reactogenicity, with C5a and C3a promoting inflammation via their receptors. TLR4 and C3aR/C5aR activation converge on MAPKs, increasing cytokine production by APCs.

Considering that TLR signaling, specifically TLR4-dependent signal propagation, can be categorized into two main pathways, namely MyD88- and TRIF- facilitated pathways (refer to Figure 3), it is crucial to employ both adaptor proteins in reactogenicity studies and to investigate their involvement in the eLNP-mediated induction of reactogenic manifestations. Therefore, considering the involvement of these proteins in propagating pro-inflammatory signals, researchers utilized genetic ablation approaches such as MyD88 and TRIF knock-out (KO) mouse models to investigate the impact of eLNPs on TLR receptors. For instance, MyD88 KO mice showed no response to empty LNPs in terms of follicular T-helper and germinal center B-cell upregulation, indicating that the adjuvant properties and, possibly, the reactogenicity of eLNPs rely on signal transduction via MyD88 adaptors [52]. Moreover, the convergence of signaling pathways dependent on MyD88 and TRIF adaptors results in the activation of a common set of cytokines, namely tumor necrosis factor-alpha (TNF-α), interleukin 6 (IL-6), and interleukin 1 β (IL-1β). This activation occurs through the induction of nuclear translocation of transcription factors such as nuclear factor-kappa B (NF-κB) and interferon regulatory factors 3 (IRF3) and 7 (IRF7). The expression of these cytokines is further enhanced by positive feedback loops involving type I interferons and interferon-stimulated gene factors (ISGFs) (Figure 3). Consequently, this amplification of cytokine expression leads to the activation of additional effectors, ultimately resulting in the global cessation of mRNA expression and the maturation of cytokines such as IL-1β that is associated with physiological reactogenic responses such as fever and painful sensations. Importantly, within the context of investigations concerning MyD88 and TRIF adaptors in LNP reactogenicity studies, mice with a dual knockout of MyD88 and TRIF exhibited reduced expression of downstream effectors, specifically TNF-α and IL-6, in comparison with wild-type (WT) mice when exposed to mRNA-loaded LNPs [94]. The study has a limitation from the perspective of reactogenicity investigations in that it did not distinguish between the effects of mRNA-loaded LNPs and empty LNPs on the MyD88/TRIF dual KO model. This is further complicated by the fact that both TRIF and MyD88 proteins also function as adaptors to TLRs that detect nucleic acids, such as TLR3, which recognizes double-stranded RNA (dsRNA) molecules as PAMPs and DAMPs [95]. Moreover, the MyD88 adaptor is involved in signal transduction from TLR7 that is activated by single-stranded RNA (ssRNA) [89]. As such, it is unclear whether the observed response is due to the nucleic acid payload or the LNP carrier or both. A further puzzle that arises in the decoding of reactogenicity of mRNA-loaded LNPs and eLNPs is that both the induction of TLRs by nucleic acids and eLNPs result in the expression of a similar subset of cytokines and chemokines involved in reactogenic symptoms. Additionally, multiple positive feedback loops and feeder pathways can exacerbate the expression of reactogenicity-related effectors.

Cytokine-dependent reactogenic manifestation can be exacerbated following complement cascade activation, where pro-inflammatory effects of complement effector molecules acting on their respective receptors result in the upregulation of IL-6, TNF-α, and IL-1β expression (Figure 3). The anaphylatoxins, C5a and C3a, are produced through proteolytic processes during the complement cascade activation, which involves the previously mentioned liposome-dependent activation of the classical, mannose-binding lectin, and properdin-mediated complement pathways [57–61,96]. The administration of LNPs possibly results in similar activation patterns, resulting in the generation of C3a and C5a effectors through the action of proteolytic convertases [97,98]. While functioning as anaphylatoxins, attracting innate and adaptive immune cells, and promoting the maturation of adaptive immune cells, C3a and C5a also interact with the C3a receptor (C3aR) and the C5a receptor (C5aR), propagating and amplifying the TLR-dependent inflammatory cascade [99–105]. For instance, the activation of TLR4 and C3aR/C5aR converges to the same mitogen-activated protein kinases (MAPKs), leading to the nuclear translocation of NF-κB, which results in a significant upregulation of IL-6, TNF-α, and IL-1β by antigen-presenting cells (APCs) [106,107].

5. Enhanced Cytokine Gene Expression in Response to eLNP Administration

Reactogenic symptoms such as fever, chills, and localized inflammation at the injection site of the LNP-based vaccines are known to be driven by cytokine expression in the resident and migratory immune cells attracted to the injection site [108]. Recent research shed light on the mechanisms underlying these reactogenic manifestations, revealing that they are driven by certain cytokines, including IL-6, IL-1β, and TNF-α [109]. These cytokines are part of the body's natural immune response and are responsible for inducing inflammation and fever, which help to mobilize the immune system to fight off the perceived target pathogen. The regulation of pro-inflammatory cytokine expression is tightly controlled by the previously mentioned transcription factors NF-κB, IRF3, and IRF7, which play crucial roles in the molecular mechanism of acute and chronic inflammation (Figure 4) [110,111].

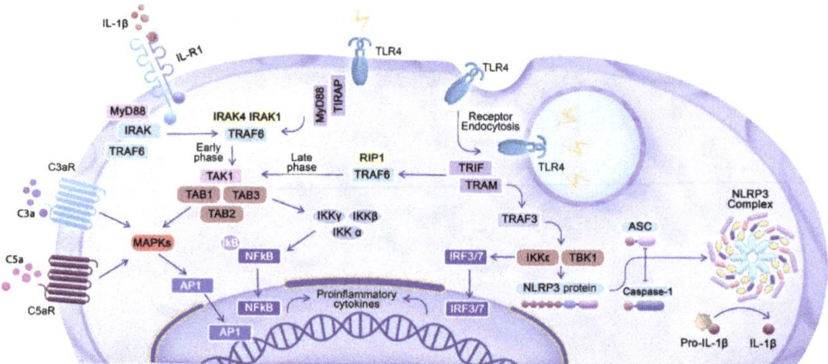

Figure 4. Integration of TLR4 signaling, inflammasome activation, and complement anaphylatoxin receptors in cytokine regulation: Upon TLR4 stimulation on the plasma membrane, a MyD88-dependent pathway is initiated, leading to the phosphorylation of interleukin-1 receptor-associated kinases (IRAKs), particularly IRAK1 and IRAK4. The recruited TNF-Receptor-Associated Factor 6 (TRAF6) undergoes ubiquitination, facilitating the formation of polyubiquitin chains that recruit transforming growth factor-β-activated kinase 1 (TAK1), TGF-beta-activated kinase 1 (MAP3K7), binding protein 1/2/3 (TAB 1/2/3), and inhibitor of nuclear factor-κB kinases (IKKs). These molecules are crucial for activating NF-κB and mitogen-activated protein kinase (MAPK) signaling. NF-κB translocates to the nucleus, acting as a transcription factor for pro-inflammatory cytokines such as TNF-α, IL-1β, and IL-6, signifying completion of the "early phase" of NF-κB activation. Activation of TLR4 in the endosome triggers a TRIF-dependent pathway, where translocating chain-associating membrane protein (TRAM) serves as an adaptor molecule connecting TLR4 and TRIF. TRAF6, recruited via TRIF, undergoes ubiquitination and interacts with receptor-interacting serine/threonine-protein kinase 1 (RIP1), facilitating the recruitment and activation of IKK for the "late phase" of NF-κB activation. Regardless of MyD88 or TRIF dependence, TLR activation induces NF-κB nuclear translocation, resulting in the expression of cytokines such as TNF-α, IL-6, IL-1β, and others, with temporal variations. Additionally, TNF-Receptor-Associated Factor 3 (TRAF3) interacts with TRIF and recruits TANK-binding kinase 1 protein (TBK1) and IκB kinase epsilon (IKKε) kinase, which phosphorylate and activate IRF3/7. IRF3/7 translocates to the nucleus, promoting the expression of type I interferons. Post-translational modifications are necessary to activate pro-IL-1β, with caspase-1 and apoptosis-associated speck-like protein containing CARD (ASC) adaptor activation by the NOD-, LRR-, and pyrin-domain-containing protein 3 (NLRP3) inflammasome complex playing a key role in this process. TRAF3, through IKKε and TBK1, can interact with NLRP3 inflammasome components in certain cellular contexts. Activated IL-1β, via interaction with IL-1R, can upregulate NF-κB nuclear translocation via a MyD88-dependent mechanism. Furthermore, C3aR and C5aR receptors ligated by C3a and C5a complement anaphylatoxins, lead to activation of the AP-1 and NF-κB transcription factors, either by interacting with MAPKs or IKKs, further propagating pro-inflammatory cytokine expression.

The activation of transcription factors IRF3/7 is governed by the TRIF-dependent signaling via TLR4 upon ligation by eLNPs and via TLR3 upon ligation by dsRNA structures as integral components of secondary mRNA confirmations. [50,112,113]. The activation through the phosphorylation and subsequent nuclear translocation of IRF3/7 results in the expression of interferon β (IFN-β) and interferon-stimulated genes factors (ISGFs). Moreover, TLR stimulation with the subsequent MyD88-dependent signal transduction results in the expression and phosphorylation of another transcription factor, NF-κB, indicating the initiation of the "early" NF-κB pathway [114]. The phosphorylated NF-κB protein translocates to the nucleus, where it acts as a transcription factor to regulate the expression of pro-inflammatory effector molecules, including TNF-α, IL-1β, and IL-6 [110]. Together with IRF activation, the TRIF-dependent signaling pathway also guides the "late" activation of NF-κB, further emphasizing the convergence of TRIF- and MyD88-dependent pathways [114]. The converging nature of these pathways is elucidated in Figure 4. Overall, the pathway involving TLR activation leading to NF-κB nuclear translocation, regardless of whether it is MyD88- or TRIF-dependent, leads to the expression of cytokines such as TNF-α, IL-6, interleukin 8 (IL-8), IL-1β, and others, although the timing of their expression differs. In this context, the mechanism of transcriptional activation of IL-1β is somewhat complicated, because the interleukin-1 receptor (IL-1R) requires MyD88 as an adaptor molecule to transmit signals following IL-1R ligation by IL-1β (Figure 4) [115]. Therefore, the expression of *IL1β* in cells and tissues that encounter eLNPs presents the challenge of how the initial TLR-dependent expression of *IL1β* can be distinguished from its subsequent expression that is self-potentiated by IL-1β binding to IL-1R. Furthermore, at the protein level, post-translational modifications are necessary to activate the precursor of IL-1β, pro-IL-1β, and release the mature, biologically active form of IL-1β. Proteolytic activation of IL-1β is induced by the enzyme caspase-1 that is activated by the multi-protein complex inflammasome, NLRP3, which is assembled in response to TLR activation (Figure 4) [116]. Once activated, caspase-1 cleaves pro-IL-1β into its mature, active IL-1β form, which can then be secreted by the cell to exert its pro-inflammatory effects. In summary, the ligation of TLRs with the subsequent activation of different signaling pathways leads to the expression and post-translational activation of cytokines, including IFN-β, IL-6, TNF-α, and IL-1β, which are commonly used as outcome measures to study eLNP-induced reactogenicity.

The upregulation of pro-inflammatory cytokines in response to eLNP treatment has been studied in both ex vitro experiments and in vivo murine studies, with results showing increased expression over time and across different proprietary lipid formulations. eLNPs containing Acuitas' proprietary lipids were assessed in ex vitro experiments with human PBMCs and in in vivo murine studies [50,52]. Expression of IL-1β and IL-6 was upregulated in monocytes and increased in a time-dependent manner after treatment with eLNPs [50]. Furthermore, Tahtinen et al. and Alameh et al. showed that the eLNPs containing SM-102 utilized in the Moderna COVID-19 vaccine and eLNPs containing the Alnylam ionizable lipid led to an increase in IL-1β levels in purified monocytes and draining lymph node lysate, respectively [52,53]. Levels of IL-1β and IL-6 were also increased in the sera of mice treated with eLNPs containing the MC3 and YK009 ionizable lipids compared with a control group treated with phosphate-buffered saline (PBS) [46]. Furthermore, serum TNF-α in this study was higher in mice treated with MC3 eLNPs than with mRNA-containing MC3 LNPs in the first 6 h post-treatment, although no information was provided about dosing considerations of eLNPs in comparison with mRNA–LNPs [46]. Interestingly, in contrast to TNF-α, levels of both IL-1β and IL-6 were increased in the eLNP treatment group, similarly to the mRNA-loaded LNP treatment group [46]. Parhiz et al. also found that MC3 eLNPs upregulated serum IL-6 in mice but were less reactogenic in terms of IL-6 levels compared with C12-200 ionizable-lipid-containing eLNPs [56]. In contrast, Tahtinen et al. reported that MC3 eLNPs did not change IL-1β levels; however, the doses of eLNPs administered to the mice were not reported in the study [53]. Sedic et al. found no change in IL-6 and TNF-α expression in rats subjected to MC3 eLNPs in comparison with the control group [49].

Despite the limited availability of data concerning eLNP reactogenicity in inflamed tissues, there is evidence indicating that pre-treatment with lipopolysaccharide (LPS), which is known to induce a TLR4-dependent innate immune response and acute inflammation, exacerbates existing inflammation following subsequent eLNP administration [56]. The exacerbation of inflammation induced by LPS may arise from various factors, such as heightened eLNP internalization or the self-potentiation of chemokine and cytokine expression via parallel or converging reactogenic pathways induced by LPS and eLNPs. Furthermore, LPS induces not only peripheral inflammation but also hypothalamic inflammation, thereby introducing a brain axis that leads to the induction of sickness behavior components, such as fatigue, fever, weight loss, decreased food intake, and anhedonia [117–119]. These findings emphasize the need to mitigate the reactogenic effects of LNPs to ensure their safe and effective application.

Abundant evidence from the studies demonstrates the utilization of not only diverse ionizable lipids but also different doses, emphasizing the significance of a comprehensive assessment of these factors to gain a more informed understanding of their impact on therapeutic applications. Table 2 showcases a selection of representative studies that vividly demonstrate the significant differences in eLNP doses employed. It emphasizes the wide range of doses utilized in the administered formulations. Therefore, the introduction of standardization in the doses and dosage regimens of eLNPs is crucial for facilitating a comparative evaluation of eLNP reactogenicity. Furthermore, standardization is particularly important for evaluating the safety profile of eLNPs to identify potential adverse reactions and to determine the optimal dose range for clinical use. Since pre-existing inflammation can increase the risk of adverse reactions to eLNPs, utilizing standardized dosing in research settings could help to identify the optimal dose range for minimizing the risk of exacerbating inflammation or of inducing further damage to cells and tissues.

6. LNP-Inducible Expression of Cytokines Modulating Sickness Behavior

The physiologic responses to eLNPs include a typical sickness response, consisting of attenuation of food intake and loss of body weight (Figure 5). This is driven, at least partially, by the action of pro-inflammatory cytokines on the hypothalamic centers regulating appetite and metabolism. Cytokines such as IL-6, IL-1β, and TNF-α play a role in the negative regulation of body weight in rodents as part of their sickness behavior in response to inflammatory conditions [120–125]. IL-6 is mainly expressed by innate immune cells, such as monocytes, but it is also produced by skeletal muscle and adipose tissues and has both pro- and anti-inflammatory effects [126–129]. In terms of body weight regulation, IL-6 exhibits a biphasic effect, where acute elevation of IL-6 levels decreases food intake and increases energy expenditure, while chronic elevation of IL-6 levels is associated with increased body weight and insulin resistance [123,130]. IL-1β is produced by a variety of cells, including innate immune cells such as macrophages, monocytes, and dendritic cells, and is known to be a potent pro-inflammatory cytokine [131,132]. Both IL-6 and IL-1β act on the hypothalamus, a key regulatory center in the brain that controls feeding behavior and energy expenditure [133]. IL-6 acts on the hypothalamus to increase the expression of anorexigenic (appetite-reducing) neuropeptides [134,135]. Although IL-1β increases the expression of orexigenic (appetite-stimulating) neuropeptides, such as neuropeptide Y (NPY) and agouti-related protein (AgRP), its potent induction of hypothalamic inflammation leads to a reduction in food intake and a consequent decrease in body weight [136,137].

The findings suggest that the elevated levels of IL-6 and IL-1β induced by eLNPs lead to decreased body weight through the modulation of hypothalamic function. IL-6 and IL-1β were shown to be increased at both the mRNA and protein levels in mice treated with eLNPs containing non-disclosed proprietary ionizable lipids [23]. Importantly, IL-6 and IL-1β overexpression was also associated with a decrease in murine body weight [23]. Of note, the authors also observed high mortality at the 10 µg eLNP dose delivered intranasally in this study, with just 20% survival on day 1 post-treatment [23]. Therefore, the observed weight reduction could be due to TLR-dependent septic shock involving a cytokine storm with the possible overexpression of IL-6, IL-1β, and TNF-α, as discussed in [138]. Importantly, the results of studies utilizing MyD88/TRIF KO mice that were administered mRNA–LNP injections suggest that MyD88/TRIF dual KO mice did not exhibit weight loss [94]. These findings suggest that effector molecules produced due to the LNP activation of TRIF- or MyD88-dependent reactogenic pathways play a pivotal role in inducing sickness behavior. Therefore, incorporating food intake and body weight as key indicators of systemic reactogenicity in the routine evaluation of eLNP is crucial, as they not only form an integral part of sickness behavior but are also paramount in assessing the efficacy and safety of LNP therapies for conditions that afflict patients' frailty, such as cancer and other chronic diseases.

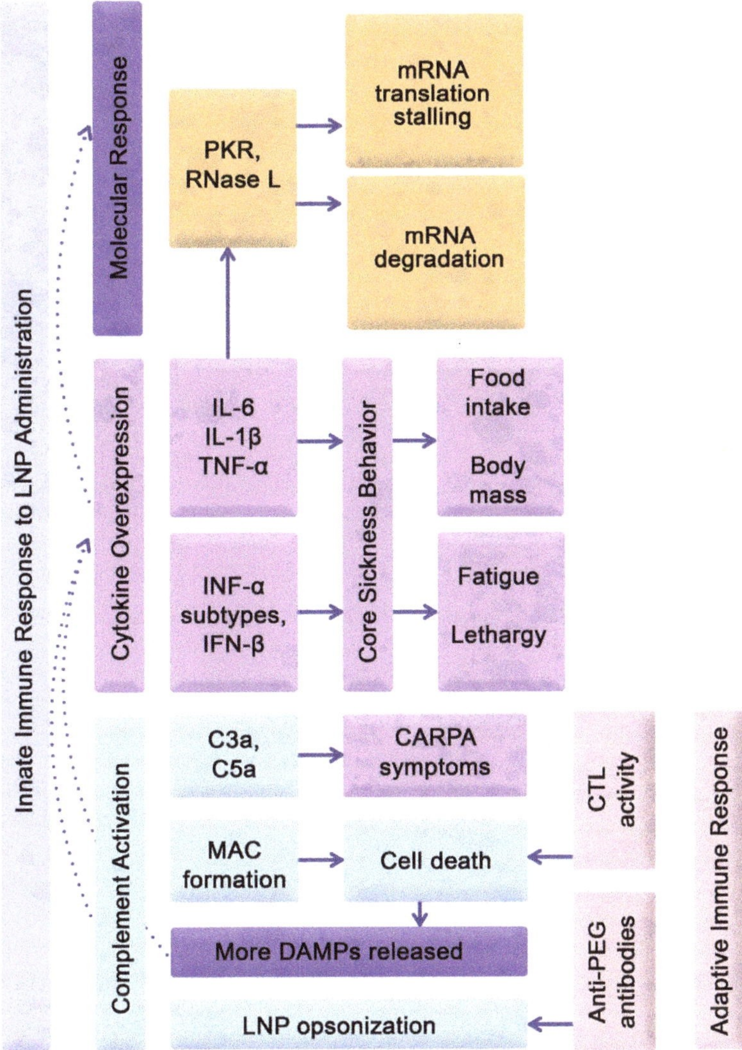

Figure 5. Mechanistic insights into reactogenic manifestations and therapeutic challenges in LNP administration: Complex mechanisms underlie reactogenic manifestations of LNP administration. Expression of cytokines, including IL-6, IL-1B, TNF-a, and interferons, initiate core sickness behaviors such as decreased food-motivated behaviors, fatigue, and lethargy. Concurrent LNP-dependent complement

activation can result in CARPA symptoms, including anaphylaxis, chills, headache, and cardiopulmonary distress. Moreover, complement activation-dependent MAC formation potentially eliminates cells that are actively internalizing LNPs, leading to the release of additional DAMP signals and additional cytokine expression. CTLs also contribute to removing cells presenting LNP-related antigens from the treated cell pool. Complement opsonization of LNPs, along with anti-PEG antibodies, may increase systemic and local reactogenicity by sequestering particles and reduce their therapeutic efficacy. Additionally, activated PKR and RNase L enzymes can hinder mRNA translation or degrade the mRNA therapeutic payload, further decreasing the therapeutic efficacy.

Together with a decrease in food-motivated behavior, fatigue is an important indicator of the severity of the reactogenic insult (Figure 5). Type I and Type II interferons play a critical role in developing disease-associated and iatrogenic fatigue syndromes [139–144]. Hence, the assessment of interferon expression holds significant importance due to their role in causing symptomatic reactogenic manifestations, including fatigue, in response to mRNA–LNP formulations. This is particularly relevant in the context of COVID-19 vaccine administration, where fatigue is a frequent side effect [145,146]. The role of interferons, along with other pro-inflammatory cytokines, is considered significant in both localized and systemic inflammation and in the development of fever [147]. Type I interferons, including IFN-α subtypes and IFN-β, are expressed as part of the pro-inflammatory cascade induced by unmodified mRNA acting on TLR3, TLR7, and TLR9 and by eLNPs acting on TLR2 or TLR4 [50,148,149]. Interferon-gamma (IFN-γ), or type II interferon, has lower pro-inflammatory potency and is important for the induction of adaptive immunity against intracellular pathogens [150]. Liang et al. reported that, in contrast to mRNA-loaded LNPs, eLNPs do not increase Type I IFN-inducible myxovirus resistance gene A (MxA) expression, which is used as a marker for the induction of endogenous type I interferons [48]. However, in the study by Connors et al., protein levels of IFNα and IFNγ were significantly increased after 24 h of Acuitas eLNP stimulation [50]. Connors et al. also report that eLNPs induced increased levels of phosphorylated IRF7, leading to the expression of ISGs [50]. Although there is a slight increase in IRF7 activation when TLR4 is ligated, significant activation only occurs when TLR7 or TLR9 are engaged, such as in the case of an LNP-encapsulated payload of nucleic acids acting on these receptors [149].

7. Reactogenicity Interference with Translation of mRNA Delivered by LNP Carriers

The immune response triggered by the injection of mRNA–LNP formulations can result in the downregulation of protein translation from the delivered mRNA, which limits the efficacy of mRNA-based therapies (Figure 5) [151,152]. The production of pro-inflammatory effector molecules downregulates expression of the delivered mRNA through various mechanisms, including the inhibition of translation initiation and the degradation of mRNA [153,154]. The immune system may recognize the eLNP carriers or eLNP structural components as a threat and mount an immune response, even in the absence of an mRNA payload. Significantly, compelling evidence suggests that mRNA–LNP formulations exhibit a substantial abundance of eLNPs that lack the incorporation of any therapeutic payload [45]. Hence, it is imperative to explore the reactogenic effects of eLNPs that may trigger immune responses and ultimately diminish mRNA expression in order to ensure optimal protein expression.

The delivery of mRNA using LNPs was observed to result in reduced mRNA translation when mice were simultaneously exposed to mild doses of LPS [152]. This finding holds significance as both eLNPs and LPS are capable of binding to TLR4. Lokugamage et al. further showed that administering a TLR4 inhibitor increased mRNA translation; however, it did not fully restore it to the levels observed in the absence of LPS treatment [152]. Furthermore, TLR4 activation by mRNA–LNPs themselves led to a decrease in mRNA translation. Importantly, the reduction in mRNA expression was not attributed to a decline in the particle endocytosis or endosomal escape of LNPs, but rather to the action of RNA-dependent protein kinase R (PKR) subsequent to TLR4 ligation. PKR, which reduces mRNA translation in the cell, is an intermediary component downstream of TLR signaling that, upon activation, phosphorylates eukaryotic initiation factor 2 (eIF2) [16,155,156]. This phosphorylation event prevents the recruitment of the initiator transfer RNA (tRNA) to the ribosome and the activation of eIF2 by binding to guanosine triphosphate (GTP), thereby inhibiting the initiation of translation [156–159]. Furthermore, one of the innate immune mechanisms by which effector molecules such as TNF-α, IL-1 family cytokines, type I IFNs, and other pro-inflammatory cytokines can inhibit translation initiation is by controlling the phosphorylation of the alpha subunit of eIF2, eIF2α [159,160]. Consequently, the initial event of TLR4 ligation, along with the subsequent expression of downstream molecules such as TNF-α, members of the IL-1 family, and type I interferons, contributes to the decreased expression of both therapeutic mRNA and the entire pool of mRNA within the cell as part of a reactogenic outcome.

In addition to inhibiting translation initiation, cytokines can also induce the degradation of mRNA molecules (Figure 5). One mechanism by which this occurs is through the activation of ribonuclease L (RNase L), an enzyme that degrades mRNA in response to exogenous nucleic acid insults, such as those arising from viral infection [161]. The activation of RNase L by pro-inflammatory cytokines can lead to both viral and host mRNA degradation, thereby reducing the overall level of mRNAs available for translation [162,163]. Moreover, pro-inflammatory cytokines can activate signaling pathways that lead to the induction of cell death, which also contributes to the downregulation of mRNA expression by the cells actively internalizing mRNA–LNP formulations [164]. Despite the low-reactogenicity modified mRNA formulations used in clinical practice, [17,18] the use of eLNP carriers may still cause reactogenic manifestations and subsequently lead to cytokine-dependent downregulation of mRNA expression.

The reduction in exogenous mRNA expression can be further modulated by activating complement and adaptive immunity by actively removing the cells internalizing mRNA–LNPs. Activation of the complement pathway by LNPs can initiate the formation of membrane attack complexes (MACs), which often inflict cellular damage. The formation of MACs as a result of activation through classical, mannose-binding lectin, and properdin-mediated complement pathways [165] not only poses a direct threat to the targeted cells but can also impact the uptake and internalization of LNP formulations, leading to a decrease in their therapeutic effectiveness. Additionally, anti-PEG antibodies and complement effector molecules play a critical role in the opsonization of LNPs, resulting in their accelerated clearance from the system and subsequently reducing their therapeutic efficacy. Furthermore, PEG incorporated into the LNP coating induces an anaphylactoid, complement-activation-related pseudoallergy (CARPA) rection [166,167]. CARPA is a harmful immune reaction triggered by the activation of the complement system, leading to adverse symptoms and potentially life-threatening complications in response to certain medications or therapeutic agents [166,168]. In their study, Ndeupen et al. put forth the hypothesis that PEGylated lipids present in LNPs may elicit CARPA in individuals who possess pre-existing PEG-specific antibodies. These antibodies could arise from the previous administration of mRNA–LNP formulations, including COVID-19 vaccines [23]. Of significant importance, extensive evidence exists regarding the activation of the adaptive immune system by LNP delivery, resulting in the generation of antibodies against immunogenic LNP components, including the formation of anti-PEG antibodies [20,169].

Furthermore, the activation of cytotoxic T lymphocyte (CTL) cells and their accumulation in draining lymph nodes adjacent to the xenobiotic injection site can lead to the destruction of cells such as APCs that have taken up LNPs containing the immunogenic components (Figure 5). Consequently, CTLs can facilitate an increase in the clearance of PEGylated LNPs, thereby causing a further decrease in the expression of the delivered mRNA. The actions of CTLs are indeed advantageous in therapeutic approaches that utilize mRNA–LNPs as cancer vaccines. The delivery of therapeutic mRNA–LNPs can lead to the expression of novel antigens in cancer cells that is potentiated by a triggered immune response [170]. However, this approach may be counterproductive in mRNA therapeutics aimed at applications beyond the elimination of diseased cells. These immune responses highlight the immunogenic potential of LNP bridging to reactogenic manifestations and emphasize the need for careful evaluation and monitoring of immune reactions in LNP-based therapeutic applications.

8. Reactogenicity Interference with Multiple Injections of Lipid Nanoparticle Formulations

Similar to the immune system's ability to interfere with mRNA translation after a single injection, there is growing apprehension regarding the possibility of decreased mRNA expression in response to repeated administrations or after prior exposure to mRNA–LNP formulations. This phenomenon can be attributed to the recognition of the LNP delivery system as a foreign entity by the adaptive immune system, leading to an immediate immune response that may result in mRNA degradation prior to its translation into proteins. As the utilization of mRNA vaccines and therapeutics continues to expand, it is imperative to gain a comprehensive understanding of the potential long-term ramifications that may arise from repeated administrations. If repeated injections or pre-exposure to LNPs lead to a decrease in mRNA expression, it could impact the efficacy of these treatments and may require changes to their dosing, dosage, or delivery methods. Therefore, understanding the potential risks associated with repeated administration of mRNA–LNPs is important to improve the safety and efficacy of mRNA-based therapies.

Despite the limited amount of research on the pre-exposure to mRNA–LNP formulations decreasing mRNA expression, the available evidence suggests that there are significant implications for understanding its impact. In a study aiming to express an mRNA-encoded antigen, Qin et al. reported that pre-exposure to eLNPs or mRNA-loaded LNPs decreased the response in terms of both antibody production and germinal center B-cell expansion [54]. Further, upon administering mRNA–LNPs repeatedly, there was an observed transition in LNP distribution from the liver to the spleen after the third successive injection [171]. This observation was attributed to increased internalization of LNPs by splenic APCs, possibly recognizing the protein corona surrounding LNPs. Additionally, exposure of LNPs to plasma from LNP-immunized mice revealed the enhancement of immunoglobulins attached to the protein corona encircling the LNPs [171]. In line with prior research, the opsonizing immunoglobulins detected in this study included antibodies against PEG [171]. These findings suggest that the LNP carriers themselves, and not the mRNA payload, play a crucial role in the immune elimination of mRNA–LNP formulations. Of note, the physical characteristics of LNPs and their interactions with serum proteins can be altered by employing diverse ionizable lipid components, leading to variations in LNP accumulation across different tissues, such as liver, spleen, and lung [172]. Hence, the redistribution of LNPs following multiple injections may depend on the composition of the LNPs themselves.

In addition to stimulating adaptive immunity, pre-exposure to LNP formulations can also alter the innate immune response, which could aggravate mRNA elimination, decreasing its expression. For instance, the use of the BNT162b2 mRNA–LNP formulation as a vaccine resulted in the upregulation of pro-inflammatory and IFN-stimulated genes such as the chemokine CXCL10 and the cytokine IL-6 in monocytes [173]. These effects were more pronounced after the booster vaccination with BNT162b2 than after the initial vaccination [173]. Despite these findings, mRNA–LNP-based vaccines continue to play a crucial role in the ongoing battle against the COVID-19 pandemic, and their success provides a foundation for developing novel and innovative mRNA–LNP formulations for the treatment of various other diseases.

9. Conclusions and Next Steps in eLNP Reactogenicity Research

While LNP-mediated delivery of nucleic acid therapeutics offers substantial potential for disease prevention and treatment, optimizing their formulation to minimize side effects and reactogenicity is crucial. Furthermore, caution should be exercised when administering mRNA–LNP-based therapies to individuals with pre-existing chronic inflammation, as

LNP reactogenicity may exacerbate the underlying inflammatory conditions. Additionally, even in healthy individuals, reactogenicity could pose a risk to the effectiveness of mRNA translation and may hinder the repeated administration of mRNA therapeutics. The current understanding of the effects of LNP composition, associated temporal kinetics, chronic dosage, and dosing on their ability to evoke reactogenic manifestations is still evolving, and further investigations are needed to develop safe and effective LNP carrier formulations.

Future studies should focus on elucidating the mechanisms of LNP-induced inflammation, as well as on identifying ways to mitigate their reactogenicity. For instance, temporal kinetics is an important consideration when studying eLNP reactogenicity, since the prolonged presence of LNP carriers can cause toxicity and interfere with the efficacy of the therapy. Therefore, the optimal timing and frequency of administration of LNP-based therapies must be carefully evaluated to minimize the risk of adverse reactions. The dose of LNP carriers and density of the mRNA payload distribution per particle is another factor that needs to be optimized for the desired therapeutic effect, especially in the setting of chronic administration. In addition, it is worth noting that variations in ionizable lipids, mRNA cargo, and PEG coating can significantly impact the reactogenicity of LNP carriers. Therefore, the standardization and optimization of LNP carrier formulations in reactogenicity studies can significantly enhance both their safety and effectiveness, paving the way for developing new treatments.

Author Contributions: Conceptualization, D.L.M., O.T. and T.K.; methodology, T.K.; resources, O.R.T., D.L.M. and O.T.; writing—original draft preparation, T.K.; writing—review and editing, T.K., A.S.M., P.D., A.L.S., O.R.T., G.S., O.T. and D.L.M.; visualization, T.K.; supervision, D.L.M. and O.T.; project administration, T.K.; funding acquisition, D.L.M. and O.T. All authors have read and agreed to the published version of the manuscript.

Funding: This publication was supported by the National Cancer Institute of the National Institutes of Health under Award Numbers R37CA234006 and R01CA237569, OHSU Knight Cancer Institute, and Friends of Doernbecher. Support was also received from the College of Pharmacy at Oregon State University, Papé Family Pediatric Research Institute at Oregon Health & Science University, and an ARCS Scholarship (The Karen Irons Medicis Memorial Scholar Award, Diane and Dick Alexander). Additionally, the project described was supported by the National Center for Advancing Translational Sciences, National Institutes of Health, through Grant Award Number TL1TR002371. The funding sources were not involved in study design; in the collection, analysis and interpretation of data; in the writing of the manuscript; and in the decision to submit the article for publication.

Institutional Review Board Statement: Not applicable.

Informed Consent Statement: Not applicable.

Data Availability Statement: Data sharing is not applicable.

Conflicts of Interest: D.L.M. is a consultant for Pfizer, Inc. and Alkermes, Inc. D.L.M. is a consultant, has received grant funding, is the Chief Medical Officer, and has equity in Endevica Bio, Inc. The other authors declare no competing interests.

Abbreviations

AP-1	Activator Protein 1
ASC	Apoptosis-Associated Speck-Like Protein Containing CARD
C3a	Complement Component 3a
C3aR	C3a Receptor
C5a	Complement Component 5a
C5aR	C5a Receptor
CARPA	Complement-Activation-Related Pseudoallergy
CTL	Cytotoxic T Lymphocytes
DAMPs	Danger-Associated Molecular Patterns
dsRNA	Double-stranded RNA

ELISA	Enzyme-Linked Immunosorbent Assay
eLNP	Empty Lipid Nanoparticle
eIF2	Eukaryotic Initiation Factor 2
FDA	Food and Drug Administration
GFP	Green Fluorescent Protein
IFN	Interferon
IL	Interleukin
IL-1β	Interleukin 1 β
IL-1R	Interleukin-1 Receptor
IL-6	Interleukin 6
IRAKs	Interleukin-1-Receptor-Associated Kinases
IRF	Interferon Regulatory Factor
KO	Knock-Out
LNP	Lipid Nanoparticle
MAC	Membrane Attack Complex
MAPKs	Mitogen-Activated Protein Kinases
MC3	Dlin-MC3-DMA
MyD88	Myeloid Differentiation Primary Response 88
N/P ratio	Nitrogen-to-phosphate ratio
NLRP3	NOD-, LRR-, and Pyrin Domain-Containing Protein 3
NF-κB	Nuclear Factor-Kappa B
PAMP	Pathogen-Associated Molecular Pattern
PBMCs	Peripheral Blood Mononuclear Cells
PEG	Polyethylene Glycol
PKR	Protein Kinase R
RBC	Red Blood Cell
TAK1	Transforming Growth Factor-β-Activated Kinase 1
TBK1	TANK-Binding Kinase 1
TLR	Toll-Like Receptor
TLR4	Toll-Like Receptor 4
TRAF6	TNF-Receptor-Associated Factor 6
TRAM	Translocating Chain-Associating Membrane Protein
TRIF	TIR-Domain-Containing Adaptor-Inducing Interferon-β
WT	Wild-Type
WBC	White Blood Cell

References

1. Patra, J.K.; Das, G.; Fraceto, L.F.; Campos, E.V.R.; del Pilar Rodriguez-Torres, M.; Acosta-Torres, L.S.; Diaz-Torres, L.A.; Grillo, R.; Swamy, M.K.; Sharma, S.; et al. Nano Based Drug Delivery Systems: Recent Developments and Future Prospects. *J. Nanobiotechnol.* **2018**, *16*, 71. [CrossRef] [PubMed]
2. Pelaz, B.; Alexiou, C.; Alvarez-Puebla, R.A.; Alves, F.; Andrews, A.M.; Ashraf, S.; Balogh, L.P.; Ballerini, L.; Bestetti, A.; Brendel, C.; et al. Diverse Applications of Nanomedicine. *ACS Nano* **2017**, *11*, 2313–2381. [CrossRef] [PubMed]
3. Polack, F.P.; Thomas, S.J.; Kitchin, N.; Absalon, J.; Gurtman, A.; Lockhart, S.; Perez, J.L.; Pérez Marc, G.; Moreira, E.D.; Zerbini, C.; et al. Safety and Efficacy of the Bnt162b2 Mrna COVID-19 Vaccine. *N. Engl. J. Med.* **2020**, *383*, 2603–2615. [CrossRef] [PubMed]
4. Walsh, E.E.; Frenck, R.W., Jr.; Falsey, A.R.; Kitchin, N.; Absalon, J.; Gurtman, A.; Lockhart, S.; Neuzil, K.; Mulligan, M.J.; Bailey, R.; et al. Safety and Immunogenicity of Two Rna-Based COVID-19 Vaccine Candidates. *N. Engl. J. Med.* **2020**, *383*, 2439–2450. [CrossRef]
5. Verbeke, R.; Lentacker, I.; De Smedt, S.C.; Dewitte, H. Three Decades of Messenger Rna Vaccine Development. *Nano Today* **2019**, *28*, 100766. [CrossRef]
6. Baden, L.R.; El Sahly, H.M.; Essink, B.; Kotloff, K.; Frey, S.; Novak, R.; Diemert, D.; Spector, S.A.; Rouphael, N.; Creech, C.B.; et al. Efficacy and Safety of the Mrna-1273 SARS-CoV-2 Vaccine. *N. Engl. J. Med.* **2021**, *384*, 403–416. [CrossRef]
7. Sahin, U.; Muik, A.; Derhovanessian, E.; Vogler, I.; Kranz, L.M.; Vormehr, M.; Baum, A.; Pascal, K.; Quandt, J.; Maurus, D.; et al. COVID-19 Vaccine Bnt162b1 Elicits Human Antibody and T(H)1 T Cell Responses. *Nature* **2020**, *586*, 594–599. [CrossRef]
8. Sasso, J.M.; Ambrose, B.J.B.; Tenchov, R.; Datta, R.S.; Basel, M.T.; DeLong, R.K.; Zhou, Q.A. The Progress and Promise of RNA Medicine—An Arsenal of Targeted Treatments. *J. Med. Chem.* **2022**, *65*, 6975–7015. [CrossRef]
9. Jackson, L.A.; Anderson, E.J.; Rouphael, N.G.; Roberts, P.C.; Makhene, M.; Coler, R.N.; McCullough, M.P.; Chappell, J.D.; Denison, M.R.; Stevens, L.J.; et al. An Mrna Vaccine against SARS-CoV-2—Preliminary Report. *N. Engl. J. Med.* **2020**, *383*, 1920–1931. [CrossRef]

10. Matsumura, T.; Takano, T.; Takahashi, Y. Immune Responses Related to the Immunogenicity and Reactogenicity of COVID-19 Mrna Vaccines. *Int. Immunol.* **2022**, *35*, 213–220. [CrossRef]

11. Watad, A.; De Marco, G.; Mahajna, H.; Druyan, A.; Eltity, M.; Hijazi, N.; Haddad, A.; Elias, M.; Zisman, D.; Naffaa, M.E.; et al. Immune-Mediated Disease Flares or New-Onset Disease in 27 Subjects Following Mrna/DNA SARS-CoV-2 Vaccination. *Vaccines* **2021**, *9*, 435. [CrossRef]

12. Chen, Y.; Xu, Z.; Wang, P.; Li, X.; Shuai, Z.; Ye, D.; Pan, H. New-Onset Autoimmune Phenomena Post-COVID-19 Vaccination. *Immunology* **2022**, *165*, 386–401. [CrossRef]

13. Ouldali, N.; Bagheri, H.; Salvo, F.; Antona, D.; Pariente, A.; Leblanc, C.; Tebacher, M.; Micallef, J.; Levy, C.; Cohen, R.; et al. Hyper Inflammatory Syndrome Following COVID-19 Mrna Vaccine in Children: A National Post-Authorization Pharmacovigilance Study. *Lancet Reg. Health Eur.* **2022**, *17*, 100393. [CrossRef]

14. Hermann, E.A.; Lee, B.; Balte, P.P.; Xanthakis, V.; Kirkpatrick, B.D.; Cushman, M.; Oelsner, E. Association of Symptoms after COVID-19 Vaccination with Anti–SARS-CoV-2 Antibody Response in the Framingham Heart Study. *JAMA Netw. Open* **2022**, *5*, e2237908. [CrossRef]

15. Sprent, J.; King, C. COVID-19 Vaccine Side Effects: The Positives About Feeling Bad. *Sci. Immunol.* **2021**, *6*, eabj9256. [CrossRef]

16. Anderson, B.R.; Muramatsu, H.; Nallagatla, S.R.; Bevilacqua, P.C.; Sansing, L.H.; Weissman, D.; Karikó, K. Incorporation of Pseudouridine into Mrna Enhances Translation by Diminishing Pkr Activation. *Nucleic Acids Res.* **2010**, *38*, 5884–5892. [CrossRef]

17. Karikó, K.; Buckstein, M.; Ni, H.; Weissman, D. Suppression of Rna Recognition by Toll-Like Receptors: The Impact of Nucleoside Modification and the Evolutionary Origin of Rna. *Immunity* **2005**, *23*, 165–175. [CrossRef]

18. Karikó, K.; Ni, H.; Capodici, J.; Lamphier, M.; Weissman, D. mRNA Is an Endogenous Ligand for Toll-Like Receptor 3. *J. Biol. Chem.* **2004**, *279*, 12542–12550. [CrossRef]

19. Buschmann, M.D.; Carrasco, M.J.; Alishetty, S.; Paige, M.; Alameh, M.G.; Weissman, D. Nanomaterial Delivery Systems for Mrna Vaccines. *Vaccines* **2021**, *9*, 65. [CrossRef]

20. Ju, Y.; Carreño, J.M.; Simon, V.; Dawson, K.; Krammer, F.; Kent, S.J. Impact of Anti-Peg Antibodies Induced by SARS-CoV-2 Mrna Vaccines. *Nat. Rev. Immunol.* **2022**, *23*, 135–136. [CrossRef]

21. Hause, A.M.; Baggs, J.; Marquez, P.; Abara, W.E.; Baumblatt, J.; Blanc, P.G.; Su, J.R.; Hugueley, B.; Parker, C.; Myers, T.R.; et al. Safety Monitoring of COVID-19 Mrna Vaccine Second Booster Doses among Adults Aged ≥50 Years—United States, March 29, 2022–July 10, 2022. *MMWR* **2022**, *71*, 971. [CrossRef] [PubMed]

22. Mulligan, M.J.; Lyke, K.E.; Kitchin, N.; Absalon, J.; Gurtman, A.; Lockhart, S.; Neuzil, K.; Raabe, V.; Bailey, R.; Swanson, K.A.; et al. Phase I/II Study of COVID-19 RNA Vaccine Bnt162b1 in Adults. *Nature* **2020**, *586*, 589–593. [CrossRef] [PubMed]

23. Ndeupen, S.; Qin, Z.; Jacobsen, S.; Bouteau, A.; Estanbouli, H.; Igyártó, B.Z. The Mrna-Lnp Platform's Lipid Nanoparticle Component Used in Preclinical Vaccine Studies Is Highly Inflammatory. *iScience* **2021**, *24*, 103479. [CrossRef] [PubMed]

24. Cafri, G.; Gartner, J.J.; Zaks, T.; Hopson, K.; Levin, N.; Paria, B.C.; Parkhurst, M.R.; Yossef, R.; Lowery, F.J.; Jafferji, M.S.; et al. mRNA Vaccine-Induced Neoantigen-Specific T Cell Immunity in Patients with Gastrointestinal Cancer. *J. Clin. Investig.* **2020**, *130*, 5976–5988. [CrossRef] [PubMed]

25. Aldosari, B.N.; Alfagih, I.M.; Almurshedi, A.S. Lipid Nanoparticles as Delivery Systems for RNA-Based Vaccines. *Pharmaceutics* **2021**, *13*, 206. [CrossRef]

26. Samaridou, E.; Heyes, J.; Lutwyche, P. Lipid Nanoparticles for Nucleic Acid Delivery: Current Perspectives. *Adv. Drug Deliv. Rev.* **2020**, *154–155*, 37–63. [CrossRef]

27. Cheng, X.; Lee, R.J. The Role of Helper Lipids in Lipid Nanoparticles (Lnps) Designed for Oligonucleotide Delivery. *Adv. Drug Deliv. Rev.* **2016**, *99 Pt A*, 129–137. [CrossRef]

28. Patel, S.; Ashwanikumar, N.; Robinson, E.; Xia, Y.; Mihai, C.; Griffith, J.P.; Hou, S.; Esposito, A.A.; Ketova, T.; Welsher, K.; et al. Naturally-Occurring Cholesterol Analogues in Lipid Nanoparticles Induce Polymorphic Shape and Enhance Intracellular Delivery of Mrna. *Nat. Commun.* **2020**, *11*, 983. [CrossRef]

29. Holland, J.W.; Hui, C.; Cullis, P.R.; Madden, T.D. Poly(Ethylene Glycol)–Lipid Conjugates Regulate the Calcium-Induced Fusion of Liposomes Composed of Phosphatidylethanolamine and Phosphatidylserine. *Biochemistry* **1996**, *35*, 2618–2624. [CrossRef]

30. Kalyanram, P.; Puri, A.; Gupta, A. Thermotropic Effects of Pegylated Lipids on the Stability of Hpph-Encapsulated Lipid Nanoparticles (Lnp). *J. Therm. Anal. Calorim.* **2022**, *147*, 6337–6348. [CrossRef]

31. Judge, A.; McClintock, K.; Phelps, J.R.; MacLachlan, I. Hypersensitivity and Loss of Disease Site Targeting Caused by Antibody Responses to Pegylated Liposomes. *Mol. Ther.* **2006**, *13*, 328–337. [CrossRef]

32. Albertsen, C.H.; Kulkarni, J.A.; Witzigmann, D.; Lind, M.; Petersson, K.; Simonsen, J.B. The Role of Lipid Components in Lipid Nanoparticles for Vaccines and Gene Therapy. *Adv. Drug Deliv. Rev.* **2022**, *188*, 114416. [CrossRef]

33. Akinc, A.; Maier, M.A.; Manoharan, M.; Fitzgerald, K.; Jayaraman, M.; Barros, S.; Ansell, S.; Du, X.; Hope, M.J.; Madden, T.D.; et al. The Onpattro Story and the Clinical Translation of Nanomedicines Containing Nucleic Acid-Based Drugs. *Nat. Nanotechnol.* **2019**, *14*, 1084–1087. [CrossRef]

34. Suzuki, Y.; Ishihara, H. Difference in the Lipid Nanoparticle Technology Employed in Three Approved Sirna (Patisiran) and Mrna (COVID-19 Vaccine) Drugs. *Drug Metab. Pharmacokinet.* **2021**, *41*, 100424. [CrossRef]

35. Paloncýová, M.; Čechová, P.; Šrejber, M.; Kührová, P.; Otyepka, M. Role of Ionizable Lipids in SARS-CoV-2 Vaccines as Revealed by Molecular Dynamics Simulations: From Membrane Structure to Interaction with Mrna Fragments. *J. Phys. Chem. Lett.* **2021**, *12*, 11199–11205. [CrossRef]

36. Suzuki, T.; Suzuki, Y.; Hihara, T.; Kubara, K.; Kondo, K.; Hyodo, K.; Yamazaki, K.; Ishida, T.; Ishihara, H. Peg Shedding-Rate-Dependent Blood Clearance of Pegylated Lipid Nanoparticles in Mice: Faster Peg Shedding Attenuates Anti-Peg Igm Production. *Int. J. Pharm.* **2020**, *588*, 119792. [CrossRef]

37. McSweeney, M.D.; Shen, L.; DeWalle, A.C.; Joiner, J.B.; Ciociola, E.C.; Raghuwanshi, D.; Macauley, M.S.; Lai, S.K. Pre-Treatment with High Molecular Weight Free Peg Effectively Suppresses Anti-Peg Antibody Induction by Peg-Liposomes in Mice. *J. Control. Release* **2021**, *329*, 774–781. [CrossRef]

38. Chen, B.-M.; Cheng, T.-L.; Roffler, S.R. Polyethylene Glycol Immunogenicity: Theoretical, Clinical, and Practical Aspects of Anti-Polyethylene Glycol Antibodies. *ACS Nano* **2021**, *15*, 14022–14048. [CrossRef]

39. Lutz, J.; Lazzaro, S.; Habbeddine, M.; Schmidt, K.E.; Baumhof, P.; Mui, B.L.; Tam, Y.K.; Madden, T.D.; Hope, M.J.; Heidenreich, R.; et al. Unmodified mRNA in Lnps Constitutes a Competitive Technology for Prophylactic Vaccines. *NPJ Vaccines* **2017**, *2*, 29. [CrossRef]

40. Richner, J.M.; Himansu, S.; Dowd, K.A.; Butler, S.L.; Salazar, V.; Fox, J.M.; Julander, J.G.; Tang, W.W.; Shresta, S.; Pierson, T.C.; et al. Modified Mrna Vaccines Protect against Zika Virus Infection. *Cell* **2017**, *168*, 1114–1125.e10. [CrossRef]

41. Freyn, A.W.; da Silva, J.R.; Rosado, V.C.; Bliss, C.M.; Pine, M.; Mui, B.L.; Tam, Y.K.; Madden, T.D.; Ferreira, L.C.d.S.; Weissman, D.; et al. A Multi-Targeting, Nucleoside-Modified Mrna Influenza Virus Vaccine Provides Broad Protection in Mice. *Mol. Ther.* **2020**, *28*, 1569–1584. [CrossRef] [PubMed]

42. Corbett, K.S.; Flynn, B.; Foulds, K.E.; Francica, J.R.; Boyoglu-Barnum, S.; Werner, A.P.; Flach, B.; O'Connell, S.; Bock, K.W.; Minai, M.; et al. Evaluation of the Mrna-1273 Vaccine against SARS-CoV-2 in Nonhuman Primates. *N. Engl. J. Med.* **2020**, *383*, 1544–1555. [CrossRef] [PubMed]

43. Rauch, S.; Roth, N.; Schwendt, K.; Fotin-Mleczek, M.; Mueller, S.O.; Petsch, B. mRNA-Based SARS-CoV-2 Vaccine Candidate Cvncov Induces High Levels of Virus-Neutralising Antibodies and Mediates Protection in Rodents. *NPJ Vaccines* **2021**, *6*, 57. [CrossRef] [PubMed]

44. Kalnin, K.V.; Plitnik, T.; Kishko, M.; Zhang, J.; Zhang, D.; Beauvais, A.; Anosova, N.G.; Tibbitts, T.; DiNapoli, J.; Ulinski, G.; et al. Immunogenicity and Efficacy of Mrna COVID-19 Vaccine Mrt5500 in Preclinical Animal Models. *NPJ Vaccines* **2021**, *6*, 61. [CrossRef] [PubMed]

45. Li, S.; Hu, Y.; Li, A.; Lin, J.; Hsieh, K.; Schneiderman, Z.; Zhang, P.; Zhu, Y.; Qiu, C.; Kokkoli, E.; et al. Payload Distribution and Capacity of Mrna Lipid Nanoparticles. *Nat. Commun.* **2022**, *13*, 5561. [CrossRef]

46. Long, J.; Yu, C.; Zhang, H.; Cao, Y.; Sang, Y.; Lu, H.; Zhang, Z.; Wang, X.; Wang, H.; Song, G.; et al. Novel Ionizable Lipid Nanoparticles for SARS-CoV-2 Omicron Mrna Delivery. *Adv. Healthc. Mater.* **2023**, *12*, 2202590. [CrossRef]

47. Pardi, N.; Tuyishime, S.; Muramatsu, H.; Kariko, K.; Mui, B.L.; Tam, Y.K.; Madden, T.D.; Hope, M.J.; Weissman, D. Expression Kinetics of Nucleoside-Modified mRNA Delivered in Lipid Nanoparticles to Mice by Various Routes. *J. Control. Release* **2015**, *217*, 345–351. [CrossRef]

48. Liang, F.; Lindgren, G.; Lin, A.; Thompson, E.A.; Ols, S.; Röhss, J.; John, S.; Hassett, K.; Yuzhakov, O.; Bahl, K.; et al. Efficient Targeting and Activation of Antigen-Presenting Cells In vivo after Modified Mrna Vaccine Administration in Rhesus Macaques. *Mol. Ther.* **2017**, *25*, 2635–2647. [CrossRef]

49. Sedic, M.; Senn, J.J.; Lynn, A.; Laska, M.; Smith, M.; Platz, S.J.; Bolen, J.; Hoge, S.; Bulychev, A.; Jacquinet, E.; et al. Safety Evaluation of Lipid Nanoparticle-Formulated Modified Mrna in the Sprague-Dawley Rat and Cynomolgus Monkey. *Vet. Pathol.* **2018**, *55*, 341–354. [CrossRef]

50. Connors, J.; Joyner, D.; Mege, N.J.; Cusimano, G.M.; Bell, M.R.; Marcy, J.; Taramangalam, B.; Kim, K.M.; Lin, P.J.C.; Tam, Y.K.; et al. Lipid Nanoparticles (Lnp) Induce Activation and Maturation of Antigen Presenting Cells in Young and Aged Individuals. *Commun. Biol.* **2023**, *6*, 188. [CrossRef]

51. Maier, M.A.; Jayaraman, M.; Matsuda, S.; Liu, J.; Barros, S.; Querbes, W.; Tam, Y.K.; Ansell, S.M.; Kumar, V.; Qin, J.; et al. Biodegradable Lipids Enabling Rapidly Eliminated Lipid Nanoparticles for Systemic Delivery of Rnai Therapeutics. *Mol. Ther.* **2013**, *21*, 1570–1578. [CrossRef]

52. Alameh, M.-G.; Tombácz, I.; Bettini, E.; Lederer, K.; Ndeupen, S.; Sittplangkoon, C.; Wilmore, J.R.; Gaudette, B.T.; Soliman, O.Y.; Pine, M.; et al. Lipid Nanoparticles Enhance the Efficacy of Mrna and Protein Subunit Vaccines by Inducing Robust T Follicular Helper Cell and Humoral Responses. *Immunity* **2021**, *54*, 2877–2892.e7. [CrossRef]

53. Tahtinen, S.; Tong, A.-J.; Himmels, P.; Oh, J.; Paler-Martinez, A.; Kim, L.; Wichner, S.; Oei, Y.; McCarron, M.J.; Freund, E.C.; et al. Il-1 and Il-1ra Are Key Regulators of the Inflammatory Response to Rna Vaccines. *Nat. Immunol.* **2022**, *23*, 532–542. [CrossRef]

54. Qin, Z.; Bouteau, A.; Herbst, C.; Igyártó, B.Z. Pre-Exposure to Mrna-Lnp Inhibits Adaptive Immune Responses and Alters Innate Immune Fitness in an Inheritable Fashion. *PLoS Pathog.* **2022**, *18*, e1010830. [CrossRef]

55. Pardi, N.; Hogan, M.J.; Naradikian, M.S.; Parkhouse, K.; Cain, D.W.; Jones, L.; Moody, M.A.; Verkerke, H.P.; Myles, A.; Willis, E.; et al. Nucleoside-Modified Mrna Vaccines Induce Potent T Follicular Helper and Germinal Center B Cell Responses. *J. Exp. Med.* **2018**, *215*, 1571–1588. [CrossRef]

56. Parhiz, H.; Brenner, J.S.; Patel, P.N.; Papp, T.E.; Shahnawaz, H.; Li, Q.; Shi, R.; Zamora, M.E.; Yadegari, A.; Marcos-Contreras, O.A.; et al. Added to Pre-Existing Inflammation, Mrna-Lipid Nanoparticles Induce Inflammation Exacerbation (Ie). *J. Control. Release* **2022**, *344*, 50–61. [CrossRef]

57. Bradley, A.J.; Brooks, D.E.; Norris-Jones, R.; Devine, D.V. C1q Binding to Liposomes Is Surface Charge Dependent and Is Inhibited by Peptides Consisting of Residues 14-26 of the Human C1qa Chain in a Sequence Independent Manner. *Biochim. Biophys. Acta* **1999**, *1418*, 19–30. [CrossRef]

58. Moghimi, S.M.; Hamad, I. Liposome-Mediated Triggering of Complement Cascade. *J. Liposome Res.* **2008**, *18*, 195–209. [CrossRef]
59. Szebeni, J.; Baranyi, L.; Savay, S.; Milosevits, J.; Bodo, M.; Bunger, R.; Alving, C.R. The Interaction of Liposomes with the Complement System: In Vitro and in Vivo Assays. *Methods Enzymol.* **2003**, *373*, 136–154. [CrossRef]
60. Szebeni, J.; Wassef, N.; Hartman, K.; Rudolph, A.; Alving, C. Complement Activation in Vitro by the Red Cell Substitute, Liposome-Encapsulated Hemoglobin: Mechanism of Activation and Inhibition by Soluble Complement Receptor Type 1. *Transfusion* **1997**, *37*, 150–159. [CrossRef]
61. Neun, B.W.; Ilinskaya, A.N.; Dobrovolskaia, M.A. Analysis of Complement Activation by Nanoparticles. *Methods Mol. Biol.* **2018**, *1682*, 149–160. [CrossRef] [PubMed]
62. Pannuzzo, M.; Esposito, S.; Wu, L.-P.; Key, J.; Aryal, S.; Celia, C.; Di Marzio, L.; Moghimi, S.M.; Decuzzi, P. Overcoming Nanoparticle-Mediated Complement Activation by Surface Peg Pairing. *Nano Lett.* **2020**, *20*, 4312–4321. [CrossRef] [PubMed]
63. Alving, C.R.; Swartz, G.M., Jr. Antibodies to Cholesterol, Cholesterol Conjugates and Liposomes: Implications for Atherosclerosis and Autoimmunity. *Crit. Rev. Immunol.* **1991**, *10*, 441–453. [PubMed]
64. Alving, C.R.; Kinsky, S.C.; Haxby, J.A.; Kinsky, C.B. Antibody Binding and Complement Fixation by a Liposomal Model Membrane. *Biochemistry* **1969**, *8*, 1582–1587. [CrossRef] [PubMed]
65. La-Beck, N.M.; Islam, R.; Markiewski, M.M. Nanoparticle-Induced Complement Activation: Implications for Cancer Nanomedicine. *Front. Immunol.* **2020**, *11*, 603039. [CrossRef]
66. Longmire, M.; Choyke, P.L.; Kobayashi, H.; El-Boubbou, K.; Tang, X.; Loc, W.S.; Dong, C.; Matters, G.L.; Butler, P.J.; Kester, M.; et al. Clearance Properties of Nano-Sized Particles and Molecules as Imaging Agents: Considerations and Caveats. *Nanomedicine* **2008**, *3*, 703–717. [CrossRef]
67. Sturgill, M.G.; Lambert, G.H. Xenobiotic-Induced Hepatotoxicity: Mechanisms of Liver Injury and Methods of Monitoring Hepatic Function. *Clin. Chem.* **1997**, *43*, 1512–1526. [CrossRef]
68. Werner, M.; Costa, M.J.; Mitchell, L.G.; Nayar, R. Nephrotoxicity of Xenobiotics. *Clin. Chim. Acta* **1995**, *237*, 107–154. [CrossRef]
69. Shi, C.; Pamer, E.G. Monocyte Recruitment during Infection and Inflammation. *Nat. Rev. Immunol.* **2011**, *11*, 762–774. [CrossRef]
70. Kolaczkowska, E.; Kubes, P. Neutrophil Recruitment and Function in Health and Inflammation. *Nat. Rev. Immunol.* **2013**, *13*, 159–175. [CrossRef]
71. Beyrau, M.; Bodkin, J.V.; Nourshargh, S. Neutrophil Heterogeneity in Health and Disease: A Revitalized Avenue in Inflammation and Immunity. *Open Biol.* **2012**, *2*, 120134. [CrossRef]
72. Eash, K.J.; Greenbaum, A.M.; Gopalan, P.K.; Link, D.C. Cxcr2 and Cxcr4 Antagonistically Regulate Neutrophil Trafficking from Murine Bone Marrow. *J. Clin. Investig.* **2010**, *120*, 2423–2431. [CrossRef]
73. Summers, C.; Rankin, S.M.; Condliffe, A.M.; Singh, N.; Peters, A.M.; Chilvers, E.R. Neutrophil Kinetics in Health and Disease. *Trends Immunol.* **2010**, *31*, 318–324. [CrossRef]
74. Köhler, A.; De Filippo, K.; Hasenberg, M.; van den Brandt, C.; Nye, E.; Hosking, M.P.; Lane, T.E.; Männ, L.; Ransohoff, R.M.; Hauser, A.E.; et al. G-Csf-Mediated Thrombopoietin Release Triggers Neutrophil Motility and Mobilization from Bone Marrow via Induction of Cxcr2 Ligands. *Blood* **2011**, *117*, 4349–4357. [CrossRef]
75. Hwang, T.-L.; Hsu, C.-Y.; Aljuffali, I.A.; Chen, C.-H.; Chang, Y.-T.; Fang, J.-Y. Cationic Liposomes Evoke Proinflammatory Mediator Release and Neutrophil Extracellular Traps (Nets) toward Human Neutrophils. *Colloids Surf. B Biointerfaces* **2015**, *128*, 119–126. [CrossRef]
76. Hwang, T.-L.; Aljuffali, I.A.; Hung, C.-F.; Chen, C.-H.; Fang, J.-Y. The Impact of Cationic Solid Lipid Nanoparticles on Human Neutrophil Activation and Formation of Neutrophil Extracellular Traps (Nets). *Chem. Biol. Interact.* **2015**, *235*, 106–114. [CrossRef]
77. Lin, M.-H.; Lin, C.-F.; Yang, S.-C.; Hung, C.-F.; Fang, J.-Y. The Interplay between Nanoparticles and Neutrophils. *J. Biomed. Nanotechnol.* **2018**, *14*, 66–85. [CrossRef]
78. Liu, Y.; Cao, Z.-T.; Xu, C.-F.; Lu, Z.-D.; Luo, Y.-L.; Wang, J. Optimization of Lipid-Assisted Nanoparticle for Disturbing Neutrophils-Related Inflammation. *Biomaterials* **2018**, *172*, 92–104. [CrossRef]
79. Wynn, T.A.; Chawla, A.; Pollard, J.W. Macrophage Biology in Development, Homeostasis and Disease. *Nature* **2013**, *496*, 445–455. [CrossRef]
80. Serbina, N.V.; Jia, T.; Hohl, T.M.; Pamer, E.G. Monocyte-Mediated Defense against Microbial Pathogens. *Annu. Rev. Immunol.* **2008**, *26*, 421–452. [CrossRef]
81. Hughes, C.E.; Nibbs, R.J.B. A Guide to Chemokines and Their Receptors. *FEBS J.* **2018**, *285*, 2944–2971. [CrossRef] [PubMed]
82. Gustafson, H.H.; Holt-Casper, D.; Grainger, D.W.; Ghandehari, H. Nanoparticle Uptake: The Phagocyte Problem. *Nano Today* **2015**, *10*, 487–510. [CrossRef] [PubMed]
83. Owens, D.E., III; Peppas, N.A. Opsonization, Biodistribution, and Pharmacokinetics of Polymeric Nanoparticles. *Int. J. Pharm.* **2006**, *307*, 93–102. [CrossRef] [PubMed]
84. Ohno, K.; Akashi, T.; Tsujii, Y.; Yamamoto, M.; Tabata, Y. Blood Clearance and Biodistribution of Polymer Brush-Afforded Silica Particles Prepared by Surface-Initiated Living Radical Polymerization. *Biomacromolecules* **2012**, *13*, 927–936. [CrossRef]
85. Cai, D.; Gao, W.; Li, Z.; Zhang, Y.; Xiao, L.; Xiao, Y. Current Development of Nano-Drug Delivery to Target Macrophages. *Biomedicines* **2022**, *10*, 1203. [CrossRef]
86. Lonez, C.; Bessodes, M.; Scherman, D.; Vandenbranden, M.; Escriou, V.; Ruysschaert, J.-M. Cationic Lipid Nanocarriers Activate Toll-Like Receptor 2 and Nlrp3 Inflammasome Pathways. *Nanomedicine* **2014**, *10*, 775–782. [CrossRef]
87. O'Neill, L.A.J.; Bowie, A.G. The Family of Five: Tir-Domain-Containing Adaptors in Toll-Like Receptor Signalling. *Nat. Rev. Immunol.* **2007**, *7*, 353–364. [CrossRef]

88. Murphy, J.E.; Padilla, B.E.; Hasdemir, B.; Cottrell, G.S.; Bunnett, N.W. Endosomes: A Legitimate Platform for the Signaling Train. *Proc. Natl. Acad. Sci. USA* **2009**, *106*, 17615–17622. [CrossRef]

89. Yamamoto, M.; Sato, S.; Hemmi, H.; Hoshino, K.; Kaisho, T.; Sanjo, H.; Takeuchi, O.; Sugiyama, M.; Okabe, M.; Takeda, K.; et al. Role of Adaptor Trif in the Myd88-Independent Toll-Like Receptor Signaling Pathway. *Science* **2003**, *301*, 640–643. [CrossRef]

90. Huotari, J.; Helenius, A. Endosome Maturation. *EMBO J.* **2011**, *30*, 3481–3500. [CrossRef]

91. Patel, S.; Kim, J.; Herrera, M.; Mukherjee, A.; Kabanov, A.V.; Sahay, G. Brief Update on Endocytosis of Nanomedicines. *Adv. Drug Deliv. Rev.* **2019**, *144*, 90–111. [CrossRef]

92. Herrera, M.; Kim, J.; Eygeris, Y.; Jozic, A.; Sahay, G. Illuminating Endosomal Escape of Polymorphic Lipid Nanoparticles That Boost Mrna Delivery. *Biomater. Sci.* **2021**, *9*, 4289–4300. [CrossRef]

93. Hui, S.; Langner, M.; Zhao, Y.; Ross, P.; Hurley, E.; Chan, K. The Role of Helper Lipids in Cationic Liposome-Mediated Gene Transfer. *Biophys. J.* **1996**, *71*, 590–599. [CrossRef]

94. Tregoning, J.S.; Stirling, D.C.; Wang, Z.; Flight, K.E.; Brown, J.C.; Blakney, A.K.; McKay, P.F.; Cunliffe, R.F.; Murugaiah, V.; Fox, C.B.; et al. Formulation, Inflammation, and Rna Sensing Impact the Immunogenicity of Self-Amplifying Rna Vaccines. *Mol. Ther. Nucleic Acids* **2023**, *31*, 29–42. [CrossRef]

95. Chattopadhyay, S.; Sen, G.C. dsRNA-activation of TLR3 and RLR signaling: Gene induction-dependent and independent effects. *J. Interferon Cytokine Res.* **2014**, *34*, 427–436. [CrossRef]

96. Merle, N.S.; Noe, R.; Halbwachs-Mecarelli, L.; Fremeaux-Bacchi, V.; Roumenina, L.T. Complement System Part II: Role in Immunity. *Front. Immunol.* **2015**, *6*, 257. [CrossRef]

97. Noris, M.; Remuzzi, G. Overview of Complement Activation and Regulation. *Semin. Nephrol.* **2013**, *33*, 479–492. [CrossRef]

98. Szebeni, J.; Muggia, F.; Gabizon, A.; Barenholz, Y. Activation of Complement by Therapeutic Liposomes and Other Lipid Excipient-Based Therapeutic Products: Prediction and Prevention. *Adv. Drug Deliv. Rev.* **2011**, *63*, 1020–1030. [CrossRef]

99. Aksamit, R.R.; Falk, W.; Leonard, E.J. Chemotaxis by Mouse Macrophage Cell Lines. *J. Immunol.* **1981**, *126*, 2194–2199. [CrossRef]

100. Lett-Brown, M.A.; Leonard, E.J. Histamine-Induced Inhibition of Normal Human Basophil Chemotaxis to C5a. *J. Immunol.* **1977**, *118*, 815–818. [CrossRef]

101. Peng, Q.; Li, K.; Patel, H.; Sacks, S.H.; Zhou, W. Dendritic Cell Synthesis of C3 Is Required for Full T Cell Activation and Development of a Th1 Phenotype. *J. Immunol.* **2006**, *176*, 3330–3341. [CrossRef] [PubMed]

102. Ehrengruber, M.U.; Geiser, T.; Deranleau, D.A. Activation of Human Neutrophils by C3a and C5a. Comparison of the Effects on Shape Changes, Chemotaxis, Secretion, and Respiratory Burst. *FEBS Lett.* **1994**, *346*, 181–184. [CrossRef] [PubMed]

103. Lalli, P.N.; Strainic, M.G.; Lin, F.; Medof, M.E.; Heeger, P.S. Decay Accelerating Factor Can Control T Cell Differentiation into Ifn-Gamma-Producing Effector Cells via Regulating Local C5a-Induced Il-12 Production. *J. Immunol.* **2007**, *179*, 5793–5802. [CrossRef] [PubMed]

104. Markiewski, M.M.; DeAngelis, R.A.; Benencia, F.; Ricklin-Lichtsteiner, S.K.; Koutoulaki, A.; Gerard, C.; Coukos, G.; Lambris, J.D. Modulation of the Antitumor Immune Response by Complement. *Nat. Immunol.* **2008**, *9*, 1225–1235. [CrossRef] [PubMed]

105. Hartmann, K.; Henz, B.M.; Krüger-Krasagakes, S.; Köhl, J.; Burger, R.; Guhl, S.; Haase, I.; Lippert, U.; Zuberbier, T. C3a and C5a Stimulate Chemotaxis of Human Mast Cells. *Blood* **1997**, *89*, 2863–2870. [CrossRef]

106. Asgari, E.; Le Friec, G.; Yamamoto, H.; Perucha, E.; Sacks, S.S.; Köhl, J.; Cook, H.T.; Kemper, C. C3a Modulates Il-1β Secretion in Human Monocytes by Regulating Atp Efflux and Subsequent Nlrp3 Inflammasome Activation. *Blood* **2013**, *122*, 3473–3481. [CrossRef]

107. Takabayashi, T.; Vannier, E.; Clark, B.D.; Margolis, N.H.; Dinarello, C.A.; Burke, J.F.; Gelfand, J.A. A New Biologic Role for C3a and C3a Desarg: Regulation of Tnf-Alpha and Il-1 Beta Synthesis. *J. Immunol.* **1996**, *156*, 3455–3460. [CrossRef]

108. Kumar, S.; Basu, M.; Ghosh, P.; Ansari, A.; Ghosh, M.K. COVID-19: Clinical Status of Vaccine Development to Date. *Br. J. Clin. Pharmacol.* **2023**, *89*, 114–149. [CrossRef]

109. Hervé, C.; Laupeze, B.; Del Giudice, G.; Didierlaurent, A.M.; Da Silva, F.T. The How's and What's of Vaccine Reactogenicity. *NPJ Vaccines* **2019**, *4*, 39. [CrossRef]

110. Hayden, M.S.; West, A.P.; Ghosh, S. Nf-Kappab and the Immune Response. *Oncogene* **2006**, *25*, 6758–6780. [CrossRef]

111. Negishi, H.; Taniguchi, T.; Yanai, H. The Interferon (Ifn) Class of Cytokines and the Ifn Regulatory Factor (Irf) Transcription Factor Family. *Cold Spring Harb. Perspect. Biol.* **2018**, *10*, a028423. [CrossRef]

112. Tanaka, T.; Legat, A.; Adam, E.; Steuve, J.; Gatot, J.-S.; Vandenbranden, M.; Ulianov, L.; Lonez, C.; Ruysschaert, J.-M.; Muraille, E.; et al. Dic14-Amidine Cationic Liposomes Stimulate Myeloid Dendritic Cells through Toll-Like Receptor 4. *Eur. J. Immunol.* **2008**, *38*, 1351–1357. [CrossRef]

113. Verbeke, R.; Hogan, M.J.; Loré, K.; Pardi, N. Innate Immune Mechanisms of Mrna Vaccines. *Immunity* **2022**, *55*, 1993–2005. [CrossRef]

114. Kawai, T.; Akira, S. Signaling to Nf-Kappab by Toll-Like Receptors. *Trends Mol. Med.* **2007**, *13*, 460–469. [CrossRef]

115. Medzhitov, R.; Preston-Hurlburt, P.; Kopp, E.; Stadlen, A.; Chen, C.; Ghosh, S.; Janeway, C.A., Jr. Myd88 Is an Adaptor Protein in the Htoll/Il-1 Receptor Family Signaling Pathways. *Mol. Cell* **1998**, *2*, 253–258. [CrossRef]

116. Kelley, N.; Jeltema, D.; Duan, Y.; He, Y. The Nlrp3 Inflammasome: An Overview of Mechanisms of Activation and Regulation. *Int. J. Mol. Sci.* **2019**, *20*, 3328. [CrossRef]

117. Frenois, F.; Moreau, M.; O'connor, J.; Lawson, M.; Micon, C.; Lestage, J.; Kelley, K.W.; Dantzer, R.; Castanon, N. Lipopolysaccharide Induces Delayed Fosb/Deltafosb Immunostaining within the Mouse Extended Amygdala, Hippocampus and Hypothalamus, That Parallel the Expression of Depressive-Like Behavior. *Psychoneuroendocrinology* **2007**, *32*, 516–531. [CrossRef]
118. Burfeind, K.G.; Michaelis, K.A.; Marks, D.L. The Central Role of Hypothalamic Inflammation in the Acute Illness Response and Cachexia. *Semin. Cell Dev. Biol.* **2016**, *54*, 42–52. [CrossRef]
119. Engström, L.; Ruud, J.; Eskilsson, A.; Larsson, A.; Mackerlova, L.; Kugelberg, U.; Qian, H.; Vasilache, A.M.; Larsson, P.; Engblom, D.; et al. Lipopolysaccharide-Induced Fever Depends on Prostaglandin E2 Production Specifically in Brain Endothelial Cells. *Endocrinology* **2012**, *153*, 4849–4861. [CrossRef]
120. Timper, K.; Denson, J.L.; Steculorum, S.M.; Heilinger, C.; Engström-Ruud, L.; Wunderlich, C.M.; Rose-John, S.; Wunderlich, F.T.; Brüning, J.C. Il-6 Improves Energy and Glucose Homeostasis in Obesity via Enhanced Central Il-6 Trans-Signaling. *Cell Rep.* **2017**, *19*, 267–280. [CrossRef]
121. Wallenius, K.; Wallenius, V.; Sunter, D.; Dickson, S.L.; Jansson, J.-O. Intracerebroventricular Interleukin-6 Treatment Decreases Body Fat in Rats. *Biochem. Biophys. Res. Commun.* **2002**, *293*, 560–565. [CrossRef] [PubMed]
122. Petruzzelli, M.; Schweiger, M.; Schreiber, R.; Campos-Olivas, R.; Tsoli, M.; Allen, J.; Swarbrick, M.; Rose-John, S.; Rincon, M.; Robertson, G.; et al. A Switch from White to Brown Fat Increases Energy Expenditure in Cancer-Associated Cachexia. *Cell Metab.* **2014**, *20*, 433–447. [CrossRef] [PubMed]
123. Wallenius, V.; Wallenius, K.; Ahrén, B.; Rudling, M.; Carlsten, H.; Dickson, S.L.; Ohlsson, C.; Jansson, J.-O. Interleukin-6-Deficient Mice Develop Mature-Onset Obesity. *Nat. Med.* **2002**, *8*, 75–79. [CrossRef] [PubMed]
124. Nov, O.; Shapiro, H.; Ovadia, H.; Tarnovscki, T.; Dvir, I.; Shemesh, E.; Kovsan, J.; Shelef, I.; Carmi, Y.; Voronov, E.; et al. Interleukin-1β Regulates Fat-Liver Crosstalk in Obesity by Auto-Paracrine Modulation of Adipose Tissue Inflammation and Expandability. *PLoS ONE* **2013**, *8*, e53626. [CrossRef]
125. Konsman, J.P.; Parnet, P.; Dantzer, R. Cytokine-Induced Sickness Behaviour: Mechanisms and Implications. *Trends Neurosci.* **2002**, *25*, 154–159. [CrossRef]
126. Tanaka, T.; Narazaki, M.; Kishimoto, T. Il-6 in Inflammation, Immunity, and Disease. *Cold Spring Harb. Perspect. Biol.* **2014**, *6*, a016295. [CrossRef]
127. Han, M.S.; White, A.; Perry, R.J.; Camporez, J.-P.; Hidalgo, J.; Shulman, G.I.; Davis, R.J. Regulation of Adipose Tissue Inflammation by Interleukin 6. *Proc. Natl. Acad. Sci. USA* **2020**, *117*, 2751–2760. [CrossRef]
128. Kistner, T.M.; Pedersen, B.K.; Lieberman, D.E. Interleukin 6 as an Energy Allocator in Muscle Tissue. *Nat. Metab.* **2022**, *4*, 170–179. [CrossRef]
129. Mohamed-Ali, V.; Goodrick, S.; Rawesh, A.; Katz, D.R.; Miles, J.M.; Yudkin, J.S.; Klein, S.; Coppack, S.W. Subcutaneous Adipose Tissue Releases Interleukin-6, but Not Tumor Necrosis Factor-A, in Vivo. *J. Clin. Endocrinol. Metab.* **1997**, *82*, 4196–4200. [CrossRef]
130. López-Ferreras, L.; Longo, F.; Richard, J.E.; Eerola, K.; Shevchouk, O.T.; Tuzinovic, M.; Skibicka, K.P. Key Role for Hypothalamic Interleukin-6 in Food-Motivated Behavior and Body Weight Regulation. *Psychoneuroendocrinology* **2021**, *131*, 105284. [CrossRef]
131. A Dinarello, C. Biologic Basis for Interleukin-1 in Disease. *Blood* **1996**, *87*, 2095–2147. [CrossRef]
132. Ren, K.; Torres, R. Role of Interleukin-1beta during Pain and Inflammation. *Brain Res. Rev.* **2009**, *60*, 57–64. [CrossRef]
133. Ahima, R.S.; Antwi, D.A. Brain Regulation of Appetite and Satiety. *Endocrinol. Metab. Clin. N. Am.* **2008**, *37*, 811–823. [CrossRef]
134. Katahira, M.; Iwasaki, Y.; Aoki, Y.; Oiso, Y.; Saito, H. Cytokine Regulation of the Rat Proopiomelanocortin Gene Expression in Att-20 Cells. *Endocrinology* **1998**, *139*, 2414–2422. [CrossRef]
135. Pereda, M.P.; Lohrer, P.; Kovalovsky, D.; Castro, C.P.; Goldberg, V.; Losa, M.; Chervín, A.; Berner, S.; Molina, H.; Stalla, G.K.; et al. Interleukin-6 Is Inhibited by Glucocorticoids and Stimulates Acth Secretion and Pomc Expression in Human Corticotroph Pituitary Adenomas. *Exp. Clin. Endocrinol. Diabetes* **2000**, *108*, 202–207. [CrossRef]
136. Laddha, N.C.; Dwivedi, M.; Mansuri, M.S.; Singh, M.; Patel, H.H.; Agarwal, N.; Shah, A.M.; Begum, R. Association of Neuropeptide Y (Npy), Interleukin-1b (Il1b) Genetic Variants and Correlation of Il1b Transcript Levels with Vitiligo Susceptibility. *PLoS ONE* **2014**, *9*, e107020. [CrossRef]
137. Braun, T.P.; Zhu, X.; Szumowski, M.; Scott, G.D.; Grossberg, A.J.; Levasseur, P.R.; Graham, K.; Khan, S.; Damaraju, S.; Colmers, W.F.; et al. Central Nervous System Inflammation Induces Muscle Atrophy via Activation of the Hypothalamic–Pituitary–Adrenal Axis. *J. Exp. Med.* **2011**, *208*, 2449–2463. [CrossRef]
138. Kumar, V. Toll-Like Receptors in Sepsis-Associated Cytokine Storm and Their Endogenous Negative Regulators as Future Immunomodulatory Targets. *Int. Immunopharmacol.* **2020**, *89 Pt B*, 107087. [CrossRef]
139. Yang, T.; Yang, Y.; Wang, D.; Li, C.; Qu, Y.; Guo, J.; Shi, T.; Bo, W.; Sun, Z.; Asakawa, T. The Clinical Value of Cytokines in Chronic Fatigue Syndrome. *J. Transl. Med.* **2019**, *17*, 213. [CrossRef]
140. Trask, P.C.; Paterson, A.G.; Esper, P.; Pau, J.; Redman, B. Longitudinal Course of Depression, Fatigue, and Quality of Life in Patients with High Risk Melanoma Receiving Adjuvant Interferon. *Psycho-Oncology* **2004**, *13*, 526–536. [CrossRef]
141. Kirkwood, J.M.; Bender, C.; Agarwala, S.; Tarhini, A.; Shipe-Spotloe, J.; Smelko, B.; Donnelly, S.; Stover, L.; Goh, B.-C.; Lee, S.-C.; et al. Mechanisms and Management of Toxicities Associated with High-Dose Interferon Alfa-2b Therapy. *Clin. Oncol.* **2002**, *20*, 3703–3718. [CrossRef] [PubMed]
142. Malik, U.R.; Makower, D.F.; Wadler, S. Interferon-Mediated Fatigue. *CA Cancer J. Clin.* **2001**, *92*, 1664–1668. [CrossRef]

143. Russell, A.; Hepgul, N.; Nikkheslat, N.; Borsini, A.; Zajkowska, Z.; Moll, N.; Forton, D.; Agarwal, K.; Chalder, T.; Mondelli, V.; et al. Persistent Fatigue Induced by Interferon-Alpha: A Novel, Inflammation-Based, Proxy Model of Chronic Fatigue Syndrome. *Psychoneuroendocrinology* **2019**, *100*, 276–285. [CrossRef] [PubMed]

144. Rönnblom, L.; Leonard, D. Interferon Pathway in Sle: One Key to Unlocking the Mystery of the Disease. *Lupus Sci. Med.* **2019**, *6*, e000270. [CrossRef]

145. Dighriri, I.M.; Alhusayni, K.M.; Mobarki, A.Y.; Aljerary, I.S.; Alqurashi, K.A.; Aljuaid, F.A.; Alamri, K.A.; Mutwalli, A.A.; Maashi, N.A.; Aljohani, A.M.; et al. Pfizer-Biontech COVID-19 Vaccine (Bnt162b2) Side Effects: A Systematic Review. *Cureus* **2022**, *14*, e23526. [CrossRef]

146. Rabail, R.; Ahmed, W.; Ilyas, M.; Rajoka, M.S.R.; Hassoun, A.; Khalid, A.R.; Khan, M.R.; Aadil, R.M. The Side Effects and Adverse Clinical Cases Reported after COVID-19 Immunization. *Vaccines* **2022**, *10*, 488. [CrossRef]

147. Teijaro, J.R.; Farber, D.L. COVID-19 Vaccines: Modes of Immune Activation and Future Challenges. *Nat. Rev. Immunol.* **2021**, *21*, 195–197. [CrossRef]

148. Dalpke, A.H.; Helm, M. RNA Mediated Toll-Like Receptor Stimulation in Health and Disease. *RNA Biol.* **2012**, *9*, 828–842. [CrossRef]

149. Ning, S.; Pagano, J.S.; Barber, G.N. Irf7: Activation, Regulation, Modification and Function. *Genes Immun.* **2011**, *12*, 399–414. [CrossRef]

150. Ivashkiv, L.B. Ifnγ: Signalling, Epigenetics and Roles in Immunity, Metabolism, Disease and Cancer Immunotherapy. *Nat. Rev. Immunol.* **2018**, *18*, 545–558. [CrossRef]

151. Delehedde, C.; Even, L.; Midoux, P.; Pichon, C.; Perche, F. Intracellular Routing and Recognition of Lipid-Based Mrna Nanoparticles. *Pharmaceutics* **2021**, *13*, 945. [CrossRef]

152. Lokugamage, M.P.; Gan, Z.; Zurla, C.; Levin, J.; Islam, F.Z.; Kalathoor, S.; Sato, M.; Sago, C.D.; Santangelo, P.J.; Dahlman, J.E. Mild Innate Immune Activation Overrides Efficient Nanoparticle-Mediated Rna Delivery. *Adv. Mater.* **2020**, *32*, e1904905. [CrossRef]

153. Duan, L.-J.; Wang, Q.; Zhang, C.; Yang, D.-X.; Zhang, X.-Y. Potentialities and Challenges of Mrna Vaccine in Cancer Immunotherapy. *Front. Immunol.* **2022**, *13*, 923647. [CrossRef]

154. Barbier, A.J.; Jiang, A.Y.; Zhang, P.; Wooster, R.; Anderson, D.G. The Clinical Progress of Mrna Vaccines and Immunotherapies. *Nat. Biotechnol.* **2022**, *40*, 840–854. [CrossRef]

155. García, M.A.; Gil, J.; Ventoso, I.; Guerra, S.; Domingo, E.; Rivas, C.; Esteban, M. Impact of Protein Kinase Pkr in Cell Biology: From Antiviral to Antiproliferative Action. *Microbiol. Mol. Biol. Rev.* **2006**, *70*, 1032–1060. [CrossRef]

156. Goh, K.C.; Deveer, M.J.; Williams, B.R. The Protein Kinase Pkr Is Required for P38 Mapk Activation and the Innate Immune Response to Bacterial Endotoxin. *EMBO J.* **2000**, *19*, 4292–4297. [CrossRef]

157. Ito, T.; Yang, M.; May, W.S. Rax, a Cellular Activator for Double-Stranded RNA-Dependent Protein Kinase during Stress Signaling. *J. Biol. Chem.* **1999**, *274*, 15427–15432. [CrossRef]

158. Nakamura, T.; Furuhashi, M.; Li, P.; Cao, H.; Tuncman, G.; Sonenberg, N.; Gorgun, C.Z.; Hotamisligil, G.S. Double-Stranded RNA-Dependent Protein Kinase Links Pathogen Sensing with Stress and Metabolic Homeostasis. *Cell* **2010**, *140*, 338–348. [CrossRef]

159. Liu, Y.; Wang, M.; Cheng, A.; Yang, Q.; Wu, Y.; Jia, R.; Liu, M.; Zhu, D.; Chen, S.; Zhang, S.; et al. The Role of Host Eif2α in Viral Infection. *Virol. J.* **2020**, *17*, 112. [CrossRef]

160. Jiang, H.-Y.; Wek, S.A.; McGrath, B.C.; Scheuner, D.; Kaufman, R.J.; Cavener, D.R.; Wek, R.C.; Rademakers, S.; Volker, M.; Hoogstraten, D.; et al. Phosphorylation of the Alpha Subunit of Eukaryotic Initiation Factor 2 Is Required for Activation of Nf-Kappab in Response to Diverse Cellular Stresses. *Mol. Cell. Biol.* **2003**, *23*, 5651–5663. [CrossRef]

161. Burke, J.M.; Moon, S.L.; Matheny, T.; Parker, R. Rnase L Reprograms Translation by Widespread Mrna Turnover Escaped by Antiviral Mrnas. *Mol. Cell* **2019**, *75*, 1203–1217.e5. [CrossRef] [PubMed]

162. Gusho, E.; Baskar, D.; Banerjee, S. New Advances in Our Understanding of the "Unique" Rnase L in Host Pathogen Interaction and Immune Signaling. *Cytokine* **2020**, *133*, 153847. [CrossRef] [PubMed]

163. Burke, J.M.; Ripin, N.; Ferretti, M.B.; Clair, L.A.S.; Worden-Sapper, E.R.; Salgado, F.; Sawyer, S.L.; Perera, R.; Lynch, K.W.; Parker, R. Rnase L Activation in the Cytoplasm Induces Aberrant Processing of Mrnas in the Nucleus. *PLoS Pathog.* **2022**, *18*, e1010930. [CrossRef] [PubMed]

164. Green, D.R.; Ferguson, T.; Zitvogel, L.; Kroemer, G. Immunogenic and Tolerogenic Cell Death. *Nat. Rev. Immunol.* **2009**, *9*, 353–363. [CrossRef]

165. Dunkelberger, J.R.; Song, W.-C. Complement and Its Role in Innate and Adaptive Immune Responses. *Cell Res.* **2010**, *20*, 34–50. [CrossRef]

166. Szebeni, J. Complement Activation-Related Pseudoallergy: A New Class of Drug-Induced Acute Immune Toxicity. *Toxicology* **2005**, *216*, 106–121. [CrossRef]

167. Kozma, G.T.; Shimizu, T.; Ishida, T.; Szebeni, J. Anti-Peg Antibodies: Properties, Formation, Testing and Role in Adverse Immune Reactions to Pegylated Nano-Biopharmaceuticals. *Adv. Drug Deliv. Rev.* **2020**, *154–155*, 163–175. [CrossRef]

168. Szebeni, J.; Simberg, D.; González-Fernández, A.; Barenholz, Y.; Dobrovolskaia, M.A. Roadmap and Strategy for Overcoming Infusion Reactions to Nanomedicines. *Nat. Nanotechnol.* **2018**, *13*, 1100–1108. [CrossRef]

169. Ju, Y.; Lee, W.S.; Pilkington, E.H.; Kelly, H.G.; Li, S.; Selva, K.J.; Wragg, K.M.; Subbarao, K.; Nguyen, T.H.O.; Rowntree, L.C.; et al. Anti-Peg Antibodies Boosted in Humans by SARS-CoV-2 Lipid Nanoparticle Mrna Vaccine. *ACS Nano* **2022**, *16*, 11769–11780. [CrossRef]
170. Oberli, M.A.; Reichmuth, A.M.; Dorkin, J.R.; Mitchell, M.J.; Fenton, O.S.; Jaklenec, A.; Anderson, D.G.; Langer, R.; Blankschtein, D. Lipid Nanoparticle Assisted Mrna Delivery for Potent Cancer Immunotherapy. *Nano Lett.* **2017**, *17*, 1326–1335. [CrossRef]
171. Bevers, S.; Kooijmans, S.A.; Van de Velde, E.; Evers, M.J.; Seghers, S.; Gitz-Francois, J.J.; van Kronenburg, N.C.; Fens, M.H.; Mastrobattista, E.; Hassler, L.; et al. mRNA-Lnp Vaccines Tuned for Systemic Immunization Induce Strong Antitumor Immunity by Engaging Splenic Immune Cells. *Mol. Ther.* **2022**, *30*, 3078–3094. [CrossRef]
172. Dilliard, S.A.; Cheng, Q.; Siegwart, D.J. On the Mechanism of Tissue-Specific Mrna Delivery by Selective Organ Targeting Nanoparticles. *Proc. Natl. Acad. Sci. USA* **2021**, *118*, e2109256118. [CrossRef]
173. Yamaguchi, Y.; Kato, Y.; Edahiro, R.; Søndergaard, J.N.; Murakami, T.; Amiya, S.; Nameki, S.; Yoshimine, Y.; Morita, T.; Takeshima, Y.; et al. Consecutive Bnt162b2 Mrna Vaccination Induces Short-Term Epigenetic Memory in Innate Immune Cells. *J. Clin. Investig.* **2022**, *7*, e163347. [CrossRef]

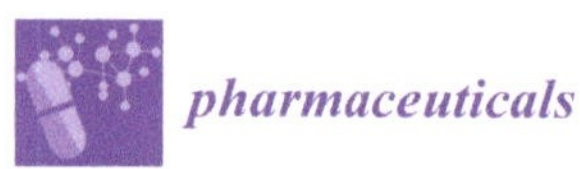

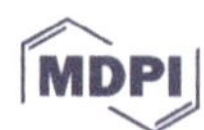

Review

Advances with Lipid-Based Nanosystems for siRNA Delivery to Breast Cancers

Md Abdus Subhan [1,2,*], Nina Filipczak [3,*] and Vladimir P. Torchilin [3,4,*]

1 Department of Chemistry, ShahJalal University of Science and Technology, Sylhet 3114, Bangladesh
2 Division of Nephrology, University of Rochester Medical Center, School of Medicine and Dentistry, 601 Elmwood Ave, Box 675, Rochester, NY 14642, USA
3 Center for Pharmaceutical Biotechnology and Nanomedicine, Department of Pharmaceutical Sciences, Northeastern University, Boston, MA 02115, USA
4 Department of Chemical Engineering, Northeastern University, Boston, MA 02115, USA
* Correspondence: subhan-che@sust.edu (M.A.S.); nina.filipczak@gmail.com (N.F.); v.torchilin@northeastern.edu (V.P.T.)

Abstract: Breast cancer is the most frequently diagnosed cancer among women. Breast cancer is also the key reason for worldwide cancer-related deaths among women. The application of small interfering RNA (siRNA)-based drugs to combat breast cancer requires effective gene silencing in tumor cells. To overcome the challenges of drug delivery to tumors, various nanosystems for siRNA delivery, including lipid-based nanoparticles that protect siRNA from degradation for delivery to cancer cells have been developed. These nanosystems have shown great potential for efficient and targeted siRNA delivery to breast cancer cells. Lipid-based nanosystems remain promising as siRNA drug delivery carriers for effective and safe cancer therapy including breast cancer. Lipid nanoparticles (LNPs) encapsulating siRNA enable efficient and specific silencing of oncogenes in breast tumors. This review discusses a variety of lipid-based nanosystems including cationic lipids, sterols, phospholipids, PEG-lipid conjugates, ionizable liposomes, exosomes for effective siRNA drug delivery to breast tumors, and the clinical translation of lipid-based siRNA nanosystems for solid tumors.

Keywords: lipid NPs; breast cancer; siRNA delivery; gene silencing; personalized therapy

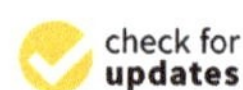

Citation: Subhan, M.A.; Filipczak, N.; Torchilin, V.P. Advances with Lipid-Based Nanosystems for siRNA Delivery to Breast Cancers. *Pharmaceuticals* **2023**, *16*, 970. https://doi.org/10.3390/ph16070970

Academic Editors: Ana Catarina Silva, João Nuno Moreira and José Manuel Sousa Lobo

Received: 13 May 2023
Revised: 1 July 2023
Accepted: 4 July 2023
Published: 6 July 2023

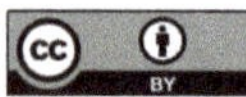

1. Introduction

Breast cancer is the most frequent type of cancer in women and is the main cause of cancer death, accounting for 2.08 million new patients and 0.67 million deaths every year [1]. Breast cancer has become the most prevalent form of cancer globally, surpassing lung cancer in 2020. It is also the most diagnosed cancer among women in the United States. It is a leading cause of cancer-related deaths in less developed nations and ranks as the second highest cause of cancer-related deaths in American women. In 2020, approximately 2.3 million women worldwide were diagnosed with breast cancer, resulting in 685,000 fatalities. Shockingly, every 14 s, a woman somewhere in the world receives a breast cancer diagnosis. Overall, breast cancer is the most frequently occurring cancer in women worldwide, being the top diagnosis in 140 out of 184 countries. It represents a quarter of all cancers affecting women globally. In the United States, breast cancer is the second most common cancer among women, following nonmelanoma skin cancer. In 2023, an estimated 300,590 people in the U.S. will receive a breast cancer diagnosis, with 297,790 of them being women, making it the most prevalent cancer among American women. Furthermore, in 2023, an estimated 2800 men will also be diagnosed with breast cancer in the U.S. [2]. Currently, breast cancer treatment is focused primarily on neoadjuvant or adjuvant therapy, surgery, and radiation therapy. Systemic therapy for breast cancer includes chemotherapy, hormonal therapy, targeted therapy, and immunotherapy. Breast cancer patient survival depends on the stage of disease, metastatic progression, and development of drug resistance [3–5]. Cancer cells demonstrate proliferative signaling, evasion of growth suppression, inhibition of programmed cell death, rapid angiogenesis, and stimulate invasion as well as metastasis. The cancer cells also can reprogram energy metabolism and evade immune responses. The reprogramming of energy metabolism and evasion of immune responses by cancer cells is enabled by genome instability and mutations. Thus, cancer qualifies as a heterogeneous disease. Breast cancers with their diverse diagnostic landscapes may influence clinical behavior and patient survival. Personalized therapies for breast cancers have been focused on targeting proteins and signaling pathways emphasizing the significance of novel molecular targets, utilization of efficient delivery tools, and early and accurate detection to enhance breast cancer therapy [1]. In the realm of breast cancer therapy, several specific small interfering RNA (siRNA) molecules have been investigated for their potential therapeutic applications. For instance, siRNA targeting the oncogene HER2 (human epidermal growth factor receptor 2) has been explored as a strategy to downregulate HER2 expression and inhibit the proliferation of HER2-positive breast cancer cells [6]. Additionally, siRNA targeting genes involved in cell cycle regulation, such as cyclin-dependent kinases (CDKs) and checkpoint proteins, have shown promise for the modulation of cell growth and induction of apoptosis in breast cancer cells [7,8]. Furthermore, siRNA molecules targeting angiogenesis-related factors, such as vascular endothelial growth factor (VEGF), have been investigated for inhibition of tumor vascularization to impair tumor growth in breast cancer [9]. siRNAs used in breast cancer therapy can be classified into different categories based on their structure and mode of action as shown in Figure 1. These examples illustrate the potential of siRNA-based therapies in breast cancer, providing targeted approaches to silence specific genes or pathways involved in cancer progression.

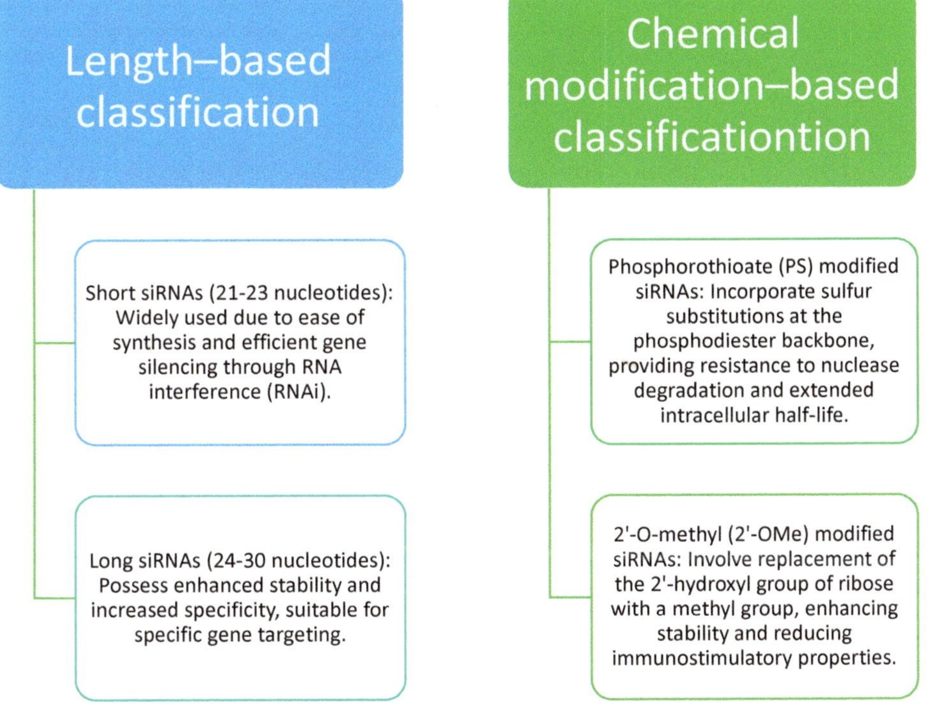

Figure 1. Classification of siRNAs used in breast cancer therapy [10].

Lipid-based nanosystems have served as promising siRNA drug delivery carriers for effective and safe cancer therapy [1]. SiRNAs are a small class of dsRNAs, consisting of 19 to 21 nucleotides. siRNAs impede gene expression and protein synthesis via complementary binding to their target mRNA, and they activate their target gene silencing through RNAi [11]. The potency of siRNAs may increase with length. A study demonstrated that a 27-nucleotide siRNA may be 100 times more potent than a conventional 21-neucleotide siRNA [12].

In recent years, lipidic nanosystems (Table 1) have emerged as promising vehicles for the delivery of small interfering RNA (siRNA). The physicochemical properties of lipidic systems play a crucial role in their effectiveness as carriers for siRNA delivery. One important property is the size and surface charge of the lipid nanoparticles. Generally, smaller nanoparticles have shown enhanced cellular uptake and improved penetration into tissues, making them desirable for efficient siRNA delivery [13]. Additionally, the surface charge of lipid nanoparticles influences their stability, interaction with biological barriers, and cellular internalization. Cationic lipids used in lipidic systems provide a positive charge, facilitating complex formation with negatively charged siRNA and promoting cellular uptake [14,15]. However, it is important to strike a balance, as excessive positive charge can lead to cytotoxicity and non-specific interactions. Hence, optimizing the surface charge of lipidic systems is crucial for achieving efficient and safe siRNA delivery. Another important physicochemical property is the lipid composition of the nanoparticle formulation. Lipidic systems for siRNA delivery often incorporate a mixture of lipids to modify desired properties. The selection of lipids influences the stability, encapsulation efficiency, and release profile of siRNA. For instance, the choice of lipids with appropriate hydrophobicity and chain length can improve the stability and loading capacity of siRNA in the lipidic system. Additionally, incorporating lipids with fusogenic properties can aid in endosomal escape, enabling effective siRNA release into the cytoplasm [16]. Furthermore, the inclusion of PEGylated lipids can enhance the stability and circulation time of lipid nanoparticles, reducing their clearance by the immune system [17]. Therefore, careful consideration of lipid composition is essential to optimize the physicochemical properties of lipidic systems for efficient siRNA delivery.

Table 1. Examples of lipid nanocarriers used for delivery of siRNA.

Lipid Nanocarrier Type	Lipids Used	Active Moiety Delivered	Key Conclusions	References
Lipid Nanoparticles (LNPs)	Ionizable cationic lipids (e.g., DOTAP, DLin-MC3-DMA) and helper lipids (e.g., cholesterol, PEG-lipids)	siRNA (Small interfering RNA)	LNPs effectively encapsulated siRNA and protected it from degradation. The formulation demonstrated high stability, efficient cellular uptake, and endosomal escape. LNPs efficiently delivered siRNA to target cells and achieved significant gene silencing, offering promising potential for therapeutic applications.	[18,19]
Solid Lipid Nanoparticles (SLNs)	Solid lipids (e.g., stearic acid, glyceryl monostearate) and surfactants (e.g., Tween, Span)	siRNA	SLNs provided a stable and biocompatible platform for siRNA delivery. The formulation protected siRNA from enzymatic degradation and facilitated cellular uptake. SLNs demonstrated effective gene silencing in vitro and in vivo, highlighting their potential as siRNA delivery systems.	[20]
Liposomes	Cationic lipids (e.g., DOTAP, DODAB) and neutral lipids (e.g., phosphatidylcholine)	siRNA	Liposomes efficiently encapsulated siRNA and protected it from nuclease degradation. The cationic lipids facilitated cellular uptake and endosomal escape of siRNA. Liposomal siRNA delivery showed effective gene silencing in target cells, making liposomes a promising option for siRNA therapeutics.	[21–23]
Cationic Lipid-DNA Complexes (lipoplexes)	Cationic lipids (e.g., Lipofectamine, Polyethylenimine) and plasmid DNA	siRNA or gene encoding siRNA	Cationic lipids formed stable complexes with siRNA or plasmid DNA and facilitated their cellular uptake. Lipoplexes efficiently delivered siRNA or gene encoding siRNA, resulting in effective gene silencing or knockdown of the target gene. Lipoplexes showed potential for siRNA-based therapeutics and gene therapy applications.	[12,24]
Ethosomes	Phospholipids (e.g., phosphatidylcholine) and ethanol	siRNA	Ethosomes provided enhanced permeation of siRNA through the skin or mucosal barriers. The formulation improved siRNA stability and promoted efficient delivery into target cells. Ethosomes showed potential for transdermal or mucosal siRNA delivery, offering opportunities for local or systemic treatments.	[25]

The first generation of lipid-based nanosystems employed cationic liposomes to encapsulate and protect siRNA molecules. Cationic liposomes possess a positive charge, enabling electrostatic interaction with the negatively charged siRNA, forming stable complexes that facilitate cellular uptake and endosomal escape. One such example is the widely utilized lipofectamine-based system, which combines cationic lipids with siRNA, leading to efficient gene silencing [26]. However, these early lipid-based nanosystems revealed challenges such as poor stability, limited siRNA loading capacity, and potential cytotoxicity.

To overcome these limitations, the second generation of lipidic nanosystems introduced the concept of lipid nanoparticles LNPs. LNPs are comprised of a lipid bilayer encapsulating the siRNA payload and often contain additional components, such as polyethylene glycol (PEG) and targeting ligands. These components enhance stability, circulation time, and specific delivery to the target cells or tissues. Notably, LNPs incorporating ionizable cationic lipids have shown remarkable success in siRNA delivery. For instance, the FDA-approved lipid nanoparticle system, Onpattro, utilizes an ionizable lipid formulation to effectively deliver siRNA targeting transthyretin (TTR) for the treatment of hereditary ATTR amyloidosis [27]. The second-generation lipidic nanosystems represent a significant advancement in siRNA delivery, addressing previous challenges and exhibiting improved therapeutic potential. Lipid nanoparticles act to reduce biological barriers to siRNA delivery, degradation by nuclease, and intracellular trafficking. LNPs may offer potential advantages including enhanced bioavailability, increasing aqueous solubility to reduce cellular clearance time, improving receptor specificity, and targeting drugs to exact tissue.

LNPs fabricated using well-tolerated components can be prepared on a large scale and can be sterilized and lyophilized, providing storage stability. They are also biocompatible and biodegradable, similarly to liposomes. The LNPs are composed mainly of phospholipids, organized in a bi-layered structure. LNPs form vesicles in the presence of water, increasing the solubility and stability of anticancer drugs when loaded into the carrier [28]. The LNP-based vehicles can encapsulate both soluble and insoluble drugs [29]. In addition to phospholipids, other compounds, including cholesterol, may be loaded onto the carriers. Cholesterol, in the LNP-based vehicles, reduces the membrane fluidity of the NPs, enhances its penetrability to insoluble drugs, and improves their stability in the circulation [28].

siRNA delivery of LNPs encapsulating siRNA facilitates effective and specific silencing of oncogenes, such as the tyrosine kinase receptors (TKRs) expressed on cancer cells since they are recognized as regulators of oncogenesis [30]. The most frequently utilized nanosystems for siRNA drug delivery include cationic, ionizable, neutral liposomes, exosomes, and other synthetic nanocarriers. These are simply prepared liposome-based delivery systems that have several benefits for in vitro and in vivo delivery of siRNA.

The innate immune system provides a first line, and the adaptive immune system provides a second line, of the body's defense [1]. The size of the LNP determines the Th1 response (IFNγ production) and Th2 response (IL-4 production). Particles of 40 to 50 nm improved Th1 stimulation, while larger-sized (>100 nm) particles activated the Th2 response [31]. The white blood cells and erythrocytes interact with LNPs depending on their various characteristics. These may affect the delivery of LNPs forming aggregates with the abundant erythrocytes, which may be toxic to immune cells [32]. The geometry of the LNPs may also influence the cellular internalization. The rod-like LNPs are internalized by the leukocytes with high efficiency, followed by spherical- and cylindrical-like NPs. However, cube-like LNPs are internalized less efficiently [32]. Cationic NPs can interact with cell membranes. However, cationic liposomes may increase immunotoxicity by activation of neutrophils and by prompting oxidative stress. Anionic LNPs have less favorable interactions with cell membranes due to repulsive forces and may exhibit poor cellular internalization [33]. Leukocytes-LNP interactions are beneficial because the resultant system crosses physiological barriers and moves into tumor niches [34].

Cationic liposomes are suitable for encapsulating therapeutic siRNA. The incorporated siRNAs within cationic liposomes demonstrate a superior uptake by the target cells through endocytosis. To target the desired cells effectively, ligand binding to the cell surface receptors of target cells was merged with the cationic coat of the liposome [35]. The fabrication of lipid-based nanocarriers has received much consideration due to the progress of systems for delivering siRNA to the cytoplasm of the tumor cells, protecting them from the circulatory environment that provides resistance to nucleases, overcoming immune responses enabling sufficient delivery to cancer cells [36].

The efficiency of LNPs for the delivery of siRNAs targeting CDK4 was evaluated in a study by Wang et al. [37]. The results of the study demonstrated that LNP-siRNA prompted efficient gene silencing compared to lipofectamine in MDA-MB-468-triple-negative breast cancer (TNBC) cells and triggered G_1 phase cell cycle arrest. CDK4 inhibited cell cycle and proliferation in cancer cells. The advances in siRNA-based selective inhibiting agents targeting CDK4 may be an effective approach for breast cancer therapy.

Lipid-coated calcium phosphate NPs loaded with siRNA promoted the siRNA delivery to TNBC cells. The NPs accumulated in tumor cells because of the enhanced permeability and retention (EPR) effect and the ability of siRNA drugs to target cancer cells. LNPs coated with calcium phosphate were utilized for the delivery of a mixture of siRNAs targeting genes required for cell survival [38]. The outcomes indicated an improved cellular uptake and hindrance of TNBC MDA-MB-468 cells.

Effective delivery of chemotherapeutics and therapeutic siRNA has significant possible benefits. A co-delivery system consisting of paclitaxel (PTX) and siRNA coupled to LNPs significantly inhibited cancer cells utilizing targeted siRNA therapy [39]. Micellar LNPs carrying both PTX and siRNA targeting polo-like kinase 1 (PLK1) demonstrated synergistic tumor reduction in a xenograft murine model of MDA-MB-435s (a model cell line often used for the study of breast cancer) cells [40]. PLK1 is often overexpressed on breast cancer cell lines. Concurrent delivery of siRNA and chemotherapeutic drugs using cationic liposomes is an effective delivery system to target PLK1 [41,42]. The simultaneous delivery of PTX and PLK1 siRNA synergistically enhanced apoptotic MCF-7 cells and decreased angiogenesis. This combination delivery method demonstrated noteworthy benefits over single therapies using either PTX or siRNA [41]. Similarly, delivery of doxorubicin (Dox) with siRNA liposomes is a frequently used approach in cancer therapy [42].

The tumor inhibitory effect of siRNA loaded into liposomes targeting VEGF was effective against SKBR3 breast cancer cells compared to a commercial transfecting system, metafectene [43]. A polycation liposome encapsulating calcium phosphate (PLCP) NPs facilitated endosomal escape. The silencing function of PLCP/VEGF siRNA complexes was two times greater in MCF-7 cells compared to a commercial transfecting agent in an in vivo study using a xenograft model of MCF-7 cells. Additionally, a synergistic tumor hindrance effect was detected in tumor cells co-treated with doxorubicin in a mouse model. This study demonstrated that the PLCP/VEGF siRNA delivery system targeting VEGF is a promising approach to inhibit angiogenesis in breast tumors [44].

Ionizable liposomes with vincristine at a drug lipid ratio of 1:1 was tested in a breast cancer model [45]. In another study, ionizable liposomes conjugated to lipocalin 2(Lcn2) siRNA was used to inhibit the metastatic MDA-MB-436 and MDA-MB-231 breast cancer cell lines. The results indicated that the liposomal Lnc2 siRNA system can be effective in reducing breast cancer progression [46].

Cationic porphyrin lipid microbubbles loaded with hypoxia-inducible factor-1α siRNA along with photodynamic therapy were utilized for the treatment of TNBC, monitored using ultrasound imaging. HIF-1α siRNA down-regulated the HIF-1α expression, which was facilitated by the hypoxic tumor conditions or Ros generated during PDT. This approach improved PDT efficacy and reduced tumor development [47].

Lipid-coated calcium phosphate nanoparticles (LCP NPs) are a biocompatible, multifunctional efficient delivery system for cancer therapy. BsAb conjugated with LCP NPs targeted EGFR on MDA-MB-468 cells. These multifunctional LCP-BsA NPs were efficiently taken up by the tumor tissue. The integration of CD (cell death) siRNA and photothermal (ICG) therapy utilizing LCP-BsAb NPs hindered tumor growth in vivo in a mouse model [48,49].

The LNP surface was modified with HB-EGF antibody to target breast cancer [50,51]. HB-EGF is a ligand that binds to the EGF receptor (EGFR). TNBC tumors over-express HB-EGF [52]. Utilization of anti-HB-EGF antibody-modified LNP enhanced the siRNA delivery to breast tumors after intravenous injections. TNBC is a refractory disease with a poor prognosis. Nanomaterials such as functionalized mesoporous silica, chitosan-layered gold NPs, and cationic LNPs are utilized for siRNA delivery via an EPR effect [53–55]. However, active targeting may be utilized to deliver the LNPs containing siRNA to inhibit TNBC growth. TNBC growth was hindered by silencing PLK1 protein expression in tumors after intravenous injection of anti-HB-EGF antibody-modified LNPs incorporating siRNA against PLK1. This antibody alteration approach is an innovative strategy for the therapy of TNBC tumors [20].

Exosomes can be used as carriers for siRNA. Exosomes generated by the recipient's own cells may be a prospective and safe carrier for siRNA delivery [56,57]. The surface of the exosomes can be modified with suitable ligands to improve the selectivity for target cells. Artificial exosomes or exosome mimetics may be advantageous for tissue-specific efficient delivery of siRNA [20]. Further, exosome-modified liposomes may be utilized for the targeted delivery of siRNA drugs for anticancer immunotherapy [58].

Major barriers to siRNA delivery that target an adequate dose to the tumor will enhance its internalization into tumor cells. Its release into the cytoplasm can be reduced with a complex comprising siRNA, cationic lipids, and pH-responsive peptide suitable for tumor uptake enhancement through focused ultrasound (FUS). The system offers efficient siRNA encapsulation, nuclease protection, endosomal escape, and effective gene silencing. Both lipid and ternary (lipid: peptide: siRNA complexes prepared with NIR fluorescently labeled siRNA) accumulate in tumors following FUS treatment. As a result, combining a well-designed lipid: peptide: siRNA complex with FUS therapy provides a prospective approach to achieve effective gene delivery in vivo and gene silencing [59].

Lyotropic mesophase LNPs consisting of an internal cubic phase nanostructure are known as cubosomes. In recent years, cubosomes have garnered attention as a promising drug delivery carrier for cancer therapy [60–63]. Cubosomes have many advantages over liposomes. Drug-loaded cubosomes can be utilized for cancer treatment. A cubosome functionalizing with HA to target CD44, which is highly expressed in TNBC cells, was utilized to incorporate siRNA to target breast cancer cells [62,63].

The siRNA drug was formulated with cationic lipid-assisted PEG-PLA NPs to target cyclin-dependent kinase 1 for TNBC therapy. The NPs inhibited c-myc overexpressing TNBC cells by reducing CDK-1 expression [64,65]. Further, aptamer-guided siRNA NPs targeting CD44 expression in TNBC were prepared [65]. The results of the study demonstrated that the drug exhibited improved anticancer effects against TNBC [65,66].

2. Recent Development of Lipid and Lipidoid-Based NPs for siRNA Delivery for Cancer Therapy

Advancements in understanding the molecular targets of cancer have opened the way for personalized therapy, which has overcome the complex and asymptomatic nature of various cancers. Targeted therapy, which interferes with specific molecular targets, has replaced the traditional approach of developing new chemotherapeutics. Over the past few decades, various molecules, such as tyrosine inhibitors, small molecule drug conjugates, serine/threonine inhibitors, and monoclonal antibodies, have been used to develop targeted anti-cancer therapies. Although these molecules have been effective, challenges related to protein stability remain.

2.1. RNAi Therapy: Challenges and Advantages

However, RNA interference has revolutionized targeted therapies by using non-coding RNAs to silence gene expression in various cells. Despite the existence of various options for gene silencing, such as TALENs and CRISPR/Cas, RNA interference remains the preferred option due to its precise mechanism, high potential, high specificity of gene silencing, and minimal off-target effects [67]. The main challenge associated with siRNA-based therapies for cancer and other diseases is delivering siRNA to the target cells in vivo in an effective manner. Successful use of siRNA-based drugs in the fight against cancer requires effective gene silencing in cancer cells. For effective siRNA delivery, the ideal systemic siRNA delivery system should possess several characteristics. These include biocompatibility, biodegradability, non-immunogenicity, protection of siRNA from serum nucleases during circulation and endosome release, avoidance of rapid hepatic or renal clearance, and promotion of siRNA delivery to target cells while avoiding normal tissues. Therefore, an in vivo, systemic siRNA delivery system should aim to increase the serum half-life of the siRNA, promote its distribution to target tissues, promote cellular uptake with intracytoplasmic release without degradation, and avoid off-target gene silencing activity. Several siRNA delivery systems have been developed for cancer therapy, including chemical modifications of siRNA, lipid-based delivery systems, polymer-based delivery systems, conjugate delivery systems, co-delivery of siRNA and anticancer drugs, and inorganic nanoparticles such as quantum dots, carbon nanotubes, and gold nanoparticles [68]. These modifications help address the problems associated with naked siRNA, such as serum stability, clearance of large molecular mass material, high toxicity, ligand-receptor interaction, vascular permeability to reach cancer tissues, and renal clearance as shown in Figure 2.

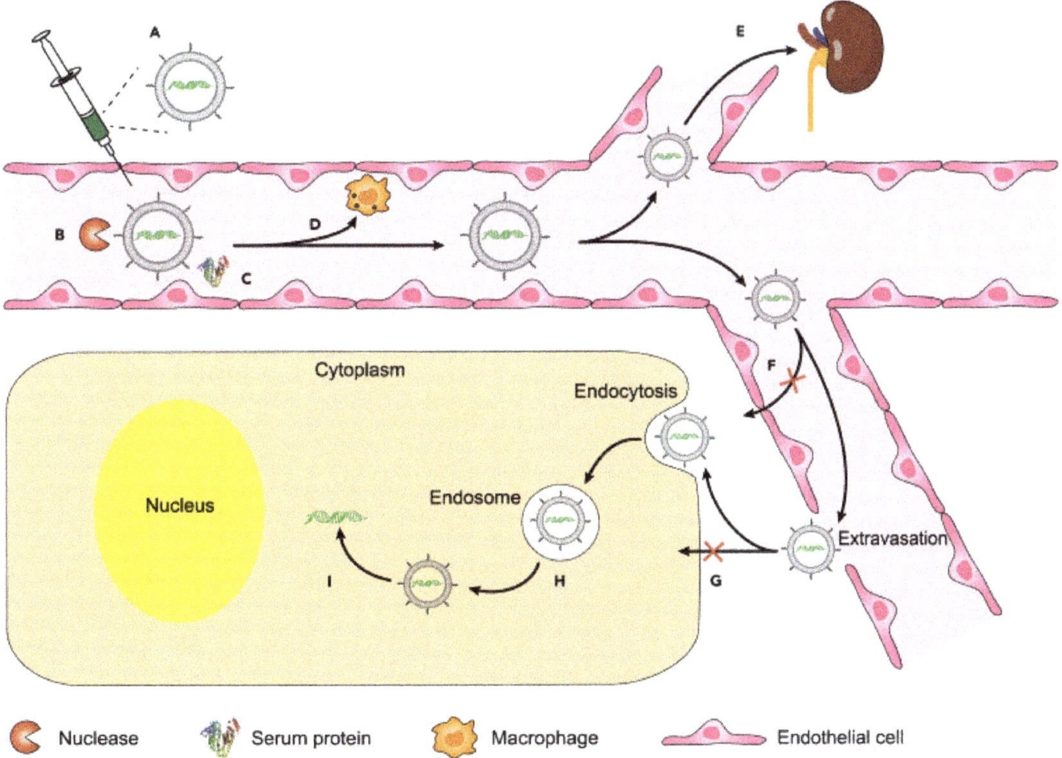

Figure 2. Challenges in in vivo delivery of RNA therapeutics using nanoparticles. (**A**) Spontaneous hydrolysis of RNAs. (**B**) Nuclease-mediated degradation. (**C**) Protein adsorption. (**D**) Immune recognition and clearance. (**E**) Renal clearance. (**F**) Endothelial barrier. (**G**) Cell membrane barrier. (**H**) Endosomal barrier. (**I**) Insufficient cargo release. Adapted from [69] with copyright permissions.

However, achieving these benefits from a single modification is difficult, as siRNA delivery systems interact with various components. Poorly designed modifications can lead to problems such as a high positive charge on the surface of nanoparticles, which may cause unfavorable aggregation with erythrocytes [70,71].

2.2. Nanoparticles

RNAi-based cancer therapies have led to the use of nanoparticles as delivery molecules, which enhance transportation efficiency due to the EPR effect. However, preclinical characterization of the nanocarrier and studies on the release mechanism for loaded non-coding RNAs by these carriers must be analyzed before these molecules are taken into clinical trials [72].

Preclinical studies that evaluate the rate, range, and perpetuation of silencing as well as the timeframe of delivery of the carriers to the tumor site are crucial for improving siRNA delivery [70]. In recent years, there has been growing interest in the use of lipid and lipidoid-based nanoparticles (NPs) for the delivery of small interfering RNAs as a potential cancer therapy. siRNA is an encouraging therapeutic agent that can silence specific genes involved in cancer growth and progression, but its clinical utility has been limited by challenges in delivering it to cancer cells. Lipid and lipidoid-based NPs have emerged as an approach for delivering siRNA to cancer cells due to their biocompatibility, biodegradability, and ability to encapsulate and protect siRNA from degradation. Several lipid-based NPs have been developed for siRNA delivery in cancer therapy. Five major nanomaterial-based delivery platforms now include lipid, peptide, polymer, biomembrane, and inorganic NPs. Among various NPs, liposomes, exosomes, and lipid-like NPs are major categories that have attracted significant interest since the introduction of a cationic liposome formulated with 1,2-di-O-octadecyl-3-trimethylammonium propane (DOTMA) for therapeutic mRNA delivery into mammalian cells in 1989 [73]. Lipid-based drug delivery systems have several advantages including FDA approval, simplicity of the preparation, good biocompatibility, low immunogenicity, and high transfection efficiency. Lately, new ionizable lipids have been designed to replace the traditionally used cationic lipids to reduce toxicity without compromising transfection efficacy (Table 2). These ionizable lipids contain three moieties and have an optimal pKa value of 6.2–6.5, allowing for efficient encapsulation of RNAs into nanoparticles while maintaining neutrality at physiological pH and becoming protonated at lower cell pH to facilitate endosomal escape [74,75].

Table 2. Examples of lipids commonly used in delivery systems for siRNA [20,69].

Group of Lipids/Lipidoids	Examples
Cationic lipids	DOTAP, DOTMA, DC-6-14
Ionizable lipids/lipidoids	A6, A18-Iso-5-2DC18, 98N$_{12}$-5, DLin-MC3-DMA, Lin-DMA, DODAP, DLin-KC2-DMA, DLin-MC3-DMA, YSK05, YSK13, CL4H6.
Sterols	Cholesterol, DC-cholesterol, Sitosterol
PEG-lipid conjugates	DSPE-PEG, DMG-PEG
Phospholipids	DOPE, DSPC, DSPC

The choice of a lipid-based nanosystem for siRNA delivery depends on several factors, including the physicochemical properties of siRNA, the desired release kinetics, and the route of administration. The most natural and biocompatible vehicles that can be used for nucleic acid delivery are exosomes.

2.2.1. Exosomes

Exosomes are endogenous vesicles that have recently received much attention in the field of small interfering RNA delivery research. They are seen to be safe and efficient carriers. Exosomes used as siRNA carriers are preferably self-derived from exosome-producing cells to keep low immunogenicity. Although the use of exosomes as siRNA carriers is still under investigation, it has been reported that exosomes taken from human serum can be loaded with siRNA by electroporation and introduced into human lymphocytes and monocytes [76]. Similarly, liposomes are considered safe, biocompatible, and effective delivery systems for siRNA. They are spherical vesicles composed of phospholipids that can encapsulate siRNA.

2.2.2. Liposomes

Liposomes also offer the possibility of co-delivering multiple drugs with different properties, such as hydrophilic and hydrophobic drugs, within the same particle. This can reduce the frequency of drug administration, which can improve patient compliance and reduce potential side effects [77,78]. Despite their advantages, liposomes also have some limitations, such as poor stability in biological fluids, susceptibility to opsonization by serum proteins, and potential toxicity associated with the use of certain lipid components. Thus, ongoing research continues to address these issues and explore new strategies to improve the clinical efficacy and safety of liposomal drug delivery systems [78,79].

2.2.3. Solid Lipid Nanoparticles

Another commonly used delivery system is called the solid lipid nanoparticle (SLN). Those carrier systems are composed of natural lipids that are stabilized by surfactants in an aqueous solution, which distinguishes them from liposomes. SLNs are created using solid lipids such as glycerides, fatty acids, or waxes. By contrast, nanostructured lipid carriers (NLC) use a combination of solid and liquid lipids (oils) that form a solid blend at body temperature. The addition of oil prevents the formation of perfect lipid crystals, creating imperfections that increase the drug-loading capacity and physical stability of the lipid matrix [80,81]. Cationic compounds, typically lipids, are also used to let the negatively charged nucleic acids form a complex at the surface of the particle [82].

2.2.4. Lipid-Polymer Nanoparticles

Another interesting delivery system uses lipid-polymer nanoparticles. LPNs are composed of a lipid bilayer and a polymer core that can enhance siRNA encapsulation and stability [83]. Lipidoid-based NPs are a newer class of NPs that have shown promise for siRNA delivery due to their ability to form stable complexes with siRNA molecules and efficiently deliver them to target cells. Lipidoids are modified lipids that can form NPs through self-assembly with siRNA. Lipidoid-based NPs have been shown to effectively deliver siRNA to cancer cells in preclinical models and have several advantages over traditional lipid-based NPs, including improved stability and reduced toxicity [83,84]. Despite the promising results of these preclinical studies, there are still challenges to be addressed in the development of lipid and lipidoid-based NPs for siRNA delivery for cancer therapy. These challenges include improving the stability and targeting efficiency of NPs, minimizing side effects, and optimizing the dosing and administration of NPs [20].

2.3. Targeted Therapy

The targeted delivery of drug nanoparticles to a specific site of action is crucial for effective treatment with minimal side effects. Passive targeting utilizes the enhanced permeation and retention effect, which occurs in many solid tumors due to leaky vascular blood vessels and incomplete lymphatic systems. Nanoparticles can accumulate in these incomplete vascular systems, and modifying their surfaces with hydrophilic macromolecules such as PEG can further optimize this effect. PEGylation can increase the stability of nanoparticles in biological fluids and reduce aggregation during storage and during in vivo application [85]. The main challenge is to design nanocarriers that can specifically recognize and target molecules presented on the tumor cell surface. Several different types of nanoparticles have been designed to meet this challenge, including nanoparticles that react to light, ultrasound, or heat to release the contents and disrupt cancer cells. Moreover, nanoparticles can be designed to carry multiple drugs simultaneously [86]. An alternate way to precisely transport the siRNA to the targeted site requires functionalization of the NPs' surface by using various ligands. Consequently, structures presented on the cells' surface or in tissues can be specifically targeted with proper ligands attached to the surface of the NPs [87]. The most used ligands include aptamers, small molecules, antibodies, peptides, polysaccharides, receptors, or antibody fragments. It has been proven that surface modification is a key factor affecting the binding and uptake of the nanoparticles once they reach the target site [88]. However, the effectiveness of active targeting is not so impressive, since studies have shown that only a small percentage of injected nanoparticles typically reach the tumor tissue. Despite this, surface functionalization can significantly influence the binding and uptake of nanoparticles by target tissues and can lead to improved therapeutic effects. It has been demonstrated that less than 1% of the administered nanoparticles can accumulate at the target site [89]. These findings imply that higher delivery efficiency is crucial for the achievement of lower NP dosages and reducing the cost of treatment where the current nanoparticles production cost is high. In addition, the remaining molecules that do not accumulate at the target tissue (~99%) are deposited in peripheral tissues, creating a risk of side effects. Finally, this very low delivery rate highlights an understanding that the exact delivery process is still unclear and further knowledge and research are needed to improve the delivery rate well above ~1% [89,90].

3. Promising Lipid-Based Nanosystems for siRNA Drug Delivery to Breast Cancer

Breast cancer is a complex and heterogeneous disease that poses significant challenges for treatment. Small interfering RNAs are a potent therapeutic approach that can silence specific genes involved in tumor growth and progression. However, the delivery of siRNAs to breast cancer cells remains a major obstacle. To overcome these challenges, researchers have developed various nanosystems for siRNA delivery, including lipid-based nanoparticles to protect it from degradation and deliver it to cancer cells. These nanosystems have shown great potential for efficient and targeted siRNA delivery to breast cancer cells [91,92].

3.1. Liposomes

One promising lipid-based nanosystem for siRNA delivery to breast cancer uses liposomes. Cationic liposomes have a positive charge that can interact with the negatively charged siRNA molecules to form stable complexes. These complexes enter cancer cells through endocytosis and release siRNA into the cytoplasm, where it can silence specific genes involved in tumor growth and progression. The formulation of cationic liposomes affects their physical and chemical properties, which in turn affects their ability to form stable complexes with siRNA, protect siRNA from degradation in the blood stream, and deliver siRNA into target cells. Factors that can affect the formulation of cationic liposomes include the type and concentration of cationic lipid used, the presence of helper lipids, the ratio of cationic lipid to siRNA, the method of preparation, and the size and surface charge of the resulting liposomes [93]. Liposomes also offer an option of co-delivery of the anticancer drug and nucleic acid. Recently, paclitaxel (PTX) and siRNA (siPlk1) were co-encapsulated using cationic liposomes (CLs) to estimate the anticancer activity of the developed formulations using MDA-MB-231 and MCF-7 cell lines. The developed formulation showed sustained drug release for up to 168 h and significantly increased the biological half-life of PTX when compared to the marketed PTX formulation and enhanced its anticancer activity [94]. To counteract PTX resistance and enhance the anticancer effects of PTX, another nanosystem was created that consisted of a redox-sensitive cationic oligopeptide lipid (LHSSG2C14), a natural soybean phosphatidylcholine (SPC), and cholesterol. This liposome-based system, called PTX/siRNA/SS-L, delivers both PTX and anti-survivin siRNA, which specifically downregulates survivin overexpression. The increased expression of survivin in breast cancer cells is a significant contributor to the resistance of breast cancer cells to paclitaxel. The PTX/siRNA/SS-L system was found to have high encapsulation efficiency and released both PTX and siRNA quickly in response to redox changes. In vitro studies on 4T1 breast cancer cells showed that PTX/siRNA/SS-L exhibited elevated cellular uptake, endosomal escape, lower survivin expression, reduced cell viability and wound healing rate, and higher apoptosis rate. Moreover, in vivo experiments with 4T1 tumor-bearing mice demonstrated that PTX/siRNA/SS-L exhibited lower toxicity and inhibited tumor growth and pulmonary metastasis [95]. Another approach used to improve paclitaxel activity was to develop liposomes co-encapsulating paclitaxel, crizotinib (CRI), and Bcl-xL siRNA [96]. A different approach utilizing liposomes for targeted delivery of siRNAs into breast cancer has also been applied. Phage display was used to identify the most selective and specific ligands that can deliver nanocarriers to the tumor. The targeted liposomes, loaded with siRNA, were obtained by fusion of two types of liposomes: one containing siRNA and fusion phage protein (pVIII coat protein), and the other a MCF-7 cell-targeting peptide (DMPGTVLP). The presence of two fused proteins in the final liposomal formulation was further confirmed by Western blotting. Significantly downregulated PRDM14 gene expression followed by decreased PRDM14 protein synthesis in the target MCF-7 cells was also observed indicating that this approach has the potential for development as a new anticancer siRNA-based targeted nanomedicine [97]. The targeted liposomal system that encapsulated Lcn2 siRNA for selective targeting of MCF-7 and MDA-MB-231 cell lines was recently developed. The overexpression of Lcn2 in metastatic breast cancer promotes cancer progression by enhancing tumor angiogenesis and inducing epithelial-to-mesenchymal transition. The liposomes were PEGylated and decorated with octreotide peptide, which binds to somatostatin receptors overexpressed on breast cancer cells. The optimized liposomes had a mean size of 152 nm, a PDI of 0.13, a zeta potential of 4.10 mV, and high entrapment and loading efficiencies of 69.5% and 7.8%, respectively. In vitro studies showed that the OCT-targeted liposomes achieved approximately 55–60% silencing of Lcn2 mRNA. Additionally, the liposomes exhibited in vitro anti-angiogenic activity by reducing VEGF-A and HUVEC migration levels in the MCF-7 and MDA-MB-231 cells, suggesting their potential utility in inhibiting angiogenesis in MBC [98]. Liposomal drug delivery systems can also combine chemo- and immunotherapy as well as targeting as shown in Figure 3. Cationic liposomes conjugated with two DNA aptamers (called Aptm[DOX/IDO1]) to target cancer cells with the anticancer drug DOX and IDO1 siRNA, which reverses the immunosuppressive tumor microenvironment (TME). Aptm[DOX/IDO1] specifically delivered cargos to target sites via receptor-mediated endocytosis with aptamer-ligand binding. It demonstrated that the developed platform inhibits tumor metastasis by specifically targeting and efficiently delivering anticancer drugs to metastatic cancer cells via systemic circulation. Aptm[DOX/IDO1] effectively facilitated an immune response by inducing ICD and suppressing IDO1, promoting tumor regression in a subcutaneous breast cancer model mouse. The formulation has many advantages including site-specific drug delivery and accumulation in the targeted area, inhibition of PD-1/PD-L1 interaction, and inhibition of tumor metastasis by targeting circulating metastatic cancer cells [99]. To modulate the tumor immune microenvironment, pH-sensitive liposomes modified with cRGD and loaded with anemoside B4 (AB4) and programmed cell death ligand 1 (PD-L1) small interfering RNA (siP) were recently developed. This approach successfully co-delivered both AB4 and siP with good stability and targeted distribution in tumors, leading to improved immunosuppression and attenuation of tumor growth in two animal models. The results showed that cRGD surface modification of liposomes enhances cellular uptake and liposomes accumulation in the tumor tissue, followed by tumor growth inhibition against lung and breast cancer in vivo. Additionally, the co-delivery of AB4 and siP in AB4/siP-c-L resulted in the silencing of the PD-L1 gene and changes in the tumor microenvironment, which allowed the immune system to react better against cancer and induced long-term memory effects. This targeted nanovesicle approach has great potential for clinical application and offers a well-controlled design for investigating the effectiveness of combining herbal monomer components with various immunotherapies such as vaccines, cytokines, and antibodies [100].

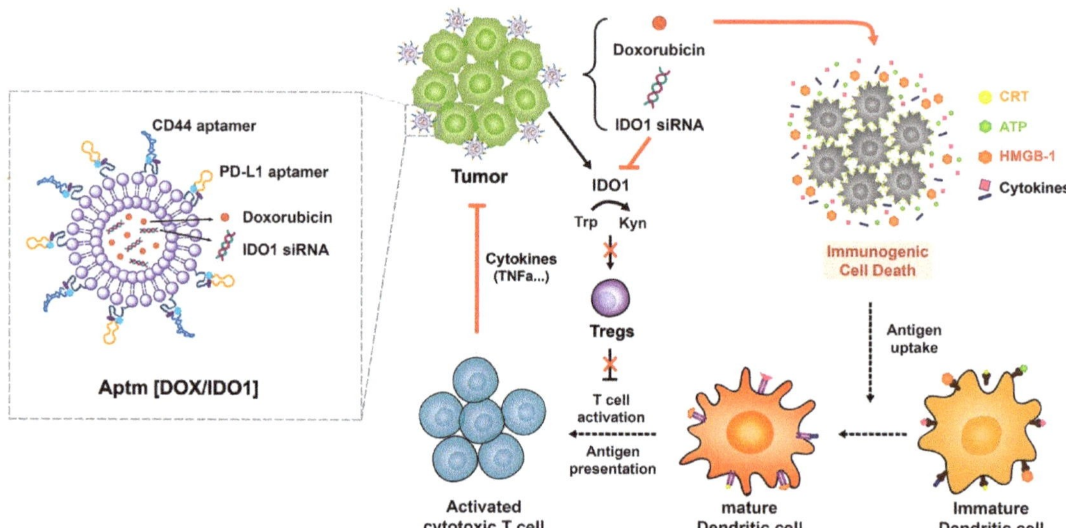

Figure 3. Aptamer-conjugated liposome for immunogenic chemotherapy with reversal of immuno-suppression. Adapted from [99] with copyright permissions.

3.2. Lipid Nanoparticles

The concept of electrostatic encapsulation of siRNA was also utilized in developing other nanocarriers, including cationic solid lipid nanoparticles (cSLN). The cSLN, based on 1,2-dioleoyl-sn-glycero-3-ethylphosphocholine, were prepared using emulsification solidification methods and characterized by paclitaxel and siRNA encapsulation efficiency. The use of cSLN increased the cellular uptake of fluorescently labeled dsRNA in human epithelial carcinoma (KB) cells. For the co-delivery of therapeutic siRNA, the human MCL1-specific siRNA (siMCL1) was complexed with PcSLN. In KB cells treated with siMCL1 complexed to PcSLN, MCL1 mRNA levels were significantly reduced and in vitro anticancer effects in KB cells were observed. Additionally, intratumoral injection of PcSLN complexed with siMCL1 significantly inhibited tumor growth in KB cell-xenografted mice [39].

Another promising lipid-based nanosystem for siRNA delivery to breast cancer includes LPNs. LPNs combine the advantages of both liposomes and polymers to achieve efficient siRNA delivery. The lipid bilayer can protect siRNA from degradation and enhance cellular uptake, while the polymer core can enhance siRNA encapsulation and stability. A recent study demonstrated the potential of LPNs for targeted siRNA delivery to breast cancer cells. Hybrid nanoparticles (HNPs) were created using a tri-block copolymer of PLA-PEG-PLA and DDAB cationic lipids. The method for preparing HNPs/siRNA complexes was simple and efficient, utilizing electrostatic interactions with lipids likely occurring at the interface of the hydrophilic shell and hydrophobic core. The HNPs demonstrated excellent biocompatibility, were easily internalized by MCF7 cells, successfully delivered siRNA into cells, and significantly and specifically downregulated the targeted IGF-1R gene [101]. Thus, these HNPs acting as siRNA delivery vehicles led to successful in vitro gene silencing and hold potential for use as effective nanomaterials for siRNA delivery with potential for reduced side effects in vivo. Recently, hybrid nanoparticles composed of phospholipids and PAMAM dendrimers were also developed to reverse multidrug resistance in cancer. The downregulation of P-glycoprotein (P-gp) using small interfering RNA (siRNA) was observed in breast (MDA-MB-231 and MCF-7) cancer cell lines. Nanoparticles containing generation 4 (G4) polyamidoamine (PAMAM)-PEG2k-DOPE and PEG5k-DOPE were surface modified with monoclonal antibody 2C5 (mAb 2C5) to target cancer cells. This active targeting of tumors results in increased drug and siRNA accumulation at the tumor site, thus minimizing off-target effects. In vitro studies have shown that the micelles have a higher cellular association and effectiveness [102,103]. Another targeted siRNA therapy for triple-negative breast cancer was developed using cationic lipid-assisted poly(ethylene glycol)-b-poly(d,l-lactide) (PEG-PLA) nanoparticles as the carrier. The study showed that only in TNBC cells that overexpress c-Myc, delivery of siRNA targeting cyclin-dependent kinase 1 (CDK1) with the carrier (NPsiCDK1), induced cell death through RNAi-mediated CDK1 expression inhibition, which indicates the synthetic lethality between c-Myc and CDK1 in TNBC cells. The NPsiCDK1 also suppressed tumor growth in mice bearing SUM149 and BT549 xenografts with no systemic toxicity or activation of the innate immune response, demonstrating the therapeutic potential of such nanoparticles loaded with siCDK1 for c-Myc overexpressed TNBC [64].

In summary, lipid-based nanosystems are a promising approach for siRNA delivery to breast cancer. These nanosystems can encapsulate siRNA, protect it from degradation, and deliver it to cancer cells. Nowadays, research on siRNA delivery to cancer focuses on combining multiple strategies to utilize the advantages of different delivery systems and to thus minimize the off-target effect. However further research is needed to optimize these lipid-based nanosystems for clinical translation.

4. Lipid-Based Nanosystems in Clinical Development for siRNA Drug Delivery to Breast Cancer

Lipid-based NPs have demonstrated promising outcomes in clinic and clinical trials [104–106]. siRNA-based drug delivery strategies signify an avenue for more effective and less toxic cancer therapy compared to chemotherapy. siRNA drugs may be applied in combination with standard therapy approaches to create a personalized and effective therapy result for breast cancer patients [107]. siRNA drugs could be utilized integrated with chemotherapy or immunotherapy to minimize systemic toxicity to improve the efficacy of siRNAs targeting resistance pathways in tumor cells [20,68,108].

The phase I trial investigated the best dose and side effects of EphA2-targeted DOPC (1,2-dioleoyl-sn-glycero-3-phosphatidylcholine) encapsulated siRNA (EphA2 siRNA for the treatment of patients with metastatic, advanced, and recurrent solid tumors. EphA2 siRNA reduced tumor growth by downregulating the gene that causes tumor growth. EphA2 siRNA was delivered using neutral liposomes. By intravenous injection in patients with advanced, metastatic, recurrent solid tumors, it may be applied for breast cancer treatment [108,109].

In 2014, a liposomal siRNA drug Atu027 was produced by Silence Therapeutics GmbH, targeting protein kinase 3. This siRNA drug was evaluated in a dose-escalation phase I clinical trial and resulted in disease stabilization in 41% of patients [110].

A lipid-based drug with two siRNAs targeting both VEGF and kinase spindle protein (KSP) (known as ALN-VSP) was tested on 41 patients with solid tumors in a phase I study. From a safety viewpoint, ALN-VSP was generally well tolerated and favorable. The result was promising with most of the patients having stabilized disease for approximately 8–12 months [111].

Another lipid-based siRNA drug called EnCore lipid NPs (DCR-PHXC-101) has been developed. DCR-PHXC-101 downregulates the expression of the transcription factor Myc, which is overexpressed in many solid tumors including breast cancer in a Phase 1 dose-escalation study [112]. Several lipid-based siRNA drugs in different phases of clinical trials for the treatment of solid tumors may be applied for breast cancer therapy (Table 3) [20,108].

Table 3. Lipid-based siRNA drugs are in different phases of clinical trials for the treatment of solid tumors.

siRNA Drug	Delivery System	Target	Cancer Type	Phase, Status	Company	NCT	Ref.
siRNA-EphA2	Liposomes	EphA2	Advanced Solid tumors	I, Active, Not Recruiting	M.D. Anderson Cancer Center	01591356	[113]
DCR-PHXC-101	Lipid-based NPs	Myc	Solid tumors	Terminated	Dicerna Pharmaceuticals	02110563	[114]
Atu027	Liposomes	Protein kinase 3	Solid tumors	I, Completed	Silence Therapeutics GmbH	00938574	[110]
ALN-VSP	Lipid-based NPs	VEGF, KSP	Solid tumors	I, completed Completed	Alnylam Pharmaceuticals	00882180 01158079	[115,116]
TKM-080301	Lipid NPs	PLK1	Advanced Solid tumors	II, completed	Arbutus Biopharma Corporation	01262235 02191878	[117,118]

For clinical evaluation of siRNA-based therapy, clinical trials must monitor and provide data on RNA-NP pharmacokinetics/pharmacodynamics, dosage and dose frequency, administration route, immunogenicity, bioavailability, biodistribution, biodegradation, and elimination pathway for FDA review as well as the physiochemical properties of the RNA-NP, including charge, size, and how it reacts to environmental factors such as pH, salt concentration, and temperature. In addition, the manufacturing processes and controls, such as stability, sensitivity, and purity/quality of the RNA-NPs during production and storage, must be assessed. The RNA-NP's safety and efficacy depend on the targeted disease, but the treatment should have a significant therapeutic effect with minimal adverse side effects. Due to the extensive preclinical and clinical assessments required, along with the variation in acceptable efficacy and safety parameters, the number of FDA-approved RNA-NPs is currently limited [119–121].

Despite these challenges, three RNA-NPs have successfully met these requirements and gained FDA approval for public use in the United States. One of these is Onpattro® (or patisiran), developed by Alnylam Pharmaceuticals Inc., which treats polyneuropathy associated with autosomal dominant hereditary transthyretin amyloidosis (hATTR). Onpattro® consists of liposome-encapsulated siRNA that inhibits the expression of transthyretin (TTR), a protein released by the liver to transport thyroid hormone, which can undergo mutations causing hATTR [122]. Onpattro® liposomes contain DLin-MC3-DMA (MC3), cholesterol, 1,2-distearoyl-sn-glycero-3-phosphocholine (DSPC), and PEG, with a diameter range of 60–100 nm [123]. After intravenous (IV) administration, Onpattro® NPs localize in the liver via the RES, where they release siRNA in hepatocytes to inhibit TTR production and secretion. A crucial factor contributing to Onpattro's® success is the incorporation of the pH-sensitive ionizable lipid MC3. As the pKa of MC3 is ~6.5, matching the pH of the late endosome/lysosome, the liposome can fuse to the endosomal membrane after uptake and release therapeutic siRNA into the cytoplasm [124]. However, the need for IV infusion every three weeks limits the ease and widespread use of this RNA-NP therapy, even though it can suppress TTR expression by >80% [121,124].

While a few RNA-NPs have demonstrated success in clinical settings, most RNA-NPs do not progress through or complete clinical trials due to safety concerns and toxicity observed in both non-human primates and humans. To address these challenges and enhance the successful translation of RNA-NPs into clinical applications, there is a need for reliable methods to effectively and stably incorporate RNA, ensuring a low surface charge post-incorporation. Additionally, RNA-NPs should possess high stability, have a diameter of less than 100 nm to facilitate optimal cellular uptake, and be manufactured through established, large-scale, sterile processes [27].

5. Conclusions and Future Perspective

Breast cancer therapy utilizing lipid-based nanosystems significantly improves the delivery of siRNA to tumor cells. This approach has important advantages such as low therapeutic doses, reduced cytotoxicity to healthy cells, and inhibition of resistance to chemotherapy. Lipid-based nanosystems delivering siRNA to tumor cells can regulate the expression levels of genes associated with cell growth, proliferation, cell death, invasion, and metastasis. Fabrication of novel lipid-based siRNA nanosystems and novel targeting ligands may enhance breast cancer therapy as well as treatments for other diseases [125].

Recently, four siRNA drugs (patisiran, givosiran, lumasiran, and inclisiran) have received FDA approval for various diseases. siRNA drugs are in various phases of clinical trials based on different delivery systems and have been used to cover a wide range of pathologies including breast cancer [126].

Lipid nanosystems have enhanced the therapeutic potential of siRNA in several cancers including breast cancer. LNPs such as liposomes SLN, NLS, and NEs are suitable for incorporation of the siRNA. LNPs have efficiently delivered the siRNA drugs by stabilizing nucleic acid, extending the use of siRNA for numerous applications, and enhancing therapy for breast cancer. For further improvement in bioavailability, enhanced circulation in the blood, delivery to the target organ, surface functionalization of LNPs such as PEGylation, and introduction of surface ligands on the LNPs have all been effective approaches. Engineered strategies to 'shed' the incorporated targeting/functional moieties may improve the therapeutic effects once the carrier reaches its target [18].

Bone marrow deposition of LNPs utilized to treat solid tumors may prompt immune activation that could contribute to the antitumor effect and hinder the biodistribution of LNPs to tumors and reduce the therapeutic effect from immune activation [18].

siRNA-loaded NPs have shown promise due to their potential for gene silencing effects in cancer therapy. However, monitoring of in vivo release and distribution of siRNA is still challenging. To improve monitoring, the use of different imaging techniques, such as fluorescence imaging and CT imaging, may be an effective approach [127].

The LNP consisting of ionizable lipid, helper lipid, cholesterol, and PEG-encored lipid can stably encapsulate siRNA and improve release into the cytoplasm. Recently, noteworthy advancements were made in LNP research starting from the modification of LNP constituents, their formulation, and their application in breast cancer therapy to create a desirable composition and size, with a high siRNA encapsulation efficiency and a saleable product [128].

Lipid-based nanosystems are a promising strategy for siRNA delivery to breast tumors. These nanosystems can encapsulate siRNA efficiently, shield it from degradation, and deliver it effectively to cancer cells. Research focusing on siRNA delivery to breast tumors in a combination of multiple modalities to utilize the advantages of different delivery systems minimizing the off-target effects can combat breast cancer to save lives by reducing mortality rates.

Lipid-based nanocarriers such as SLNPs, liposomes, NLCs, and conjugates may be developed specifically for enhanced siRNA delivery and improved in vivo efficacy. Lipid-based NPs utilized for therapeutic approaches for siRNA delivery may be effectively used for targeting specific genetic elements of breast and other cancer cells leading to precise and efficient killing of cancer cells to inhibit gene expression or translation of cancer-allied proteins, reducing cell proliferation and tumor growth. This approach may improve greatly the stability and circulation time of siRNA molecules in the body, permitting more efficient therapeutic targeting of cancer cells with a potential to regulate the tumor microenvironment with decreased tumor immunosuppression.

Author Contributions: M.A.S. conceived idea and designed the study. M.A.S. and N.F. prepared the manuscript and revised it. V.P.T. contributed to manuscript revisions and supervised the overall study. All authors have read and agreed to the published version of the manuscript.

Funding: This research received no external funding.

Institutional Review Board Statement: Not applicable.

Informed Consent Statement: Not applicable.

Data Availability Statement: Not applicable.

Acknowledgments: William Hartner of CPBN, Northeastern University, Boston, MA, USA is gratefully acknowledged for his help during the preparation of the manuscript.

Conflicts of Interest: The authors declare no conflict of interest.

References

1. Silva-Cázares, M.B.; Saavedra-Leos, M.Z.; Jordan-Alejandre, E.; Nuñez-Olvera, S.I.; Cómpean-Martínez, I.; López-Camarillo, C. Lipid-based nanoparticles for the therapeutic delivery of non-coding RNAs in breast cancer (Review). *Oncol. Rep.* **2020**, *44*, 2353–2363. [CrossRef] [PubMed]
2. Breast Cancer Statistics and Resources. Available online: https://www.bcrf.org/breast-cancer-statistics-and-resources/ (accessed on 7 June 2023).
3. Bray, F.; Ferlay, J.; Soerjomataram, I.; Siegel, R.L.; Torre, L.A.; Jemal, A. Global cancer statistics 2018: GLOBOCAN estimates of incidence and mortality worldwide for 36 cancers in 185 countries. *CA Cancer J. Clin.* **2018**, *68*, 394–424. [CrossRef] [PubMed]
4. Cronin, K.A.; Lake, A.J.; Scott, S.; Sherman, R.L.; Noone, A.M.; Howlader, N.; Henley, S.J.; Anderson, R.N.; Firth, A.U.; Ma, J.; et al. Annual Report to the Nation on the Status of Cancer, part I: National cancer statistics. *Cancer* **2018**, *124*, 2785–2800. [CrossRef] [PubMed]
5. Miller, K.D.; Nogueira, L.; Mariotto, A.B.; Rowland, J.H.; Yabroff, K.R.; Alfano, C.M.; Jemal, A.; Kramer, J.L.; Siegel, R.L. Cancer treatment and survivorship statistics, 2019. *CA Cancer J. Clin.* **2019**, *69*, 363–385. [CrossRef]
6. Faltus, T.; Yuan, J.; Zimmer, B.; Krämer, A.; Loibl, S.; Kaufmann, M.; Strebhardt, K. Silencing of the HER2/neu gene by siRNA inhibits proliferation and induces apoptosis in HER2/neu-overexpressing breast cancer cells. *Neoplasia* **2004**, *6*, 786–795. [CrossRef]
7. Parmar, M.B.; Aliabadi, H.M.; Mahdipoor, P.; Kucharski, C.; Maranchuk, R.; Hugh, J.C.; Uludağ, H. Targeting Cell Cycle Proteins in Breast Cancer Cells with siRNA by Using Lipid-Substituted Polyethylenimines. *Front. Bioeng. Biotechnol.* **2015**, *3*, 14. [CrossRef]
8. Johnson, N.; Shapiro, G.I. Cyclin-dependent kinases (cdks) and the DNA damage response: Rationale for cdk inhibitor-chemotherapy combinations as an anticancer strategy for solid tumors. *Expert Opin. Ther. Targets* **2010**, *14*, 1199–1212. [CrossRef]
9. Ayoub, N.M.; Jaradat, S.K.; Al-Shami, K.M.; Alkhalifa, A.E. Targeting Angiogenesis in Breast Cancer: Current Evidence and Future Perspectives of Novel Anti-Angiogenic Approaches. *Front. Pharmacol.* **2022**, *13*, 838133. [CrossRef]
10. Kobayashi, Y.; Fukuhara, D.; Akase, D.; Aida, M.; Ui-Tei, K. siRNA Seed Region Is Divided into Two Functionally Different Domains in RNA Interference in Response to 2′-OMe Modifications. *ACS Omega* **2022**, *7*, 2398–2410. [CrossRef]
11. Abdelrahim, M.; Safe, S.; Baker, C.; Abudayyeh, A. RNAi and cancer: Implications and applications. *J. RNAi Gene Silenc.* **2006**, *2*, 136–145.
12. Ewert, K.K.; Zidovska, A.; Ahmad, A.; Bouxsein, N.F.; Evans, H.M.; McAllister, C.S.; Samuel, C.E.; Safinya, C.R. Cationic liposome-nucleic acid complexes for gene delivery and silencing: Pathways and mechanisms for plasmid DNA and siRNA. *Top. Curr. Chem.* **2010**, *296*, 191–226. [CrossRef]
13. Barua, S.; Mitragotri, S. Challenges associated with Penetration of Nanoparticles across Cell and Tissue Barriers: A Review of Current Status and Future Prospects. *Nano Today* **2014**, *9*, 223–243. [CrossRef] [PubMed]
14. Sun, D.; Lu, Z.R. Structure and Function of Cationic and Ionizable Lipids for Nucleic Acid Delivery. *Pharm. Res.* **2023**, *40*, 27–46. [CrossRef] [PubMed]
15. Schroeder, A.; Levins, C.G.; Cortez, C.; Langer, R.; Anderson, D.G. Lipid-based nanotherapeutics for siRNA delivery. *J. Intern. Med.* **2010**, *267*, 9–21. [CrossRef] [PubMed]
16. Hald Albertsen, C.; Kulkarni, J.A.; Witzigmann, D.; Lind, M.; Petersson, K.; Simonsen, J.B. The role of lipid components in lipid nanoparticles for vaccines and gene therapy. *Adv. Drug Deliv. Rev.* **2022**, *188*, 114416. [CrossRef]
17. Suk, J.S.; Xu, Q.; Kim, N.; Hanes, J.; Ensign, L.M. PEGylation as a strategy for improving nanoparticle-based drug and gene delivery. *Adv. Drug Deliv. Rev.* **2016**, *99*, 28–51. [CrossRef]
18. Kalita, T.; Dezfouli, S.A.; Pandey, L.M.; Uludag, H. siRNA Functionalized Lipid Nanoparticles (LNPs) in Management of Diseases. *Pharmaceutics* **2022**, *14*, 2520. [CrossRef] [PubMed]
19. Jung, H.N.; Lee, S.Y.; Lee, S.; Youn, H.; Im, H.J. Lipid nanoparticles for delivery of RNA therapeutics: Current status and the role of in vivo imaging. *Theranostics* **2022**, *12*, 7509–7531. [CrossRef] [PubMed]
20. Yonezawa, S.; Koide, H.; Asai, T. Recent advances in siRNA delivery mediated by lipid-based nanoparticles. *Adv. Drug Deliv. Rev.* **2020**, *154–155*, 64–78. [CrossRef]
21. Sato, Y.; Hatakeyama, H.; Sakurai, Y.; Hyodo, M.; Akita, H.; Harashima, H. A pH-sensitive cationic lipid facilitates the delivery of liposomal siRNA and gene silencing activity in vitro and in vivo. *J. Control. Release* **2012**, *163*, 267–276. [CrossRef]
22. Tenchov, R.; Bird, R.; Curtze, A.E.; Zhou, Q. Lipid Nanoparticles—From Liposomes to mRNA Vaccine Delivery, a Landscape of Research Diversity and Advancement. *ACS Nano* **2021**, *15*, 16982–17015. [CrossRef] [PubMed]

23. Hou, X.; Zaks, T.; Langer, R.; Dong, Y. Lipid nanoparticles for mRNA delivery. *Nat. Rev. Mater.* **2021**, *6*, 1078–1094. [CrossRef] [PubMed]

24. Gujrati, M.; Malamas, A.; Shin, T.; Jin, E.; Sun, Y.; Lu, Z.-R. Multifunctional Cationic Lipid-Based Nanoparticles Facilitate Endosomal Escape and Reduction-Triggered Cytosolic siRNA Release. *Mol. Pharm.* **2014**, *11*, 2734–2744. [CrossRef] [PubMed]

25. Singh, P.; Muhammad, I.j.; Nelson, N.E.; Tran, K.T.M.; Vinikoor, T.; Chorsi, M.T.; D'Orio, E.; Nguyen, T.D. Transdermal delivery for gene therapy. *Drug Deliv. Transl. Res.* **2022**, *12*, 2613–2633. [CrossRef]

26. Yang, J.P.; Huang, L. Time-dependent maturation of cationic liposome-DNA complex for serum resistance. *Gene Ther.* **1998**, *5*, 380–387. [CrossRef]

27. Akinc, A.; Maier, M.A.; Manoharan, M.; Fitzgerald, K.; Jayaraman, M.; Barros, S.; Ansell, S.; Du, X.; Hope, M.J.; Madden, T.D.; et al. The Onpattro story and the clinical translation of nanomedicines containing nucleic acid-based drugs. *Nat. Nanotechnol.* **2019**, *14*, 1084–1087. [CrossRef]

28. Del Pozo-Rodríguez, A.; Solinís, M.; Rodríguez-Gascón, A. Applications of lipid nanoparticles in gene therapy. *Eur. J. Pharm. Biopharm.* **2016**, *109*, 184–193. [CrossRef]

29. Yingchoncharoen, P.; Kalinowski, D.S.; Richardson, D.R. Lipid-Based Drug Delivery Systems in Cancer Therapy: What Is Available and What Is Yet to Come. *Pharmacol. Rev.* **2016**, *68*, 701–787. [CrossRef]

30. Hashemi, M.; Kalalinia, F. Application of encapsulation technology in stem cell therapy. *Life Sci.* **2015**, *143*, 139–146. [CrossRef]

31. Reichmuth, A.M.; Oberli, M.A.; Jaklenec, A.; Langer, R.; Blankschtein, D. mRNA vaccine delivery using lipid nanoparticles. *Ther. Deliv.* **2016**, *7*, 319–334. [CrossRef]

32. de la Harpe, K.M.; Kondiah, P.P.D.; Choonara, Y.E.; Marimuthu, T.; du Toit, L.C.; Pillay, V. The Hemocompatibility of Nanoparticles: A Review of Cell-Nanoparticle Interactions and Hemostasis. *Cells* **2019**, *8*, 1209. [CrossRef]

33. Buzea, C.; Pacheco, I.I.; Robbie, K. Nanomaterials and nanoparticles: Sources and toxicity. *Biointerphases* **2007**, *2*, MR17–MR71. [CrossRef] [PubMed]

34. Huang, Y.; Gao, X.; Chen, J. Leukocyte-derived biomimetic nanoparticulate drug delivery systems for cancer therapy. *Acta Pharm. Sin. B* **2018**, *8*, 4–13. [CrossRef] [PubMed]

35. Huynh, A.B.; Madu, C.O.; Lu, Y. siRNA: A Promising New Tool for Future Breast Cancer Therapy. *Oncomedicine* **2018**, *3*, 74–81. [CrossRef]

36. Singh, A.; Trivedi, P.; Jain, N.K. Advances in siRNA delivery in cancer therapy. *Artif. Cells Nanomed. Biotechnol.* **2018**, *46*, 274–283. [CrossRef]

37. Wang, X.; Yu, B.; Wu, Y.; Lee, R.J.; Lee, L.J. Efficient down-regulation of CDK4 by novel lipid nanoparticle-mediated siRNA delivery. *Anticancer Res.* **2011**, *31*, 1619–1626.

38. Tang, J.; Howard, C.B.; Mahler, S.M.; Thurecht, K.J.; Huang, L.; Xu, Z.P. Enhanced delivery of siRNA to triple negative breast cancer cells in vitro and in vivo through functionalizing lipid-coated calcium phosphate nanoparticles with dual target ligands. *Nanoscale* **2018**, *10*, 4258–4266. [CrossRef]

39. Yu, Y.H.; Kim, E.; Park, D.E.; Shim, G.; Lee, S.; Kim, Y.B.; Kim, C.W.; Oh, Y.K. Cationic solid lipid nanoparticles for co-delivery of paclitaxel and siRNA. *Eur. J. Pharm. Biopharm.* **2012**, *80*, 268–273. [CrossRef]

40. Sun, T.M.; Du, J.Z.; Yao, Y.D.; Mao, C.Q.; Dou, S.; Huang, S.Y.; Zhang, P.Z.; Leong, K.W.; Song, E.W.; Wang, J. Simultaneous delivery of siRNA and paclitaxel via a "two-in-one" micelleplex promotes synergistic tumor suppression. *ACS Nano* **2011**, *5*, 1483–1494. [CrossRef]

41. Yu, S.; Bi, X.; Yang, L.; Wu, S.; Yu, Y.; Jiang, B.; Zhang, A.; Lan, K.; Duan, S. Co-Delivery of Paclitaxel and PLK1-Targeted siRNA Using Aptamer-Functionalized Cationic Liposome for Synergistic Anti-Breast Cancer Effects In Vivo. *J. Biomed. Nanotechnol.* **2019**, *15*, 1135–1148. [CrossRef]

42. Wang, W.; Shao, A.; Zhang, N.; Fang, J.; Ruan, J.J.; Ruan, B.H. Cationic Polymethacrylate-Modified Liposomes Significantly Enhanced Doxorubicin Delivery and Antitumor Activity. *Sci. Rep.* **2017**, *7*, 43036. [CrossRef]

43. Golkar, N.; Samani, S.M.; Tamaddon, A.M. Data on cell growth inhibition induced by anti-VEGF siRNA delivered by Stealth liposomes incorporating G2 PAMAM-cholesterol versus Metafectene® as a function of exposure time and siRNA concentration. *Data Brief* **2016**, *8*, 1018–1023. [CrossRef] [PubMed]

44. Chen, J.; Sun, X.; Shao, R.; Xu, Y.; Gao, J.; Liang, W. VEGF siRNA delivered by polycation liposome-encapsulated calcium phosphate nanoparticles for tumor angiogenesis inhibition in breast cancer. *Int. J. Nanomed.* **2017**, *12*, 6075–6088. [CrossRef] [PubMed]

45. Johnston, M.J.; Semple, S.C.; Klimuk, S.K.; Edwards, K.; Eisenhardt, M.L.; Leng, E.C.; Karlsson, G.; Yanko, D.; Cullis, P.R. Therapeutically optimized rates of drug release can be achieved by varying the drug-to-lipid ratio in liposomal vincristine formulations. *Biochim. Biophys. Acta* **2006**, *1758*, 55–64. [CrossRef] [PubMed]

46. Guo, P.; You, J.O.; Yang, J.; Jia, D.; Moses, M.A.; Auguste, D.T. Inhibiting metastatic breast cancer cell migration via the synergy of targeted, pH-triggered siRNA delivery and chemokine axis blockade. *Mol. Pharm.* **2014**, *11*, 755–765. [CrossRef]

47. Sun, S.; Xu, Y.; Fu, P.; Chen, M.; Sun, S.; Zhao, R.; Wang, J.; Liang, X.; Wang, S. Ultrasound-targeted photodynamic and gene dual therapy for effectively inhibiting triple negative breast cancer by cationic porphyrin lipid microbubbles loaded with HIF1α-siRNA. *Nanoscale* **2018**, *10*, 19945–19956. [CrossRef]

48. Tang, J.; Li, B.; Howard, C.B.; Mahler, S.M.; Thurecht, K.J.; Wu, Y.; Huang, L.; Xu, Z.P. Multifunctional lipid-coated calcium phosphate nanoplatforms for complete inhibition of large triple negative breast cancer via targeted combined therapy. *Biomaterials* **2019**, *216*, 119232. [CrossRef]

49. Ghasemiyeh, P.; Mohammadi-Samani, S. Solid lipid nanoparticles and nanostructured lipid carriers as novel drug delivery systems: Applications, advantages and disadvantages. *Res. Pharm. Sci.* **2018**, *13*, 288–303. [CrossRef]

50. Okamoto, A.; Asai, T.; Kato, H.; Ando, H.; Minamino, T.; Mekada, E.; Oku, N. Antibody-modified lipid nanoparticles for selective delivery of siRNA to tumors expressing membrane-anchored form of HB-EGF. *Biochem. Biophys. Res. Commun.* **2014**, *449*, 460–465. [CrossRef]

51. Okamoto, A.; Asai, T.; Hirai, Y.; Shimizu, K.; Koide, H.; Minamino, T.; Oku, N. Systemic Administration of siRNA with Anti-HB-EGF Antibody-Modified Lipid Nanoparticles for the Treatment of Triple-Negative Breast Cancer. *Mol. Pharm.* **2018**, *15*, 1495–1504. [CrossRef]

52. Yotsumoto, F.; Oki, E.; Tokunaga, E.; Maehara, Y.; Kuroki, M.; Miyamoto, S. HB-EGF orchestrates the complex signals involved in triple-negative and trastuzumab-resistant breast cancer. *Int. J. Cancer* **2010**, *127*, 2707–2717. [CrossRef] [PubMed]

53. Shen, J.; Liu, H.; Mu, C.; Wolfram, J.; Zhang, W.; Kim, H.C.; Zhu, G.; Hu, Z.; Ji, L.N.; Liu, X.; et al. Multi-step encapsulation of chemotherapy and gene silencing agents in functionalized mesoporous silica nanoparticles. *Nanoscale* **2017**, *9*, 5329–5341. [CrossRef] [PubMed]

54. Yang, Z.; Liu, T.; Xie, Y.; Sun, Z.; Liu, H.; Lin, J.; Liu, C.; Mao, Z.W.; Nie, S. Chitosan layered gold nanorods as synergistic therapeutics for photothermal ablation and gene silencing in triple-negative breast cancer. *Acta Biomater.* **2015**, *25*, 194–204. [CrossRef] [PubMed]

55. Parvani, J.G.; Gujrati, M.D.; Mack, M.A.; Schiemann, W.P.; Lu, Z.R. Silencing β3 Integrin by Targeted ECO/siRNA Nanoparticles Inhibits EMT and Metastasis of Triple-Negative Breast Cancer. *Cancer Res.* **2015**, *75*, 2316–2325. [CrossRef]

56. Wahlgren, J.; De, L.K.T.; Brisslert, M.; Vaziri Sani, F.; Telemo, E.; Sunnerhagen, P.; Valadi, H. Plasma exosomes can deliver exogenous short interfering RNA to monocytes and lymphocytes. *Nucleic Acids Res.* **2012**, *40*, e130. [CrossRef]

57. Kamerkar, S.; LeBleu, V.S.; Sugimoto, H.; Yang, S.; Ruivo, C.F.; Melo, S.A.; Lee, J.J.; Kalluri, R. Exosomes facilitate therapeutic targeting of oncogenic KRAS in pancreatic cancer. *Nature* **2017**, *546*, 498–503. [CrossRef]

58. Yang, Y.; Wang, Q.; Zou, H.; Chou, C.K.; Chen, X. Exosome-Modified Liposomes Targeted Delivery of Thalidomide to Regulate Treg Cells for Antitumor Immunotherapy. *Pharmaceutics* **2023**, *15*, 1074. [CrossRef]

59. Abuhelal, S.; Centelles, M.N.; Wright, M.; Mason, A.J.; Thanou, M. Development of Cationic Lipid LAH4-L1 siRNA Complexes for Focused Ultrasound Enhanced Tumor Uptake. *Mol. Pharm.* **2023**, *20*, 2341–2351. [CrossRef]

60. Nguyen, T.H.; Hanley, T.; Porter, C.J.; Larson, I.; Boyd, B.J. Phytantriol and glyceryl monooleate cubic liquid crystalline phases as sustained-release oral drug delivery systems for poorly water-soluble drugs II. In-vivo evaluation. *J. Pharm. Pharmacol.* **2010**, *62*, 856–865. [CrossRef]

61. Karami, Z.; Hamidi, M. Cubosomes: Remarkable drug delivery potential. *Drug Discov. Today* **2016**, *21*, 789–801. [CrossRef]

62. Pramanik, A.; Xu, Z.; Ingram, N.; Coletta, P.L.; Millner, P.A.; Tyler, A.I.I.; Hughes, T.A. Hyaluronic-Acid-Tagged Cubosomes Deliver Cytotoxics Specifically to CD44-Positive Cancer Cells. *Mol. Pharm.* **2022**, *19*, 4601–4611. [CrossRef] [PubMed]

63. Pramanik, A.; Xu, Z.; Shamsuddin, S.H.; Khaled, Y.S.; Ingram, N.; Maisey, T.; Tomlinson, D.; Coletta, P.L.; Jayne, D.; Hughes, T.A.; et al. Affimer Tagged Cubosomes: Targeting of Carcinoembryonic Antigen Expressing Colorectal Cancer Cells Using In Vitro and In Vivo Models. *ACS Appl. Mater. Interfaces* **2022**, *14*, 11078–11091. [CrossRef] [PubMed]

64. Liu, Y.; Zhu, Y.H.; Mao, C.Q.; Dou, S.; Shen, S.; Tan, Z.B.; Wang, J. Triple negative breast cancer therapy with CDK1 siRNA delivered by cationic lipid assisted PEG-PLA nanoparticles. *J. Control. Release* **2014**, *192*, 114–121. [CrossRef] [PubMed]

65. Pradhan, R.; Dey, A.; Taliyan, R.; Puri, A.; Kharavtekar, S.; Dubey, S.K. Recent Advances in Targeted Nanocarriers for the Management of Triple Negative Breast Cancer. *Pharmaceutics* **2023**, *15*, 246. [CrossRef] [PubMed]

66. Alshaer, W.; Hillaireau, H.; Vergnaud, J.; Mura, S.; Deloménie, C.; Sauvage, F.; Ismail, S.; Fattal, E. Aptamer-guided siRNA-loaded nanomedicines for systemic gene silencing in CD-44 expressing murine triple-negative breast cancer model. *J. Control. Release* **2018**, *271*, 98–106. [CrossRef]

67. Mansoori, B.; Sandoghchian Shotorbani, S.; Baradaran, B. RNA interference and its role in cancer therapy. *Adv. Pharm. Bull.* **2014**, *4*, 313–321. [CrossRef]

68. Mainini, F.; Eccles, M.R. Lipid and Polymer-Based Nanoparticle siRNA Delivery Systems for Cancer Therapy. *Molecules* **2020**, *25*, 2692. [CrossRef]

69. Han, X.; Mitchell, M.J.; Nie, G. Nanomaterials for Therapeutic RNA Delivery. *Matter* **2020**, *3*, 1948–1975. [CrossRef]

70. Kumar, A.; Singam, A.; Swaminathan, G.; Killi, N.; Tangudu, N.K.; Jose, J.; Gundloori Vn, R.; Dinesh Kumar, L. Combinatorial therapy using RNAi and curcumin nano-architectures regresses tumors in breast and colon cancer models. *Nanoscale* **2022**, *14*, 492–505. [CrossRef]

71. Juliano, R.L. The delivery of therapeutic oligonucleotides. *Nucleic Acids Res.* **2016**, *44*, 6518–6548. [CrossRef]

72. Xin, Y.; Huang, M.; Guo, W.W.; Huang, Q.; Zhang, L.Z.; Jiang, G. Nano-based delivery of RNAi in cancer therapy. *Mol. Cancer* **2017**, *16*, 134. [CrossRef] [PubMed]

73. Malone, R.W.; Felgner, P.L.; Verma, I.M. Cationic liposome-mediated RNA transfection. *Proc. Natl. Acad. Sci. USA* **1989**, *86*, 6077–6081. [CrossRef] [PubMed]

74. Semple, S.C.; Klimuk, S.K.; Harasym, T.O.; Dos Santos, N.; Ansell, S.M.; Wong, K.F.; Maurer, N.; Stark, H.; Cullis, P.R.; Hope, M.J.; et al. Efficient encapsulation of antisense oligonucleotides in lipid vesicles using ionizable aminolipids: Formation of novel small multilamellar vesicle structures. *Biochim. Biophys. Acta BBA-Biomembr.* **2001**, *1510*, 152–166. [CrossRef] [PubMed]

75. Jayaraman, M.; Ansell, S.M.; Mui, B.L.; Tam, Y.K.; Chen, J.; Du, X.; Butler, D.; Eltepu, L.; Matsuda, S.; Narayanannair, J.K.; et al. Maximizing the Potency of siRNA Lipid Nanoparticles for Hepatic Gene Silencing In Vivo. *Angew. Chem. Int. Ed.* **2012**, *51*, 8529–8533. [CrossRef]

76. Zhou, Y.; Zhou, G.; Tian, C.; Jiang, W.; Jin, L.; Zhang, C.; Chen, X. Exosome-mediated small RNA delivery for gene therapy. *WIREs RNA* **2016**, *7*, 758–771. [CrossRef]

77. Elouahabi, A.; Ruysschaert, J.M. Formation and intracellular trafficking of lipoplexes and polyplexes. *Mol. Ther.* **2005**, *11*, 336–347. [CrossRef]

78. Sarisozen, C.; Salzano, G.; Torchilin, V.P. Recent advances in siRNA delivery. *Biomol. Concepts* **2015**, *6*, 321–341. [CrossRef]

79. Ozpolat, B.; Sood, A.K.; Lopez-Berestein, G. Liposomal siRNA nanocarriers for cancer therapy. *Adv. Drug Deliv. Rev.* **2014**, *66*, 110–116. [CrossRef]

80. Gasco, M.R. Lipid nanoparticles: Perspectives and challenges. *Adv. Drug Deliv. Rev.* **2007**, *59*, 377–378. [CrossRef]

81. Müller, R.H. Lipid nanoparticles: Recent advances. *Adv. Drug Deliv. Rev.* **2007**, *59*, 375–376. [CrossRef]

82. Jorge, A.; Pais, A.; Vitorino, C. Targeted siRNA Delivery Using Lipid Nanoparticles. *Methods Mol. Biol.* **2020**, *2059*, 259–283. [CrossRef] [PubMed]

83. Hadinoto, K.; Sundaresan, A.; Cheow, W.S. Lipid-polymer hybrid nanoparticles as a new generation therapeutic delivery platform: A review. *Eur. J. Pharm. Biopharm.* **2013**, *85*, 427–443. [CrossRef] [PubMed]

84. Li, Y.; Jarvis, R.; Zhu, K.; Glass, Z.; Ogurlu, R.; Gao, P.; Li, P.; Chen, J.; Yu, Y.; Yang, Y.; et al. Protein and mRNA Delivery Enabled by Cholesteryl-Based Biodegradable Lipidoid Nanoparticles. *Angew. Chem. Int. Ed. Engl.* **2020**, *59*, 14957–14964. [CrossRef]

85. Subhan, M.A.; Yalamarty, S.S.K.; Filipczak, N.; Parveen, F.; Torchilin, V.P. Recent Advances in Tumor Targeting via EPR Effect for Cancer Treatment. *J. Pers. Med.* **2021**, *11*, 571. [CrossRef]

86. Ball, R.L.; Hajj, K.A.; Vizelman, J.; Bajaj, P.; Whitehead, K.A. Lipid Nanoparticle Formulations for Enhanced Co-Delivery of siRNA and mRNA. *Nano Lett.* **2018**, *18*, 3814–3822. [CrossRef] [PubMed]

87. Press, A.T.; Traeger, A.; Pietsch, C.; Mosig, A.; Wagner, M.; Clemens, M.G.; Jbeily, N.; Koch, N.; Gottschaldt, M.; Bézière, N.; et al. Cell type-specific delivery of short interfering RNAs by dye-functionalised theranostic nanoparticles. *Nat. Commun.* **2014**, *5*, 5565. [CrossRef] [PubMed]

88. Bartlett, D.W.; Su, H.; Hildebrandt, I.J.; Weber, W.A.; Davis, M.E. Impact of tumor-specific targeting on the biodistribution and efficacy of siRNA nanoparticles measured by multimodality in vivoimaging. *Proc. Natl. Acad. Sci. USA* **2007**, *104*, 15549–15554. [CrossRef] [PubMed]

89. Wilhelm, S.; Tavares, A.J.; Dai, Q.; Ohta, S.; Audet, J.; Dvorak, H.F.; Chan, W.C.W. Analysis of nanoparticle delivery to tumours. *Nat. Rev. Mater.* **2016**, *1*, 16014. [CrossRef]

90. Gabel, M.; Knauss, A.; Fischer, D.; Neurath, M.F.; Weigmann, B. Surface Design Options in Polymer- and Lipid-Based siRNA Nanoparticles Using Antibodies. *Int. J. Mol. Sci.* **2022**, *23*, 13929. [CrossRef]

91. Chadar, R.; Afsana; Kesharwani, P. Nanotechnology-based siRNA delivery strategies for treatment of triple negative breast cancer. *Int. J. Pharm.* **2021**, *605*, 120835. [CrossRef]

92. Ashique, S.; Almohaywi, B.; Haider, N.; Yasmin, S.; Hussain, A.; Mishra, N.; Garg, A. siRNA-based nanocarriers for targeted drug delivery to control breast cancer. *Adv. Cancer Biol.-Metastasis* **2022**, *4*, 100047. [CrossRef]

93. Hattori, Y.; Tang, M.; Torii, S.; Tomita, K.; Sagawa, A.; Inoue, N.; Yamagishi, R.; Ozaki, K.I. Optimal combination of cationic lipid and phospholipid in cationic liposomes for gene knockdown in breast cancer cells and mouse lung using siRNA lipoplexes. *Mol. Med. Rep.* **2022**, *26*, 253. [CrossRef] [PubMed]

94. Bulbake, U.; Kommineni, N.; Bryszewska, M.; Ionov, M.; Khan, W. Cationic liposomes for co-delivery of paclitaxel and anti-Plk1 siRNA to achieve enhanced efficacy in breast cancer. *J. Drug Deliv. Sci. Technol.* **2018**, *48*, 253–265. [CrossRef]

95. Chen, X.; Zhang, Y.; Tang, C.; Tian, C.; Sun, Q.; Su, Z.; Xue, L.; Yin, Y.; Ju, C.; Zhang, C. Co-delivery of paclitaxel and anti-survivin siRNA via redox-sensitive oligopeptide liposomes for the synergistic treatment of breast cancer and metastasis. *Int. J. Pharm.* **2017**, *529*, 102–115. [CrossRef] [PubMed]

96. Li, M.; Li, S.; Li, Y.; Li, X.; Yang, G.; Li, M.; Xie, Y.; Su, W.; Wu, J.; Jia, L.; et al. Cationic liposomes co-deliver chemotherapeutics and siRNA for the treatment of breast cancer. *Eur. J. Med. Chem.* **2022**, *233*, 114198. [CrossRef]

97. Bedi, D.; Musacchio, T.; Fagbohun, O.A.; Gillespie, J.W.; Deinnocentes, P.; Bird, R.C.; Bookbinder, L.; Torchilin, V.P.; Petrenko, V.A. Delivery of siRNA into breast cancer cells via phage fusion protein-targeted liposomes. *Nanomedicine* **2011**, *7*, 315–323. [CrossRef]

98. Gote, V.; Pal, D. Octreotide-Targeted Lcn2 siRNA PEGylated Liposomes as a Treatment for Metastatic Breast Cancer. *Bioengineering* **2021**, *8*, 44. [CrossRef]

99. Kim, M.; Lee, J.S.; Kim, W.; Lee, J.H.; Jun, B.-H.; Kim, K.-S.; Kim, D.-E. Aptamer-conjugated nano-liposome for immunogenic chemotherapy with reversal of immunosuppression. *J. Control. Release* **2022**, *348*, 893–910. [CrossRef]

100. Li, X.; Zhou, X.; Liu, J.; Zhang, J.; Feng, Y.; Wang, F.; He, Y.; Wan, A.; Filipczak, N.; Yalamarty, S.S.K.; et al. Liposomal Co-delivery of PD-L1 siRNA/Anemoside B4 for Enhanced Combinational Immunotherapeutic Effect. *ACS Appl. Mater. Interfaces* **2022**, *14*, 28439–28454. [CrossRef]

101. Monirinasab, H.; Asadi, H.; Rostamizadeh, K.; Esmaeilzadeh, A.; Khodaei, M.; Fathi, M. Novel lipid-polymer hybrid nanoparticles for siRNA delivery and IGF-1R gene silencing in breast cancer cells. *J. Drug Deliv. Sci. Technol.* **2018**, *48*, 96–105. [CrossRef]

102. Yalamarty, S.S.K.; Filipczak, N.; Li, X.; Pathrikar, T.V.; Cotter, C.; Torchilin, V.P. Co-Delivery of siRNA and Chemotherapeutic Drug Using 2C5 Antibody-Targeted Dendrimer-Based Mixed Micelles for Multidrug Resistant Cancers. *Pharmaceutics* **2022**, *14*, 1470. [CrossRef] [PubMed]

103. Pan, J.; Mendes, L.P.; Yao, M.; Filipczak, N.; Garai, S.; Thakur, G.A.; Sarisozen, C.; Torchilin, V.P. Polyamidoamine dendrimers-based nanomedicine for combination therapy with siRNA and chemotherapeutics to overcome multidrug resistance. *Eur. J. Pharm. Biopharm.* **2019**, *136*, 18–28. [CrossRef] [PubMed]

104. Thi, T.T.H.; Suys, E.J.A.; Lee, J.S.; Nguyen, D.H.; Park, K.D.; Truong, N.P. Lipid-Based Nanoparticles in the Clinic and Clinical Trials: From Cancer Nanomedicine to COVID-19 Vaccines. *Vaccines* **2021**, *9*, 359. [CrossRef] [PubMed]

105. Namiot, E.D.; Sokolov, A.V.; Chubarev, V.N.; Tarasov, V.V.; Schiöth, H.B. Nanoparticles in Clinical Trials: Analysis of Clinical Trials, FDA Approvals and Use for COVID-19 Vaccines. *Int. J. Mol. Sci.* **2023**, *24*, 787. [CrossRef]

106. Marques, A.C.; Costa, P.C.; Velho, S.; Amaral, M.H. Lipid Nanoparticles Functionalized with Antibodies for Anticancer Drug Therapy. *Pharmaceutics* **2023**, *15*, 216. [CrossRef]

107. Eljack, S.; David, S.; Chourpa, I.; Faggad, A.; Allard-Vannier, E. Formulation of Lipid-Based Nanoparticles for Simultaneous Delivery of Lapatinib and Anti-Survivin siRNA for HER2+ Breast Cancer Treatment. *Pharmaceuticals* **2022**, *15*, 1452. [CrossRef]

108. Huang, J.; Xiao, K. Nanoparticles-Based Strategies to Improve the Delivery of Therapeutic Small Interfering RNA in Precision Oncology. *Pharmaceutics* **2022**, *14*, 1586. [CrossRef]

109. Wagner, M.J.; Mitra, R.; McArthur, M.J.; Baze, W.; Barnhart, K.; Wu, S.Y.; Rodriguez-Aguayo, C.; Zhang, X.; Coleman, R.L.; Lopez-Berestein, G.; et al. Preclinical Mammalian Safety Studies of EPHARNA (DOPC Nanoliposomal EphA2-Targeted siRNA). *Mol. Cancer Ther.* **2017**, *16*, 1114–1123. [CrossRef]

110. Schultheis, B.; Strumberg, D.; Santel, A.; Vank, C.; Gebhardt, F.; Keil, O.; Lange, C.; Giese, K.; Kaufmann, J.; Khan, M.; et al. First-in-human phase I study of the liposomal RNA interference therapeutic Atu027 in patients with advanced solid tumors. *J. Clin. Oncol.* **2014**, *32*, 4141–4148. [CrossRef]

111. Tabernero, J.; Shapiro, G.I.; LoRusso, P.M.; Cervantes, A.; Schwartz, G.K.; Weiss, G.J.; Paz-Ares, L.; Cho, D.C.; Infante, J.R.; Alsina, M.; et al. First-in-humans trial of an RNA interference therapeutic targeting VEGF and KSP in cancer patients with liver involvement. *Cancer Discov.* **2013**, *3*, 406–417. [CrossRef]

112. Tolcher, A.W.; Papadopoulos, K.P.; Patnaik, A.; Rasco, D.W.; Martinez, D.; Wood, D.L.; Fielman, B.; Sharma, M.; Janisch, L.A.; Brown, B.D.; et al. Safety and activity of DCR-MYC, a first-in-class Dicer-substrate small interfering RNA (DsiRNA) targeting MYC, in a phase I study in patients with advanced solid tumors. *J. Clin. Oncol.* **2015**, *33*, 11006. [CrossRef]

113. EphA2 siRNA in Treating Patients with Advanced or Recurrent Solid Tumors. Available online: https://classic.clinicaltrials.gov/ct2/show/NCT01591356 (accessed on 7 June 2023).

114. *Phase I, Multicenter, Cohort Dose Escalation Trial to Determine the Safety, Tolerance, and Maximum Tolerated Dose of DCR-MYC, a Lipid Nanoparticle (LNP)-Formulated Small Inhibitory RNA (siRNA) Oligonucleotide Targeting MYC, in Patients with Refractory Locally Advanced or Metastatic Solid Tumor Malignancies, Multiple Myeloma, or Lymphoma*; Adis International Ltd.: Auckland, New Zealand, 2017.

115. Dose Escalation Trial to Evaluate the Safety, Tolerability, Pharmacokinetics and Pharmacodynamics of Intravenous ALN-VSP02 in Patients with Advanced Solid Tumors with Liver Involvement. Available online: https://classic.clinicaltrials.gov/ct2/show/NCT00882180 (accessed on 7 June 2023).

116. Multi-Center, Open Label, Extension Study of ALN-VSP02 in Cancer Patients Who Have Responded to ALN-VSP02 Treatment. Available online: https://classic.clinicaltrials.gov/ct2/show/NCT01158079 (accessed on 7 June 2023).

117. El Dika, I.; Lim, H.Y.; Yong, W.P.; Lin, C.C.; Yoon, J.H.; Modiano, M.; Freilich, B.; Choi, H.J.; Chao, T.Y.; Kelley, R.K.; et al. An Open-Label, Multicenter, Phase I, Dose Escalation Study with Phase II Expansion Cohort to Determine the Safety, Pharmacokinetics, and Preliminary Antitumor Activity of Intravenous TKM-080301 in Subjects with Advanced Hepatocellular Carcinoma. *Oncologist* **2019**, *24*, 747-e218. [CrossRef] [PubMed]

118. A Dose Finding Study of TKM-080301 Infusion in Neuroendocrine Tumors (NET) and Adrenocortical Carcinoma (ACC) Patients. Available online: https://classic.clinicaltrials.gov/ct2/show/NCT01262235 (accessed on 7 June 2023).

119. Mahase, E. FDA allows drugs without proven clinical benefit to languish for years on accelerated pathway. *BMJ* **2021**, *374*, n1898. [CrossRef] [PubMed]

120. Brown, D.G.; Wobst, H.J. A Decade of FDA-Approved Drugs (2010–2019): Trends and Future Directions. *J. Med. Chem.* **2021**, *64*, 2312–2338. [CrossRef]

121. Lim, S.A.; Cox, A.; Tung, M.; Chung, E.J. Clinical progress of nanomedicine-based RNA therapies. *Bioact. Mater.* **2022**, *12*, 203–213. [CrossRef]

122. Urits, I.; Swanson, D.; Swett, M.C.; Patel, A.; Berardino, K.; Amgalan, A.; Berger, A.A.; Kassem, H.; Kaye, A.D.; Viswanath, O. A Review of Patisiran (ONPATTRO®) for the Treatment of Polyneuropathy in People with Hereditary Transthyretin Amyloidosis. *Neurol. Ther.* **2020**, *9*, 301–315. [CrossRef]

123. European Medicines Agency. Available online: https://www.ema.europa.eu/en/medicines/human/EPAR/onpattro (accessed on 1 July 2023).

124. Zhang, X.; Goel, V.; Attarwala, H.; Sweetser, M.T.; Clausen, V.A.; Robbie, G.J. Patisiran Pharmacokinetics, Pharmacodynamics, and Exposure-Response Analyses in the Phase 3 APOLLO Trial in Patients With Hereditary Transthyretin-Mediated (hATTR) Amyloidosis. *J. Clin. Pharmacol.* **2020**, *60*, 37–49. [CrossRef]

125. Ebenezer, O.; Comoglio, P.; Wong, G.K.; Tuszynski, J.A. Development of Novel siRNA Therapeutics: A Review with a Focus on Inclisiran for the Treatment of Hypercholesterolemia. *Int. J. Mol. Sci.* **2023**, *24*, 4019. [CrossRef]

126. Friedrich, M.; Aigner, A. Therapeutic siRNA: State-of-the-Art and Future Perspectives. *BioDrugs* **2022**, *36*, 549–571. [CrossRef]

127. Sun, L.; Zhang, J.; Zhou, J.E.; Wang, J.; Wang, Z.; Luo, S.; Wang, Y.; Zhu, S.; Yang, F.; Tang, J.; et al. Monitoring the in vivo siRNA release from lipid nanoparticles based on the fluorescence resonance energy transfer principle. *Asian J. Pharm. Sci.* **2023**, *18*, 100769. [CrossRef]

128. Seo, H.; Jeon, L.; Kwon, J.; Lee, H. High-Precision Synthesis of RNA-Loaded Lipid Nanoparticles for Biomedical Applications. *Adv. Healthc. Mater.* **2023**, *12*, e2203033. [CrossRef] [PubMed]

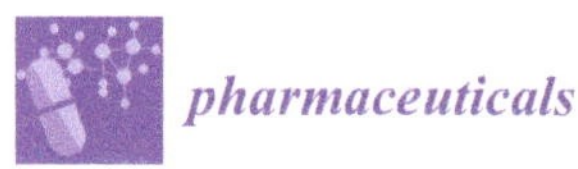

pharmaceuticals

MDPI

Review

Recent Progress of Solid Lipid Nanoparticles and Nanostructured Lipid Carriers as Ocular Drug Delivery Platforms

Viliana Gugleva * and Velichka Andonova

Department of Pharmaceutical Technologies, Faculty of Pharmacy, Medical University of Varna, 55 Marin Drinov Str., 9000 Varna, Bulgaria
* Correspondence: viliana.gugleva@mu-varna.bg

Abstract: Sufficient ocular bioavailability is often considered a challenge by the researchers, due to the complex structure of the eye and its protective physiological mechanisms. In addition, the low viscosity of the eye drops and the resulting short ocular residence time further contribute to the observed low drug concentration at the target site. Therefore, various drug delivery platforms are being developed to enhance ocular bioavailability, provide controlled and sustained drug release, reduce the number of applications, and maximize therapy outcomes. Solid lipid nanoparticles (SLNs) and nanostructured lipid carriers (NLCs) exhibit all these benefits, in addition to being biocompatible, biodegradable, and susceptible to sterilization and scale-up. Furthermore, their successive surface modification contributes to prolonged ocular residence time (by adding cationic compounds), enhanced penetration, and improved performance. The review highlights the salient characteristics of SLNs and NLCs concerning ocular drug delivery, and updates the research progress in this area.

Keywords: lipid nanoparticles; mucoadhesion; ocular bioavailability; surface modification

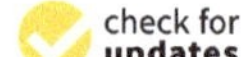

Citation: Gugleva, V.; Andonova, V. Recent Progress of Solid Lipid Nanoparticles and Nanostructured Lipid Carriers as Ocular Drug Delivery Platforms. *Pharmaceuticals* **2023**, *16*, 474. https://doi.org/10.3390/ph16030474

Academic Editors: Ana Catarina Silva, João Nuno Moreira and José Manuel Sousa Lobo

Received: 14 February 2023
Revised: 12 March 2023
Accepted: 20 March 2023
Published: 22 March 2023

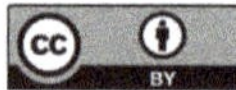

1. Introduction

According to World Health Organization, the prevalence of eye conditions is expected to increase in the following years as a result of population aging, the associated rise of non-communicable diseases (diabetes, cardiovascular diseases), along with various lifestyle factors, such as an unhealthy diet, smoking, extensive usage of digital devices, etc. [1–4]. Furthermore, a recent analysis for the Global Burden of Disease Study forecasts that by 2050, around 474 million people will suffer from moderate to severe visual impairments, among which 61 million will develop complete blindness [5]. Although the human eye is one of the most accessible organs in terms of drug application, efficient ocular delivery is still a goal to be achieved. Possible explanations lie in the anatomical and physiological characteristics of the eyeball and its protective mechanisms, as well as in the technological properties of the ocular formulations [6]. According to location, the human eye may be distinguished into two segments: anterior, presented by the cornea, conjunctiva, iris, ciliary body, lens, and aqueous humor, and posterior, consisting of the sclera, choroid, retina, vitreous humor, and optic nerve [7,8]. The preferred route of administration in ophthalmology—topical instillation—provides the possibility for treatment of anterior segment diseases such as blepharitis, dry eye disease, conjunctivitis, ocular infections or injuries [9], however, reaching the posterior part of the eye and ensuring sufficient therapeutic concentration thereby is still a challenge. Eye drops, representing the majority of ophthalmic formulations, are relatively easy for self-administration, characterized by high patient approval, cost-effectiveness, and well-established formulation and manufacturing processes [10]. Their main limitations include their intrinsic low viscosity, a short ocular contact time, and the relatively large volume of applied drops, often leading to drug loss via physiological pathways [11–13].

Additionally, ocular defense mechanisms such as reflex blinking, tear turnover, nasolacrimal drainage, and static and dynamic anatomical barriers further hinder drug absorption, resulting in less than 5% of the instilled dose attaining deeper ocular tissues [14,15]. In ocular surface diseases, drug bioavailability may be partially improved through modulating the formulations' viscosity, by including viscosity enhancers or using in situ gel-forming systems/semisolid dosage forms [16]. However, this strategy does not apply to posterior segment diseases. Unfortunately, diseases affecting the back part of the eye, e.g., age-related macular degeneration, diabetic retinopathy, and glaucoma, may often cause visual impairment or blindness unless treated efficiently [17,18]. The therapy of posterior segment eye diseases usually includes intravitreal injections, which enable drug delivery to the vitreous cavity. However, the invasive nature of this approach and the potential associated complications (e.g., endophthalmitis, retinal detachment) determine the low patient compliance [19,20]. Reaching the posterior segment via the peroral or intravenous route has also been associated with limited therapeutic success, due to the presence of blood–ocular barriers (the blood–retinal barrier, in particular), in addition to the potential risk of occurrence of side effects [21]. Altogether, these factors determine the necessity of further progress in the field of ocular delivery by improving the technological characteristics of conventional ophthalmic formulations, exploring advanced drug delivery systems, or combining both strategies.

Various nanoscale drug delivery systems, such as liposomes [22,23], niosomes [24,25], solid lipid/polymeric nanoparticles [26–29], nanostructured lipid carriers [30,31], nanomicelles [32,33], microemulsions [34,35], and dendrimers [36], have been successfully developed for ocular delivery purposes, and have been reported to achieve enhanced bioavailability, sustained and controlled drug release, and a reduction in the number of applications, as well as side effects. SLNs and NLCs raise great interest due to their excellent biocompatibility and tolerability, tunable physiochemical characteristics, and scaling-up capabilities [37–39]. Developed for the first in the 1990s by Professor Müller and Professor Gasco, SLNs represent a mixture of solids at ambient temperature and and lipids at physiological temperatures, dispersed in an aqueous phase containing surfactants [40,41]. Approximately 10 years later, a second generation of lipid nanoparticles was proposed—NLCs,—which additionally include liquid lipid(s) in their structure [42,43]. Both drug delivery systems are feasible carriers for hydrophilic and hydrophobic drugs. They are characterized by their long-term stability and favored uptake through biological membranes, owing to their lipid nature and nano dimensions [44,45]. The possibilities to impart mucoadhesiveness by surface coating with various polymers, or by incorporating them into semisolid/in situ gelling/formulations, further promotes their beneficial effects in ocular therapeutics.

The current review aimed to summarize the recent research progress of solid lipid nanoparticles and nanostructured lipid carriers in ocular delivery. In the first part, the anatomical and physiological features of the human eye and potential delivery routes have been discussed. The second part provides an overview of the specific characteristics of SLNs and NLCs, with respect to their compositions, suitable physicochemical properties tailored for effective ocular delivery, surface modification strategies, and sterilization feasibility. Recent advances in this area have also been outlined.

2. Eye Anatomy, Barriers and Routes in Ocular Drug Delivery

Generally, human eye structures are distinguished according to their location in the eyeball, where the eye is divided into two segments (anterior and posterior) (Figure 1A), or according to their functionalities, where it is divided into three different layers—an outer (fibrous), middle (vascular) and inner (neuronal) coat [46]. The outer layer (fibrous tunic) consists of the cornea (at its front) and sclera, occupying five-sixths of the coat [47]. Its main functions are related to maintaining the shape of the eyeball, and providing protection to the inner ocular tissues [48]. The middle layer, also referred to as uvea, is composed of the iris and the ciliary body (in the anterior), and the choroid, forming the posterior uvea (Figure 1) [49]. The retina represents the innermost layer, which is involved in the visual perception process by converting light energy into neuronal signals, which are transmitted to the visual cortex of the brain by the optic nerve [50,51].

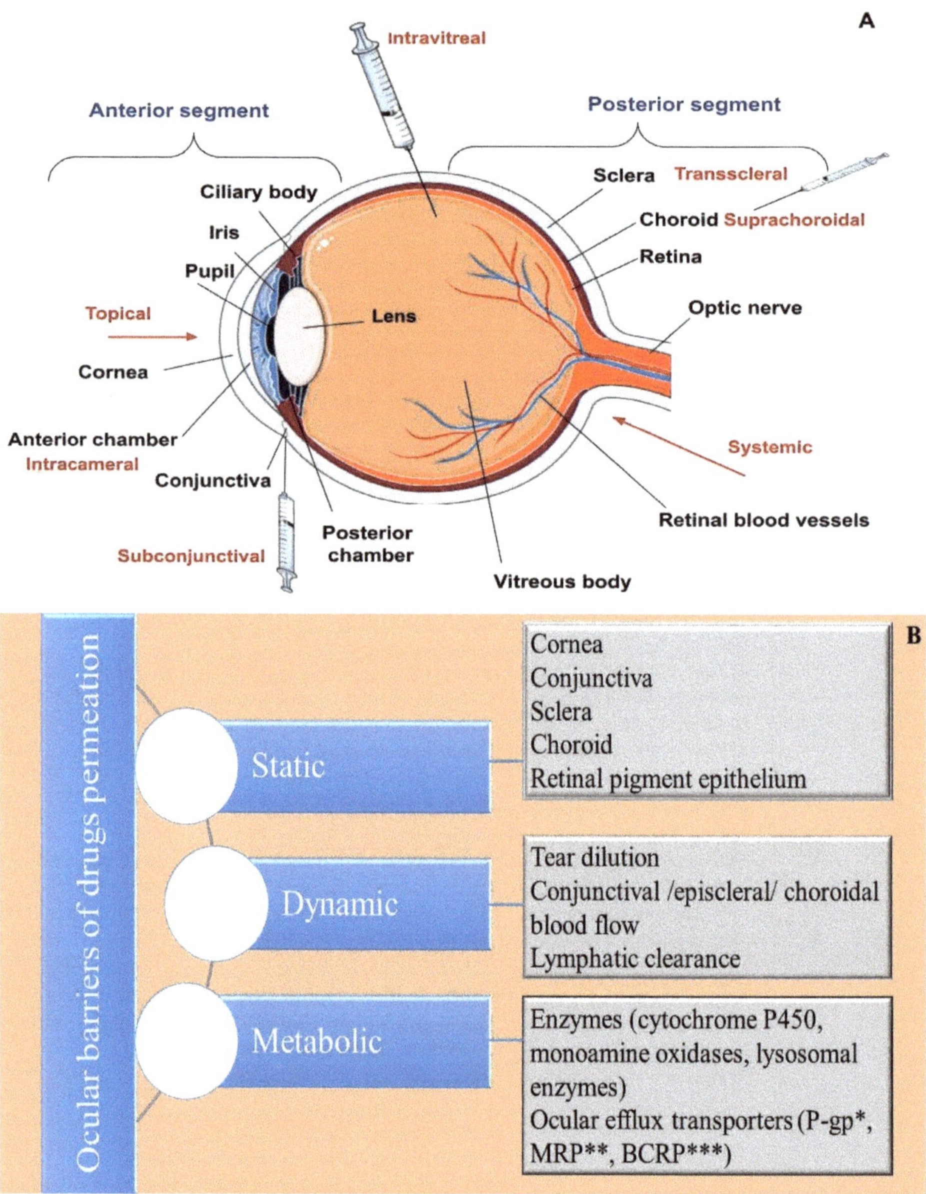

Figure 1. An overview of (**A**) ocular anatomy and routes for administration. (**B**) Ocular drug delivery barriers. * P-glycoprotein; ** Multidrug-resistant protein; *** Breast cancer resistance protein.

For better perception, the anatomical and physiological features of the human eye will be discussed from the anterior to posterior segment.

2.1. Anterior Segment of the Eye

2.1.1. Tear Film

The tear film is the first hindrance for topically applied drugs, often referred to as a dynamic (physiological) ocular barrier (Figure 1B) due to its high turnover rate, (0.5–2.2 µL/min), determining a short ocular residence time, and limited drug penetration ability [9,52,53]. Spread onto the corneal and conjunctival epithelium, it provides a smooth and lubricated optical surface, prevents the occurrence of infections due to its antimicrobial compounds (lysozyme, lactoferrin, lipocalin), or by washing out foreign substances, and supplies oxygen and nutrients to the cornea [54]. Traditionally, the tear film is described as a three-layered structure—an outer lipid layer produced by the Meibomian glands, a middle aqueous layer, and an inner mucous layer secreted predominantly by the conjunctival goblet cells [55]. However, a more recent theory considers that the tear film consists of two layers—an outer lipid layer and an inner muco-aqueous, gel-like layer [55–57]. Regarding ocular delivery, both layers exhibit barrier functions, the lipid one for hydrophilic drugs and the muco-aqueous layer for hydrophobic drugs [58]. Other precorneal factors negatively influencing ocular bioavailability include drug binding with proteins/mucin in the tear film, as well as drug loss via nasolacrimal drainage [53]. The latter is affected by the volume of applied drops (larger volumes correspond to more significant loss) and the blink reflex [9,12].

2.1.2. Cornea

The cornea is the main route for drug absorption after topical instillation, often referred to as a static (anatomical) barrier (Figure 1B). It is a transparent, highly specialized, avascular structure comprising six layers: the corneal epithelium, Bowman's layer, stroma, Dua's layer, Descemet's membrane, and endothelium [59,60]. Among these, the epithelium, the stroma, and the endothelium have a primary role in the drug/nanocarrier transport. Corneal epithelium is a five to seven-layered structure, composed of squamous, wing and basal cells [61]. Its lipophilic nature, and the existing intercellular tight junctions (zonula occludens) hinder the entry of hydrophilic substances and macromolecules [14,62]. Additionally, the presence of efflux transporters, such as breast cancer resistance protein (BCRP), multidrug resistance-associated proteins (MRPs), P-glycoprotein (P-gp), and enzymes (e.g., cytochrome P450), acting as metabolic barriers, may further decrease ocular drug bioavailability [58,63,64]. Beneath the epithelium is the stroma, which occupies approximately 90% of the corneal thickness [65]. It is a hydrophilic, gel-like structure made of collagen fibrils and mucopolysaccharides, and represents the main obstacle for the permeation of lipophilic compounds [66]. The corneal endothelium is a single layer composed of hexagonal-shaped cells involved in water transport towards the anterior chamber, as well as the maintenance of corneal transparency [67]. Unlike the epithelial layer, the endothelial junctions are considered "leaky" and enable the transport of macromolecules [11]. In general, drugs are transported across the cornea via transcellular (for lipophilic compounds) and paracellular (for hydrophilic molecules) pathways [68]. Factors affecting corneal absorption include a drug's molecular weight (compounds up to 500 Da are able to permeate across the epithelium), lipophilicity (facilitated for lipophilic compounds; preferably log D values of 2–3), degree of ionization (non-ionized forms penetrate more easily), and the charge of the ionized species (facilitated penetration of cationic molecules) [21,69–71].

2.1.3. Conjunctiva

The conjunctiva is a transparent mucous membrane, which overlays the anterior ocular surface and the interior of the eyelids. It is involved in the production of mucus and the maintenance of the tear film, ensuring the lubrication of the eye, and also preventing the entrance of exogenous substances or microorganisms [53,72]. The conjunctiva may be divided into three areas: the bulbar conjunctiva, covering the anterior part of the sclera; the conjunctival fornices, forming the cul-de-sac; the palpebral conjunctiva located on the posterior eyelid's surface [50]. Generally, the cul-de-sac is estimated to retain a volume of up to 30 µL—a capacity insufficient to preserve the entire volume of an applied drop (most often in the range of 40–70 µL), which leads to partial drug loss immediately after instillation [67]. The conjunctiva is considered to be more permeable when compared to the cornea, especially in terms of hydrophilic compounds, due to the wider intercellular spaces between the junctions in its structure, allowing for the passage of larger compounds (5000–10,000 Da), as well as owing to its bigger surface area. Nevertheless, conjunctival drug absorption is considered ineffective, mainly due to its high vascularity [71,73,74]. Conjunctival blood and lymph circulation functions as a dynamic barrier, leading to drug clearance and systemic absorption, hence the observed low drug concentration in the anterior chamber. Additionally, the existing transporters (amino acids transporters, P-gp) acting as efflux pumps further contribute to this process [63,75].

2.1.4. Iris

The iris is a circular, colored, contractile structure, which surrounds an aperture in its center (the pupil) (Figure 1A). It regulates the constriction or dilation of the pupil according to the light intensity, via parasympathetic/sympathetic activation, respectively [76]. It contains pigmented epithelial cells in its structure, enabling drug accumulation and altering its pharmacokinetics [77]. The melanin-containing cells in the eye (localized to the iris/ciliary body at the front and in the choroid/retinal pigment epithelium in the posterior) can bind drug molecules via electrostatic and van der Waals forces, as well as by charge interactions. The formed complex may be considered a "reservoir", releasing drugs at a slow rate, therefore, it can also be used in a drug-targeting approach to achieve prolonged action in the corresponding (pigmented) ocular areas [78–80].

2.1.5. Ciliary Body

The ciliary body is part of the middle (vascular) layer in the eye and is involved in the maintenance of the shape of the lens via the ciliary muscle, and in the production of aqueous humor [53,81]. Furthermore, the ciliary epithelium and the endothelial cells of the iris blood vessels form the *blood–aqueous barrier (BAB)*, which prevents molecules' entrance from systemic circulation to the aqueous humor [82]. The tight junctions in its structure limit the paracellular transport of large hydrophilic molecules, unlike small lipophilic compounds, which can penetrate via the transcellular pathway, and are subsequently eliminated by the uveal blood flow and aqueous humor turnover [49,78,83,84]. Alternatively, the elimination of hydrophilic compounds from the anterior chamber is carried out solely by the aqueous humor through Schlemm's canal, which determines their slower clearance [67,78].

2.1.6. Lens

The lens is located behind the iris and the pupil (Figure 1A), and is characterized by its transparent appearance, biconvex shape, great index of refraction, and high concentration of proteins in its structure (i.e., crystallins). Its main functions include light transmission and focusing it onto the retina to obtain a distinct image [85,86].

2.2. Posterior Segment of the Eye

The sclera, the choroid, and the retinal pigment epithelium (RPE) represent the posterior static ocular barriers used for drug delivery [63].

2.2.1. Sclera

The sclera is a white, dense tissue, made of collagen fibers (predominantly type I, and <5% type III) and proteoglycans [87]. The porous areas within the collagenous, aqueous medium determine the relatively easy passage of hydrophilic molecules when compared to hydrophobic ones. In addition to drugs' lipo/hydrophilicity, other physicochemical characteristics, such as their charge, molecular weight, and molecular radius, also influence scleral permeability [19]. The proteoglycan matrix, negatively charged at physiological pH, hinders the permeation of positively charged compounds as a result of the electrostatic interactions in between [88]. Regarding the impact of molecular weight/radius, studies showed that molecules up to 70 kDa are able to permeate across the sclera [89], and there is an inverse relationship between radius and drug permeability—smaller molecules penetrate more easily [88].

2.2.2. Choroid

The choroid is a thin, vascularized, pigmented tissue, involved in the transport of nutrients and oxygen to the retina [90,91]. Concerning drug delivery, it may be considered as both a static and dynamic barrier (Figure 1B), the latter owing to its high blood flow rate, determining rapid drug elimination [7,92]. Choroidal blood vessels are characterized by fenestrated walls, which enable drugs to reach the extravascular space of the choroid. Still, their further distribution towards the retina is limited by the presence of the blood–retinal barrier (BRB) [14,78].

2.2.3. Retina

The retina is a thin, transparent tissue lining the inner ocular surface [50]. It is characterized by a complex structure—histologically, it can be divided into ten layers. The outermost layer, the retinal pigment epithelium, represents a significant barrier to ocular drug delivery, due to the existing tight junctions between the epithelial cells, hindering paracellular drug transport [93,94]. The retinal pigment epithelium participates in the formation of the *blood–retinal barrier* (the outer BRB), whereas the retinal capillary endothelial cells constitute the inner BRB [95].

2.2.4. Vitreous Body

The vitreous body is a clear, avascular gel-like substance occupying the majority of the eyeball (Figure 1A) [96]. It performs several important functions, including maintaining the shape of the eyeball, acting as a shock absorber, protecting the retina from mechanical stress, and participating in light transmission towards the retina [97]. The vitreous body may be also considered as an area for drug delivery to the posterior eye segment. Intravitreal permeation depends on drugs' physicochemical characteristics, such as their charge (facilitated for negatively charged molecules, which do not interact electrostatically with the negatively charged vitreous humor constituents), size (small molecules diffuse easily), and lipophilicity (easier when compared to hydrophilic drugs). The last two parameters also influence drug clearance—larger and hydrophilic molecules are characterized by a longer half-life, due to their elimination via the anterior route (through the aqueous humor), in contrast to small lipophilic compounds, which are cleared via the posterior route (crossing the BRB) [19,21,69].

2.3. Alternative Routes of Ocular Delivery

The complex anatomical and physiological features of the eye elucidate the challenges in ocular drug delivery from a physiological point of view. To achieve higher therapeutic concentrations in the posterior segment, alternative routes of administration have been exploited, the most common of which are presented in Table 1. However, most of them (excluding the oral route) are invasive, and are not applicable by the patients themselves, therefore, research efforts are focused on the elaboration of advanced drug delivery platforms, aiming to improve drug bioavailability and therapeutic outcomes for both anterior and posterior eye segment diseases.

Table 1. Alternative routes of ocular drug delivery.

Alternative Route	Specifics	Benefits	Limitations	References
Sub-conjunctival (SC)	SC route includes SC injections, administered in the lower or upper fornix, as well as instillation of SC implants; Clinical indications include corneal/scleral lesions, glaucoma, cytomegalovirus rhinitis.	Possibility to ensure high local drug concentration; Improved penetration of water-soluble drugs due to the bypassing of the corneal epithelium.	Conjunctival and choroidal blood/lymphatic flow; Temporary pain at the injection site; Local irritations.	[98,99]
Intracameral (IC)	Injections applied in the anterior chamber, often as a prevention of postoperative endophthalmitis after cataract surgery; Delivery of antibiotics, steroids, anesthetics.	Lower drug concentration needed; Decreased side effects vs. topical steroid application; Increased anesthesia during surgery when co-administered with topical anesthetics.	Potential complications, such as toxic anterior segment syndrome, corneal endothelial toxicity.	[100–102]
Transscleral	Drug delivery to the posterior segment of the eye; The sclera is thinnest around the equator, therefore, it is the preferred area for injection.	Obviates the corneal and conjunctival barrier; Less-invasive procedure compared to intravitreal injections.	Static barriers (sclera, choroid, retina) and dynamic barriers (choroidal blood flow) reduce drug bioavailability; Necessity of high doses.	[84,99,103]
Supra-choroidal (SC)	Drug injection under the choroid, targeting the following areas: choroid and retina; Microneedles have also been used for drug deposition into the SC space; Clinical indications include: posterior uveitis, macular edema.	Obviates the sclera and improves drug bioavailability within the choroid and retina; Effective for the delivery of small molecules; Lower risk of intraocular pressure spikes.	Choroidal circulation; Risk of occurrence of choroidal hemorrhage or detachment.	[99,104,105]
Intravitreal (IV)	Direct injection to the vitreous body targeting posterior eye segment; Drug delivery of vascular endothelial growth factor (VEGF) inhibitors, antibiotics, corticosteroids; IV injections are applied in the therapy of age-related macular degeneration, cytomegalovirus retinitis, diabetic macular edema, retinal vein occlusions.	Bypasses the BRB; Provides high local therapeutic concentration and prolonged drug levels; Reduced systemic side effects.	Repetitive instillations lead to serious ocular complications and patient non-compliance. Eye discomfort and pain were reported following IV injections.	[53,106]
Systemic/Oral	Drugs are administered orally or intravenously; Therapeutic applications include: scleritis, cytomegalovirus retinitis.	Acceptance by the patients.	Low bioavailability (<2%)—barrier role of BAB, BRB; Necessity of high doses, corresponding to increased risk of side effects.	[107]

3. Feasibility of Lipid Nanoparticles in Ophthalmology

Lipid-based drug delivery systems, such as nanoemulsions, liposomes, niosomes, cubosomes, and lipid nanoparticles, have attracted an enormous scientific interest, due to their biocompatibility, biodegradability, and tolerability [108]. An excellent review summarizing the feasibility of all the aforementioned lipid-based nanocarriers in ophthalmology is provided here [109]. Emerging initially as an alternative to liposomes in terms of their superior physical stability, cost-effective process and materials, as well as being alternatives to polymeric nanoparticles, due to the absence of toxic degradation products, [37] SLNs have been explored as drug delivery systems for various routes of application—dermal [110,111], ocular [112,113], pulmonary [114], parenteral [115], nasal [116], and oral [117]. Another advantageous characteristic of the lipid nanocarriers is the possibility of encapsulating more than one therapeutic agent, leading to the elaboration of dual or multidrug lipid nanoparticles, characterized by a synergetic effect and improved therapeutic performance [118]. In ophthalmology, in particular, SLNs and the second-generation lipid particles—NLCs—are considered especially beneficial due to their ability to provide sustained drug release by acting as drug depot formulations, and enhance corneal penetration due to the corresponding activity of non-ionic surfactants included in their structure [119,120]. The latter may further contribute towards an improved ocular bioavailability, by opening the tight junctions between corneal epithelial cells, facilitating paracellular drug transport, and by inhibiting P-glycoprotein activity, limiting drug efflux [121–123].

The lipid nanoparticles' transcorneal penetration mechanism has been studied by Nagai et al., according to which the process is implemented via energy-dependent endocytosis. The authors proposed three endocytosis pathways (clathrin-dependent, caveolae-dependent and macropinocytosis) as possible mechanisms for penetration of indomethacin-loaded nanoparticles, with an emphasis on the caveolae-dependent endocytosis [124]. Undoubtedly, nanoparticles' permeation and internalization are highly affected by their physicochemical characteristics, such as size, size distribution pattern, zeta potential, and subsequent surface modification. Generally, nanoparticles up to 200 nm are reported to penetrate across the cornea [125]. In the case of periocular application, the excessive downsizing of their dimensions (e.g., ≈20 nm) may lead to their rapid clearance, as reported by Amritte et al. [126]. In their study Niamprem et al. investigated the penetration of fluorescent dye (Nile red)-loaded NLCs across porcine cornea, as a function of their size and surface modifications. According to the authors, NLCs with a size of 40 nm exhibited enhanced penetration when compared to larger (150 nm) nanoparticles.

Regarding their internalization, non-modified NLCs had a higher uptake in porcine corneal epithelial cells than PEG- and stearylamine-modified nanocarriers. The latter may be attributed to their superior mucoadhesive properties, arising from hydrogen boding between PEG molecules and mucin glycoproteins, or from ionic interactions between cationic stearylamine and anionic groups present in mucin regions [127].

Ocular drug delivery is also affected by the zeta potential of the nanocarriers. Positive values contribute to an increased ocular contact time, as a result of the occurred electrostatic interactions with the negatively charged corneal epithelium [125]. Regarding zeta potential's impact on the colloidal stability of the nanocarriers, generally, absolute values of 30 mV are considered to be sufficient to provide repulsion between the nanoparticles in the dispersion and prevent their aggregation [128].

3.1. Lipid Nanoparticles—Structural Features and Recent Progress in Ocular Therapeutics

According to their main structural components, lipid nanoparticles may be distinguished into solid lipid nanoparticles (composed of solid-state lipids under ambient and physiological conditions) and nanostructured lipid carriers (additionally containing liquid lipids in their composition). In both cases, the lipid constituents are dispersed in an aqueous medium stabilized by surfactants [108]. Their specific structures and types are illustrated in Figure 2.

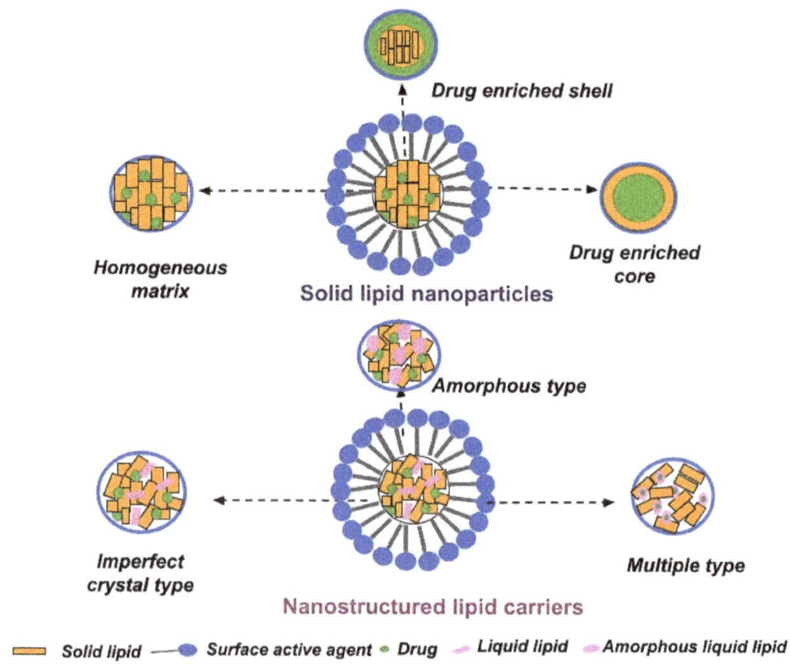

Figure 2. Different types of solid lipid nanoparticles and nanostructured lipid carriers.

3.1.1. Solid Lipid Nanoparticles

Solid lipid nanoparticles are generally sphere-shaped colloidal systems, ranging between 50 and 1000 nm, and have been successfully explored as carriers for both hydrophilic and hydrophobic drugs [129]. The most frequently used solid lipids for their preparation include *triglycerides* (tristearin (Dynasan 118), tripalmitin (Dynasan 116), trimyristin (Dynasan 114)), a *mixture or mixtures of mono-, di- and triglycerides* (glyceryl behenate (Compritol 888 ATO), glyceryl palmitostearate (Precirol ATO 5)), *waxes* (beeswax, carnauba wax), *fatty acids* (lauric/stearic/myristic acid), and the corresponding *fatty alcohols* [130,131].

The chemical structure of lipids has a major impact on their physicochemical properties and delivery process of the nanoparticles, as reported by several studies. Boonme et al. investigated the effect of different lipids (glyceryl trimyristate, glyceryl tripalmitate, glyceryl tristearate, stearic acid, glyceryl monostearate) on the characteristics of SLNs obtained by the microemulsion technique. The selected lipids differ in the number of C atoms of the fatty acids chains, as well as their polarity. According to the obtained results, lipid polarity influences the capability to obtain microemulsions—the formation of such was reported in three of the studied formulations (comprising glyceryl monostearate, stearic acid and glyceryl trimyristate). This may be related to the absence of polar functional groups in the structure of glyceryl tripalmitate/glyceryl tristearate, as well as to their long (C-16/C-18) chains, determining large molecular volumes unable to penetrate into the hydrophobic region of the surfactant interface. The number of carbon atoms of the fatty acid residue also affects nanoparticle size—the smallest diameter was observed in the glyceryl trimyristate-based formulation, as a result of the shorter carbon chain (14 C atoms vs. C18 atoms) facilitating its penetration into the surfactant's interface [132]. Palival et al. investigated the influence of several solid lipids (stearic acid, glycerol monostearate, tristearin, and Compritol 888 ATO) on the properties of methotrexate-loaded SLNs intended for oral delivery. According to the obtained results, the highest entrapment efficacy was reported for the Compritol 888-based SLNs, which may be related to the drug interchain intercalation [133].

The appropriate selection of a solid lipid or lipid mixture is an important subject, as it impacts the physicochemical characteristics (size, drug loading capacity), as well as drug release and storage stability, of the nanocarriers. Important issues to be considered during (pre)formulation studies include the solubility of drug in the lipid matrix, drug/lipid compatibility, and the lipid(s) crystalline behavior [134,135]. Based on the structural organization and drug location within the nanoparticles, three types of SLNs can be distinguished, as illustrated in Figure 2.

The *homogenous matrix model* is characterized by a uniformly allocated drug within the lipid matrix (molecularly dissolved or in form of amorphous clusters), mainly produced via the high-pressure homogenization method. The homogenous matrix particles result from the agitation of the dispersed drug in bulk lipid (when the cold technique is applied) or from the crystallization of cooled liquid droplets, in the case of hot homogenization. The latter is suitable for highly lipophilic drugs, without the necessity of using solubilizing agents [136].

The *drug-enriched shell model* involves predominantly localizing the drug in the outer shell of the nanoparticles, arising from phase separation and drug migration during the cooling stage of the process. Fast cooling induces the lipid in the center to precipitate, whereas the drug concentration in the residual liquid lipid increases, forming the outer shell. This model is characterized by fast drug release [137].

The *drug-enriched core model* is characterized by a high drug concentration in the melted lipid, leading to supersaturation of the drug and its precipitation during the cooling phase before lipid recrystallization. Further cooling subsequently leads to lipid recrystallization, and to the formation of a membrane overlaying the drug-enriched core [138].

In addition to the lipid constituents, a SLN formulation also contains surfactants, which facilitate the dispersion of lipids within the aqueous medium and stabilize the system by reducing the interfacial tension between both immiscible phases [139]. Generally, surfactants are included in the composition up to 5%*w/w*, and their selection is based upon several considerations, such as hydrophilic–lipophilic balance (HLB value), the route of administration of SLNs, safety profile, and compatibility with the other excipients [135,140]. In SLNs, intended for ophthalmic applications, the most-often included surfactants are non-ionic, such as polyoxyethylene sorbitan fatty acid esters (Polysorbates/Tweens), polyoxyethylene/polyoxypropylene block copolymers (Poloxamers/Pluronic), and amphoteric molecules, e.g., soy lecithin, due to their superior safety profiles compared to their anionic or cationic counterparts [119,131].

In their study, Silva et al., 2019 investigated the cytotoxicity of SLNs, containing the cationic surfactants cetyltrimethylammonium bromide (CTAB) and dimethyldioctadecylammonium bromide (DDAB), against five human cell lines of different origin. According to the obtained results CTAB-containing SLNs exhibited superior cytotoxicity in comparison to DDAB-SLNs, as the experimental concentration is closer to the critical micellar concentration of CTAB (the latter is related to cell lysis) [141].

SLNs may also contain cryoprotectants (e.g., trehalose, sorbitol, mannitol), in case the nanoparticles are subjected to lyophilization [142], as well as surface-modifying additives, such as polyethylene glycol, to confer stealth properties of the nanocarriers [143], or selective ligands, antibodies, etc., to provide targeted delivery [144,145]. In ocular therapeutics, SLNs are often modified using polyethylene glycol to improve their pharmacokinetic profile, or are coated with mucoadhesive polymers (e.g., chitosan), aiming to prolong their precorneal residence time [146,147].

In their study, Eid et al. investigated the impact of PEGylation and chitosan coating on the ocular bioavailability of ofloxacin-loaded SLNs. The addition of PEG stearate to the compositions determined higher transcorneal permeability, with a moderate effect on the mucoadhesion, in contrast to chitosan, which exerted the opposite effects. Ultimately, the developed PEGylated chitosan-coated SLNs improved the ocular bioavailability of ofloxacin by increasing the drug concentration in rabbits' eyes two- to three-fold when compared to the plain drug [148]. The PEGylation approach was also adopted by Dang et al., who developed a PEGylated SLNs-laden contact lens, characterized by an enhanced latanoprost-loading capacity, smaller sizes (compared to non-PEGylated SLNs), and sustained drug release up to 96 h [149].

The development of *hybrid drug-delivery platforms* based on nanocarriers and a vehicle (semisolid formulations, in situ gels, contact lens) is an advantageous strategy for ocular delivery purposes, as it exploits the beneficial effects of both systems. In their study, Sun and Hu developed tacrolimus-loaded SLNs that were thermosensitive in situ gel, which were characterized by suitable gelling and rheological characteristics (gelation temperature 32 °C, pseudoplastic behavior), sustained drug release and improved pharmacodynamic effects when compared to the free drug and tacrolimus-loaded SLNs [150]. Improved biopharmaceutical and therapeutic outcomes were reported also for mizolastine-loaded hydrogel SLNs, manifesting in sustained drug release (up to 30 h) and reduced symptoms of allergic conjunctivitis in rabbits' eyes [151].

Another beneficial SLN-based delivery strategy implemented in ocular therapeutics is the elaboration of dual solid lipid nanoparticles, as reported by Carbone et al. [152]. The authors aimed to improve the effectiveness of *Candida albicans* mycosis treatment by combining the antimycotic effect of clotrimazole and the antioxidant activity of alpha-lipoic acid. SLN as a delivery platform enabled the simultaneous loading of both drugs, and determined slow and controlled drug release, without an initial burst effect. The latter was achieved due to the successful incorporation of both drugs within the inner lipid matrix, and not on the nanoparticles' surface [152].

An overview of the developed SLNs for ocular delivery purposes is provided in Table 2.

Table 2. Recent progress of SLNs for ophthalmic application (5 years' overview).

Composition	Drug/Disease	Method of Preparation	Physicochemical Characteristics	Results	References
Tripalmitin Tween 80 Glycerol	Econazole/ *Fungal keratitis*	Microemulsion method	Size 19.05 ± 0.28 nm PDI 0.21 ± 0.01 ζ potential −2.20 ± 0.10 mV EE = 94.18 ± 1.86%	Slow and controlled drug release (within 96 h); Improved antifungal activity; Enhanced bioavailability—drug concentration was above MIC within 3 h after application.	[153]
Precirol ATO 5 Pluronic F68 Stearyl amine	Natamycin/ *Fungal keratitis*	Hot emulsification-ultrasonication technique	Size 42 nm PDI 0.224 ζ potential 26 mV EE ≈ 85%	Prolonged drug release (within 8 h); Improved corneal penetration; Superior antifungal activity vs. free drug; Excellent ocular tolerability.	[154]
Compritol 888 ATO Stearic acid Tween 80 Soy lecithin	Isoniazid/ *Ocular tuberculosis*	Microemulsion method	Size 149.2 ± 4.9 nm PDI 0.15 ± 0.02 ζ potential −0.35 ± 0.28 mV EE = 65.2 ± 2.2%	Prolonged drug release (48 h); Enhanced corneal permeability (1.6 fold); Improved ocular bioavailability (4.2 fold) vs. drug solution.	[155]
Stearic acid Tween 80 Transcutol P	Clarithromycin/ *Bacterial endophthalmitis*	High-speed mixing and the ultrasonication method	Size 157 ± 42.4 nm PDI 0.13 ± 0.02 ζ potential −17.2 ± 3.1 mV EE = 81.3 ± 4.6	Sustained drug release (~80% in 8 h); Improved transcorneal permeation and bioavailability compared to drug solution.	[156]

Table 2. *Cont.*

Composition	Drug/Disease	Method of Preparation	Physicochemical Characteristics	Results	References
Softisan 100 (Hydrogenated Coco-Glycerides) Suppocire NB (C10–C18 Triglycerides) Tween 80 Tegin O DOTAP DDAB	Sorafenib/ *Uveal melanoma*	Phase inversion temperature method	Size 127.85 ± 1.50 nm PDI 0.215 ± 0.014 ζ potential 20 mV EE= 75.0 ± 2.1%	Sustained drug release (less than 25% of encapsulated drug released after 72 h); Good physical stability, cytocompatibility and mucoadhesive properties of elaborated SLNs.	[157]
Compritol 888ATO PEG 400 Poloxamer 188 Phospholipon 90H	Atorvastatin/ *Age-related macular degeneration*	Hot high-pressure homogenization	Size 256.3 ± 10.5 nm PDI 0.26 ± 0.02 ζ potential −2.65 mV EE= 73.1 ± 1.52%	Improved bioavailability (8-fold in aqueous humor and 12-fold in vitreous humor) vs. free drug; Proven safety in corneal/retinal cell lines; Successful delivery to the retina, confirmed by intact fluorescein-labeled SLNs.	[158]
Compritol 888 ATO/Compritol HD5 ATO Pluronic F127	Betulinic acid (BA) derivatives H3, H5 and H7/ *Retinal diseases (diabetic retinopathy, age-related macular degeneration, choroidal neovascularization)*	Microemulsion method	Size 58.5± 9.8 nm PDI 0.246 ζ potential 6.45 ± 5.58 mV EE = 75.10%	Improved drug delivery and enhanced anti-oxidative efficacy of BA derivatives; Suppressed glutamate-induced ROS production/necrosis in human Müller cells.	[159]
Gelucire 44/14 Compritol ATO 888 Tween 80	Etoposide/ *Posterior segment-related diseases (e.g., age-related macular degeneration, diabetic retinopathy)*	Melt-emulsification and ultrasonication technique	Size 239.43 ± 2.35 nm PDI 0.261 ± 0.001 EE 80.96 ± 2.21%	Sustained etoposide concentration of etoposide in vitreous body for 7 days after IV injection Better toxicological profile vs. etoposide solution.	[160]
Stearic acid Sodium taurodeoxycholate Phosphatidylcholine	Sutinib (Sb)/ *Retinal diseases (age-related macular degeneration, diabetic retinopathy, retinal vein occlusions)*	Microemulsion method	Size 140 nm PDI 0.20	Excellent tolerability profile based on in vivo study on 20 albino rabbits; After IV injections, Sb SLNs didn't cause any abnormalities in ocular morphology in contrast to polymeric nanocapsules.	[161]
Chitosan Phospholipids (Lipoid S100) Glyceryl mono-stearate Tween 80 PEG 400	Methazolamide/ *Glaucoma*	Emulsion-solvent evaporation method	Size 247.7 ± 17.3 nm PDI ζ potential 33.5 ± 3.9 mV EE = 58.5 ± 4.5%	Prolonged drug release compared to drug solution; Excellent tolerability and marked reduction in IOP vs. uncoated methazolamide SLNs.	[162]
Compritol 888 ATO Pluronic F68 Tween 80 Glycerol	Δ^9-Tetrahydrocannabinol-valine-hemisuccinate/ *Glaucoma*	Ultrasonication	Size 287.80 ± 7.35 nm PDI 0.29 ± 0.01 EE = 93.57 ± 4.68%	Greater reduction in the IOP with respect to intensity and duration compared to pilocarpine/timolol maleate eye drops; High drug concentration in the iris/ciliary body and choroid/ retina.	[163]

Legend: DDAB—Didodecyldimethylammonium bromide; DOTAP—Dioleoyl-trimethylammonium–propane chloride; EE—Entrapment efficiency; IOP—Intraocular pressure; MIC—Minimum inhibitory concentration; PDI—Polydispersity index; ROS—Reactive oxygen species.

As presented in Table 2, SLNs have been successfully exploited for both anterior and posterior eye segment diseases. The reported therapeutic results may be attributed to various factors, such as the ability of SLNs to form a depot for the prolonged release of the drug, the fluidizing effect of included surfactants on the lipid bilayers of ocular membranes, facilitating drug permeation, as well as the large surface area of nanocarriers, providing maximized contact with the ocular mucosa [163,164]. It is also worth noting the ability of SLNs to encapsulate high molecular weight compounds, such as atorvastatin [158] and natamycin [154], which are also characterized by poor solubility, therefore, their ocular delivery through conventional ophthalmic formulations would be a challenge. Encapsulation of atorvastatin in SLNs further contributed to improved drug photostability, as confirmed by the photostability studies conducted according to ICH guidelines [158]. Liang et al. also reported overcoming the unfavorable characteristics of the drug by developing econazole-loaded SLNs. The antimycotic is characterized by low aqueous solubility and strong irritation potential, which restrain its application in the therapy of ocular fungal infections. The conducted in vivo studies showed enhanced corneal permeation, and no ocular irritation with the econazole-loaded SLNs [153]. Solid lipid nanoparticles are also beneficial in the therapy of posterior segment diseases, e.g., glaucoma, as confirmed by the superior intraocular pressure reduction [162], and higher therapeutic concentration in the iris, ciliary body, and retina [163].

The pre-clinical safety of SLNs was evaluated in polymeric nanospheres and liposomes in a recent study conducted by Gomes Souza et al. The authors elaborated sunitinib-loaded nanocarriers as topical formulation strategies for corneal neovascularization treatment. The sunitinib-loaded SLNs were selected as the optimal formulation due to their excellent tolerability profile, controlled drug release, and highest corneal retention [165].

3.1.2. Nanostructured Lipid Carriers

Nanostructured lipid carriers were initially developed to surmount the limitations associated with SLNs, such as their poor drug-loading capacity, owing to their perfectly arranged crystalline structure, and their propensity towards drug expulsion during storage, resulting from lipid crystallization [37,166]. The addition of spatially incompatible liquid lipid(s) to the formulations is beneficial in two aspects, it leads to the formation of a less-ordered crystalline structure (Figure 2), ensuring extra area for drug loading, decreases the crystalline degree of the lipid matrix and averts drug expulsion [128,167]. Usually, the liquid lipid is included up to 30% of the total lipid amount in the NLCs formulations [168,169]. As such, researchers often use castor/olive/argan oil, oleic acid, Miglyol® 812 (medium-chain triglycerides), propylene glycol dicaprylocaprate—Labrafac™ PG (Gattefosse, Saint-Priest, France), or caprylocaproyl macrogol-8 glycerides—Labrasol® (Gattefosse, Saint-Priest, France) [170–172].

The selection of both solid and liquid lipids is reported to influence NLCs' size. According to Apostolou et al., NLCs comprising solid lipids, such as Precirol ATO 5 (Gattefosse, Saint-Priest, France), Compritol 888 ATO (Gattefosse, Saint-Priest, France) or Dynasan 118 (IOI Oleo GmbH, Hamburg, Germany), exhibit larger particle sizes when compared to glyceryl monostearate- and stearic acid-based nanocarriers. A possible explanation may lie in the higher molecular weight of the lipids, leading to the formation of a more complex structure, with a tendency of aggregation between the molecules, which results in an increased nanoparticle diameter [173]. Concerning the selection of liquid lipids, NLCs containing Mygliol® 812 (IOI Oleo GmbH, Hamburg, Germany) are generally characterized by larger size when compared to oleic acid or Capryol 90-containing ones (Gattefosse, Saint-Priest, France) [174–176].

NLCs can be classified into three models depending on the preparation methods, lipid matrix structure, and drug location [177].

The *imperfect type* is obtained by blending structurally different lipids, resulting in the formation of disorganized lipid matrix. The selected lipids, usually a small fraction of liquid oil mixed with larger amount of solid lipid, may differ in terms of fatty acid origin, in their carbon chain length or degree of saturation. This type of NLC is characterized by its high drug-loading capacity, proportionally related to the imperfections within the lipid matrix [178].

The *amorphous-type* NLCs are formed owing to the addition of specific lipids to the formulation, such as hydroxyoctacosanyl hydroxystearate and isopropyl myristate. These lipids contribute to the formation of a non-crystalline (amorphous) matrix, limiting drug expulsion as a result of solid lipid crystallization [143].

The *multiple-type* NLCs are oil-in-solid, fat-in-water nanocarriers, composed of numerous liquid oil nanocompartments within a solid lipid matrix, usually obtained through the hot homogenization technique. The greater amount of liquid lipid in the formulation leads to phase separation and the formation of the nanosized droplets upon the cooling phase. The multiple-type NLCs are characterized by high drug-loading capacities, due to the superior solubility of lipophilic drugs in liquid lipids compared to those in solid ones. Furthermore, the solid matrix exhibits a barrier function, limiting drug leakage and controlling the release process [178,179].

Similar to SLNs, the surface of NLCs can be modified with cationic additives (e.g., chitosan) to impart muco-adhesiveness, sustained drug release, and increased penetration, as reported by Selvaraj et al. [180], Sharma et al. [181], and Fu et al. [182]. Derivatives of chitosan (trimethyl chitosan) and chitin (chitosan oligosaccharide) have also been investigated as nanoparticle surface-coating materials, as they exhibit improved aqueous solubility at a neutral pH (including in the lacrimal fluid) and superior safety profiles compared to native chitosan, while at the same time retaining all of its beneficial characteristics (biodegradability, muco-adhesion, penetration-enhancing properties, etc.) [183,184].

Mucoadhesive NLCs have also been developed by functionalization with (3-aminomethylphenyl) boronic acid attached to chondroitin sulfate, to increase corneal residence time by specifically targeting the sialic acid residues on the ocular surface, which ultimately improves drug performance regarding dry eye disease [185]. In vivo relief of dry eye disease symptoms, accompanied by enhanced corneal retention, was also reported by Zhu et al., developing chondroitin sulfate and L-cysteine conjugate-modified dexamethasone NLCs [186].

In another study Abdelhakeem et al. elaborated on surface-modified eplerenone-loaded NLCs for the treatment of central serous chorioretinopathy. The authors evaluated the effect of three different coating polymers (hyaluronic acid, chitosan oligosaccharide lactate, and hydrogenated collagen) on the properties of the nanocarriers. The largest particle size was reported for the hyaluronic acid-coated NLCs, corresponding to the formulation's highest eplerenone entrapment efficiency and viscosity. The higher viscosity determined the superior sustained drug release from hyaluronic acid-modified NLCs compared to the other NLCs models. The selected optimal formulations (hyaluronic acid/chitosan oligosaccharide lactate-coated) were characterized by an excellent ocular tolerability, as confirmed by the Draize test [187].

Nanostructured lipid carriers have been also an integral component of *hybrid drug-delivery platforms*, recently included into thermosensitive in situ gel-forming systems [188,189]. An interesting approach is described by Yu et al. in two of their studies, elaborating on baicalin NLCs and quercetin NLCs that were subsequently incorporated into dual pH and thermosensitive in situ gels. The dual stimuli-responsive formulation was based on carboxymethyl chitosan and Poloxamer 407, cross-linked by the natural cross-linker genipin. Both hybrid, NLC-loaded, in situ gels were characterized by prolonged drug release and precorneal residence time, and improved transcorneal penetration compared to eye drops [190,191].

Dual nanostructured lipid carriers have also been developed for ocular delivery purposes. In their study Youseff et al. developed simultaneously loaded natamycin/ciprofloxacin NLCs as a drug delivery system for microbial keratitis treatment. The selection of model drugs (an antifungal agent and fluoroquinolone antibiotic) was based on the complex etiology of corneal infections (which may be caused by bacteria/fungi/protozoa, when a secondary or co-infection is present). The elaborated dual NLCs were subsequently incorporated into in situ ionic gel formulations, aiming to further enhance the therapeutic efficacy by providing prolonged ocular surface contact time [120]. Dual therapeutic synergy was exploited also by Chen and Wu when developing brinzolamide- and latanoprost-loaded NLCs for the therapy of glaucoma (details of the study are presented in Table 3) [192].

Table 3. Recent progress of NLCs for ophthalmic application (5 years' overview).

Composition	Drug/*Disease*	Method of Preparation	Physicochemical Characteristics	Results	References
Glycerol monostearate 40–55 Soy lecithin Compritol 888 ATO Cholesterol Capryol 90 Miglyol 812 N Kolliphor P 407 Kolliphor P 188 α-Tocopherol-PEG	Lactoferrin/ *Keratoconus*	Double emulsion/ solvent evaporation method.	Size 119.45 ± 11.44 nm PDI 0.151 ± 0.045 ζ potential 17.50 ± 2.53 mV EE $\approx 75\%$	Controlled release profile; Good physical stability (up to 3 months); Muco-adhesive properties (for at least 240 min); Ocular tolerability.	[193]
Labrafac lipophile WL1349 Cholesterol Tween 80	Dexamethasone (DXM)/ *Dry Eye Disease*	Solvent diffusion method	Size 19.51 ± 0.5 nm PDI 0.08 ζ potential 9.8 mV EE = $99.6 \pm 0.5\%$	Cellular internalization in HCECs and corneal distribution in ex vivo porcine cornea; Significant reduction in inflammatory cytokines (MMP-9, IL-6 and TNF-α) related to DED pathogenesis vs. free DXM.	[194]
Precirol ATO5 Capryol PGMC Stearylamine Tween 80 Poloxamer 188	Rapamycin/ *Corneal alkaline burn injury*	Emulsification solvent diffusion and evaporation method	Size 216 ± 40 nm ζ potential 14 ± 2.6 mV EE = $97.66 \pm 0.57\%$	Improved fibroblast uptake of encapsulated cargo via NLCs (1.5 times); Superior in vivo corneal healing properties of NLCs vs. control groups.	[195]
Stearic acid, oleic acid Poloxamer 407	Itraconazole/ *Fungal keratitis*	High-speed homogenization technique	Size 150.67 nm ζ potential -28 mV EE = 94.65%	Ocular safe formulation according to HET−CAM test; Enhanced antifungal activity of the NLCs compared to commercial eye drops.	[196]
PrecirolATO 5,Castor oil, Span 80, mPEG-2K-DSPE sodium salt Poloxamer 188, Tween 80, glycerin	Natamycin/ *Fungal keratitis*	High-pressure homogenization	Size 241.96 nm, PDI 0.406 EE = 95.35%	Improved in vitro transcorneal permeation and flux of formulated NT compared to drug suspension.	[197]
Glycerin monostearate Miglyol 812 N Solutol HS 15 Gelucire 44/14 Soy lecithin	Dasatinib (DAS)/ *Corneal neovascularization*	Melt-emulsification method	Size 78.53 ± 0.36 nm PDI 0.21 ± 0.01 ζ potential -29.6 ± 1.0 mV EE = $97.71\% \pm 0.89\%$	Enhanced solubility of DAS (1200-fold) after inclusion in NLCs; Inhibition of the development of CNV and associated corneal pathological alterations in a mouse model of CNV.	[198]
Monolaurin Capryol-90 Cremophor RH40 Transcutol P Glycerin	Sorafenib/ *Corneal neovascularization*	Microemulsion method	Size 111.87 ± 0.93 nm PDI 0.15 ± 0.01 ζ potential -0.35 ± 0.08 mV EE = $99.20 \pm 0.86\%$	Excellent ocular tolerability (in vivo test on rabbits), non-toxic in HCEC; Approximately 6.7- and 1.3-fold higher drug concentrations in rabbit cornea and conjunctiva vs. free drug.	[199]
Compritol 888 ATO Apifil (PEG-8 beeswax) Miglyol 812N Labrasol, Kolliphor EL Cremophor RH60	Dexamethasone/ *Ophthalmic inflammatory diseases, severe uveitis*	Ultrasonication method	Size 92.18 ± 0.49 nm PDI 0.12 ± 0.02 ζ potential -7.62 ± 0.26, EE = 88.31%	Good ocular tolerability; Ability to penetrate across the cornea; High concentration of NLCs in the stroma, according to porcine corneal penetration study.	[171]

Table 3. *Cont.*

Capmul MCM C10 Soya lecithin Captex 200 P Transcutol P Polysorbate 80 Stearylamine	Triamcinolone acetonide/ *Uveitis*	Hot microemulsion method	Size 198.95 $\pm$ 12.82 nm PDI 0.326 $\pm$ 0.04 ζ potential 35.8 $\pm$ 1.94 mV EE = 88.14 $\pm$ 3.03 %	Sustained drug release (84% within 24 h); Ex vivo corneal permeation of 51%; Biocompatible and ocular tolerable formulation (HET-CAM test).	[200]
Cholesterol Stearic acid Stearylamine Oleic acid Labrafil M 1944 Tween 80	Vancomycin (VMC)/ *Bacterial endophthalmitis*	Cold homogenization technique	Size 96.40 $\pm$ 0.71 nm PDI 0.352 $\pm$ 0.011 ζ potential 29.7 $\pm$ 0.47 mV, EE = 74.80 $\pm$ 4.30%	Improved transcorneal penetration; Biocompatible, non-irritant formulation (in vitro RBC hemolytic assay); Enhanced (3-fold) intravitreal VMC concentration after topical application compared to drug solution.	[201]
Miglyol 812 Compritol 888 ATO Lutrol F68	Palmitoylethanolamide (PEA)/ *Retinal diseases (diabetic retinopathy, glaucoma)*	High shear homogenization	Size 208.6 $\pm$ 10.2 nm PDI 0.18 ζ potential > 20 mV	Improved ocular bioavailability: 40% and 100% higher PEA levels in vitreous body and retina compared to free drug.	[202]
Glyceryl monostearate Labrafil M 2125 CS Tween 80 Transcutol HP Chitosan	5-Fluorouracil (5-FU)/ *Diabetic retinopathy*	Melt emulsification-ultrasonication method	Size 163.2 $\pm$ 2.3 nm PDI 0.28 $\pm$ 1.52 ζ potential 21.4 $\pm$ 0.5 mV EE = 85.0 $\pm$ 0.2 %	Higher and sustained 5-FU release vs. free drug; Non-irritant formulations; Antiangiogenic effect confirmed by in vivo study in a diabetic retinopathy rat model.	[181]
Capryol 90 Softisan 100 Tween 80	Diosmin/ *Diabetic retinopathy*	Melt emulsification method and ultrasonication	Size 83.58 $\pm$ 0.77 nm PDI 0.263 $\pm$ 0.067 ζ potential -18.5 ± 0.60 mV EE = 99.53$\pm$ 2.50	Very good physical stability of NLCs up to 60 days; Cytocompatibility assessed on ARPE-19 cells, Cytoprotective effects.	[203]
Compritol 888 ATO Miglyol 812 Lutrol F68	Mangiferin (MNG)/ *Oxidative stress related diseases, macular degeneration, diabetic retinopathy*	High shear homogenization and ultrasound	Size 148.9 $\pm$ 0.1 nm PDI 0.21 $\pm$ 0.02 ζ potential -23.5 ± 0.2 mV, EE $\approx$ 92%	Higher antioxidant activity of MNG NLCs vs. free compound according to ORAC assay; Non-irritant formulations according to HET$-$CAM Assay.	[204]
Glyceryl monostearate Castor oil Poloxamer 188	Brimonidine/ *Glaucoma, ocular hypertension*	High shear homogenization	Size 151.97 $\pm$1.98 nm PDI 0.230 $\pm$ 0.01 ζ potential -44.2 ± 7.81 mV EE = 83.631 $\pm$ 0.495%	Improved permeability compared to analogous model SLNs; Highest reduction in the IOP in rabbits (vs. SLNs and free drug).	[172]
Captex 200P (propylene glycol dicaprate) Soya lecithin Capmul® MCM C10 (glyceryl monocaprate) Tween 80 Transcutol P Stearylamine Captex 200P	Brinzolamide (Brla) Latanoprost (Ltp)/ *Glaucoma*	Hot microemulsion method	Size165.28 $\pm$ 2.36 nm PDI 0.31 $\pm$ 0.015 ζ potential 35.33 $\pm$ 0.37 mV EE = 97.5 $\pm$ 2.16%	Adequate transcorneal permeation (Brla and Ltp levels after 24 h were $\approx$82% and $\approx$84%, respectively); Effective reduction of IOP in rats' eyes with laser-induced glaucoma.	[192]

Legend: ARPE—Human retinal pigment epithelial cell line, CNV—Corneal neovascularization, DED—Dry eye disease, HCEC—Human corneal epithelial cell lines, HET$-$CAM—Hen's egg test on chorioallantoic membrane, IL-6—Interleukin-6, MMP—Matrix metalloproteinases, mPEG-2K-DSPE sodium salt—N-(Carbonyl-methoxypolyethylenglycol-2000)-1,2-distearoyl-sn-glycero-3-phosphoethanolamine sodium salt, ORAC—Oxygen radical absorbance capacity, TNF-α—Tumor necrosis factor α.

Further overview of the recent progress of NLCs in ocular therapeutics is shown in Table 3.

Nanostructured lipid carriers are feasible delivery systems for both drugs and biologically active compounds, as illustrated in Table 3. Polyphenolic compounds are well-known for their antioxidant effects, which would be highly beneficial in the therapy of ocular degenerative diseases. However, these phytochemicals are usually characterized by poor aqueous solubility and an unfavorable pharmacokinetic profile, as reported for diosmin [203] and mangiferin [204]. Their encapsulation in NLCs led to an improvement of their disadvantageous physicochemical properties (e.g., low aqueous solubility), and further contributed to superior antioxidant activity (in the case of the mangiferin-loaded NLCs) and cytoprotective effects (for diosmin-loaded NLCs). Other beneficial outcomes following drug loading into NLCs include superior chemical/photo stability, estimated by the rapamycin-loaded NLCs [195], as well as the pronounced enhancement of the solubility of dasatinib upon encapsulation. The latter further contributes to the observed higher anti-proliferation and anti-migration effects [198].

In addition to the conventional topical application, NLCs have been formulated for periocular administration (transscleral delivery), as reported by González-Fernández et al. The authors prepared dexamethasone acetate-loaded NLCs intended for the treatment of posterior eye segment diseases (e.g., macular edema, age-related macular degeneration). The encapsulated prodrug acetate ester provided sustained drug release as a result of the required enzymatic conversion step, and enhanced scleral/choroidal permeability [205].

3.2. Sterilization Feasibility of SLNs and NLCs

Owing to their compositional similarities, NLCs and SLNs can be prepared by identical methods, such as high-pressure homogenization (hot/cold option), high-speed homogenization and/or ultrasonication, solvent emulsification/evaporation, microemulsion, phase inversion techniques, and the solvent injection method [143]. A comprehensive description of the various preparation methods has been detailed by Gordillo-Galeano and Mora-Huertas [131], Khairnar et al. [206] and Duong et al. [207]. However, of great importance for ocular application is one of the post-production steps, namely, the sterilization feasibility.

Techniques such as heat sterilization (autoclaving), sterile filtration and gamma irradiation have been used as *sterilization methods* for SLNs and NLCs intended for ophthalmic application. The selection of the specific method is based on several considerations, such as drug heat stability, composition constituents (melting point of lipids, choice of surfactants), nanoparticle size, and the viscosity of the solution in case of sterile filtration [83,162,208]. *Autoclaving* is the most commonly exploited technique for the sterilization of lipid nanoparticles in ophthalmology, however, with controversial results regarding its impact on the physiochemical characteristics of the nanocarriers. According to some reports, there is no significant change in the particle size [158,172,209] or entrapment efficiency [158] of developed lipid nanocarriers before and after sterilization, in contrast to others, which established an increase in particle size in the micrometer range [210]. The latter may be ascribed to the compromised surfactant film properties, as well as to the melting of lipids at 121 °C, leading to the formation of an o/w emulsion. During the successive cooling and lipid recrystallization, no energy input (i.e., homogenization) was applied to the system, resulting in the increase of particle size [210]. In their study Youshia et al. investigated the influence of autoclaving and *sterilization by gamma irradiation* on the physicochemical parameters of methazolamide-loaded cationic NLCs. According to the results, NLCs subjected to heat sterilization were characterized by significantly lower entrapment efficiency and zeta potential values. At the same time an increase in the particle size and polydispersity index was observed. On the contrary, gamma radiation did not induce significant alterations in the particles size, size distribution pattern, or in the degree of methazolamide entrapment [211]. However, one of the main limitations of this method is the formation of free radicals, therefore, subsequent studies need to be performed, in order to evaluate the chemical stability of the components. Additionally, different strategies may be applied to mitigate the adverse effects of radiation, such as adjustment of the applied dose, lyophilization of the samples, and the use of suitable (endure to γ-radiation) excipients [208].

Sterile filtration has also been exploited as a sterilization approach for lipid nanoparticles used in ophthalmic application, as described by Bonaccorso et al. [157]. The authors investigated the influence of different types of membranes (polypropylene, polyethylene sulfone, polyvinylidene fluoride; pore size of 0.22 µm) on the filtration feasibility of sorafenib-loaded SLNs. The obtained results showed that polypropylene and polyethylene sulfone filters restrain the filtration process by retaining the nanoparticles within the membrane, unlike the polyvinylidene fluoride membrane, which enables SLNs' passage. Furthermore, the obtained SLN suspension after filtration was characterized by unaltered physiochemical parameters [157].

3.3. Clinical Application of SLNs and NLCs in Ocular Therapeutics

Several lipid-based ophthalmic nanocarriers have been successfully implemented into clinical practice, such as Visudyne® (Novartis Pharma AG, Basel, Switzerland), a liposomal verteporfine nanoformulation intended for the therapy of age-related macular degeneration, Durezol® (Alcon, Geneva, Switzerland), a difluprednate nanoemulsion for ocular inflammation treatment, and Restasis® (AbbVie, North Chicago, IL, USA), a cyclosporine nanoemulsion intended for the therapy of dry eye disease [212,213]. However, regardless of the positive outcomes garnered from conducted studies, currently, there are no SLN- or NLC-based ophthalmic formulations that have been translated into clinical applications or marketed. A search through the website www.clinicaltrials.gov (accessed on 1 March 2023) using the keyword "solid lipid nanoparticles" resulted in 10 studies, whereas the keyword "nanostructured lipid carriers" led to 2 results. Currently, none of these trials are related to ocular delivery purposes. Further details are provided in Table S1.

4. Conclusions and Prospects

Solid lipid nanoparticles and nanostructured lipid carriers have shown significant potential for effective ocular drug delivery, as confirmed by the findings summarized in this review. Their advantageous characteristics such as biodegradability, biocompatibility, owing to the generally recognized as safe (GRAS) lipid constituents, and their possibility to provide controlled and sustained drug release, to improve transcorneal penetration and enhance ocular bioavailability, determine their increasing progress in ocular therapeutics. Furthermore, the surface of both types of nanocarriers can be modified to improve their pharmacokinetic characteristics, impart mucoadhesive properties, prolong corneal residence time, and enhance their therapeutic efficacy. The latter can also be achieved by incorporating them into semisolid/in situ gelling formulations and contact lenses (i.e., hybrid delivery systems), which is another promising research direction and would be of great benefit, especially in case of ocular surface diseases. Drug delivery to the posterior segment of the eye can also be accomplished via SLNs and NLCs by proper adjustment of the formulation-related parameters (lipid constituents/surfactant(s) selection; tuning particles' size into the desired nano range), which would be of great significance in the therapy of vision-threatening diseases. However, despite all the promising outcomes from conducted studies, the research progress has not been implemented into clinical application yet. Some of the challenges related to this matter include the possibility of developing reproducible batches of lipid nanoparticles, which exhibit sufficient colloidal stability during storage. In this regard, the implementation of quality-by-design (QbD) approach during the (pre)formulation stage is a feasible strategy, as it provides the possibility to obtain a final product with predictable quality attributes, which would benefit and facilitate nanocarriers' subsequent commercialization [214]. Ocular toxicity is another critical issue to be considered during the development of ophthalmic formulations. According to the findings from the reviewed articles, SLNs and NLCs showed no level of toxicity (based on in vitro or in vivo studies), however, further studies are needed to evaluate their long-term toxicity, as well as their fate after application in vivo [215]. Regarding their clinical application approval, it is crucial to establish unified protocols evaluating their safety and effectiveness [107]. Based on the promising results from the conducted studies, it can be concluded that the potential of SLNs and NLCs should be fully deployed in the near future.

Supplementary Materials: The following supporting information can be downloaded at: https://www.mdpi.com/article/10.3390/ph16030474/s1, Table S1. Solid lipid nanoparticles and nanostructured lipid carriers in clinical trials (terminated studies and studies with unknown status are excluded).

Author Contributions: Conceptualization, V.G. and V.A.; methodology, V.G. and V.A.; investigation, V.G. and V.A.; writing—original draft preparation, V.G. and V.A.; writing—review and editing, V.A.; visualization, V.G.; supervision, V.A.; project administration, V.A. All authors have read and agreed to the published version of the manuscript.

Funding: This research received no external funding.

Institutional Review Board Statement: Not applicable.

Informed Consent Statement: Not applicable.

Data Availability Statement: Data sharing not applicable.

Conflicts of Interest: The authors declare no conflict of interest.

References

1. World Health Organization. *World Report on Vision*; World Health Organization: Geneva, Switzerland, 2019; ISBN 9789241516570.
2. Usgaonkar, U.; Shet Parkar, S.R.; Shetty, A. Impact of the use of digital devices on eyes during the lockdown period of COVID-19 pandemic. *Ind. J. Ophthalmol.* **2021**, *69*, 1901–1906. [CrossRef]
3. Shalini, S.; Ipsita, P.; Abhay, P.; Pandey, A.K. Life style disorders in ophthalmology and their management. *Environ. Conserv. J.* **2019**, *20*, 67–72.
4. García-Marqués, J.V.; Talens-Estarelles, C.; García-Lázaro, S.; Wolffsohn, J.S.; Cerviño, A. Systemic, environmental and lifestyle risk factors for dry eye disease in a mediterranean caucasian population. *Cont. Lens Anterior Eye.* **2022**, *45*, 101539. [CrossRef] [PubMed]
5. Bourne, R.R.A.; Steinmetz, J.D.; Flaxman, S.; Briant, P.S.; Taylor, H.R.; Resnikoff, S.; Casson, R.J.; Abdoli, A.; Gharbieh, E.A.; Afshin, A.; et al. Trends in prevalence of blindness and distance and near vision impairment over 30 years: An analysis for the Global Burden of Disease Study. *Lancet Glob. Health.* **2021**, *9*, e130–e143. [CrossRef]
6. Gote, V.; Sikder, S.; Sicotte, J.; Pal, D. Ocular Drug Delivery: Present Innovations and Future Challenges. *J. Pharmacol. Exp. Ther.* **2019**, *370*, 602–624. [CrossRef]
7. Patel, A.; Cholkar, K.; Agrahari, V.; Mitra, A.K. Ocular drug delivery systems: An overview. *World J. Pharmacol.* **2013**, *2*, 47–64. [CrossRef] [PubMed]
8. Nayak, K.; Misra, M. A review on recent drug delivery systems for posterior segment of eye. *Biomed. Pharmacother.* **2018**, *107*, 1564–1582. [CrossRef]
9. Bachu, R.D.; Chowdhury, P.; Al-Saedi, Z.H.F.; Karla, P.K.; Boddu, S.H.S. Ocular Drug Delivery Barriers-Role of Nanocarriers in the Treatment of Anterior Segment Ocular Diseases. *Pharmaceutics* **2018**, *10*, 28. [CrossRef]
10. Wilson, C.G. Ophthalmic Formulation. In *Specialized Pharmaceutical Formulation: The Science and Technology of Dosage Forms*, 1st ed.; Tovey, G.D., Ed.; Royal Society of Chemistry: London, UK, 2022; pp. 1–44.
11. Kuno, N.; Fujii, S. Recent Advances in Ocular Drug Delivery Systems. *Polymers* **2011**, *3*, 193–221. [CrossRef]
12. Jünemann, A.G.M.; Chorągiewicz, T.; Ozimek, M.; Grieb, P.; Rejdak, R. Drug bioavailability from topically applied ocular drops. Does drop size matter? *Ophthalmol. J.* **2016**, *1*, 29–35. [CrossRef]
13. Taghe, S.; Mirzaeei, S. Preparation and characterization of novel, mucoadhesive ofloxacin nanoparticles for ocular drug delivery. *Braz. J. Pharm. Sci.* **2019**, *55*, e17105. [CrossRef]
14. Gaudana, R.; Ananthula, H.K.; Parenky, A.; Mitra, A.K. Ocular drug delivery. *AAPS J.* **2010**, *12*, 348–360. [CrossRef]
15. Baranowski, P.; Karolewicz, B.; Gajda, M.; Pluta, J. Ophthalmic drug dosage forms: Characterisation and research methods. *Sci. World J.* **2014**, *2014*, 861904. [CrossRef]
16. Wu, Y.; Liu, Y.; Li, X.; Kebebe, D.; Zhang, B.; Ren, J.; Lu, J.; Li, J.; Du, S.; Liu, Z. Research progress of in-situ gelling ophthalmic drug delivery system. *Asian J. Pharm. Sci.* **2019**, *14*, 1–15. [CrossRef]
17. Bastawrous, A.; Burgess, P.I.; Mahdi, A.M.; Kyari, F.; Burton, M.J.; Kuper, H. Posterior segment eye disease in sub-Saharan Africa: Review of recent population-based studies. *Trop. Med. Int. Health.* **2014**, *19*, 600–609. [CrossRef]
18. Tóth, G.; Szabó, D.; Sándor, G.L.; Nagy, Z.Z.; Limburg, H.; Németh, J. Hátsószegmens-betegségek okozta látásromlás és vakság Magyarországon az 50 évnél idosebb korú lakosság körében [Visual impairment and blindness caused by posterior segment diseases in Hungary in people aged 50 years and older]. *Orv. Hetil.* **2022**, *163*, 624–630. [CrossRef]

19. Varela-Fernández, R.; Díaz-Tomé, V.; Luaces-Rodríguez, A.; Conde-Penedo, A.; García-Otero, X.; Luzardo-Álvarez, A.; Fernández-Ferreiro, A.; Otero-Espinar, F.J. Drug Delivery to the Posterior Segment of the Eye: Biopharmaceutic and Pharmacokinetic Considerations. *Pharmaceutics* **2020**, *12*, 269. [CrossRef] [PubMed]

20. Otero-Espinar, F.J.; Fernández-Ferreiro, A.; González-Barcia, M.; Blanco-Méndez, J.; Luzardo, A. Stimuli sensitive ocular drug delivery systems. In *Drug Targeting and Stimuli Sensitive Drug Delivery Systems*, 1st ed.; Grumezescu, A., Ed.; Elsevier: Amsterdam, The Netherlands, 2018; pp. 211–270.

21. Sánchez-López, E.; Espina, M.; Doktorovova, S.; Souto, E.B.; García, M.L. Lipid nanoparticles (SLN, NLC): Overcoming the anatomical and physiological barriers of the eye—Part I—Barriers and determining factors in ocular delivery. *Eur. J. Pharm. Biopharm.* **2017**, *110*, 70–75. [CrossRef] [PubMed]

22. Dos Santos, G.A.; Ferreira-Nunes, R.; Dalmolin, L.F.; Dos Santos Ré, A.C.; Anjos, J.L.V.; Mendanha, S.A.; Aires, C.P.; Lopez, R.F.V.; Cunha-Filho, M.; Gelfuso, G.M.; et al. Besifloxacin liposomes with positively charged additives for an improved topical ocular delivery. *Sci. Rep.* **2020**, *10*, 19285. [CrossRef]

23. Chen, X.; Wu, J.; Lin, X.; Wu, X.; Yu, X.; Wang, B.; Xu, W. Tacrolimus Loaded Cationic Liposomes for Dry Eye Treatment. *Front. Pharmacol.* **2022**, *13*, 838168. [CrossRef] [PubMed]

24. Fathalla, D.; Fouad, E.A.; Soliman, G.M. Latanoprost niosomes as a sustained release ocular delivery system for the management of glaucoma. *Drug Dev. Ind. Pharm.* **2020**, *46*, 806–813. [CrossRef] [PubMed]

25. El-Nabarawi, M.A.; Abd El Rehem, R.T.; Teaima, M.; Abary, M.; El-Mofty, H.M.; Khafagy, M.M.; Lotfy, N.M.; Salah, M. Natamycin niosomes as a promising ocular nanosized delivery system with ketorolac tromethamine for dual effects for treatment of candida rabbit keratitis; in vitro/in vivo and histopathological studies. *Drug Dev. Ind. Pharm.* **2019**, *45*, 922–936. [CrossRef] [PubMed]

26. Vicente-Pascual, M.; Gómez-Aguado, I.; Rodríguez-Castejón, J.; Rodríguez-Gascón, A.; Muntoni, E.; Battaglia, L.; del Pozo-Rodríguez, A.; Solinís Aspiazu, M.Á. Topical Administration of SLN-Based Gene Therapy for the Treatment of Corneal Inflammation by De Novo IL-10 Production. *Pharmaceutics* **2020**, *12*, 584. [CrossRef]

27. Wang, L.; Liu, W.; Huang, X. An approach to revolutionize cataract treatment by enhancing drug probing through intraocular cell line. *Libyan J. Med.* **2018**, *13*, 1500347. [CrossRef] [PubMed]

28. Lou, X.; Hu, Y.; Zhang, H.; Liu, J.; Zhao, Y. Polydopamine nanoparticles attenuate retina ganglion cell degeneration and restore visual function after optic nerve injury. *J. Nanobiotechnology* **2021**, *19*, 436. [CrossRef]

29. Francia, S.; Shmal, D.; Di Marco, S.; Chiaravalli, G.; Maya-Vetencourt, J.F.; Mantero, G.; Michetti, C.; Cupini, S.; Manfredi, G.; DiFrancesco, M.L.; et al. Light-induced charge generation in polymeric nanoparticles restores vision in advanced-stage retinitis pigmentosa rats. *Nat. Commun.* **2022**, *13*, 3677. [CrossRef]

30. Rincón, M.; Espinoza, L.C.; Silva-Abreu, M.; Sosa, L.; Pesantez-Narvaez, J.; Abrego, G.; Calpena, A.C.; Mallandrich, M. Quality by Design of Pranoprofen Loaded Nanostructured Lipid Carriers and Their Ex Vivo Evaluation in Different Mucosae and Ocular Tissues. *Pharmaceuticals* **2022**, *15*, 1185. [CrossRef] [PubMed]

31. Polat, H.K.; Kurt, N.; Aytekin, E.; Akdağ Çaylı, Y.; Bozdağ Pehlivan, S.; Çalış, S. Design of Besifloxacin HCl-Loaded Nanostructured Lipid Carriers: *In Vitro* and *Ex Vivo* Evaluation. *J. Ocul. Pharmacol. Ther.* **2022**, *38*, 412–423. [CrossRef]

32. Sun, L.; Zhang, M.; Shi, Y.; Fang, L.; Cao, F. Rational design of mixed nanomicelle eye drops with structural integrity investigation. *Acta Biomater.* **2022**, *141*, 164–177. [CrossRef]

33. Xu, X.; Sun, L.; Zhou, L.; Cheng, Y.; Cao, F. Functional chitosan oligosaccharide nanomicelles for topical ocular drug delivery of dexamethasone. *Carbohydr. Polym.* **2020**, *227*, 115356. [CrossRef]

34. Nayak, K.; Misra, M. PEGylated microemulsion for dexamethasone delivery to posterior segment of eye. *J. Biomater. Sci. Polym. Ed.* **2020**, *31*, 1071–1090. [CrossRef] [PubMed]

35. Bachu, R.D.; Stepanski, M.; Alzhrani, R.M.; Jung, R.; Boddu, S.H.S. Development and Evaluation of a Novel Microemulsion of Dexamethasone and Tobramycin for Topical Ocular Administration. *J. Ocul. Pharmacol. Ther.* **2018**, *34*, 312–324. [CrossRef] [PubMed]

36. Bravo-Osuna, I.; Vicario-de-la-Torre, M.; Andrés-Guerrero, V.; Sánchez-Nieves, J.; Guzmán-Navarro, M.; de la Mata, F.J.; Gómez, R.; de Las Heras, B.; Argüeso, P.; Ponchel, G.; et al. Novel Water-Soluble Mucoadhesive Carbosilane Dendrimers for Ocular Administration. *Mol. Pharm.* **2016**, *13*, 2966–2976. [CrossRef]

37. Ghasemiyeh, P.; Mohammadi-Samani, S. Solid lipid nanoparticles and nanostructured lipid carriers as novel drug delivery systems: Applications, advantages and disadvantages. *Res. Pharm. Sci.* **2018**, *13*, 288–303.

38. Costa, C.P.; Barreiro, S.; Moreira, J.N.; Silva, R.; Almeida, H.; Sousa Lobo, J.M.; Silva, A.C. In Vitro Studies on Nasal Formulations of Nanostructured Lipid Carriers (NLC) and Solid Lipid Nanoparticles (SLN). *Pharmaceuticals* **2021**, *14*, 711. [CrossRef]

39. Nguyen, V.H.; Thuy, V.N.; Van, T.V.; Dao, A.H.; Lee, B.-J. Nanostructured lipid carriers and their potential applications for versatile drug delivery via oral administration. *OpenNano* **2022**, *8*, 100064. [CrossRef]

40. Czajkowska-Kośnik, A.; Szekalska, M.; Winnicka, K. Nanostructured lipid carriers: A potential use for skin drug delivery systems. *Pharmacol. Rep.* **2019**, *71*, 156–166. [CrossRef]

41. Musielak, E.; Feliczak-Guzik, A.; Nowak, I. Optimization of the Conditions of Solid Lipid Nanoparticles (SLN) Synthesis. *Molecules* **2022**, *27*, 2202. [CrossRef] [PubMed]

42. Poonia, N.; Kharb, R.; Lather, V.; Pandita, D. Nanostructured lipid carriers: Versatile oral delivery vehicle. *Future Sci. OA* **2016**, *2*, FSO135. [CrossRef]

43. Abo El-Enin, H.A.; Elkomy, M.H.; Naguib, I.A.; Ahmed, M.F.; Alsaidan, O.A.; Alsalahat, I.; Ghoneim, M.M.; Eid, H.M. Lipid Nanocarriers Overlaid with Chitosan for Brain Delivery of Berberine via the Nasal Route. *Pharmaceuticals* **2022**, *15*, 281. [CrossRef]
44. Mirchandani, Y.; Patravale, V.B.; Brijesh, S. Solid lipid nanoparticles for hydrophilic drugs. *J. Control Release.* **2021**, *335*, 457–464. [CrossRef] [PubMed]
45. Neves, A.R.; Queiroz, J.F.; Weksler, B.; Romero, I.A.; Couraud, P.O.; Reis, S. Solid lipid nanoparticles as a vehicle for brain-targeted drug delivery: Two new strategies of functionalization with apolipoprotein E. *Nanotechnology* **2015**, *26*, 495103. [CrossRef] [PubMed]
46. Lee, W.J. Eye. In *Vitamin C in Human Health and Disease*, 1st ed.; Lee, W.J., Ed.; Springer: Dordrecht, The Netherlands, 2019; pp. 177–182.
47. Watson, P.G.; Young, R.D. Scleral structure, organisation and disease. A review. *Exp. Eye Res.* **2004**, *78*, 609–623. [CrossRef] [PubMed]
48. Sridhar, M.S. Anatomy of cornea and ocular surface. *Indian J. Ophthalmol.* **2018**, *66*, 190–194. [CrossRef]
49. Labelle, P. The Eye. In *Pathologic Basis of Veterinary Disease*, 6th ed.; Zachary, J.F., Ed.; Elsevier: Amsterdam, The Netherlands, 2017; pp. 1265–1318.e1.
50. Moiseev, R.V.; Morrison, P.W.J.; Steele, F.; Khutoryanskiy, V.V. Penetration Enhancers in Ocular Drug Delivery. *Pharmaceutics* **2019**, *11*, 321. [CrossRef]
51. Salazar, J.J.; Ramírez, A.I.; De Hoz, R.; Salobrar-Garcia, E.; Rojas, P.; Fernández-Albarral, J.A.; López-Cuenca, I.; Rojas, B.; Triviño, A.; Ramírez, J.M. *Anatomy of the Human Optic Nerve: Structure and Function*; Ferreri, F.M., Ed.; IntechOpen: London, UK, 2018; pp. 1–46.
52. Lin, S.; Ge, C.; Wang, D.; Xie, Q.; Wu, B.; Wang, J.; Nan, K.; Zheng, Q.; Chen, W. Overcoming the Anatomical and Physiological Barriers in Topical Eye Surface Medication Using a Peptide-Decorated Polymeric Micelle. *ACS Appl. Mater. Interfaces* **2019**, *11*, 39603–39612. [CrossRef] [PubMed]
53. Xu, X.; Zuo, Y.Y. Nanomedicine for Ocular Drug Delivery. In *Nanomedicine*, 1st ed.; Gu, N., Ed.; Springer: Singapore, 2022; pp. 755–786.
54. McDermott, A.M. Antimicrobial Compounds in Tears. *Exp. Eye Res.* **2013**, *117*, 53–61. [CrossRef]
55. Kopacz, D.; Niezgoda, Ł.; Fudalej, E.; Nowak, A.; Maciejewicz, P. Tear film—Physiology and Disturbances in Various Diseases and Disorders. In *Ocular Surface Diseases—Some Current Date on Tear Film Problem and Keratoconic Diagnosis*, 1st ed.; Kopacz, D., Ed.; IntechOpen: London, UK, 2021; pp. 1–17.
56. Willcox, M.D.P.; Argüeso, P.; Georgiev, G.A.; Holopainen, J.M.; Laurie, G.W.; Millar, T.J.; Papas, E.B.; Rolland, J.P.; Schmidt, T.A.; Stahl, U.; et al. TFOS DEWS II Tear Film Report. *Ocul. Surf.* **2017**, *15*, 366–403. [CrossRef] [PubMed]
57. Yang, Y.; Lockwood, A. Topical ocular drug delivery systems: Innovations for an unmet need. *Exp. Eye Res.* **2022**, *218*, 109006. [CrossRef]
58. Jumelle, C.; Gholizadeh, S.; Annabi, N.; Dana, R. Advances and limitations of drug delivery systems formulated as eye drops. *J. Control Release.* **2020**, *321*, 1–22. [CrossRef]
59. Shafaie, S.; Hutter, V.; Cook, M.T.; Brown, M.B.; Chau, D.Y.S. In Vitro Cell Models for Ophthalmic Drug Development Applications. *Biores. Open Access.* **2016**, *5*, 94–108. [CrossRef]
60. Peris-Martínez, C.; García-Domene, M.C.; Penadés, M.; Luque, M.J.; Fernández-López, E.; Artigas, J.M. Spectral Transmission of the Human Corneal Layers. *J. Clin. Med.* **2021**, *10*, 4490. [CrossRef] [PubMed]
61. Ruan, Y.; Jiang, S.; Musayeva, A.; Pfeiffer, N.; Gericke, A. Corneal Epithelial Stem Cells-Physiology, Pathophysiology and Therapeutic Options. *Cells* **2021**, *10*, 2302. [CrossRef] [PubMed]
62. Shastri, D.H.; Silva, A.C.; Almeida, H. Ocular Delivery of Therapeutic Proteins: A Review. *Pharmaceutics* **2023**, *15*, 205. [CrossRef]
63. Wang, R.; Gao, Y.; Liu, A.; Zhai, G. A review of nanocarrier-mediated drug delivery systems for posterior segment eye disease: Challenges analysis and recent advances. *J. Drug Target* **2021**, *29*, 687–702. [CrossRef] [PubMed]
64. Nakano, M.; Lockhart, C.M.; Kelly, E.J.; Rettie, A.E. Ocular cytochrome P450s and transporters: Roles in disease and endobiotic and xenobiotic disposition. *Drug Metab. Rev.* **2014**, *46*, 247–260. [CrossRef] [PubMed]
65. Lagali, N. Corneal Stromal Regeneration: Current Status and Future Therapeutic Potential. *Curr. Eye Res.* **2020**, *45*, 278–290. [CrossRef]
66. Morrison, P.W.; Khutoryanskiy, V.V. Advances in ophthalmic drug delivery. *Ther. Deliv.* **2014**, *5*, 1297–1315. [CrossRef]
67. Agrahari, V.; Mandal, A.; Agrahari, V.; Trinh, H.M.; Joseph, M.; Ray, A.; Hadji, H.; Mitra, R.; Pal, D.; Mitra, A.K. A comprehensive insight on ocular pharmacokinetics. *Drug Deliv. Transl. Res.* **2016**, *6*, 735–754. [CrossRef]
68. Pak, J.; Chen, Z.J.; Sun, K.; Przekwas, A.; Walenga, R.; Fan, J. Computational Modeling of Drug Transport Across the In Vitro Cornea. *Comput. Biol. Med.* **2018**, *92*, 139–146. [CrossRef]
69. Löscher, M.; Seiz, C.; Hurst, J.; Schnichels, S. Topical Drug Delivery to the Posterior Segment of the Eye. *Pharmaceutics* **2022**, *14*, 134. [CrossRef]
70. Harikumar, S.I.; Sonia, A. Nanotechnological approaches in Ophthalmic delivery systems. *Int. J. Drug Dev. Res.* **2011**, *3*, 9–19.
71. Kwatra, D.; Mitra, A.K. Drug delivery in ocular diseases: Barriers and strategies. *World J. Pharmacol.* **2013**, *2*, 78–83. [CrossRef]
72. Akhter, M.H.; Ahmad, I.; Alshahrani, M.Y.; Al-Harbi, A.I.; Khalilullah, H.; Afzal, O.; Altamimi, A.S.A.; Najib Ullah, S.N.M.; Ojha, A.; Karim, S. Drug Delivery Challenges and Current Progress in Nanocarrier-Based Ocular Therapeutic System. *Gels* **2022**, *8*, 82. [CrossRef] [PubMed]

73. de Oliveira, I.F.; Barbosa, E.J.; Peters, M.C.C.; Henostroza, M.A.B.; Yukuyama, M.N.; Dos Santos Neto, E.; Löbenberg, R.; Bou-Chacra, N. Cutting-edge advances in therapy for the posterior segment of the eye: Solid lipid nanoparticles and nanostructured lipid carriers. *Int. J. Pharm.* **2020**, *589*, 119831. [CrossRef]

74. Pescina, S.; Lucca, L.G.; Govoni, P.; Padula, C.; Favero, E.D.; Cantù, L.; Santi, P.; Nicoli, S. Ex Vivo Conjunctival Retention and Transconjunctival Transport of Poorly Soluble Drugs Using Polymeric Micelles. *Pharmaceutics* **2019**, *11*, 476. [CrossRef] [PubMed]

75. Hosoya, K.; Lee, V.H.; Kim, K.J. Roles of the conjunctiva in ocular drug delivery: A review of conjunctival transport mechanisms and their regulation. *Eur. J. Pharm. Biopharm.* **2005**, *60*, 227–240. [CrossRef]

76. Szabadi, E. Functional Organization of the Sympathetic Pathways Controlling the Pupil: Light-Inhibited and Light-Stimulated Pathways. *Front. Neurol.* **2018**, *9*, 1069. [CrossRef]

77. Jakubiak, P.; Cantrill, C.; Urtti, A.; Alvarez-Sánchez, R. Establishment of an In vitro-In vivo Correlation for Melanin Binding and the Extension of the Ocular Half-Life of Small-Molecule Drugs. *Mol. Pharm.* **2019**, *16*, 4890–4901. [CrossRef]

78. Tangri, P.; Khurana, S. Basics of ocular drug delivery systems. *Int. J. Res. Pharm. Biomed. Sci.* **2011**, *2*, 1541–1552.

79. Rimpelä, A.K.; Reinisalo, M.; Hellinen, L.; Grazhdankin, E.; Kidron, H.; Urtti, A.; Del Amo, E.M. Implications of melanin binding in ocular drug delivery. *Adv. Drug Deliv. Rev.* **2018**, *126*, 23–43. [CrossRef]

80. Rimpelä, A.K.; Hagström, M.; Kidron, H.; Urtti, A. Melanin targeting for intracellular drug delivery: Quantification of bound and free drug in retinal pigment epithelial cells. *J. Control Release* **2018**, *283*, 261–268. [CrossRef] [PubMed]

81. Achouri, D.; Alhanout, K.; Piccerelle, P.; Andrieu, V. Recent advances in ocular drug delivery. *Drug Dev. Ind. Pharm.* **2013**, *39*, 1599–1617. [CrossRef] [PubMed]

82. Dubald, M.; Bourgeois, S.; Andrieu, V.; Fessi, H. Ophthalmic Drug Delivery Systems for Antibiotherapy—A Review. *Pharmaceutics* **2018**, *10*, 10. [CrossRef] [PubMed]

83. Seyfoddin, A.; Shaw, J.; Al-Kassas, R. Solid lipid nanoparticles for ocular drug delivery. *Drug Deliv.* **2010**, *7*, 467–489. [CrossRef]

84. Ali, J.; Fazil, M.; Qumbar, M.; Khan, N.; Ali, A. Colloidal drug delivery system: Amplify the ocular delivery. *Drug Deliv.* **2014**, *23*, 700–716.

85. Hejtmancik, J.F.; Shiels, A. Overview of the Lens. *Prog. Mol. Biol. Transl. Sci.* **2015**, *134*, 119–127.

86. Ruan, X.; Liu, Z.; Luo, L.; Liu, Y. The structure of the lens and its associations with the visual quality. *BMJ Open Ophthalmol.* **2020**, *5*, e000459. [CrossRef]

87. Coudrillier, B.; Pijanka, J.; Jefferys, J.; Sorensen, T.; Quigley, H.A.; Boote, C.; Nguyen, T.D. Collagen structure and mechanical properties of the human sclera: Analysis for the effects of age. *J. Biomech. Eng.* **2015**, *137*, 410061–4100614. [CrossRef]

88. Alshaikh, R.A.; Waeber, C.; Ryan, K.B. Polymer based sustained drug delivery to the ocular posterior segment: Barriers and future opportunities for the treatment of neovascular pathologies. *Adv. Drug Deliv. Rev.* **2022**, *187*, 114342. [CrossRef]

89. Yadav, D.; Varma, L.T.; Yadav, K. Drug Delivery to Posterior Segment of the Eye: Conventional Delivery Strategies, Their Barriers, and Restrictions. In *Drug Delivery for the Retina and Posterior Segment Disease*, 1st ed.; Patel, J.K., Sutariya, V., Kanwar, J.R., Pathak, Y.V., Eds.; Springer: Cham, Switzerland, 2018; pp. 51–67.

90. Djigo, A.D.; Bérubé, J.; Landreville, S.; Proulx, S. Characterization of a tissue-engineered choroid. *Acta Biomater.* **2019**, *84*, 305–316. [CrossRef]

91. Hurley, J.B. Retina Metabolism and Metabolism in the Pigmented Epithelium: A Busy Intersection. *Annu. Rev. Vis. Sci.* **2021**, *7*, 665–692. [CrossRef] [PubMed]

92. Del Amo, E.M.; Rimpelä, A.K.; Heikkinen, E.; Kari, O.K.; Ramsay, E.; Lajunen, T.; Schmitt, M.; Pelkonen, L.; Bhattacharya, M.; Richardson, D.; et al. Pharmacokinetic aspects of retinal drug delivery. *Prog. Retin. Eye Res.* **2017**, *57*, 134–185. [CrossRef]

93. Naylor, A.; Hopkins, A.; Hudson, N.; Campbell, M. Tight Junctions of the Outer Blood Retina Barrier. *Int. J. Mol. Sci.* **2019**, *21*, 211. [CrossRef]

94. Willermain, F.; Libert, S.; Motulsky, E.; Salik, D.; Caspers, L.; Perret, J.; Delporte, C. Origins and consequences of hyperosmolar stress in retinal pigmented epithelial cells. *Front. Physiol.* **2014**, *5*, 199. [CrossRef] [PubMed]

95. Díaz-Coránguez, M.; Ramos, C.; Antonetti, D.A. The inner blood-retinal barrier: Cellular basis and development. *Vision Res.* **2017**, *139*, 123–137. [CrossRef]

96. Asencio-Duran, M.; Dabad-Moreno, J.; Vicandi-Plaza, B.; Muñoz, M.; Capote-Díez, M.; Santisteban, G. The Vitreous Body and Its Role in the Diagnosis of Eye Pathologies. *Med. Res. Arch.* **2021**, *9*, 9. [CrossRef]

97. Mishra, D.; Gade, S.; Glover, K.; Sheshala, R.; Singh, T.R.R. Vitreous Humor: Composition, Characteristics and Implication on Intravitreal Drug Delivery. *Curr. Eye Res.* **2022**, *48*, 208–218. [CrossRef]

98. Stevens, S. Administering a subconjunctival injection. *Community Eye Health J.* **2009**, *22*, 15.

99. Rafiei, F.; Tabesh, H.; Farzad, F. Sustained subconjunctival drug delivery systems: Current trends and future perspectives. *Int. Ophthalmol.* **2020**, *40*, 2385–2401. [CrossRef]

100. Nebbioso, M.; Livani, M.L.; Santamaria, V.; Librando, A.; Sepe, M. Intracameral lidocaine as supplement to classic topical anesthesia for relieving ocular pain in cataract surgery. *Int. J. Ophthalmol.* **2018**, *11*, 1932–1935.

101. Alghamdi, E.A.S.; Al Qahtani, A.Y.; Sinjab, M.M.; Alyahya, K.M. Intracameral Injections. In *Extemporaneous Ophthalmic Preparations*, 1st ed.; Alghamdi, E.A.S., Al Qahtani, A.Y., Sinjab, M.M., Alyahya, K.M., Eds.; Springer: Cham, Switzerland, 2020; pp. 67–68.

102. Shah, T.J.; Conway, M.D.; Peyman, G.A. Intracameral dexamethasone injection in the treatment of cataract surgery induced inflammation: Design, development, and place in therapy. *Clin. Ophthalmol.* **2018**, *12*, 2223–2235. [CrossRef]

103. Adrianto, M.F.; Annuryanti, F.; Wilson, C.G.; Sheshala, R.; Thakur, R.R.S. In vitro dissolution testing models of ocular implants for posterior segment drug delivery. *Drug Deliv. Transl. Res.* **2022**, *12*, 1355–1375. [CrossRef] [PubMed]

104. Marashi, A.; Zazo, A. Suprachoroidal injection of triamcinolone acetonide using a custom-made needle to treat diabetic macular edema post pars plana vitrectomy: A case series. *J. Int. Med. Res.* **2022**, *50*, 1–10. [CrossRef]

105. Chiang, B.; Jung, J.H.; Prausnitz, M.R. The suprachoroidal space as a route of administration to the posterior segment of the eye. *Adv. Drug Deliv. Rev.* **2018**, *126*, 58–66. [CrossRef]

106. Martin, D.F. Evolution of Intravitreal Therapy for Retinal Diseases-From CMV to CNV: The LXXIV Edward Jackson Memorial Lecture. *Am. J. Ophthalmol.* **2018**, *191*, xli–lviii. [CrossRef] [PubMed]

107. Gorantla, S.; Rapalli, V.K.; Waghule, T.; Singh, P.P.; Dubey, S.K.; Saha, R.N.; Singhvi, G. Nanocarriers for ocular drug delivery: Current status and translational opportunity. *RSC Adv.* **2020**, *10*, 27835–27855. [CrossRef]

108. Peng, C.; Kuang, L.; Zhao, J.; Ross, A.E.; Wang, Z.; Ciolino, J.B. Bibliometric and visualized analysis of ocular drug delivery from 2001 to 2020. *J. Control Release.* **2022**, *345*, 625–645. [CrossRef]

109. Das, B.; Nayak, A.K.; Mallick, S. Lipid-based nanocarriers for ocular drug delivery: An updated review. *J. Drug Deliv. Sci. Technol.* **2022**, *76*, 103780. [CrossRef]

110. Shahraeini, S.S.; Akbari, J.; Saeedi, M.; Morteza-Semnani, K.; Abootorabi, S.; Dehghanpoor, M.; Rostamkalaei, S.S.; Nokhodchi, A. Atorvastatin Solid Lipid Nanoparticles as a Promising Approach for Dermal Delivery and an Anti-inflammatory Agent. *AAPS PharmSciTech.* **2020**, *21*, 263. [CrossRef] [PubMed]

111. Essaghraoui, A.; Belfkira, A.; Hamdaoui, B.; Nunes, C.; Lima, S.A.C.; Reis, S. Improved Dermal Delivery of Cyclosporine A Loaded in Solid Lipid Nanoparticles. *Nanomaterials* **2019**, *9*, 1204. [CrossRef]

112. Kakkar, S.; Singh, M.; Mohan Karuppayil, S.; Raut, J.S.; Giansanti, F.; Papucci, L.; Schiavone, N.; Nag, T.C.; Gao, N.; Yu, F.X.; et al. Lipo-PEG nano-ocular formulation successfully encapsulates hydrophilic fluconazole and traverses corneal and non-corneal path to reach posterior eye segment. *J. Drug Target* **2021**, *29*, 631–650. [CrossRef]

113. Gómez-Aguado, I.; Rodríguez-Castejón, J.; Beraza-Millor, M.; Vicente-Pascual, M.; Rodríguez-Gascón, A.; Garelli, S.; Battaglia, L.; del Pozo-Rodríguez, A.; Solinís, M.Á. mRNA-Based Nanomedicinal Products to Address Corneal Inflammation by Interleukin-10 Supplementation. *Pharmaceutics* **2021**, *13*, 1472. [CrossRef] [PubMed]

114. Wang, J.L.; Hanafy, M.S.; Xu, H.; Leal, J.; Zhai, Y.; Ghosh, D.; Williams, R.O., III; Smyth, H.D.C.; Cui, Z. Aerosolizable siRNA-encapsulated solid lipid nanoparticles prepared by thin-film freeze-drying for potential pulmonary delivery. *Int. J. Pharm.* **2021**, *596*, 120215. [CrossRef] [PubMed]

115. Elbrink, K.; Van Hees, S.; Chamanza, R.; Roelant, D.; Loomans, T.; Holm, R.; Kiekens, F. Application of solid lipid nanoparticles as a long-term drug delivery platform for intramuscular and subcutaneous administration: In vitro and in vivo evaluation. *Eur. J. Pharm. Biopharm.* **2021**, *163*, 158–170. [CrossRef]

116. Khanna, K.; Sharma, N.; Rawat, S.; Khan, N.; Karwasra, R.; Hasan, N.; Kumar, A.; Jain, G.K.; Nishad, D.K.; Khanna, S.; et al. Intranasal solid lipid nanoparticles for management of pain: A full factorial design approach, characterization & Gamma Scintigraphy. *Chem. Phys. Lipids* **2021**, *236*, 105060. [CrossRef]

117. Parvez, S.; Yadagiri, G.; Gedda, M.R.; Singh, A.; Singh, O.P.; Verma, A.; Sundar, S.; Mudavath, S.L. Modified solid lipid nanoparticles encapsulated with Amphotericin B and Paromomycin: An effective oral combination against experimental murine visceral leishmaniasis. *Sci. Rep.* **2020**, *10*, 12243. [CrossRef]

118. Angelova, A.; Angelov, B. Dual and multi-drug delivery nanoparticles towards neuronal survival and synaptic repair. *Neural Regen Res.* **2017**, *12*, 886–889. [CrossRef]

119. Sahoo, R.K.; Biswas, N.; Guha, A.; Sahoo, N.; Kuotsu, K. Nonionic surfactant vesicles in ocular delivery: Innovative approaches and perspectives. *Biomed Res. Int.* **2014**, *2014*, 263604. [CrossRef]

120. Youssef, A.A.A.; Dudhipala, N.; Majumdar, S. Dual Drug Loaded Lipid Nanocarrier Formulations for Topical Ocular Applications. *Int. J. Nanomed.* **2022**, *17*, 2283–2299. [CrossRef] [PubMed]

121. Alvi, M.M.; Chatterjee, P. A prospective analysis of co-processed non-ionic surfactants in enhancing permeability of a model hydrophilic drug. *AAPS PharmSciTech.* **2014**, *15*, 339–353. [CrossRef] [PubMed]

122. Jacob, S.; Nair, A.B.; Shah, J.; Gupta, S.; Boddu, S.H.S.; Sreeharsha, N.; Joseph, A.; Shinu, P.; Morsy, M.A. Lipid Nanoparticles as a Promising Drug Delivery Carrier for Topical Ocular Therapy—An Overview on Recent Advances. *Pharmaceutics* **2022**, *14*, 533. [CrossRef] [PubMed]

123. Malvajerd, S.S.; Azadi, A.; Izadi, Z.; Kurd, M.; Dara, T.; Dibaei, M.; Zadeh, M.S.; Javar, H.A.; Hamidi, M. Brain delivery of curcumin using solid lipid nanoparticles and nanostructured lipid carriers: Preparation, optimization, and pharmacokinetic evaluation. *ACS Chem. Neurosci.* **2019**, *10*, 728–739. [CrossRef]

124. Nagai, N.; Ogata, F.; Otake, H.; Nakazawa, Y.; Kawasaki, N. Energy-dependent endocytosis is responsible for drug transcorneal penetration following the instillation of ophthalmic formulations containing indomethacin nanoparticles. *Int. J. Nanomedicine* **2019**, *14*, 1213–1227. [CrossRef] [PubMed]

125. González-Fernández, F.M.; Bianchera, A.; Gasco, P.; Nicoli, S.; Pescina, S. Lipid-Based Nanocarriers for Ophthalmic Administration: Towards Experimental Design Implementation. *Pharmaceutics* **2021**, *13*, 447. [CrossRef]

126. Amrite, A.C.; Edelhauser, H.F.; Singh, S.R.; Kompella, U.B. Effect of circulation on the disposition and ocular tissue distribution of 20 nm nanoparticles after periocular administration. *Mol. Vis.* **2008**, *14*, 150–160.

127. Niamprem, P.; Srinivas, S.P.; Tiyaboonchai, W. Penetration of Nile red-loaded nanostructured lipid carriers (NLCs) across the porcine cornea. *Colloids Surf. B Biointerfaces.* **2019**, *176*, 371–378. [CrossRef]
128. Scioli Montoto, S.; Muraca, G.; Ruiz, M.E. Solid Lipid Nanoparticles for Drug Delivery: Pharmacological and Biopharmaceutical Aspects. *Front. Mol. Biosci.* **2020**, *7*, 587997. [CrossRef] [PubMed]
129. Duan, Y.; Dhar, A.; Patel, C.; Khimani, M.; Neogi, S.; Sharma, P.; Kumar, N.S.; Vekariya, R.L. A brief review on solid lipid nanoparticles: Part and parcel of contemporary drug delivery systems. *RSC Adv.* **2020**, *10*, 26777–26791. [CrossRef] [PubMed]
130. Attama, A.A.; Momoh, M.A.; Builders, P.F. Lipid Nanoparticulate Drug Delivery Systems: A Revolution in Dosage Form Design and Development. In *Recent Advances in Novel Drug Carrier Systems*; Sezer, A.D., Ed.; IntechOpen: London, UK, 2012; pp. 107–140.
131. Gordillo-Galeano, A.; Mora-Huertas, C.E. Solid lipid nanoparticles and nanostructured lipid carriers: A review emphasizing on particle structure and drug release. *Eur. J. Pharm. Biopharm.* **2018**, *133*, 285–308. [CrossRef]
132. Boonme, P.; Souto, E.B.; Wuttisantikul, N.; Jongjit, T.; Pichayakorn, W. Influence of lipids on the properties of solid lipid nanoparticles from microemulsion technique. *Eur. J. Lipid Sci. Technol.* **2013**, *115*, 820–824. [CrossRef]
133. Paliwal, R.; Rai, S.; Vaidya, B.; Khatri, K.; Goyal, A.K.; Mishra, N.; Mehta, A.; Vyas, S.P. Effect of lipid core material on characteristics of solid lipid nanoparticles designed for oral lymphatic delivery. *Nanomedicine* **2009**, *5*, 184–191. [CrossRef] [PubMed]
134. Cavendish, M.; Nalone, L.; Barbosa, T.; Barbosa, R.; Costa, S.; Nunes, R.; da Silva, C.F.; Chaud, M.V.; Souto, E.B.; Hollanda, L.; et al. Study of pre-formulation and development of solid lipid nanoparticles containing perillyl alcohol. *J. Therm. Anal. Calorim.* **2019**, *141*, 767–774. [CrossRef]
135. Hernández-Esquivel, R.-A.; Navarro-Tovar, G.; Zárate-Hernández, E.; Aguirre-Bañuelos, P. Solid Lipid Nanoparticles (SLN). In *Nanocomposite Materials for Biomedical and Energy Storage Applications*, 1st ed.; Sharma, A., Ed.; IntechOpen: London, UK, 2022; pp. 1–27.
136. Balamurugan, K.; Chintamani, P. Lipid nano particulate drug delivery: An overview of the emerging trend. *Pharma Innov. J.* **2018**, *7*, 779–789.
137. Müller, R.H.; Radtke, M.; Wissing, S.A. Solid lipid nanoparticles (SLN) and nanostructured lipid carriers (NLC) in cosmetic and dermatological preparations. *Adv. Drug Deliv. Rev.* **2002**, *54*, S131–S155. [CrossRef]
138. Sumera; Anwar, A.; Ovais, M.; Khan, A.; Raza, A. Docetaxel-loaded solid lipid nanoparticles: A novel drug delivery system. *IET Nanobiotechnol.* **2017**, *11*, 621–629. [CrossRef]
139. Aguirre-Ramírez, M.; Silva-Jiménez, H.; Banat, I.M.; Díaz De Rienzo, M.A. Surfactants: Physicochemical interactions with biological macromolecules. *Biotechnol. Lett.* **2021**, *43*, 523–535. [CrossRef] [PubMed]
140. Nguyen, T.-T.-L.; Duong, V.-A. Solid Lipid Nanoparticles. *Encyclopedia* **2022**, *2*, 952–973. [CrossRef]
141. Silva, A.; Martins-Gomes, C.; Coutinho, T.; Fangueiro, J.; Sanchez-Lopez, E.; Pashirova, T.; Andreani, T.; Souto, E.B. Soft Cationic Nanoparticles for Drug Delivery: Production and Cytotoxicity of Solid Lipid Nanoparticles (SLNs). *Appl. Sci.* **2019**, *9*, 4438. [CrossRef]
142. Amis, T.M.; Renukuntla, J.; Bolla, P.K.; Clark, B.A. Selection of Cryoprotectant in Lyophilization of Progesterone-Loaded Stearic Acid Solid Lipid Nanoparticles. *Pharmaceutics* **2020**, *12*, 892. [CrossRef]
143. Dhiman, N.; Awasthi, R.; Sharma, B.; Kharkwal, H.; Kulkarni, G.T. Lipid Nanoparticles as Carriers for Bioactive Delivery. *Front. Chem.* **2021**, *9*, 580118. [CrossRef]
144. Siram, K.; Karuppaiah, A.; Gautam, M.; Sankar, V. Fabrication of Hyaluronic Acid Surface Modified Solid Lipid Nanoparticles Loaded with Imatinib Mesylate for Targeting Human Breast Cancer MCF-7 Cells. *J. Clust. Sci.* **2022**, *in press.*
145. Kuo, Y.-C.; Chao, I.-W. Conjugation of melanotransferrin antibody on solid lipid nanoparticles for mediating brain cancer malignancy. *Biotechnol. Prog.* **2015**, *32*, 480–490. [CrossRef] [PubMed]
146. Onugwu, A.L.; Attama, A.A.; Nnamani, P.O.; Onugwu, S.O.; Onuigbo, E.B.; Khutoryanskiy, V.V. Development and optimization of solid lipid nanoparticles coated with chitosan and poly(2-ethyl-2-oxazoline) for ocular drug delivery of ciprofloxacin. *J. Drug Deliv. Sci.Technol.* **2022**, *74*, 103527. [CrossRef]
147. Suk, J.S.; Xu, Q.; Kim, N.; Hanes, J.; Ensign, L.M. PEGylation as a strategy for improving nanoparticle-based drug and gene delivery. *Adv. Drug Deliv. Rev.* **2016**, *99*, 28–51. [CrossRef] [PubMed]
148. Eid, H.M.; Elkomy, M.H.; El Menshawe, S.F.; Salem, H.F. Development, Optimization, and In Vitro/In Vivo Characterization of Enhanced Lipid Nanoparticles for Ocular Delivery of Ofloxacin: The Influence of Pegylation and Chitosan Coating. *AAPS PharmSciTech.* **2019**, *20*, 183. [CrossRef] [PubMed]
149. Dang, H.; Dong, C.; Zhang, L. Sustained latanoprost release from PEGylated solid lipid nanoparticle-laden soft contact lens to treat glaucoma. *Pharm. Dev. Technol.* **2022**, *27*, 127–133. [CrossRef] [PubMed]
150. Sun, K.; Hu, K. Preparation and Characterization of Tacrolimus-Loaded SLNs in situ Gel for Ocular Drug Delivery for the Treatment of Immune Conjunctivitis. *Drug Des. Devel. Ther.* **2021**, *15*, 141–150. [CrossRef]
151. El-Emam, G.A.; Girgis, G.N.; Hamed, M.F.; El-Azeem Soliman, O.A.; Abd El Gawad, A.E.G.H. Formulation and Pathohistological Study of Mizolastine–Solid Lipid Nanoparticles–Loaded Ocular Hydrogels. *Int. J. Nanomed.* **2021**, *16*, 7775–7799. [CrossRef]
152. Carbone, C.; Fuochi, V.; Zielińska, A.; Musumeci, T.; Souto, E.B.; Bonaccorso, A.; Puglia, C.; Petronio, G.P.; Furneri, P.M. Dual-drugs delivery in solid lipid nanoparticles for the treatment of *Candida albicans* mycosis. *Colloids Surf. B Biointerfaces* **2020**, *186*, 110705. [CrossRef]

153. Liang, Z.; Zhang, Z.; Yang, J.; Lu, P.; Zhou, T.; Li, J.; Zhang, J. Assessment to the Antifungal Effects in vitro and the Ocular Pharmacokinetics of Solid-Lipid Nanoparticle in Rabbits. *Int. J. Nanomed.* **2021**, *16*, 7847–7857. [CrossRef]

154. Khames, A.; Khaleel, M.A.; El-Badawy, M.F.; El-Nezhawy, A.O.H. Natamycin solid lipid nanoparticles—Sustained ocular delivery system of higher corneal penetration against deep fungal keratitis: Preparation and optimization. *Int. J. Nanomedicine* **2019**, *14*, 2515–2531. [CrossRef] [PubMed]

155. Singh, M.; Guzman-Aranguez, A.; Hussain, A.; Srinivas, C.S.; Kaur, I.P. Solid lipid nanoparticles for ocular delivery of isoniazid: Evaluation, proof of concept and in vivo safety & kinetics. *Nanomedicine* **2019**, *14*, 465–491. [PubMed]

156. Nair, A.B.; Shah, J.; Al-Dhubiab, B.E.; Jacob, S.; Patel, S.S.; Venugopala, K.N.; Morsy, M.A.; Gupta, S.; Attimarad, M.; Sreeharsha, N.; et al. Clarithromycin Solid Lipid Nanoparticles for Topical Ocular Therapy: Optimization, Evaluation and In Vivo Studies. *Pharmaceutics* **2021**, *13*, 523. [CrossRef] [PubMed]

157. Bonaccorso, A.; Pepe, V.; Zappulla, C.; Cimino, C.; Pricoco, A.; Puglisi, G.; Giuliano, F.; Pignatello, R.; Carbone, C. Sorafenib Repurposing for Ophthalmic Delivery by Lipid Nanoparticles: A Preliminary Study. *Pharmaceutics* **2021**, *13*, 1956. [CrossRef]

158. Yadav, M.; Schiavone, N.; Guzman-Aranguez, A.; Giansanti, F.; Papucci, L.; Perez de Lara, M.J.; Singh, M.; Kaur, I.P. Atorvastatin-loaded solid lipid nanoparticles as eye drops: Proposed treatment option for age-related macular degeneration (AMD). *Drug Deliv. Transl. Res.* **2020**, *10*, 919–944. [CrossRef] [PubMed]

159. Cheng, Z.; Li, Y.; Wang, K.; Zhu, X.; Tharkar, P.; Shu, W.; Zhang, T.; Zeng, S.; Zhu, L.; Murray, M.; et al. Compritol solid lipid nanoparticle formulations enhance the protective effect of betulinic acid derivatives in human Müller cells against oxidative injury. *Exp. Eye Res.* **2022**, *215*, 108906. [CrossRef]

160. Ahmad, I.; Pandit, J.; Sultana, Y.; Mishra, A.K.; Hazari, P.P.; Aqil, M. Optimization by design of etoposide loaded solid lipid nanoparticles for ocular delivery: Characterization, pharmacokinetic and deposition study. *Mater. Sci. Eng. C Mater. Biol. Appl.* **2019**, *100*, 959–970. [CrossRef]

161. Freitas, L.G.A.; Isaac, D.L.C.; Lima, E.M.; Souza, L.G.; Abud, M.A.; Reis, R.G.D.; Tannure, W.T.; Ávila, M.P. Retinal changes in rabbit after intravitreal injection of sunitinib encapsulated into solid lipid nanoparticles and polymeric nanocapsules. *Arq. Bras. Oftalmol.* **2018**, *81*, 408–413. [CrossRef]

162. Wang, F.Z.; Zhang, M.W.; Zhang, D.S.; Huang, Y.; Chen, L.; Jiang, S.M.; Shi, K.; Li, R. Preparation, optimization, and characterization of chitosan-coated solid lipid nanoparticles for ocular drug delivery. *J. Biomed. Res.* **2018**, *32*, 411–423.

163. Taskar, P.S.; Patil, A.; Lakhani, P.; Ashour, E.; Gul, W.; ElSohly, M.A.; Murphy, B.; Majumdar, S. Δ9-Tetrahydrocannabinol Derivative-Loaded Nanoformulation Lowers Intraocular Pressure in Normotensive Rabbits. *Transl. Vis. Sci. Technol.* **2019**, *8*, 15. [CrossRef] [PubMed]

164. Wang, J.; Zhao, F.; Liu, R.; Chen, J.; Zhang, Q.; Lao, R.; Wang, Z.; Jin, X.; Liu, C. Novel cationic lipid nanoparticles as an ophthalmic delivery system for multicomponent drugs: Development, characterization, in vitro permeation, in vivo pharmacokinetic, and molecular dynamics studies. *Int. J. Nanomed.* **2017**, *12*, 8115–8127. [CrossRef]

165. Gomes Souza, L.; Antonio Sousa-Junior, A.; Alves Santana Cintra, B.; Vieira Dos Anjos, J.L.; Leite Nascimento, T.; Palmerston Mendes, L.; de Souza Vieira, M.; do Nascimento Ducas, R.; Campos Valadares, M.; Antônio Mendanha, S.; et al. Pre-clinical safety of topically administered sunitinib-loaded lipid and polymeric nanocarriers targeting corneal neovascularization. *Int. J. Pharm.* **2023**, *635*, 122682. [CrossRef]

166. Jaiswal, P.; Gidwani, B.; Vyas, A. Nanostructured lipid carriers and their current application in targeted drug delivery. *Artif. Cells Nanomed. Biotechnol.* **2016**, *44*, 27–40. [CrossRef]

167. Dhiman, S.; Mishra, N.; Sharma, S. Development of PEGylated solid lipid nanoparticles of pentoxifylline for their beneficial pharmacological potential in pathological cardiac hypertrophy. *Artif. Cells Nanomed. Biotechnol.* **2016**, *44*, 1901–1908. [CrossRef]

168. Elmowafy, M.; Al-Sanea, M.M. Nanostructured lipid carriers (NLCs) as drug delivery platform: Advances in formulation and delivery strategies. *Saudi Pharm. J.* **2021**, *29*, 999–1012. [CrossRef] [PubMed]

169. Shahzadi, I.; Fürst, A.; Knoll, P.; Bernkop-Schnürch, A. Nanostructured Lipid Carriers (NLCs) for Oral Peptide Drug Delivery: About the Impact of Surface Decoration. *Pharmaceutics* **2021**, *13*, 1312. [CrossRef] [PubMed]

170. Chauhan, I.; Yasir, M.; Verma, M.; Singh, A.P. Nanostructured Lipid Carriers: A Groundbreaking Approach for Transdermal Drug Delivery. *Adv. Pharm. Bull.* **2020**, *10*, 150–165. [CrossRef] [PubMed]

171. Kiss, E.L.; Berkó, S.; Gácsi, A.; Kovács, A.; Katona, G.; Soós, J.; Csányi, E.; Gróf, I.; Harazin, A.; Deli, M.A.; et al. Design and Optimization of Nanostructured Lipid Carrier Containing Dexamethasone for Ophthalmic Use. *Pharmaceutics* **2019**, *11*, 679. [CrossRef]

172. El-Salamouni, N.S.; Farid, R.M.; El-Kamel, A.H.; El-Gamal, S.S. Effect of sterilization on the physical stability of brimonidine-loaded solid lipid nanoparticles and nanostructured lipid carriers. *Int. J. Pharm.* **2015**, *496*, 976–983. [CrossRef]

173. Apostolou, M.; Assi, S.; Fatokun, A.A.; Khan, I. The Effects of Solid and Liquid Lipids on the Physicochemical Properties of Nanostructured Lipid Carriers. *J. Pharm. Sci.* **2021**, *110*, 2859–2872. [CrossRef]

174. Malik, D.S.; Kaur, G. Nanostructured gel for topical delivery of azelaic acid: Designing, characterization, and in-vitro evaluation. *J. Drug Deliv. Sci. Technol.* **2018**, *47*, 123–136. [CrossRef]

175. Bang, K.-H.; Na, Y.-G.; Huh, H.W.; Hwang, S.-J.; Kim, M.-S.; Kim, M.; Lee, H.-K.; Cho, C.-W. The Delivery Strategy of Paclitaxel Nanostructured Lipid Carrier Coated with Platelet Membrane. *Cancers* **2019**, *11*, 807. [CrossRef] [PubMed]

176. Cao, C.; Wang, Q.; Liu, Y. Lung cancer combination therapy: Doxorubicin and β-elemene co-loaded, pH-sensitive nanostructured lipid carriers. *Drug Des. Devel. Ther.* **2019**, *13*, 1087–1098. [CrossRef]

177. Javed, S.; Mangla, B.; Almoshari, Y.; Sultan, M.; Ahsan, W. Nanostructured lipid carrier system: A compendium of their formulation development approaches, optimization strategies by quality by design, and recent applications in drug delivery. *Nanotechnol. Rev.* **2022**, *11*, 1744–1777. [CrossRef]
178. Haider, M.; Abdin, S.M.; Kamal, L.; Orive, G. Nanostructured Lipid Carriers for Delivery of Chemotherapeutics: A Review. *Pharmaceutics* **2020**, *12*, 288. [CrossRef] [PubMed]
179. Khosa, A.; Reddi, S.; Saha, R.N. Nanostructured lipid carriers for site-specific drug delivery. *Biomed. Pharmacother.* **2018**, *103*, 598–613. [CrossRef]
180. Selvaraj, K.; Kuppusamy, G.; Krishnamurthy, J.; Mahalingam, R.; Singh, S.K.; Gulati, M. Repositioning of Itraconazole for the Management of Ocular Neovascularization Through Surface-Modified Nanostructured Lipid Carriers. *Assay Drug Dev. Technol.* **2019**, *17*, 178–190. [CrossRef]
181. Sharma, D.S.; Wadhwa, S.; Gulati, M.; Kumar, B.; Chitranshi, N.; Gupta, V.K.; Alrouji, M.; Alhajlah, S.; AlOmeir, O.; Vishwas, S.; et al. Chitosan modified 5-fluorouracil nanostructured lipid carriers for treatment of diabetic retinopathy in rats: A new dimension to an anticancer drug. *Int. J. Biol. Macromol.* **2023**, *224*, 810–830. [CrossRef] [PubMed]
182. Fu, T.; Yi, J.; Lv, S.; Zhang, B. Ocular amphotericin B delivery by chitosan-modified nanostructured lipid carriers for fungal keratitis-targeted therapy. *J. Liposome Res.* **2017**, *27*, 228–233. [CrossRef]
183. Pai, R.V.; Vavia, P.R. Chitosan oligosaccharide enhances binding of nanostructured lipid carriers to ocular mucins: Effect on ocular disposition. *Int. J. Pharm.* **2020**, *577*, 119095. [CrossRef] [PubMed]
184. Li, J.; Jin, X.; Yang, Y.; Zhang, L.; Liu, R.; Li, Z. Trimethyl chitosan nanoparticles for ocular baicalein delivery: Preparation, optimization, in vitro evaluation, in vivo pharmacokinetic study and molecular dynamics simulation. *Int. J. Biol. Macromol.* **2020**, *156*, 749–761. [CrossRef]
185. Tan, G.; Li, J.; Song, Y.; Yu, Y.; Liu, D.; Pan, W. Phenylboronic acid-tethered chondroitin sulfate-based mucoadhesive nanostructured lipid carriers for the treatment of dry eye syndrome. *Acta Biomater.* **2019**, *99*, 350–362. [CrossRef]
186. Zhu, R.; Chen, W.; Gu, D.; Wang, T.; Li, J.; Pan, H. Chondroitin sulfate and L-Cysteine conjugate modified cationic nanostructured lipid carriers: Pre-corneal retention, permeability, and related studies for dry eye treatment. *Int. J. Biol. Macromol.* **2023**, *228*, 624–637. [CrossRef]
187. Abdelhakeem, E.; El-Nabarawi, M.; Shamma, R. Effective Ocular Delivery of Eplerenone Using Nanoengineered Lipid Carriers in Rabbit Model. *Int. J. Nanomed.* **2021**, *16*, 4985–5002. [CrossRef]
188. Yan, T.; Ma, Z.; Liu, J.; Yin, N.; Lei, S.; Zhang, X.; Li, X.; Zhang, Y.; Kong, J. Thermoresponsive Genistein NLC-dexamethasone-moxifloxacin multi drug delivery system in lens capsule bag to prevent complications after cataract surgery. *Sci. Rep.* **2021**, *11*, 181. [CrossRef] [PubMed]
189. Tavakoli, N.; Taymouri, S.; Saeidi, A.; Akbari, V. Thermosensitive hydrogel containing sertaconazole loaded nanostructured lipid carriers for potential treatment of fungal keratitis. *Pharm. Dev. Technol.* **2019**, *24*, 891–901. [CrossRef] [PubMed]
190. Yu, Y.; Feng, R.; Li, J.; Wang, Y.; Song, Y.; Tan, G.; Liu, D.; Liu, W.; Yang, X.; Pan, H.; et al. A hybrid genipin-crosslinked dual-sensitive hydrogel/nanostructured lipid carrier ocular drug delivery platform. *Asian J. Pharm. Sci.* **2019**, *14*, 423–434. [CrossRef] [PubMed]
191. Yu, Y.; Xu, S.; Yu, S.; Li, J.; Tan, G.; Li, S.; Pan, W. A Hybrid Genipin-Cross-Linked Hydrogel/Nanostructured Lipid Carrier for Ocular Drug Delivery: Cellular, ex Vivo, and in Vivo Evaluation. *ACS Biomater. Sci. Eng.* **2020**, *6*, 1543–1552. [CrossRef]
192. Chen, L.; Wu, R. Brinzolamide- and latanoprost-loaded nano lipid carrier prevents synergistic retinal damage in glaucoma. *Acta Biochim. Pol.* **2022**, *69*, 423–428. [CrossRef]
193. Varela-Fernández, R.; García-Otero, X.; Díaz-Tomé, V.; Regueiro, U.; López-López, M.; González-Barcia, M.; Isabel Lema, M.; Javier Otero-Espinar, F. Lactoferrin-loaded nanostructured lipid carriers (NLCs) as a new formulation for optimized ocular drug delivery. *Eur. J. Pharm. Biopharm.* **2022**, *172*, 144–156. [CrossRef]
194. Kumari, S.; Dandamudi, M.; Rani, S.; Behaeghel, E.; Behl, G.; Kent, D.; O'Reilly, N.J.; O'Donovan, O.; McLoughlin, P.; Fitzhenry, L. Dexamethasone-Loaded Nanostructured Lipid Carriers for the Treatment of Dry Eye Disease. *Pharmaceutics* **2021**, *13*, 905. [CrossRef] [PubMed]
195. Zahir-Jouzdani, F.; Khonsari, F.; Soleimani, M.; Mahbod, M.; Arefian, E.; Heydari, M.; Shahhosseini, S.; Dinarvand, R.; Atyabi, F. Nanostructured lipid carriers containing rapamycin for prevention of corneal fibroblasts proliferation and haze propagation after burn injuries: In vitro and in vivo. *J. Cell Physiol.* **2019**, *234*, 4702–4712. [CrossRef] [PubMed]
196. Kumar, M.; Tiwari, A.; Asdaq, S.M.B.; Nair, A.B.; Bhatt, S.; Shinu, P.; Al Mouslem, A.K.; Jacob, S.; Alamri, A.S.; Alsanie, W.F.; et al. Itraconazole loaded nano-structured lipid carrier for topical ocular delivery: Optimization and evaluation. *Saudi J. Biol. Sci.* **2022**, *29*, 1–10. [CrossRef] [PubMed]
197. Patil, A.; Lakhani, P.; Taskar, P.; Wu, K.W.; Sweeney, C.; Avula, B.; Wang, Y.H.; Khan, I.A.; Majumdar, S. Formulation Development, Optimization, and In Vitro-In Vivo Characterization of Natamycin-Loaded PEGylated Nano-Lipid Carriers for Ocular Applications. *J. Pharm. Sci.* **2018**, *107*, 2160–2171. [CrossRef] [PubMed]
198. Li, Q.; Yang, X.; Zhang, P.; Mo, F.; Si, P.; Kang, X.; Wang, M.; Zhang, J. Dasatinib loaded nanostructured lipid carriers for effective treatment of corneal neovascularization. *Biomater. Sci.* **2021**, *9*, 2571–2583. [CrossRef] [PubMed]
199. Luo, Q.; Yang, J.; Xu, H.; Shi, J.; Liang, Z.; Zhang, R.; Lu, P.; Pu, G.; Zhao, N.; Zhang, J. Sorafenib-loaded nanostructured lipid carriers for topical ocular therapy of corneal neovascularization: Development, in-vitro and in vivo study. *Drug Deliv.* **2022**, *29*, 837–855. [CrossRef] [PubMed]

200. Nirbhavane, P.; Sharma, G.; Singh, B.; Begum, G.; Jones, M.-C.; Rauz, S.; Vincent, R.; Denniston, A.K. Triamcinolone acetonide loaded-cationic nano-lipoidal formulation for uveitis: Evidences of improved biopharmaceutical performance and anti-inflammatory activity. *Colloids Surf. B. Biointerfaces* **2020**, *190*, 110902. [CrossRef]
201. Jounaki, K.; Makhmalzadeh, B.S.; Feghhi, M.; Heidarian, A. Topical ocular delivery of vancomycin loaded cationic lipid nanocarriers as a promising and non-invasive alternative approach to intravitreal injection for enhanced bacterial endophthalmitis management. *Eur. J. Pharm. Sci.* **2021**, *167*, 105991. [CrossRef]
202. Puglia, C.; Blasi, P.; Ostacolo, C.; Sommella, E.; Bucolo, C.; Platania, C.B.M.; Romano, G.L.; Geraci, F.; Drago, F.; Santonocito, D.; et al. Innovative Nanoparticles Enhance N-Palmitoylethanolamide Intraocular Delivery. *Front. Pharmacol.* **2018**, *9*, 285. [CrossRef]
203. Zingale, E.; Rizzo, S.; Bonaccorso, A.; Consoli, V.; Vanella, L.; Musumeci, T.; Spadaro, A.; Pignatello, R. Optimization of Lipid Nanoparticles by Response Surface Methodology to Improve the Ocular Delivery of Diosmin: Characterization and In-Vitro Anti-Inflammatory Assessment. *Pharmaceutics* **2022**, *14*, 1961. [CrossRef]
204. Santonocito, D.; Vivero-Lopez, M.; Lauro, M.R.; Torrisi, C.; Castelli, F.; Sarpietro, M.G.; Puglia, C. Design of Nanotechnological Carriers for Ocular Delivery of Mangiferin: Preformulation Study. *Molecules* **2022**, *27*, 1328. [CrossRef]
205. González-Fernández, F.M.; Delledonne, A.; Nicoli, S.; Gasco, P.; Padula, C.; Santi, P.; Sissa, C.; Pescina, S. Nanostructured Lipid Carriers for Enhanced Transscleral Delivery of Dexamethasone Acetate: Development, Ex Vivo Characterization and Multiphoton Microscopy Studies. *Pharmaceutics* **2023**, *15*, 407. [CrossRef] [PubMed]
206. Khairnar, S.V.; Pagare, P.; Thakre, A.; Nambiar, A.R.; Junnuthula, V.; Abraham, M.C.; Kolimi, P.; Nyavanandi, D.; Dyawanapelly, S. Review on the Scale-Up Methods for the Preparation of Solid Lipid Nanoparticles. *Pharmaceutics* **2022**, *14*, 1886. [CrossRef] [PubMed]
207. Duong, V.-A.; Nguyen, T.-T.-L.; Maeng, H.-J. Preparation of Solid Lipid Nanoparticles and Nanostructured Lipid Carriers for Drug Delivery and the Effects of Preparation Parameters of Solvent Injection Method. *Molecules* **2020**, *25*, 4781. [CrossRef]
208. Zielińska, A.; Soles, B.B.; Lopes, A.R.; Vaz, B.F.; Rodrigues, C.M.; Alves, T.F.R.; Klensporf-Pawlik, D.; Durazzo, A.; Lucarini, M.; Severino, P.; et al. Nanopharmaceuticals for Eye Administration: Sterilization, Depyrogenation and Clinical Applications. *Biology* **2020**, *9*, 336. [CrossRef]
209. Pardeike, J.; Weber, S.; Haber, T.; Wagner, J.; Zarfl, H.P.; Plank, H.; Zimmer, A. Development of an itraconazole-loaded nanostructured lipid carrier (NLC) formulation for pulmonary application. *Int. J. Pharm.* **2011**, *419*, 329–338. [CrossRef] [PubMed]
210. Gokce, E.H.; Sandri, G.; Bonferoni, M.C.; Rossi, S.; Ferrari, F.; Güneri, T.; Caramella, C. Cyclosporine A loaded SLNs: Evaluation of cellular uptake and corneal cytotoxicity. *Int. J. Pharm.* **2008**, *364*, 76–86. [CrossRef]
211. Youshia, J.; Kamel, A.O.; El Shamy, A.; Mansour, S. Gamma sterilization and in vivo evaluation of cationic nanostructured lipid carriers as potential ocular delivery systems for antiglaucoma drugs. *Eur. J. Pharm. Sci.* **2021**, *163*, 105887. [CrossRef]
212. Thi, T.T.H.; Suys, E.J.A.; Lee, J.S.; Nguyen, D.H.; Park, K.D.; Truong, N.P. Lipid-Based Nanoparticles in the Clinic and Clinical Trials: From Cancer Nanomedicine to COVID-19 Vaccines. *Vaccines* **2021**, *9*, 359. [CrossRef]
213. Khiev, D.; Mohamed, Z.A.; Vichare, R.; Paulson, R.; Bhatia, S.; Mohapatra, S.; Lobo, G.P.; Valapala, M.; Kerur, N.; Passaglia, C.L.; et al. Emerging Nano-Formulations and Nanomedicines Applications for Ocular Drug Delivery. *Nanomaterials* **2021**, *11*, 173. [CrossRef]
214. Buttini, F.; Rozou, S.; Rossi, A.; Zoumpliou, V.; Rekkas, D.M. The application of Quality by Design framework in the pharmaceutical development of dry powder inhalers. *Eur. J. Pharm. Sci.* **2018**, *113*, 64–76. [CrossRef] [PubMed]
215. Janagam, D.R.; Wu, L.; Lowe, T.L. Nanoparticles for drug delivery to the anterior segment of the eye. *Adv. Drug Deliv. Rev.* **2017**, *122*, 31–64. [CrossRef] [PubMed]

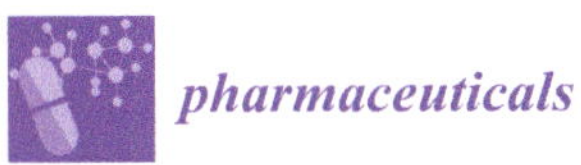

pharmaceuticals

Review

Endogenous Lipid Carriers—Bench-to-Bedside Roadblocks in Production and Drug Loading of Exosomes

Terjahna Richards, Himaxi Patel, Ketan Patel and Frank Schanne *

College of Pharmacy & Health Sciences, St. John's University, Queens, NY 11439, USA
* Correspondence: schannef@stjohns.edu

Abstract: Exosomes are cell-derived, nano-sized extracellular vesicles comprising a lipid bilayer membrane that encapsulates several biological components, such as nucleic acids, lipids, and proteins. The role of exosomes in cell–cell communication and cargo transport has made them promising candidates in drug delivery for an array of diseases. Despite several research and review papers describing the salient features of exosomes as nanocarriers for drug delivery, there are no FDA-approved commercial therapeutics based on exosomes. Several fundamental challenges, such as the large-scale production and reproducibility of batches, have hindered the bench-to-bedside translation of exosomes. In fact, compatibility and poor drug loading sabotage the possibility of delivering several drug molecules. This review provides an overview of the challenges and summarizes the potential solutions/approaches to facilitate the clinical development of exosomal nanocarriers.

Keywords: exosome; drug loading; exosomal delivery; large-scale production

1. Introduction

Exosomes, a subclass of extracellular vesicles, are lipid bilayer vesicles with an average diameter of 100 nm that are secreted by all cell types. Exosomes consist of a multitude of extracellular and intracellular bioactive compounds, which play a crucial role in cellular communication and cargo transport [1,2]. Extracellular components include tetraspanins (CD9, CD81, CD63), lipid rafts, flotillin-1, integrins, and transmembrane proteins (Figure 1A). This is in contrast with intracellular components, which include lipids, nucleic acids, and various proteins, such as cytoskeleton proteins and heat shock proteins (Figure 1A). Exosomes are produced from a specific bilayer organelle called a multivesicular body (MVB) (Figure 1B). The formation of the MVB includes several phases: (1) inward budding of the cell membrane, (2) formation of the early-sorting endosome (ESE), (3) formation of the late-sorting endosome (LSE), where exosome precursors called intraluminal vesicles (ILVs) are germinating, and (4) transformation of the LSE to a mature MVB (Figure 1B) [1,2]. Exosome biogenesis is also associated with specific sorting mechanisms, such as the endosomal sorting complex responsible for transport (ESCRT), which assists in cargo sequestration and ILV budding. The diversity shown in exosome development and characteristics aids in their isolation from other extracellular vesicles.

Exosomes possess favorable pharmacokinetic properties, biocompatibility, and tissue-targeting abilities due to their phospholipid bilayer structure and various bioactive components, such as mRNAs, microRNAs, cytokines, chemokines, and immunomodulatory compounds. Moreover, exosomes have the ability to suppress inflammation, regulate cell proliferation, and deliver biotherapeutics [3–6]. Nevertheless, the feasibility of exosomes as therapeutic agents remains limited, which may be attributed to low exosome production and poor drug loading. However, in recent years, there has been an increase in research devoted to overcoming the limitations of exosome-based therapies. The incorporation of alternative exosome sources, upstream strategies, and downstream strategies have been used to improve the yield of exosomes. Additionally, adjustments have been made to several commonly used drug-loading techniques, and new procedures have been developed

Citation: Richards, T.; Patel, H.; Patel, K.; Schanne, F. Endogenous Lipid Carriers—Bench-to-Bedside Roadblocks in Production and Drug Loading of Exosomes. *Pharmaceuticals* **2023**, *16*, 421. https://doi.org/10.3390/ph16030421

Academic Editors: Ana Catarina Silva, João Nuno Moreira and José Manuel Sousa Lobo

Received: 3 February 2023
Revised: 4 March 2023
Accepted: 7 March 2023
Published: 10 March 2023

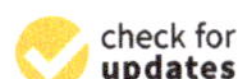

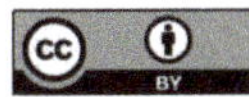

to improve the drug loading of exosomes. This review summarizes the challenges and provides potential solutions for exosome production and drug loading to facilitate the clinical development of exosome nanocarriers.

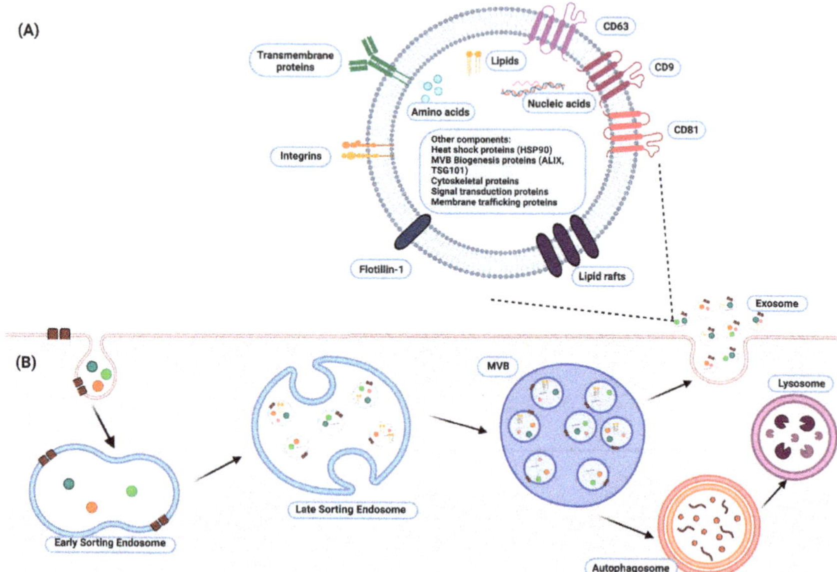

Figure 1. A schematic illustration of (**A**) the structure of a typical exosome and (**B**) the formation of exosomes. The structure of the exosome consists of intracellular (lipids, nucleic acids, and proteins) and extracellular components (tetraspanins, lipid rafts, flotillin-1, and transmembrane proteins), which assist in its characterization and many cellular functions. Exosomes are produced from a multivesicular body (MVB), which arises from a late-sorting endosome (LSE). The biogenesis of exosomes also involves specific sorting mechanisms responsible for transportation and an intraluminal vesicle (ILV) budding in the LSE. The illustration was created with BioRender.com (https://app.biorender.com; accessed on 16 January 2023).

2. Exosomal Drug Delivery: Challenges

2.1. Exosome Production and Isolation

Although exosomes have been shown to possess invaluable qualities for use in nanomedicine, their low production rate in unaltered cell cultures remains a key challenge, preventing bench-to-bedside use. In addition to the low production of exosomes, large variability in their size also exists, resulting in a lack of reproducibility in batches [1,7,8]. Consequently, the need remains to develop techniques that increase exosome production, maintain constant morphology, and limit any negative impact on cell cultures. It is worth mentioning that attention should be given to the shelf-life, stability, and storage of exosomes in their use as therapeutics.

Exosome isolation methods are important to increase the yield of exosomes. The currently available techniques for exosome isolation are based on their chemical, physical, and immunoaffinity assays and adapted from previous methods used for the isolation of viruses and other vesicles. Ultracentrifugation, the gold standard for exosome isolation, is one of the most applied techniques. However, its low recovery rate, low purity, and time-consuming process are not ideal for the implementation of exosomes in nanomedicine. Other commonly used techniques include polymer-based precipitation, ultrafiltration, size-exclusion chromatography, immunoaffinity chromatography, and microfluidics (Table 1). It is worth noting that the method of exosome isolation used may affect the yield and characteristics such as the size, structure, and biofunction of exosomes [3,9]. Thus, modifications to current methods and the development of new procedures are required to increase the yield and purity of exosomes.

Table 1. Comparison of different downstream exosome isolation techniques. The table summarizes the advantages and disadvantages of each technique and their reported exosome recovery rate.

Isolation Technique	Principle	Recovery (%)	Pros	Cons	References
Ultracentrifugation	Sedimentation rate	5–20	High sample capacity and low cost	Time-consuming and low purity	[9,10]
Density gradient ultracentrifugation	Density, size, shape	10–40	High purity and protein concentration	Long run time and low yield	[9,11,12]
Polymer-based precipitation	Sedimentation rate	90+	High yield	Low purity	[13–15]
Ultrafiltration	Size	30	Maintains integrity; simple and low-cost	Moderate purity; low yield due to exosome trapping in filter pores	[9,16,17]
Size-exclusion chromatography	Size	40–80	High purity, integrity, and functionality; reduction of exosome aggregation	Low extraction volume	[9,18]
Immunoaffinity chromatography	Surface marker	90+	Maintain integrity	Low capacity and low yield	[9,19,20]
Microfluidics	Surface marker	40–90	Low cost and low input sample required	Low sample capacity; cargo may be modified	[9,21,22]
Magnetic bead isolation	Surface marker	80+	Maintain integrity	Possible impurities	[23,24]

Preservation is important for maintaining the biological functions of exosomes and ensuring the ease of their transportation and clinical use [2,25]. Currently, there are various techniques used to improve the storage, shelf-life, and stability of exosomes. These include freeze-drying, spray-drying, and cryopreservation [2]. Freeze-drying, which is divided into three stages—pre-freezing, sublimation drying, and analytical drying, leads to the cooling of liquid components, followed by freezing. Exosomes that are stored using this method maintain their original activity but are exposed to membrane damage. Spray-drying involves the use of atomization pressure and hot air for the storage of exosomes, which may affect the stability of these extracellular vesicles. Cryopreservation, which is conducted at −80 °C, is the most commonly used method [2]. It enables the short-term storage of exosomes through the reduction of biochemical activity so that functional stability can be maintained. Furthermore, several studies have suggested that the addition of cryoprotectants, such as trehalose or DMSO, is mildly protective in maintaining exosome ability [2,26]. Despite these benefits, cryopreservation is associated with membrane destabilization and protein degradation, which may affect the therapeutic function of exosomes. In addition, the storage of exosomes for four days at −80 °C has been noted to affect their morphology, and at 28 days, their biological activity starts to be affected [2,27,28]. Therefore, further analysis of the storage, stability, and shelf-life of exosomes is of utmost importance.

2.2. Exosome Drug Loading

In addition to low production and reproducibility, another key challenge in the use of exosomes in nanomedicine is poor drug loading. Exosomes have shown favorable biocompatibility and therapeutic targeting abilities, thus making them valuable as a potential drug delivery tool. However, several factors, such as the exosome size, the pharmacokinetics of the drug, and the drug size, may hinder the efficiency of drug loading and require more specialized techniques [6,8,29,30]. For example, an exosome of a larger size may be loaded with a drug more easily than one with a smaller size. Moreover, a lipid-soluble drug may be loaded more quickly than a water-soluble drug. The exosomal structure, coupled with a therapeutic drug, requires careful consideration in the drug-loading process. Thus, new and improved procedures should be developed to enhance the effectiveness of exosome drug loading.

Drug-loading techniques can be categorized based on the time of implementation—pre-secretory or post-secretory [2]. Pre-secretory drug loading involves the loading of drugs before the development of the exosome, whereas post-secretory refers to drug loading after exosome development. Most drug-loading techniques are post-secretory and include sonication, electroporation, passive incubation, and the freeze–thaw cycle (Table 2).

Table 2. A list of the different exosome drug-loading techniques and their advantages and disadvantages.

Methods	Principle	Advantages	Disadvantages	References
Pre-secretory Drug Loading				
Co-incubation	Drug incubated with parent cell	Easy; effective in hydrophobic drugs	Low loading efficacy; possible drug toxicity	[31]
Gene editing	Editing of genes	Overexpression of specific molecules	Low loading efficacy; possible toxicity	[32]
Post-Secretory Drug Loading				
Sonication	Mechanical shear force decreases membrane integrity	Large amount of drug loaded	Possible damage to intracellular components and integrity	[3,33,34]
Electroporation	High-voltage electric charge decreases membrane integrity	Effective loading of hydrophilic drugs and nucleic acids	Possible aggregation; low loading efficacy	[35]
Passive incubation	Passive diffusion	Effective loading of hydrophobic drugs; does not affect exosome integrity	Not useful for hydrophilic drugs; low drug-loading capacity	[3,34,36–39]
Freeze–thaw	Repeated freeze–thaw cycles to decrease membrane integrity	Easy process	Low loading efficacy; possible aggregation and inactivation	[3,40]
Nanoporation	Nanosecond electrical pulse decreases membrane integrity	Effective loading of small molecules	Possible aggregation	[41,42]
Saponin treatment	Formation of porous structure on exosome membrane	Increased loading capacity compared to electroporation	May cause hemolysis in vivo; requires further purification	[3,43]
Extrusion	Mechanical stress decreases membrane integrity	Provides uniform distribution	May damage membrane; possible drug leakage	[3,44]

The advantages and disadvantages of each drug-loading technique (Table 2) depend on the experimental settings, type of drug, and source of exosomes. Passive incubation, for example, is a simple technique that involves the incubation of purified exosomes with drugs to allow for incorporation into the exosome membrane [36,38,45]. For example, the small molecule doxorubicin was passively loaded into exosomes by Wei et al. for osteosarcoma treatment [46]. Passive incubation is primarily used due to its excellent performance in the incorporation of hydrophobic compounds, such as curcumin [38]. Hydrophobic compounds can interact with the lipid bilayer of the exosome more effectively than hydrophilic compounds, and thus, can be incorporated into the exosome. The loading of hydrophilic compounds can be enhanced with the addition of the mild surfactant saponin, which, according to studies, induces transient membrane destabilization and can be used for the loading of large compounds (>200 kDa) [3,43]. However, the use of saponins may also affect biomolecules, and thus, requires purification before clinical use. Mechanical methods, such as sonication, nanoporation, and electroporation have been shown to successfully load small molecules and macromolecules into exosomes [8,30,47,48]. Research conducted by C Liu et al., for example, incorporated one of the mechanical techniques, i.e., microfluidic sonication, to effectively load PLGA into exosomes isolated from a human lung carcinoma cell line (A549) [33]. In addition, a study by Rodriguez-Morales et al. used electroporation to effectively produce insulin-loaded exosomes for the treatment of diabetes mellitus [35]. It is worth noting that these post-secretory drug-loading techniques may affect the proteins and nucleic acid drugs that are incorporated into the exosome and the structure of the exosome. The complexity of some of these methods, such as nanoporation, may render large-scale use in a clinical setting difficult. Consequently, there is a great need for effective drug-loading techniques that can be implemented on a large-scale in nanomedicine.

3. Exosomal Drug Delivery: Solutions

3.1. Exosome Production and Isolation

For the use of exosomes in a clinical setting, large-scale production is required. Research has identified the important areas that should be considered in addressing this issue. These include the selection of exosome sources and modifications (upstream and/or downstream) (Figure 2).

3.1.1. Source Selection

Exosomes can be produced from human and non-human sources. Human sources involve exosome production and isolation from the cells and fluids of the body. For example, stem cells have been shown to increase exosome production and provide larger-sized extracellular vesicles—a characteristic important for effective drug loading [49–51]. Research by Haraszti et. al. noted that human umbilical cord stem cells produce approximately four-fold larger-sized exosomes than bone marrow mesenchymal stem cells [52]. Other cell types need to be studied to evaluate exosome production and the therapeutic ability of these extracellular vesicles. This may prove to be beneficial in increasing exosome yield and improving reproducibility across batches.

The non-human sources, which arose from the increasing demand for exosome-based therapeutics, include prokaryotes (Gram-positive bacteria and Gram-negative bacteria) [53–55], bovine milk [38,56], parasitic helminths [57], plants [58], and protists [59,60]. Compared to human sources, these types of exosome sources are versatile, and hence, more easily altered in upstream and downstream modifications than the human sources. Their versatility is beneficial to the large-scale production and use of exosomes in vaccines, therapeutics, and drug delivery. For example, the vesicles of the Gram-negative *Neisseria meningitidis* were approved for use in vaccines [61]. However, a critical setback is that these exosomes can be immunogenic or allergenic depending on the administration route, dosage, and dose frequency. Furthermore, several studies have noted that the variability in the upstream and downstream modifications used to generate these exosomes introduces experimental bias, which consequently, affects the immunological outcomes [54,55]. In general, it can be stated that the source from which exosomes are derived may affect their production and properties, which may cause variable therapeutic outcomes in production. As a result, careful consideration should be taken in selecting the appropriate source.

3.1.2. Upstream Modifications

Exosome production can be influenced by modifications to the cell culture conditions. This may include appropriate cell selection and changes to the culture medium, the environmental parameters, and the method of cultivation. However, the alteration of cell culture conditions may affect the structure of exosomes and the productivity of the cultured cells.

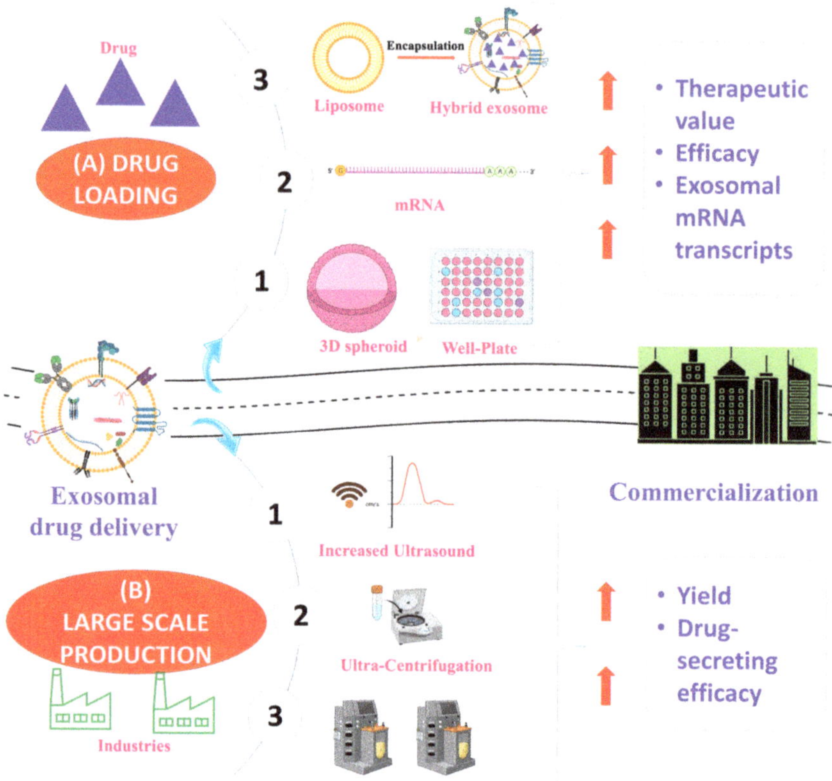

Figure 2. Key challenges in exosome production—(**A**) drug loading and (**B**) exosome production—are summarized. The therapeutic value and efficacy of the drug loading of exosomes can be improved through several methods, including the use of exosome–liposome hybrids and gene editing. The yield and drug-secreting efficacy of exosome production can be improved through ultrasound, ultracentrifugation, and the use of bioreactors. Improvements in drug loading and exosome production aid in the commercialization of exosome-based therapeutics. The illustration was created with BioRender.com (https://app.biorender.com; accessed on 16 January 2023).

Soluble Factors

The addition of soluble factors to the cell culture medium can be used to increase exosome production (Table 3). Bioactive cytokines, such as lipopolysaccharide (LPS) [62], N-methyldopamine [63], norepinephrine [63], serotonin [64], adiponectin [65], adenosine triphosphate (ATP) [66], Wnt3a [67], calcium (Ca^{2+}) ionophores [64], and plant ceramide [68] have been used in research to increase exosome production (Table 3). Furthermore, the upregulation of NadB, syndecan 4, and six-transmembrane epithelial antigen of prostate 3 (STEAP3) has increased the exosomes produced in cell cultures [7,69,70]. Research has shown that the genetic overexpressions of tetraspanin CD9 and hypoxia-induced factor 1α (HIFα) have increased exosome production by 2.4- and 2.2-fold, respectively [71–73]. However, the property and therapeutic efficacy of exosomes may be affected by the use of soluble factors. As a result, there is hesitancy in the use of soluble factors to preserve the cell culture environment.

Table 3. Comparison of different upstream modifications for increased exosome production and their reported fold increase and effects.

Upstream Modifications	Fold Increase	Alterations and Effects	References
Soluble Factors			
Lipopolysaccharide (LPS)	1.37	Upregulation of let-7b increased immunotherapeutic effect	[62]
N-methyldopamine and norepinephrine	3	No significant change	[63]
Serotonin and calcium	2–2.5	-	[64]
Adiponectin	3	Present in exosomes	[65]
ATP	4	No significant change	[66]
Wnt3a	-	Present in exosomes; increased neuroprotective abilities	[67]
Plant ceramide	2.5	-	[68]
Chemical/physical stimulation			
Hypoxia	1.5	Dependent on cell type; increased expression of nucleic acids and proteins	[71,72,74,75]
Serum deprivation	Varies	Decreased exosome protein content	[52,76]
Flow/stretch	37	Over 200 proteins expressed differently from typical exosomes	[77,78]
High-frequency ultrasound	8–10	Increased exosome protein content	[79]
3D cultivation			
3D spheroid culture	2–3	-	[80]
Microcarrier-based suspension	20; 140 with tangential flow system	No significant change	[52,81–83]
3D print fibrillar scaffold with perfusion system	100	Decreased exosome protein content	[84]
Low-shear unsubmerged 3D-printed polylactic acid lattice matrix	2	Maintained protein expression	[85]
Biomaterials			
Nitric oxide-releasing polymer	Not significant	Enhanced pro-angiogenic activity	[86]
Lithium-incorporated bioactive glass ceramic	Not significant	Enhanced pro-angiogenic activity	[87]
Iron-oxide coated poly-lactic-co-glycosidic acid (PLGA) nanoparticle	2	Increased antioxidant or tissue regeneration factors	[88]
Bioglass	2	Modulation of cargo through altered expression of microRNA; enhanced ability to promote vascularization	[89]
EXOtic	~6.8	-	[69]

Chemical and Physical Stimulation

Alterations to the cell culture environment may cause cellular adaptation and consequently lead to changes in the characteristics of cells, thus resulting in increased exosome production. On this basis, chemical or physical damage-mimetic micro-environments have been created to increase exosome production and subsequent therapeutic functions (Table 3).

Chemical stimulations, such as hypoxia, have been shown to produce exosomes with enhanced therapeutic effects [71,72,74,75]. Serum deprivation, another example of chemical stimulation, exhibits variable effects on exosome production. Moreover, studies have revealed that the ability of serum deprivation to increase exosome production depends on the cellular origin [76,90]. Physical simulation involving flow and stretching factors, such as bioreactors, can increase exosome production. Studies involving the use of bioreactors have shown elevated exosome production by up to 37-fold [77,78]. Ambattu et al. employed another technique, where cells were stimulated with high-frequency ultrasound, resulting in an 8-10-fold increase in exosome production [79]. It is worth noting that the use of chemical and physical stimulations may affect the cellular characteristics.

3D Culture

The mode of cultivation, such as 3D culture, can be used to expand the cell culture area, and exosome production can be increased by continually applying a shear force to the enlarged area (Table 3). Methods of 3D culture include the hanging drop in a 3D spheroid culture and the microcarrier-based suspension culture. The efficiency of the hanging-drop technique plateaued after a 2–3-fold increase [80]. The microcarrier-based suspension culture, an extensively used suitable method for 3D culture, showed increased exosome production of approximately 20-fold [81–83]. Additionally, in combination with a tangential flow filtration system, exosome production was further increased by 140-fold [52]. Recently, Patel et. al. cultured cells on a 3D-printed hollow fibrillar scaffold with a complementary perfusion system and reported a 100-fold increase in exosome production [84]. However, later experiments conducted by Patel et al. demonstrated that the structure and components of exosomes were substantially affected. It was noted that the extracellular components were significantly decreased, and the complex process of the 3D printing scaffold required special training. In another study, Burns et. al. developed a low-shear technique for 3D cell cultivation that was reported to maintain cell viability, purity, and phenotype [85]. Notably, in 3D cell cultivation, the conditions of the cell culture and the shear force applied requires careful evaluation to limit the effects on cell viability and phenotype.

Biomaterials

Biomaterials could improve exosome productivity and their therapeutic ability by creating a special microenvironment for cellular interaction. Biomaterials used in cell culture include nitric oxide-releasing polymer [86], lithium-incorporated bioactive glass ceramic [87], iron oxide-coated polylactic-co-glycolic acid (PLGA) nanoparticles [88], and bioglass [89] (Table 3). Kojima et al. showed that the application of exosomal transfer into cells (EXOtic) devices for cell culture significantly increased exosome production and their therapeutic capability [69]. The EXOtic devices also enhanced the specific mRNA packaging and the delivery of the mRNA into the cytosol of the target cells, thus facilitating efficient cellular communication. The combination of biomaterials with cultivation technologies could also be used to further enhance exosome production.

3.1.3. Downstream Modifications

To address the challenges associated with exosome isolation, new methods have been developed to improve exosome purity and achieve a greater yield. A one-step sucrose cushion ultracentrifugation was developed to improve the yield and purity of exosomes from the established ultracentrifugation. This procedure involves the addition of 30% sucrose solution followed by cell culture media, without mixing the layers [91]. Gupta et al. reported that the exosome cup-shaped morphology was greater than differential ultracentrifugation, thus demonstrating reduced size variability [91]. Modifications have also been made to other exosome isolation techniques, such as magnetic bead-based isolation and immunoaffinity chromatography. Smith et al. created a simple, size-based nanoscale deterministic lateral displacement array of microfluidic channels to collect exosomes, demonstrating ~50% recovery [92]. In a study by Z et al. an ExoSD microfluidic chip with an immunocapture-based method was developed to achieve exosome isolation [93]. The microfluidic chips reported >80% exosome recovery and >83% purity [93]. Heath et al. developed a cost-effective, high-throughput isolation technique called anion exchange chromatography to increase exosome yield [94]. Using higher flow rates and step elution, the authors utilized the net negative charge of exosomes to obtain 2.4×10^{11} exosomes, a quantity that was reported to be greater than that obtained using ultracentrifugation and tangential flow filtration [94].

Research into improving exosome isolation has also regarded the use of aptamer-based separation techniques [95,96]. Aptamers are single-stranded oligonucleotides that form distinct structures which bind to targets such as the extracellular components of exosomes (tetraspanins, transmembrane proteins). Zhang et al. developed a DNA aptamer-based magnetic isolation process to efficiently increase the yield of exosomes [97]. The process involved the addition of a biotin-labeled CD63 component to media and the subsequent separation of the labelled exosomes with streptavidin magnetic beads [97]. Another study by Song et al. also involved the use of a CD63-targeting aptamer for magnetic bead-based exosome immunoaffinity isolation [95]. Jiawei et al. developed a magnetic bead-based isolation technique in which tetraspanin markers (CD63, CD9, CD81) are combined with metal oxides for exosome isolation [24]. In addition, Zhang et al. discovered a novel three-step procedure involving PEG precipitation followed by iohexol gradient centrifugation and size exclusion chromatography for exosome enrichment and recovery [15]. Zhang et al. reported that the procedure produced high purity and yield of exosomes, resulting in 71% recovery and almost complete elimination of other lipoproteins [15]. Importantly, the modified or newly developed procedures for downstream modifications may assist in the large-scale use of exosomes as a drug delivery vehicle in a clinical setting.

3.2. Exosome Drug Loading

The clinical translation of exosomes requires reproducible and technologically accessible methods to load these extracellular vesicles with the desired drug (Figure 3). Several techniques have been modified or newly developed to assist in effective exosome drug loading, as discussed below.

3.2.1. Pre-Secretory Drug Loading

Pre-secretory drug loading can be performed in two ways: (1) the incubation of a parent cell with the drug or (2) gene editing [98]. In incubation, the drug is directly mixed with the cell culture medium. The drug is internalized into the cells and subsequently loaded into exosomes via endogenous mechanisms. This technique is more effective in hydrophobic drugs due to their ability to interact with the exosome membrane. Research has shown that drugs such as methotrexate, doxorubicin, cisplatin, and paclitaxel have been successfully taken up by parent cells and loaded into exosomes for therapeutic treatment in different cancers [8,47,99]. Additionally, Zhang et al. demonstrated the transfection of parent cells with a siRNA-targeting tyrosine kinase c-Met in the treatment of gastric cancer [100]. The exosomes extracted, which were enriched with anti-c-Met siRNA, resulted in a significant decrease in tumor growth in mouse xenograft models, thus reversing the resistance of gastric cancer cells in vitro to cisplatin. Pre-secretory drug loading can also be accomplished through gene editing by adding plasmids to parent cells to produce exosomes enriched with nucleic acids or proteins. A study done by Yuan et al. demonstrated effective loading of the potent anti-cancer tumor necrosis factor-related apoptosis-induced ligand (TRAIL), a molecule known for its poor pharmaceutics, in mesenchymal stem cell-derived exosomes [30,101]. In addition, O'Brien et al. showed that miR-134 loaded exosomes were able to successfully reduce cellular invasion and migration and had improved sensitivity to anti-Hsp90 drugs [102,103]. Recently, a study by Yang et al. revealed that gene editing, coupled with nanoporation, successfully loaded a phosphatase and TENsin homolog deleted on chromosome 10 (PTEN) mRNA [104]. According to Yang et al., when loaded into exosomes, PTEN mRNA, a common tumor suppressor gene, produced a 50-fold increase in exosomes and a 1000-fold increase in exosomal mRNA transcripts compared to other drug-loading methods [104]. The authors further pointed out that large quantities of PTEN mRNA-containing exosomes were produced, and following systemic injection, displayed an increased survival rate in PTEN-deficient glioma mouse models [104]. Importantly, a novel pre-secretory drug-loading technique was developed by Nawaz et al. using lipid nanoparticles [105]. The authors delivered a therapeutic agent, VEGF-A mRNA, via lipid nanoparticles and studied the uptake kinetics and transport of the exogenous nanoparticles [105]. The results showed that the lipid nanoparticles altered the exosomes as functional extensions to distribute the therapeutic agent among cells [105]. Additionally, the exosomes themselves increased the production of the therapeutic component and other pro-angiogenesis agents for the treatment of inflammatory cardiac conditions [105]. Of note, the cell type used affected the functionality of the exosomes, whereby cardiac progenitor cells resulted in the lowest production of inflammatory agents [105]. The pre-secretory drug-loading method and the cell type used are important factors to consider for effective drug loading and the subsequent use of exosomes in a clinical setting.

3.2.2. Post-Secretory Drug Loading

Post-secretory drug-loading methods generally work in two ways: (1) the passive incubation of the drug with the exosomes to allow the drug to attach to the exosome lipid bilayer membrane, or (2) the use of mechanical or chemical techniques to momentarily weaken the integrity of the exosome membrane to allow for the diffusion of the drug into the extracellular vesicles. With the increased interest in the use of exosomes as drug delivery tools, new approaches for post-secretory drug loading have been considered over the last few years. Wang et al. developed an acoustofluidic device, which is a combination of fluid mechanics and acoustics, to perform both exosome drug loading and encapsulation with silica nanoparticles [39,106–108]. In this single-step process, drug loading significantly improved with a reported 70% efficacy [39].

Methods based on liposome–exosome fusion have also recently been proposed [109,110]. Additionally, Li et al. successfully incubated and merged the cargo of exosomes with liposomes containing fusogenic lipids, providing an alternative approach to the efficient loading of larger molecules [110]. Liposome–exosome hybrids allow for the incorporation of drugs without compromising the exosome membrane. It combines the advantages of the liposomes (ease of drug loading) with that of the exosomes (biocompatibility and targeting abilities) for effective drug loading and delivery. In another study, Yim et al. established a unique optogenetic exosome system via optically reversible protein–protein interactions (EXPLORs) [48]. The effective loading of cargo proteins into the exosomes was demonstrated using a reversible protein–protein interaction module controlled by blue light via the exosome endogenous biogenesis pathway [48]. It was noted that the protein-loaded EXPLORs delivered to the cytosols of target cells resulted in a significant increase in the intracellular levels of cargo proteins and their functions in vitro and in vivo [48]. Osteikoetxea et al. developed a new method for the successful loading of the clustered regularly interspaced short palindromic repeats (CRISPR/Cas9) into exosomes through the reversible heterodimerization of Cas9 fusions with exosome-specific components, such as tetraspanins [111].

New drug-loading methods have also considered the use of ubiquitination tags as a sorting sequence to facilitate effective drug loading [112]. An engineered ubiquitin tag was developed, and its fusion with proteins, such as enhanced green fluorescent protein, led to the loading of proteins into the exosome [112]. Another method involving a short ubiquitin tag with specific binding to the L-domain motif of Ndfip1 resulted in the efficient loading of proteins into exosomes [32]. The use of a non-functional mutant Nef protein facilitated the sorting of proteins into exosomes through its association with the exosomal lipid–raft microdomains [112]. In addition, Sutaria et al. developed a mechanism for the effective loading of miR-199a into exosomes via the trans-activating response element sequence, trans-activator of transcription, and Lamp2a (a component responsible for the loading of proteins into exosomes) [113]. In one study, HuR, an RNA-binding protein, was fused to the tetraspanin CD9 to be localized in the exosomal lumen to facilitate the loading of miR-155 into the exosome [114]. These alternative drug-loading methods, coupled with exosome isolation methods, may assist in the large-scale use of exosomes in a clinical setting.

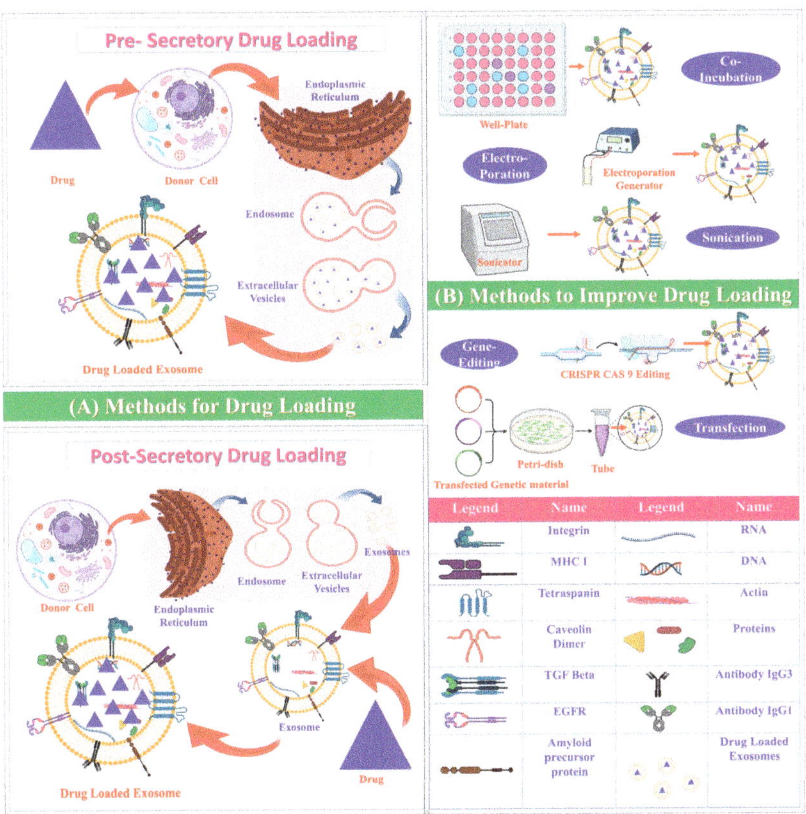

Figure 3. (**A**) Pre-secretory and post-secretory exosome drug-loading techniques and (**B**) methods of drug-loading enhancement. Pre-secretory drug loading, carried out before exosome secretion, involves (1) the incubation of the parent cell with the drug (transfection) and (2) gene editing. Post-secretory drug loading, carried out after exosome secretion, generally works in two ways: (1) passive incubation of the drug with the exosomes to allow the drug to attach to the exosome lipid bilayer membrane, or (2) the use of mechanical or chemical techniques, such as sonication and electroporation, to momentarily weaken the exosome membrane integrity to allow for the diffusion of the drug into the extracellular vesicles. The illustration was cre6ated with BioRender.com (https://app.biorender.com; accessed on 16 January 2023).

3.3. Targeted Exosome Delivery

In addition to effective drug loading, the development of targeted exosomes that are capable of high specificity and prolonged therapeutic function is of importance, as the ability of exosomes to administer the therapeutics to specific organs/tissues would reduce the possibility of undesired cellular interactions. Moreover, the administration of targeted exosomes would result in prolonged systemic circulation through the evasion of the mononuclear phagocyte system, which would aid in improving the therapeutic value of exosomes in nanomedicine. As such, a study incorporated various techniques to develop effective targeted exosomes and protection from the mononuclear phagocyte system [30]. The most common approach involves the grafting of hydrophilic polymers, such as polyethylene glycol (PEG), onto the exosome lipid bilayer membrane. The contact between exosomes and opsonin is impeded by these hydrophilic polymers, thus leading to prolonged systemic circulation. To circumvent this, Antes et al. engineered a protective 'cloaking' platform for modified exosomes to reduce their clearance by the phagocyte system [115]. However, despite its simplicity, cloaking must be done on each exosome, and as such, can be time-consuming.

Another approach to the development of targeted exosomes involves the modification of the glycan composition of the surface of exosomes, which plays an important role in uptake and cellular recognition [116]. Royo et al. reported that changes made to the sialic residues from glycoproteins produced targeted exosomes for specific organs [117]. Guo et al. developed targeted exosomes for bone tissue by the insertion of Golgi glycoprotein 1 into the exosome membrane [118]. The glycoprotein carried Wnt agonist 1, which reportedly reduced bone loss, accelerated fracture healing in colitis, and increased bone formation in mice [118]. Moreover, the presence of negatively charged phospholipids on exosomes increased their clearance through macrophages. Accordingly, research involving the blocking of the phospholipids has resulted in the prolonged circulation of exosomes.

Other approaches to improve the targeting ability of exosomes include the alterations of integrins and the use of aptamers [4]. The different integrins located on the surface of exosomes affect their pharmacokinetics and can be used to increase the accumulation of exosomes in tissues. Rana et al. were able to increase the selective uptake of exosomes in pancreatic cells by combining the protein Tspan with the extracellular exosome component integrin $\alpha4$ [119]. In addition to their use in exosome isolation, aptamers have also been shown to improve the targeting ability of exosomes. Research by Zou et al. developed aptamer-functionalized exosomes for cell-type-specific delivery of therapeutics [120]. The recognition capability of aptamers and the transport functions of exosomes were combined to effectively deliver molecular therapeutics or fluorophores to target tumor cells [120].

The incorporation of targeted exosomes with various drug-loading methods can increase the therapeutic value and efficacy of exosomes as a drug delivery tool. Liang et al. targeted colon cells specifically by fusing Her-2 to the N-terminus of Lamp2 on exosomes [121]. Following the alteration of the exosome membrane, two therapeutics—5-fluorouracil (electroporation) and miRNA-21 inhibitor (incubation)—were incorporated into the exosomes [121]. The authors noted that the method enhanced cellular uptake via the EGFR receptor-mediated endocytosis in colon cancer cells and successfully suppressed the tumor [121]. A study by Xu et al. demonstrated the specificity of kartogenin-loaded-targeted exosomes to the synovial fluid-derived mesenchymal stem cells by the addition of a specific mesenchymal stem cell-binding peptide (E7) to the exosome surface. The peptide was bound to Lamp2b, found on the surface of exosomes, and promoted mesenchymal stem cell chondrogenic differentiation and cartilage repair [122]. In a study by Jia et al., exosomes were loaded with superparamagnetic iron oxide nanoparticles and curcumin, followed by the conjugation of the exosome membrane with neuropilin-1-targeted peptides using click chemistry [123]. Through imaging and therapeutic analysis, Jia et al. reported the successful production of glioma-targeting exosomes [123]. Targeted exosomes in combination with drug-loading mechanisms are invaluable to the effective use of these extracellular vesicles as a drug delivery tool in the therapeutic treatment of various diseases in a large-scale clinical environment.

4. Conclusions

Exosomes are nanosized lipid-based extracellular vesicles that play an important role in cellular communication and cargo transport. The immunomodulatory, pharmacokinetic, and biocompatibility ability of exosomes have rendered these extracellular vesicles invaluable as a therapeutic approach for countless diseases. Studies involving the implementation of exosome-based therapies in the treatment of various diseases have shown great promise.

However, the use of exosome-based therapies in clinical settings is hindered by several challenges that require attention. One of the most significant challenges is exosome production and isolation. Importantly, exosome drug loading has proven difficult, as its effectiveness depends on the type of drug to be loaded and the source of the exosome. However, as the interest in exosomes as potential therapeutic agents grows, new mechanisms and modifications have been made to improve exosome isolation and drug loading for their possible use in nanomedicine.

Author Contributions: Conceptualization, T.R. and K.P.; writing—original draft preparation, T.R.; writing—review and editing, T.R., H.P., K.P. and F.S.; visualization, T.R. and H.P.; supervision, K.P. and F.S.; funding acquisition, K.P. and F.S. All authors have read and agreed to the published version of the manuscript.

Funding: This research received no external funding.

Institutional Review Board Statement: Not applicable.

Informed Consent Statement: Not applicable.

Data Availability Statement: Data sharing not applicable.

Acknowledgments: Publication of this article was supported by the College of Pharmacy and Health Sciences, St. John's University, New York, United States.

Conflicts of Interest: The authors declare no conflict of interest.

Abbreviations

CRISPR/CAS9	Clustered regularly interspaced short palindromic repeats-associated protein 9
ESCRT	Endosomal sorting complex required for transport
ESE	Early-sorting endosome
EXOSD	Exosome separation and detection
EXOtic	Exosomal transfer into cells
EXPLOR	Exosome system via optically reversible protein–protein interactions
HIFα	Hypoxia-induced factor α
HUR	Human antigen R
ILV	Intraluminal vesicle
LPS	Lipopolysaccharide
LSE	Late-sorting endosome
MVB	Multivesicular body
NDFIP1	Nedd4 family interacting protein 1
NEF	Negative regulatory factor
PEG	Polyethylene glycol
PLGA	Poly(lactic-co-glycolic acid)
PTEN	Phosphatase and TENsin homolog deleted on chromosome 10
STEAP3	Six-transmembrane epithelial antigen of prostate 3
TRAIL	Tumor necrosis factor-related apoptosis-induced ligand

References

1. Ha, D.; Yang, N.; Nadithe, V. Exosomes as Therapeutic Drug Carriers and Delivery Vehicles across Biological Membranes: Current Perspectives and Future Challenges. *Acta Pharm. Sin. B* **2016**, *6*, 287–296. [CrossRef] [PubMed]
2. Zhang, Y.; Bi, J.; Huang, J.; Tang, Y.; Du, S.; Li, P. Exosome: A Review of Its Classification, Isolation Techniques, Storage, Diagnostic and Targeted Therapy Applications. *Int. J. Nanomed.* **2020**, *15*, 6917–6934. [CrossRef] [PubMed]
3. Haney, M.J.; Klyachko, N.L.; Zhao, Y.; Gupta, R.; Plotnikova, E.G.; He, Z.; Patel, T.; Piroyan, A.; Sokolsky, M.; Kabanov, A.V.; et al. Exosomes as Drug Delivery Vehicles for Parkinson's Disease Therapy. *J. Control. Release* **2015**, *207*, 18–30. [CrossRef] [PubMed]
4. Elsharkasy, O.M.; Nordin, J.Z.; Hagey, D.W.; de Jong, O.G.; Schiffelers, R.M.; Andaloussi, S.E.; Vader, P. Extracellular Vesicles as Drug Delivery Systems: Why and How? *Adv. Drug Deliv. Rev.* **2020**, *159*, 332–343. [CrossRef]

5. An, Y.; Lin, S.; Tan, X.; Zhu, S.; Nie, F.; Zhen, Y.; Gu, L.; Zhang, C.; Wang, B.; Wei, W.; et al. Exosomes from Adipose-derived Stem Cells and Application to Skin Wound Healing. *Cell Prolif.* **2021**, *54*, e12993. [CrossRef]

6. Kumar, D.N.; Chaudhuri, A.; Aqil, F.; Dehari, D.; Munagala, R.; Singh, S.; Gupta, R.C.; Agrawal, A.K. Exosomes as Emerging Drug Delivery and Diagnostic Modality for Breast Cancer: Recent Advances in Isolation and Application. *Cancers* **2022**, *14*, 1435. [CrossRef]

7. Hussen, B.M.; Faraj, G.S.H.; Rasul, M.F.; Hidayat, H.J.; Salihi, A.; Baniahmad, A.; Taheri, M.; Ghafouri-Frad, S. Strategies to Overcome the Main Challenges of the Use of Exosomes as Drug Carrier for Cancer Therapy. *Cancer Cell Int.* **2022**, *22*, 323. [CrossRef]

8. Zhang, Y.; Li, J.; Gao, W.; Xie, N. Exosomes as Anticancer Drug Delivery Vehicles: Prospects and Challenges. *Front. Biosci.-Landmark* **2022**, *27*, 293. [CrossRef]

9. Ramirez, M.I.; Amorim, M.G.; Gadelha, C.; Milic, I.; Welsh, J.A.; Freitas, V.M.; Nawaz, M.; Akbar, N.; Couch, Y.; Makin, L.; et al. Technical Challenges of Working with Extracellular Vesicles. *Nanoscale* **2018**, *10*, 881–906. [CrossRef]

10. Livshits, M.A.; Khomyakova, E.; Evtushenko, E.G.; Lazarev, V.N.; Kulemin, N.A.; Semina, S.E.; Generozov, E.V.; Govorun, V.M. Isolation of Exosomes by Differential Centrifugation: Theoretical Analysis of a Commonly Used Protocol. *Sci. Rep.* **2015**, *5*, 17319. [CrossRef]

11. Li, K.; Wong, D.K.; Hong, K.Y.; Raffai, R.L. Cushioned-Density Gradient Ultracentrifugation (C-DGUC): A Refined and High Performance Method for the Isolation, Characterization, and Use of Exosomes. *Methods Mol. Biol.* **2018**, *1740*, 69–83. [CrossRef] [PubMed]

12. Onódi, Z.; Pelyhe, C.; Terézia Nagy, C.; Brenner, G.B.; Almási, L.; Kittel, Á.; Mančnek-Keber, M.; Ferdinandy, P.; Buzás, E.I.; Giricz, Z. Isolation of High-Purity Extracellular Vesicles by the Combination of Iodixanol Density Gradient Ultracentrifugation and Bind-Elute Chromatography from Blood Plasma. *Front. Physiol.* **2018**, *9*, 1479. [CrossRef] [PubMed]

13. Rider, M.A.; Hurwitz, S.N.; Meckes, D.G. ExtraPEG: A Polyethylene Glycol-Based Method for Enrichment of Extracellular Vesicles. *Sci. Rep.* **2016**, *6*, 23978. [CrossRef] [PubMed]

14. Emam, S.E.; Ando, H.; Lila, A.S.A.; Shimizu, T.; Ukawa, M.; Okuhira, K.; Ishima, Y.; Mahdy, M.A.; Ghazy, F.S.; Ishida, T. A Novel Strategy to Increase the Yield of Exosomes (Extracellular Vesicles) for an Expansion of Basic Research. *Biol. Pharm. Bull.* **2018**, *41*, 733–742. [CrossRef]

15. Zhang, X.; Borg, E.G.F.; Liaci, A.M.; Vos, H.R.; Stoorvogel, W. A Novel Three Step Protocol to Isolate Extracellular Vesicles from Plasma or Cell Culture Medium with Both High Yield and Purity. *J. Extracell. Vesicles* **2020**, *9*, 1791450. [CrossRef]

16. Benedikter, B.J.; Bouwman, F.G.; Vajen, T.; Heinzmann, A.C.A.; Grauls, G.; Mariman, E.C.; Wouters, E.F.M.; Savelkoul, P.H.; Lopez-Iglesias, C.; Koenen, R.R.; et al. Ultrafiltration Combined with Size Exclusion Chromatography Efficiently Isolates Extracellular Vesicles from Cell Culture Media for Compositional and Functional Studies. *Sci. Rep.* **2017**, *7*, 15297. [CrossRef]

17. Guerreiro, E.M.; Vestad, B.; Steffensen, L.A.; Aass, H.C.D.; Saeed, M.; Øvstebø, R.; Costea, D.E.; Galtung, H.K.; Søland, T.M. Efficient Extracellular Vesicle Isolation by Combining Cell Media Modifications, Ultrafiltration, and Size-Exclusion Chromatography. *PLoS ONE* **2018**, *13*, e0204276. [CrossRef]

18. Gámez-Valero, A.; Monguió-Tortajada, M.; Carreras-Planella, L.; Franquesa, M.; Beyer, K.; Borràs, F.E. Size-Exclusion Chromatography-Based Isolation Minimally Alters Extracellular Vesicles' Characteristics Compared to Precipitating Agents. *Sci. Rep.* **2016**, *6*, 33641. [CrossRef]

19. Sharma, P.; Ludwig, S.; Muller, L.; Hong, C.S.; Kirkwood, J.M.; Ferrone, S.; Whiteside, T.L. Immunoaffinity-Based Isolation of Melanoma Cell-Derived Exosomes from Plasma of Patients with Melanoma. *J. Extracell. Vesicles* **2018**, *7*, 1435138. [CrossRef]

20. Filipović, L.; Spasojević, M.; Prodanović, R.; Korać, A.; Matijašević, S.; Brajušković, G.; de Marco, A.; Popović, M. Affinity-Based Isolation of Extracellular Vesicles by Means of Single-Domain Antibodies Bound to Macroporous Methacrylate-Based Copolymer. *New Biotechnol.* **2022**, *69*, 36–48. [CrossRef]

21. Contreras-Naranjo, J.C.; Wu, H.-J.; Ugaz, V.M. Microfluidics for Exosome Isolation and Analysis: Enabling Liquid Biopsy for Personalized Medicine. *Lab Chip* **2017**, *17*, 3558–3577. [CrossRef] [PubMed]

22. Talebjedi, B.; Tasnim, N.; Hoorfar, M.; Mastromonaco, G.F.; De Almeida Monteiro Melo Ferraz, M. Exploiting Microfluidics for Extracellular Vesicle Isolation and Characterization: Potential Use for Standardized Embryo Quality Assessment. *Front. Vet. Sci.* **2021**, *7*, 620809. [CrossRef] [PubMed]

23. Sun, J.; Han, S.; Ma, L.; Zhang, H.; Zhan, Z.; Aguilar, H.A.; Zhang, H.; Xiao, K.; Gu, Y.; Gu, Z.; et al. Synergistically Bifunctional Paramagnetic Separation Enables Efficient Isolation of Urine Extracellular Vesicles and Downstream Phosphoproteomic Analysis. *ACS Appl. Mater. Interfaces* **2021**, *13*, 3622–3630. [CrossRef]

24. Jiawei, S.; Zhi, C.; Kewei, T.; Xiaoping, L. Magnetic Bead-Based Adsorption Strategy for Exosome Isolation. *Front. Bioeng. Biotechnol.* **2022**, *10*, 942077. [CrossRef] [PubMed]

25. Paolini, L.; Monguió-Tortajada, M.; Costa, M.; Antenucci, F.; Barilani, M.; Clos-Sansalvador, M.; Andrade, A.C.; Driedonks, T.A.P.; Giancaterino, S.; Kronstadt, S.M.; et al. Large-Scale Production of Extracellular Vesicles: Report on the "MassivEVs" ISEV Workshop. *J. Extracell. Biol.* **2022**, *1*, e63. [CrossRef]

26. Jeyaram, A.; Jay, S.M. Preservation and Storage Stability of Extracellular Vesicles for Therapeutic Applications. *AAPS J.* **2017**, *20*, 1. [CrossRef]

27. Lőrincz, Á.M.; Timár, C.I.; Marosvári, K.A.; Veres, D.S.; Otrokocsi, L.; Kittel, Á.; Ligeti, E. Effect of Storage on Physical and Functional Properties of Extracellular Vesicles Derived from Neutrophilic Granulocytes. *J. Extracell. Vesicles* **2014**, *3*, 25465. [CrossRef]

28. Maroto, R.; Zhao, Y.; Jamaluddin, M.; Popov, V.L.; Wang, H.; Kalubowilage, M.; Zhang, Y.; Luisi, J.; Sun, H.; Culbertson, C.T.; et al. Effects of Storage Temperature on Airway Exosome Integrity for Diagnostic and Functional Analyses. *J. Extracell. Vesicles* **2017**, *6*, 1359478. [CrossRef]

29. Bunggulawa, E.J.; Wang, W.; Yin, T.; Wang, N.; Durkan, C.; Wang, Y.; Wang, G. Recent Advancements in the Use of Exosomes as Drug Delivery Systems. *J. Nanobiotechnol.* **2018**, *16*, 81. [CrossRef]

30. Ferreira, D.; Moreira, J.N.; Rodrigues, L.R. New Advances in Exosome-Based Targeted Drug Delivery Systems. *Crit. Rev. Oncol./Hematol.* **2022**, *172*, 103628. [CrossRef]

31. Pascucci, L.; Coccè, V.; Bonomi, A.; Ami, D.; Ceccarelli, P.; Ciusani, E.; Viganò, L.; Locatelli, A.; Sisto, F.; Doglia, S.M.; et al. Paclitaxel Is Incorporated by Mesenchymal Stromal Cells and Released in Exosomes That Inhibit in vitro Tumor Growth: A New Approach for Drug Delivery. *J. Control. Release* **2014**, *192*, 262–270. [CrossRef] [PubMed]

32. Sterzenbach, U.; Putz, U.; Low, L.-H.; Silke, J.; Tan, S.-S.; Howitt, J. Engineered Exosomes as Vehicles for Biologically Active Proteins. *Mol. Ther.* **2017**, *25*, 1269–1278. [CrossRef] [PubMed]

33. Liu, C.; Zhang, W.; Li, Y.; Chang, J.; Tian, F.; Zhao, F.; Ma, Y.; Sun, J. Microfluidic Sonication to Assemble Exosome Membrane-Coated Nanoparticles for Immune Evasion-Mediated Targeting. *Nano Lett.* **2019**, *19*, 7836–7844. [CrossRef] [PubMed]

34. Salarpour, S.; Forootanfar, H.; Pournamdari, M.; Ahmadi-Zeidabadi, M.; Esmaeeli, M.; Pardakhty, A. Paclitaxel Incorporated Exosomes Derived from Glioblastoma Cells: Comparative Study of Two Loading Techniques. *Daru* **2019**, *27*, 533–539. [CrossRef] [PubMed]

35. Rodríguez-Morales, B.; Antunes-Ricardo, M.; González-Valdez, J. Exosome-Mediated Insulin Delivery for the Potential Treatment of Diabetes Mellitus. *Pharmaceutics* **2021**, *13*, 1870. [CrossRef]

36. Tang, M.; Chen, Y.; Li, B.; Sugimoto, H.; Yang, S.; Yang, C.; LeBleu, V.S.; McAndrews, K.M.; Kalluri, R. Therapeutic Targeting of STAT3 with Small Interference RNAs and Antisense Oligonucleotides Embedded Exosomes in Liver Fibrosis. *FASEB J.* **2021**, *35*, e21557. [CrossRef]

37. Deng, W.; Meng, Y.; Wang, B.; Wang, C.-X.; Hou, C.-X.; Zhu, Q.-H.; Tang, Y.-T.; Ye, J.-H. In Vitro Experimental Study on the Formation of MicroRNA-34a Loaded Exosomes and Their Inhibitory Effect in Oral Squamous Cell Carcinoma. *Cell Cycle* **2022**, *21*, 1775–1783. [CrossRef]

38. González-Sarrías, A.; Iglesias-Aguirre, C.E.; Cortés-Martín, A.; Vallejo, F.; Cattivelli, A.; del Pozo-Acebo, L.; Del Saz, A.; López de las Hazas, M.C.; Dávalos, A.; Espín, J.C. Milk-Derived Exosomes as Nanocarriers to Deliver Curcumin and Resveratrol in Breast Tissue and Enhance Their Anticancer Activity. *Int. J. Mol. Sci.* **2022**, *23*, 2860. [CrossRef]

39. Wang, Z.; Rich, J.; Hao, N.; Gu, Y.; Chen, C.; Yang, S.; Zhang, P.; Huang, T.J. Acoustofluidics for Simultaneous Nanoparticle-Based Drug Loading and Exosome Encapsulation. *Microsyst. Nanoeng.* **2022**, *8*, 45. [CrossRef]

40. Sato, Y.T.; Umezaki, K.; Sawada, S.; Mukai, S.; Sasaki, Y.; Harada, N.; Shiku, H.; Akiyoshi, K. Engineering Hybrid Exosomes by Membrane Fusion with Liposomes. *Sci. Rep.* **2016**, *6*, 21933. [CrossRef]

41. Yang, X.; Shi, G.; Guo, J.; Wang, C.; He, Y. Exosome-Encapsulated Antibiotic against Intracellular Infections of Methicillin-Resistant Staphylococcus Aureus. *Int. J. Nanomed.* **2018**, *13*, 8095–8104. [CrossRef] [PubMed]

42. Hao, R.; Yu, Z.; Du, J.; Hu, S.; Yuan, C.; Guo, H.; Zhang, Y.; Yang, H. A High-Throughput Nanofluidic Device for Exosome Nanoporation to Develop Cargo Delivery Vehicles. *Small* **2021**, *17*, 2102150. [CrossRef]

43. Fuhrmann, G.; Chandrawati, R.; Parmar, P.A.; Keane, T.J.; Maynard, S.A.; Bertazzo, S.; Stevens, M.M. Engineering Extracellular Vesicles with the Tools of Enzyme Prodrug Therapy. *Adv. Mater.* **2018**, *30*, 1706616. [CrossRef] [PubMed]

44. Fan, J.; Lee, C.-S.; Kim, S.; Chen, C.; Aghaloo, T.; Lee, M. Generation of Small RNA-Modulated Exosome Mimetics for Bone Regeneration. *ACS Nano* **2020**, *14*, 11973–11984. [CrossRef] [PubMed]

45. McAndrews, K.M.; Che, S.P.Y.; LeBleu, V.S.; Kalluri, R. Effective Delivery of STING Agonist Using Exosomes Suppresses Tumor Growth and Enhances Antitumor Immunity. *J. Biol. Chem.* **2021**, *296*, 100523. [CrossRef]

46. Wei, H.; Chen, J.; Wang, S.; Fu, F.; Zhu, X.; Wu, C.; Liu, Z.; Zhong, G.; Lin, J. A Nanodrug Consisting of Doxorubicin and Exosome Derived from Mesenchymal Stem Cells for Osteosarcoma Treatment in vitro. *Int. J. Nanomed.* **2019**, *14*, 8603–8610. [CrossRef] [PubMed]

47. Yang, T.; Martin, P.; Fogarty, B.; Brown, A.; Schurman, K.; Phipps, R.; Yin, V.P.; Lockman, P.; Bai, S. Exosome Delivered Anticancer Drugs Across the Blood-Brain Barrier for Brain Cancer Therapy in Danio Rerio. *Pharm. Res.* **2015**, *32*, 2003–2014. [CrossRef]

48. Yim, N.; Ryu, S.-W.; Choi, K.; Lee, K.R.; Lee, S.; Choi, H.; Kim, J.; Shaker, M.R.; Sun, W.; Park, J.-H.; et al. Exosome Engineering for Efficient Intracellular Delivery of Soluble Proteins Using Optically Reversible Protein–Protein Interaction Module. *Nat. Commun.* **2016**, *7*, 12277. [CrossRef]

49. Burrello, J.; Monticone, S.; Gai, C.; Gomez, Y.; Kholia, S.; Camussi, G. Stem Cell-Derived Extracellular Vesicles and Immune-Modulation. *Front. Cell Dev. Biol.* **2016**, *4*, 83. [CrossRef]

50. Ishiy, C.S.R.A.; Ormanji, M.S.; Maquigussa, E.; Ribeiro, R.S.; da Silva Novaes, A.; Boim, M.A. Comparison of the Effects of Mesenchymal Stem Cells with Their Extracellular Vesicles on the Treatment of Kidney Damage Induced by Chronic Renal Artery Stenosis. *Stem. Cells Int.* **2020**, *2020*, 8814574. [CrossRef]

51. Fernández-Francos, S.; Eiro, N.; Costa, L.A.; Escudero-Cernuda, S.; Fernández-Sánchez, M.L.; Vizoso, F.J. Mesenchymal Stem Cells as a Cornerstone in a Galaxy of Intercellular Signals: Basis for a New Era of Medicine. *Int. J. Mol. Sci.* **2021**, *22*, 3576. [CrossRef] [PubMed]

52. Haraszti, R.A.; Miller, R.; Stoppato, M.; Sere, Y.Y.; Coles, A.; Didiot, M.-C.; Wollacott, R.; Sapp, E.; Dubuke, M.L.; Li, X.; et al. Exosomes Produced from 3D Cultures of MSCs by Tangential Flow Filtration Show Higher Yield and Improved Activity. *Mol. Ther.* **2018**, *26*, 2838–2847. [CrossRef] [PubMed]

53. Schwechheimer, C.; Kuehn, M.J. Outer-Membrane Vesicles from Gram-Negative Bacteria: Biogenesis and Functions. *Nat. Rev. Microbiol.* **2015**, *13*, 605–619. [CrossRef] [PubMed]

54. Liu, Y.; Defourny, K.A.Y.; Smid, E.J.; Abee, T. Gram-Positive Bacterial Extracellular Vesicles and Their Impact on Health and Disease. *Front. Microbiol.* **2018**, *9*, 1502. [CrossRef]

55. Bitto, N.J.; Zavan, L.; Johnston, E.L.; Stinear, T.P.; Hill, A.F.; Kaparakis-Liaskos, M. Considerations for the Analysis of Bacterial Membrane Vesicles: Methods of Vesicle Production and Quantification Can Influence Biological and Experimental Outcomes. *Microbiol. Spectr.* **2021**, *9*, e01273-21. [CrossRef]

56. Agrawal, A.K.; Aqil, F.; Jeyabalan, J.; Spencer, W.A.; Beck, J.; Gachuki, B.W.; Alhakeem, S.S.; Oben, K.; Munagala, R.; Bondada, S.; et al. Milk-Derived Exosomes for Oral Delivery of Paclitaxel. *Nanomedicine* **2017**, *13*, 1627–1636. [CrossRef]

57. Marcilla, A.; Trelis, M.; Cortés, A.; Sotillo, J.; Cantalapiedra, F.; Minguez, M.T.; Valero, M.L.; del Pino, M.M.S.; Muñoz-Antoli, C.; Toledo, R.; et al. Extracellular Vesicles from Parasitic Helminths Contain Specific Excretory/Secretory Proteins and Are Internalized in Intestinal Host Cells. *PLoS ONE* **2012**, *7*, e45974. [CrossRef]

58. Teng, Y.; Ren, Y.; Sayed, M.; Hu, X.; Lei, C.; Kumar, A.; Hutchins, E.; Mu, J.; Deng, Z.; Luo, C.; et al. Plant-Derived Exosomal MicroRNAs Shape the Gut Microbiota. *Cell Host. Microbe* **2018**, *24*, 637–652.e8. [CrossRef]

59. Adamo, G.; Fierli, D.; Romancino, D.P.; Picciotto, S.; Barone, M.E.; Aranyos, A.; Božič, D.; Morsbach, S.; Raccosta, S.; Stanly, C.; et al. Nanoalgosomes: Introducing Extracellular Vesicles Produced by Microalgae. *J. Extracell. Vesicles* **2021**, *10*, e12081. [CrossRef]

60. Picciotto, S.; Barone, M.E.; Fierli, D.; Aranyos, A.; Adamo, G.; Božič, D.; Romancino, D.P.; Stanly, C.; Parkes, R.; Morsbach, S.; et al. Isolation of Extracellular Vesicles from Microalgae: Towards the Production of Sustainable and Natural Nanocarriers of Bioactive Compounds. *Biomater. Sci.* **2021**, *9*, 2917–2930. [CrossRef]

61. Petousis-Harris, H. Impact of Meningococcal Group B OMV Vaccines, beyond Their Brief. *Hum. Vaccines Immunother.* **2018**, *14*, 1058–1063. [CrossRef] [PubMed]

62. Ti, D.; Hao, H.; Tong, C.; Liu, J.; Dong, L.; Zheng, J.; Zhao, Y.; Liu, H.; Fu, X.; Han, W. LPS-Preconditioned Mesenchymal Stromal Cells Modify Macrophage Polarization for Resolution of Chronic Inflammation via Exosome-Shuttled Let-7b. *J. Transl. Med.* **2015**, *13*, 308. [CrossRef] [PubMed]

63. Wang, J.; Bonacquisti, E.E.; Brown, A.D.; Nguyen, J. Boosting the Biogenesis and Secretion of Mesenchymal Stem Cell-Derived Exosomes. *Cells* **2020**, *9*, 660. [CrossRef] [PubMed]

64. Glebov, K.; Löchner, M.; Jabs, R.; Lau, T.; Merkel, O.; Schloss, P.; Steinhäuser, C.; Walter, J. Serotonin Stimulates Secretion of Exosomes from Microglia Cells: Serotonin Stimulates Microglial Exosome Release. *Glia* **2015**, *63*, 626–634. [CrossRef]

65. Nakamura, Y.; Kita, S.; Tanaka, Y.; Fukuda, S.; Obata, Y.; Okita, T.; Nishida, H.; Takahashi, Y.; Kawachi, Y.; Tsugawa-Shimizu, Y.; et al. Adiponectin Stimulates Exosome Release to Enhance Mesenchymal Stem-Cell-Driven Therapy of Heart Failure in Mice. *Mol. Ther.* **2020**, *28*, 2203–2219. [CrossRef]

66. Drago, F.; Lombardi, M.; Prada, I.; Gabrielli, M.; Joshi, P.; Cojoc, D.; Franck, J.; Fournier, I.; Vizioli, J.; Verderio, C. ATP Modifies the Proteome of Extracellular Vesicles Released by Microglia and Influences Their Action on Astrocytes. *Front. Pharmacol.* **2017**, *8*, 910. [CrossRef]

67. Hooper, C.; Sainz-Fuertes, R.; Lynham, S.; Hye, A.; Killick, R.; Warley, A.; Bolondi, C.; Pocock, J.; Lovestone, S. Wnt3a Induces Exosome Secretion from Primary Cultured Rat Microglia. *BMC Neurosci.* **2012**, *13*, 144. [CrossRef]

68. Yuyama, K.; Takahashi, K.; Usuki, S.; Mikami, D.; Sun, H.; Hanamatsu, H.; Furukawa, J.; Mukai, K.; Igarashi, Y. Plant Sphingolipids Promote Extracellular Vesicle Release and Alleviate Amyloid-β Pathologies in a Mouse Model of Alzheimer's Disease. *Sci. Rep.* **2019**, *9*, 16827. [CrossRef]

69. Kojima, R.; Bojar, D.; Rizzi, G.; Hamri, G.C.-E.; El-Baba, M.D.; Saxena, P.; Ausländer, S.; Tan, K.R.; Fussenegger, M. Designer Exosomes Produced by Implanted Cells Intracerebrally Deliver Therapeutic Cargo for Parkinson's Disease Treatment. *Nat. Commun.* **2018**, *9*, 1305. [CrossRef]

70. Li, X.; Corbett, A.L.; Taatizadeh, E.; Tasnim, N.; Little, J.P.; Garnis, C.; Daugaard, M.; Guns, E.; Hoorfar, M.; Li, I.T.S. Challenges and Opportunities in Exosome Research—Perspectives from Biology, Engineering, and Cancer Therapy. *APL Bioeng.* **2019**, *3*, 011503. [CrossRef]

71. Gonzalez-King, H.; García, N.A.; Ontoria-Oviedo, I.; Ciria, M.; Montero, J.A.; Sepúlveda, P. Hypoxia Inducible Factor-1α Potentiates Jagged 1-Mediated Angiogenesis by Mesenchymal Stem Cell-Derived Exosomes. *Stem Cells* **2017**, *35*, 1747–1759. [CrossRef] [PubMed]

72. Zhang, W.; Zhou, X.; Yao, Q.; Liu, Y.; Zhang, H.; Dong, Z. HIF-1-Mediated Production of Exosomes during Hypoxia Is Protective in Renal Tubular Cells. *Am. J. Physiol. Ren. Physiol.* **2017**, *313*, F906–F913. [CrossRef]

73. Böker, K.O.; Lemus-Diaz, N.; Ferreira, R.R.; Schiller, L.; Schneider, S.; Gruber, J. The Impact of the CD9 Tetraspanin on Lentivirus Infectivity and Exosome Secretion. *Mol. Ther.* **2018**, *26*, 634. [CrossRef] [PubMed]

74. Cui, G.-H.; Wu, J.; Mou, F.-F.; Xie, W.-H.; Wang, F.-B.; Wang, Q.-L.; Fang, J.; Xu, Y.-W.; Dong, Y.-R.; Liu, J.-R.; et al. Exosomes Derived from Hypoxia-Preconditioned Mesenchymal Stromal Cells Ameliorate Cognitive Decline by Rescuing Synaptic Dysfunction and Regulating Inflammatory Responses in APP/PS1 Mice. *FASEB J.* **2018**, *32*, 654–668. [CrossRef]

75. Jiang, H.; Zhao, H.; Zhang, M.; He, Y.; Li, X.; Xu, Y.; Liu, X. Hypoxia Induced Changes of Exosome Cargo and Subsequent Biological Effects. *Front. Immunol.* **2022**, *13*, 824188. [CrossRef] [PubMed]

76. Garcia, N.A.; Ontoria-Oviedo, I.; González-King, H.; Diez-Juan, A.; Sepúlveda, P. Glucose Starvation in Cardiomyocytes Enhances Exosome Secretion and Promotes Angiogenesis in Endothelial Cells. *PLoS ONE* **2015**, *10*, e0138849. [CrossRef] [PubMed]

77. Deng, Z.; Wang, J.; Xiao, Y.; Li, F.; Niu, L.; Liu, X.; Meng, L.; Zheng, H. Ultrasound-Mediated Augmented Exosome Release from Astrocytes Alleviates Amyloid-β-Induced Neurotoxicity. *Theranostics* **2021**, *11*, 4351–4362. [CrossRef]

78. Guo, Y.; Wan, Z.; Zhao, P.; Wei, M.; Liu, Y.; Bu, T.; Sun, W.; Li, Z.; Yuan, L. Ultrasound Triggered Topical Delivery of Bmp7 MRNA for White Fat Browning Induction via Engineered Smart Exosomes. *J. Nanobiotechnol.* **2021**, *19*, 402. [CrossRef] [PubMed]

79. Ambattu, L.A.; Ramesan, S.; Dekiwadia, C.; Hanssen, E.; Li, H.; Yeo, L.Y. High Frequency Acoustic Cell Stimulation Promotes Exosome Generation Regulated by a Calcium-Dependent Mechanism. *Commun. Biol.* **2020**, *3*, 553. [CrossRef]

80. Kim, M.; Yun, H.-W.; Park, D.Y.; Choi, B.H.; Min, B.-H. Three-Dimensional Spheroid Culture Increases Exosome Secretion from Mesenchymal Stem Cells. *Tissue Eng. Regen. Med.* **2018**, *15*, 427–436. [CrossRef]

81. Cao, J.; Wang, B.; Tang, T.; Lv, L.; Ding, Z.; Li, Z.; Hu, R.; Wei, Q.; Shen, A.; Fu, Y.; et al. Three-Dimensional Culture of MSCs Produces Exosomes with Improved Yield and Enhanced Therapeutic Efficacy for Cisplatin-Induced Acute Kidney Injury. *Stem Cell Res. Ther.* **2020**, *11*, 206. [CrossRef] [PubMed]

82. Koh, B.; Sulaiman, N.; Fauzi, M.B.; Law, J.X.; Ng, M.H.; Idrus, R.B.H.; Yazid, M.D. Three Dimensional Microcarrier System in Mesenchymal Stem Cell Culture: A Systematic Review. *Cell Biosci.* **2020**, *10*, 75. [CrossRef] [PubMed]

83. Xu, C.; Zhao, J.; Li, Q.; Hou, L.; Wang, Y.; Li, S.; Jiang, F.; Zhu, Z.; Tian, L. Exosomes Derived from Three-Dimensional Cultured Human Umbilical Cord Mesenchymal Stem Cells Ameliorate Pulmonary Fibrosis in a Mouse Silicosis Model. *Stem Cell Res. Ther.* **2020**, *11*, 503. [CrossRef] [PubMed]

84. Patel, D.B.; Luthers, C.R.; Lerman, M.J.; Fisher, J.P.; Jay, S.M. Enhanced Extracellular Vesicle Production and Ethanol-Mediated Vascularization Bioactivity via a 3D-Printed Scaffold-Perfusion Bioreactor System. *Acta Biomater.* **2019**, *95*, 236–244. [CrossRef]

85. Burns, A.B.; Doris, C.; Vehar, K.; Saxena, V.; Bardliving, C.; Shamlou, P.A.; Phillips, M.I. Novel Low Shear 3D Bioreactor for High Purity Mesenchymal Stem Cell Production. *PLoS ONE* **2021**, *16*, e0252575. [CrossRef]

86. Du, W.; Zhang, K.; Zhang, S.; Wang, R.; Nie, Y.; Tao, H.; Han, Z.; Liang, L.; Wang, D.; Liu, J.; et al. Enhanced Proangiogenic Potential of Mesenchymal Stem Cell-Derived Exosomes Stimulated by a Nitric Oxide Releasing Polymer. *Biomaterials* **2017**, *133*, 70–81. [CrossRef]

87. Liu, L.; Liu, Y.; Feng, C.; Chang, J.; Fu, R.; Wu, T.; Yu, F.; Wang, X.; Xia, L.; Wu, C.; et al. Lithium-Containing Biomaterials Stimulate Bone Marrow Stromal Cell-Derived Exosomal MiR-130a Secretion to Promote Angiogenesis. *Biomaterials* **2019**, *192*, 523–536. [CrossRef]

88. Park, D.J.; Yun, W.S.; Kim, W.C.; Park, J.-E.; Lee, S.H.; Ha, S.; Choi, J.S.; Key, J.; Seo, Y.J. Improvement of Stem Cell-Derived Exosome Release Efficiency by Surface-Modified Nanoparticles. *J. Nanobiotechnol.* **2020**, *18*, 178. [CrossRef]

89. Wu, Z.; He, D.; Li, H. Bioglass Enhances the Production of Exosomes and Improves Their Capability of Promoting Vascularization. *Bioact. Mater.* **2021**, *6*, 823–835. [CrossRef]

90. Haraszti, R.A.; Miller, R.; Dubuke, M.L.; Rockwell, H.E.; Coles, A.H.; Sapp, E.; Didiot, M.-C.; Echeverria, D.; Stoppato, M.; Sere, Y.Y.; et al. Serum Deprivation of Mesenchymal Stem Cells Improves Exosome Activity and Alters Lipid and Protein Composition. *iScience* **2019**, *16*, 230–241. [CrossRef]

91. Gupta, S.; Rawat, S.; Arora, V.; Kottarath, S.K.; Dinda, A.K.; Vaishnav, P.K.; Nayak, B.; Mohanty, S. An Improvised One-Step Sucrose Cushion Ultracentrifugation Method for Exosome Isolation from Culture Supernatants of Mesenchymal Stem Cells. *Stem Cell Res. Ther.* **2018**, *9*, 180. [CrossRef] [PubMed]

92. Smith, J.T.; Wunsch, B.H.; Dogra, N.; Ahsen, M.E.; Lee, K.; Yadav, K.K.; Weil, R.; Pereira, M.A.; Patel, J.V.; Duch, E.A.; et al. Integrated Nanoscale Deterministic Lateral Displacement Arrays for Separation of Extracellular Vesicles from Clinically-Relevant Volumes of Biological Samples. *Lab Chip* **2018**, *18*, 3913–3925. [CrossRef] [PubMed]

93. Yu, Z.; Lin, S.; Xia, F.; Liu, Y.; Zhang, D.; Wang, F.; Wang, Y.; Li, Q.; Niu, J.; Cao, C.; et al. ExoSD Chips for High-Purity Immunomagnetic Separation and High-Sensitivity Detection of Gastric Cancer Cell-Derived Exosomes. *Biosens. Bioelectron.* **2021**, *194*, 113594. [CrossRef] [PubMed]

94. Heath, N.; Grant, L.; De Oliveira, T.M.; Rowlinson, R.; Osteikoetxea, X.; Dekker, N.; Overman, R. Rapid Isolation and Enrichment of Extracellular Vesicle Preparations Using Anion Exchange Chromatography. *Sci. Rep.* **2018**, *8*, 5730. [CrossRef] [PubMed]

95. Song, Z.; Mao, J.; Barrero, R.A.; Wang, P.; Zhang, F.; Wang, T. Development of a CD63 Aptamer for Efficient Cancer Immunochemistry and Immunoaffinity-Based Exosome Isolation. *Molecules* **2020**, *25*, 5585. [CrossRef]

96. Zhou, Z.; Chen, Y.; Qian, X. Target-Specific Exosome Isolation through Aptamer-Based Microfluidics. *Biosensors* **2022**, *12*, 257. [CrossRef]

97. Zhang, K.; Yue, Y.; Wu, S.; Liu, W.; Shi, J.; Zhang, Z. Rapid Capture and Nondestructive Release of Extracellular Vesicles Using Aptamer-Based Magnetic Isolation. *ACS Sens.* **2019**, *4*, 1245–1251. [CrossRef]

98. Kimiz-Gebologlu, I.; Oncel, S.S. Exosomes: Large-Scale Production, Isolation, Drug Loading Efficiency, and Biodistribution and Uptake. *J. Control. Release* **2022**, *347*, 533–543. [CrossRef]

99. Gebeyehu, A.; Kommineni, N.; Bagde, A.; Meckes, D.G.; Sachdeva, M.S. Role of Exosomes for Delivery of Chemotherapeutic Drugs. *Crit. Rev. Ther. Drug Carrier Syst.* **2021**, *38*, 53–97. [CrossRef]

100. Zhang, Q.; Zhang, H.; Ning, T.; Liu, D.; Deng, T.; Liu, R.; Bai, M.; Zhu, K.; Li, J.; Fan, Q.; et al. Exosome-Delivered c-Met SiRNA Could Reverse Chemoresistance to Cisplatin in Gastric Cancer. *Int. J. Nanomed.* **2020**, *15*, 2323–2335. [CrossRef]

101. Yuan, Z.; Kolluri, K.K.; Gowers, K.H.C.; Janes, S.M. TRAIL Delivery by MSC-Derived Extracellular Vesicles Is an Effective Anticancer Therapy. *J. Extracell. Vesicles* **2017**, *6*, 1265291. [CrossRef] [PubMed]

102. O'Brien, K.; Lowry, M.C.; Corcoran, C.; Martinez, V.G.; Daly, M.; Rani, S.; Gallagher, W.M.; Radomski, M.W.; MacLeod, R.A.F.; O'Driscoll, L. MiR-134 in Extracellular Vesicles Reduces Triple-Negative Breast Cancer Aggression and Increases Drug Sensitivity. *Oncotarget* **2015**, *6*, 32774–32789. [CrossRef] [PubMed]

103. Yuan, Y.; Wang, Q.; Cao, F.; Han, B.; Xu, L. MiRNA-134 Suppresses Esophageal Squamous Cell Carcinoma Progression by Targeting FOXM1. *Int. J. Clin. Exp. Pathol.* **2019**, *12*, 2130–2138. [PubMed]

104. Yang, Z.; Shi, J.; Xie, J.; Wang, Y.; Sun, J.; Liu, T.; Zhao, Y.; Zhao, X.; Wang, X.; Ma, Y.; et al. Large-Scale Generation of Functional MRNA-Encapsulating Exosomes via Cellular Nanoporation. *Nat. Biomed. Eng.* **2020**, *4*, 69–83. [CrossRef]

105. Nawaz, M.; Heydarkhan-Hagvall, S.; Tangruksa, B.; González-King Garibotti, H.; Jing, Y.; Maugeri, M.; Kohl, F.; Hultin, L.; Reyahi, A.; Camponeschi, A.; et al. Lipid Nanoparticles Deliver the Therapeutic VEGFA MRNA In Vitro and In Vivo and Transform Extracellular Vesicles for Their Functional Extensions. *Adv. Sci.* **2023**, 2206187. [CrossRef]

106. Wu, M.; Ozcelik, A.; Rufo, J.; Wang, Z.; Fang, R.; Jun Huang, T. Acoustofluidic Separation of Cells and Particles. *Microsyst. Nanoeng.* **2019**, *5*, 32. [CrossRef]

107. Wang, Z.; Li, F.; Rufo, J.; Chen, C.; Yang, S.; Li, L.; Zhang, J.; Cheng, J.; Kim, Y.; Wu, M.; et al. Acoustofluidic Salivary Exosome Isolation. *J. Mol. Diagn.* **2020**, *22*, 50–59. [CrossRef]

108. Fan, Y.; Wang, X.; Ren, J.; Lin, F.; Wu, J. Recent Advances in Acoustofluidic Separation Technology in Biology. *Microsyst. Nanoeng.* **2022**, *8*, 94. [CrossRef]

109. Lin, Y.; Wu, J.; Gu, W.; Huang, Y.; Tong, Z.; Huang, L.; Tan, J. Exosome–Liposome Hybrid Nanoparticles Deliver CRISPR/Cas9 System in MSCs. *Adv. Sci.* **2018**, *5*, 1700611. [CrossRef]

110. Li, L.; He, D.; Guo, Q.; Zhang, Z.; Ru, D.; Wang, L.; Gong, K.; Liu, F.; Duan, Y.; Li, H. Exosome-Liposome Hybrid Nanoparticle Codelivery of TP and MiR497 Conspicuously Overcomes Chemoresistant Ovarian Cancer. *J. Nanobiotechnol.* **2022**, *20*, 50. [CrossRef]

111. Osteikoetxea, X.; Silva, A.; Lázaro-Ibáñez, E.; Salmond, N.; Shatnyeva, O.; Stein, J.; Schick, J.; Wren, S.; Lindgren, J.; Firth, M.; et al. Engineered Cas9 Extracellular Vesicles as a Novel Gene Editing Tool. *J. Extracell. Vesicles* **2022**, *11*, e12225. [CrossRef] [PubMed]

112. Jafari, D.; Shajari, S.; Jafari, R.; Mardi, N.; Gomari, H.; Ganji, F.; Forouzandeh Moghadam, M.; Samadikuchaksaraei, A. Designer Exosomes: A New Platform for Biotechnology Therapeutics. *BioDrugs* **2020**, *34*, 567–586. [CrossRef] [PubMed]

113. Sutaria, D.S.; Jiang, J.; Elgamal, O.A.; Pomeroy, S.M.; Badawi, M.; Zhu, X.; Pavlovicz, R.; Azevedo-Pouly, A.C.P.; Chalmers, J.; Li, C.; et al. Low Active Loading of Cargo into Engineered Extracellular Vesicles Results in Inefficient MiRNA Mimic Delivery. *J. Extracell. Vesicles* **2017**, *6*, 1333882. [CrossRef] [PubMed]

114. Z, L.; X, Z.; M, W.; X, G.; L, Z.; R, S.; W, S.; Y, D.; G, Y.; L, Y. In Vitro and in Vivo RNA Inhibition by CD9-HuR Functionalized Exosomes Encapsulated with MiRNA or CRISPR/DCas9. *Nano Lett.* **2019**, *19*, 19–28. [CrossRef]

115. Antes, T.J.; Middleton, R.C.; Luther, K.M.; Ijichi, T.; Peck, K.A.; Liu, W.J.; Valle, J.; Echavez, A.K.; Marbán, E. Targeting Extracellular Vesicles to Injured Tissue Using Membrane Cloaking and Surface Display. *J. Nanobiotechnol.* **2018**, *16*, 61. [CrossRef] [PubMed]

116. Martins, Á.M.; Ramos, C.C.; Freitas, D.; Reis, C.A. Glycosylation of Cancer Extracellular Vesicles: Capture Strategies, Functional Roles and Potential Clinical Applications. *Cells* **2021**, *10*, 109. [CrossRef]

117. Royo, F.; Cossío, U.; de Angulo, A.R.; Llop, J.; Falcon-Perez, J.M. Modification of the Glycosylation of Extracellular Vesicles Alters Their Biodistribution in Mice. *Nanoscale* **2019**, *11*, 1531–1537. [CrossRef]

118. Guo, J.; Wang, F.; Hu, Y.; Luo, Y.; Wei, Y.; Xu, K.; Zhang, H.; Liu, H.; Bo, L.; Lv, S.; et al. Exosome-Based Bone-Targeting Drug Delivery Alleviates Impaired Osteoblastic Bone Formation and Bone Loss in Inflammatory Bowel Diseases. *Cell Rep. Med.* **2023**, *4*, 100881. [CrossRef]

119. Rana, S.; Yue, S.; Stadel, D.; Zöller, M. Toward Tailored Exosomes: The Exosomal Tetraspanin Web Contributes to Target Cell Selection. *Int. J. Biochem. Cell Biol.* **2012**, *44*, 1574–1584. [CrossRef]

120. Zou, J.; Shi, M.; Liu, X.; Jin, C.; Xing, X.; Qiu, L.; Tan, W. Aptamer-Functionalized Exosomes: Elucidating the Cellular Uptake Mechanism and the Potential for Cancer-Targeted Chemotherapy. *Anal. Chem.* **2019**, *91*, 2425–2430. [CrossRef]

121. Liang, G.; Zhu, Y.; Ali, D.J.; Tian, T.; Xu, H.; Si, K.; Sun, B.; Chen, B.; Xiao, Z. Engineered Exosomes for Targeted Co-Delivery of MiR-21 Inhibitor and Chemotherapeutics to Reverse Drug Resistance in Colon Cancer. *J. Nanobiotechnol.* **2020**, *18*, 10. [CrossRef] [PubMed]

122. Xu, X.; Liang, Y.; Li, X.; Ouyang, K.; Wang, M.; Cao, T.; Li, W.; Liu, J.; Xiong, J.; Li, B.; et al. Exosome-Mediated Delivery of Kartogenin for Chondrogenesis of Synovial Fluid-Derived Mesenchymal Stem Cells and Cartilage Regeneration. *Biomaterials* **2021**, *269*, 120539. [CrossRef] [PubMed]
123. Jia, G.; Han, Y.; An, Y.; Ding, Y.; He, C.; Wang, X.; Tang, Q. NRP-1 Targeted and Cargo-Loaded Exosomes Facilitate Simultaneous Imaging and Therapy of Glioma in vitro and in vivo. *Biomaterials* **2018**, *178*, 302–316. [CrossRef] [PubMed]

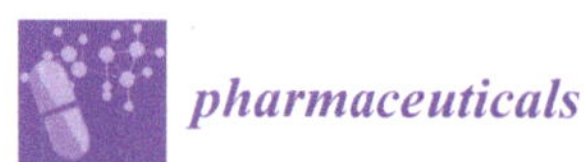

pharmaceuticals

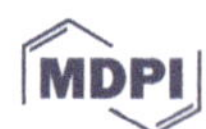

Review

Intranasal Lipid Nanoparticles Containing Bioactive Compounds Obtained from Marine Sources to Manage Neurodegenerative Diseases

Joana Torres [1,2], Inês Costa [2,3], Andreia F. Peixoto [4], Renata Silva [2,3], José Manuel Sousa Lobo [1,2] and Ana Catarina Silva [1,2,5,*]

1 UCIBIO, REQUIMTE, Laboratory of Pharmaceutical Technology/Centre of Research in Pharmaceutical Sciences, Faculty of Pharmacy, University of Porto, 4050-313 Porto, Portugal
2 Associate Laboratory i4HB-Institute for Health and Bioeconomy, Faculty of Pharmacy, University of Porto, 4050-313 Porto, Portugal
3 UCIBIO, REQUIMTE, Laboratory of Toxicology, Department of Biological Sciences, Faculty of Pharmacy, University of Porto, 4050-3131 Porto, Portugal
4 LAQV/REQUIMTE, Department of Chemistry and Biochemistry, Faculty of Sciences, University of Porto, 4169-007 Porto, Portugal
5 FP-I3ID (Instituto de Investigação, Inovação e Desenvolvimento), FP-BHS (Biomedical and Health Sciences Research Unit), Faculty of Health Sciences, University Fernando Pessoa, 4200-150 Porto, Portugal
* Correspondence: anacatsil@gmail.com

Abstract: Marine sources contain several bioactive compounds with high therapeutic potential, such as remarkable antioxidant activity that can reduce oxidative stress related to the pathogenesis of neurodegenerative diseases. Indeed, there has been a growing interest in these natural sources, especially those resulting from the processing of marine organisms (i.e., marine bio-waste), to obtain natural antioxidants as an alternative to synthetic antioxidants in a sustainable approach to promote circularity by recovering and creating value from these bio-wastes. However, despite their expected potential to prevent, delay, or treat neurodegenerative diseases, antioxidant compounds may have difficulty reaching the brain due to the need to cross the blood–brain barrier (BBB). In this regard, alternative delivery systems administered by different routes have been proposed, including intranasal administration of lipid nanoparticles, such as solid lipid nanoparticles (SLN) and nanostructured lipid carriers (NLC), which have shown promising results. Intranasal administration shows several advantages, including the fact that molecules do not need to cross the BBB to reach the central nervous system (CNS), as they can be transported directly from the nasal cavity to the brain (i.e., nose-to-brain transport). The benefits of using SLN and NLC for intranasal delivery of natural bioactive compounds for the treatment of neurodegenerative diseases have shown relevant outcomes through in vitro and in vivo studies. Noteworthy, for bioactive compounds obtained from marine bio-waste, few studies have been reported, showing the open potential of this research area. This review updates the state of the art of using SLN and NLC to transport bioactive compounds from different sources, in particular, those obtained from marine bio-waste, and their potential application in the treatment of neurodegenerative diseases.

Keywords: antioxidants; marine bio-waste; bioactive compounds; neurodegenerative diseases; nanostructured lipid carriers; NLC; solid lipid nanoparticles; SLN; intranasal administration; nose-to-brain

Citation: Torres, J.; Costa, I.; Peixoto, A.F.; Silva, R.; Sousa Lobo, J.M.; Silva, A.C. Intranasal Lipid Nanoparticles Containing Bioactive Compounds Obtained from Marine Sources to Manage Neurodegenerative Diseases. *Pharmaceuticals* **2023**, *16*, 311. https://doi.org/10.3390/ph16020311

Academic Editor: Rachel Auzély

Received: 23 January 2023
Revised: 8 February 2023
Accepted: 14 February 2023
Published: 16 February 2023

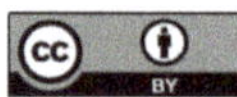

1. Introduction

In recent years, the average consumption of fish, shellfish, and crustaceans has increased significantly, as they can contribute positively to human health and well-being, when combined with a healthy lifestyle [1,2]. However, this increase in the consumption of marine organisms has led to the annual production of tens of millions of tons of solid waste resulting from their processing. Currently, the Food and Agriculture Organization of the United Nations (FAO) recognizes the environmental, social, and economic problems resulting from the landfilling of this waste [1,3,4]. To overcome this challenge, an innovative solution has been proposed, consisting of the recovery and valorization of waste resulting from the processing of marine organisms, as this bio-waste is a rich reservoir of various bio-functional components [2,5]. There are already many investigations that demonstrate the potential of using these products to obtain bioactive compounds with different activities (e.g., anticancer, antimicrobial, antioxidant, and immunomodulatory) that can be used to develop value-added products in the pharmaceutical industry for the treatment of different diseases [2–4,6,7]. For example, bioactive compounds that can be isolated from shrimp waste include the chito-oligosaccharides present in chitin or chitosan, omega-3, and astaxanthin. Salmon nasal cartilage is a valuable source of proteoglycans with anti-angiogenic activity. Fish skin is an important source of collagen, which can be hydrolyzed to bioactive peptides. Algae contain high amounts of phytonutrients, particularly those belonging to the gender *Chlorophyta*, *Rhodophyta*, and *Phaeophyta*, which are rich in dietary fibers, omega-3, β-carotene, astaxanthin, vitamin C, and other compounds beneficial to human health [3,8].

The scientific community already recognizes the extraordinary potential of bioactive compounds obtained from marine bio-waste to prevent and treat various diseases, such as those showing antioxidant activity that can prevent, delay, or treat neurodegenerative diseases. Indeed, within the circular economy paradigm, the use of this bio-waste has multiple benefits, promoting a more sustainable aquaculture and fishing industries, and reducing the impact of anthropic exploitation of marine resources [1,9–11]. However, despite the potential of these new bioactive compounds, there is still no effective therapeutic solution for neurodegenerative diseases. Researchers have been pointed that the main challenge is the difficulty for molecules to cross the blood–brain barrier (BBB) to reach the brain. Different approaches have been investigated to circumvent this problem. Among them, the use of lipid nanoparticles (i.e., solid lipid nanoparticles—SLN and nanostructured lipid carriers—NLC), administered by alternative routes, such as the intranasal (i.e., nose-to-brain route), has been described as the most promising option [12–17].

This review work begins with a description of the different pathophysiological mechanisms underlying neurodegenerative diseases, followed by the presentation of examples of bioactive compounds obtained from marine bio-waste with potential antioxidant activity in the management of these diseases. Finally, the state-of-the-art use of intranasal SLN and NLC to transport bioactive compounds directly to the brain, promoting the treatment of neurodegenerative diseases, is presented.

2. Neurodegenerative Diseases

Neurodegenerative diseases are a group of debilitating conditions that result from progressive damage inflicted on cells and nervous system, with abnormal deposition of proteins and the progressive loss of synapses and neurons [18,19]. Due to the different pathophysiological mechanisms underlying these diseases, they present a wide spectrum of clinical manifestations. With neurodegenerative disease progression, the severity of the symptoms gradually increases, resulting in a reduced ability to live independently and in a huge impact on the patients' quality of life [19].

Some examples of neurodegenerative diseases include Alzheimer's disease, vascular dementia, frontotemporal dementia, mixed dementia, and dementia with Lewy bodies, which are characterized by cognitive deficits and memory loss. On the other side, neurodegenerative diseases that mainly affect the locomotor system include Amyotrophic lateral sclerosis, Huntington's disease, Parkinson's disease, Multiple sclerosis, and Spinocerebellar ataxias [20,21]. In the present review, the most prevalent and debilitating neurodegenerative diseases will be explored, namely Alzheimer's disease, Parkinson's disease, multiple sclerosis, and amyotrophic lateral sclerosis.

Alzheimer's disease is the most common neurodegenerative disease, corresponding to 60% to 80% of cases of dementia [22]. This illness was described for the first time in

1906 by Alois Alzheimer, and is characterized by the extracellular deposition of amyloid-β (Aβ) peptide in senile plaques, by the intraneuronal accumulation of hyperphosphorylated tau protein (leading to the formation of intracellular neurofibrillary tangles), as well as by oxidative stress, neuroinflammation, ferroptosis, and synaptic loss [23,24]. The main symptoms expressed by the patients are persistent and frequent memory difficulties, vague speech, delay in performing routine activities, emotional unpredictability, and inability to understand questions and instructions [25].

Parkinson's disease is a complex neurological disease with early death of dopaminergic neurons in *substantia nigra pars compacta* and is characterized by Lewy bodies formation, oxidative stress, iron overload, mitochondrial dysfunction, ferroptosis, and neuroinflammation. It affects about 0.1–0.2% of the population, and patients experience motor symptoms such as tremor, bradykinesia, rigidity, and postural instability [26,27], and also non-motor symptoms such as depression and sleep problems [28].

Multiple sclerosis is recognized as a chronic inflammatory and demyelinating disease that affects 2.1 million people worldwide [29]. The defects in oligodendrocyte regeneration and myelin damage leads to axonal degeneration, which constitutes the main cause for the progression of the irreversible neuronal destruction that leads to permanent disability [30]. Symptoms experienced by patients include walking impairment, weakness, cognitive impairment, depression, and fatigue [31].

Amyotrophic lateral sclerosis is a neurodegenerative disease characterized by the selective dysfunction and loss of motor neurons in specific brain regions, with aggregation and accumulation of ubiquitinated proteinaceous inclusions, consequently leading to paralysis and death [32–34]. This neurodegenerative disease has an incidence of approximately 1.2–6 per 100.000 persons annually [34]. In most cases of amyotrophic lateral sclerosis, there is no family history associated, but in about 10% of cases, a dominantly inherited autosomal mutation occurs in distinct genes, such as in superoxide dismutase 1 (SOD1), C9orf72, and TAR DNA-binding protein 43 (TDP-43) genes [35]. The main symptoms are progressive muscle weakness, slowness of movements with muscle stiffness, muscle atrophy, and muscle cramps [33]. In the next sub-section, the main pathophysiological mechanisms common to these neurodegenerative diseases will be addressed.

2.1. Main Pathophysiological Mechanism Underlying Neurodegenerative Diseases

Although the mentioned neurodegenerative diseases are complex and present different symptoms and underlying mechanisms, several common mechanisms have been studied aiming to explain the development and progression of these pathologies. Figure 1 summarizes the main pathophysiological mechanisms that appear to be common to distinct neurodegenerative diseases, including oxidative stress and mitochondrial dysfunction, neuroinflammation, protein misfolding, and iron overload and ferroptosis.

2.1.1. Oxidative Stress and Mitochondrial Dysfunction

Oxidative stress is considered a state in which free radicals and their products are in excess when compared to the levels of antioxidant defenses. Under normal cellular conditions, reactive oxygen species (ROS) and reactive nitrogen species (RNS) play an important physiological role, and their intracellular concentrations are kept at low or moderate levels by an endogenous antioxidant system. When the production of ROS/RNS surpasses the capacity of the endogenous antioxidant system, the onset of several adverse mechanisms is observed, such as interaction with lipids, proteins, and DNA, which contribute to cell degeneration [36].

The brain has several features that make it very susceptible to oxidative stress [37]: (i) membrane lipids contain high levels of polyunsaturated fatty acids (PUFAs) that are the preferred substrate for lipid peroxidation; (ii) high consumption of oxygen that contributes to the generation of superoxide anions; (iii) lower concentrations of antioxidant enzymes (catalase—CAT, superoxide dismutase—SOD and glutathione peroxidase—GPx); (iv) high concentration of iron, which promotes participation in the Fenton reaction and in the generation of ROS.

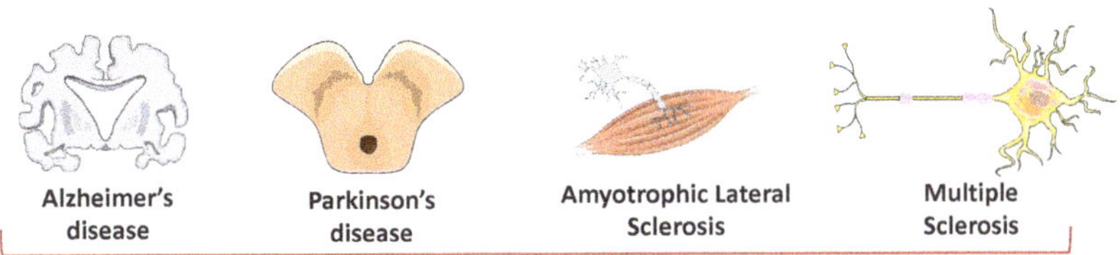

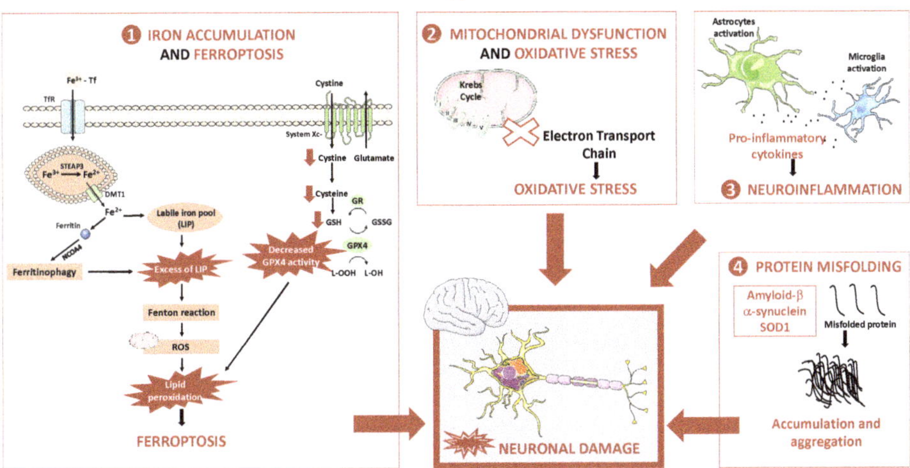

Figure 1. Common pathophysiological mechanisms underlying the most prevalent and debilitating neurodegenerative diseases. Neurodegenerative diseases are a group of debilitant conditions that result from the progressive damage inflicted to the neuronal cells and nervous system, with abnormal deposition of proteins, and with the progressive loss of synapses and neurons. Alzheimer's disease, Parkinson's disease, Amyotrophic Lateral Sclerosis, and Multiple Sclerosis are examples of complex neurodegenerative diseases sharing several common pathophysiological mechanisms, such as: (1) iron overload, (2) mitochondrial dysfunction and oxidative stress, (3) neuroinflammation, and (4) protein misfolding. Iron has essential functions in the brain and, therefore, needs to cross the blood–brain barrier (BBB) to reach this organ. The most elucidating hypothesis of the passage of iron through the luminal membrane of the capillary endothelium mainly occurs through the transferrin/transferrin receptor (Tf/TfR) pathway. This process starts with the binding of the complex ferric iron (Fe^{3+})-Tf to the extracellular portion of transferrin receptor (TfR), followed by the endocytosis of the complex, formation of endosome, and acidification of the microenvironment within endosome. Next, occurs the dissociation of iron from Tf and the reduction of ferric iron (Fe^{3+}) to Fe^{2+} by the ferrireductase six-transmembrane epithelial antigen of prostate 3 (STEAP3). Fe^{2+} accumulates in cytoplasm, forming the labile iron pool (LIP), and the excess of intracellular iron is then stored in ferritin. Ferritinophagy is defined as the autophagic degradation of ferritin, a process mediated by nuclear receptor coactivator 4 (NCOA4). Ferritin, in combination with NCOA4, is transported to the lysosomes for degradation, being then the iron released for cellular physiological activities. However, when this metal is in excess, it participates in Fenton reaction leading to a cycle between the two redox states and prompting the generation of ●OH, promoting lipid peroxidation and ferroptosis, a new type of regulated cell death. Ferroptosis is also characterized by an inhibition of System Xc-, with the consequent decrease in glutathione peroxidase 4 (GPX4) activity and promotion of lipid

peroxidation, leading to neuronal damage. Mitochondria are essential organelles for eukaryotic life, producing most of the energy or adenosine triphosphate (ATP) required by the cell, being responsible for cellular respiration and oxidative phosphorylation. Changes in the correct functioning or in structures involved in this process lead to a decrease in ATP production, to the accumulation of reactive oxygen species (ROS), and to the release of apoptosis-inducing factors, leading to oxidative stress and cell death. Neuroinflammation is another pathological mechanism present in neurodegenerative diseases, and results from the presence of chronically activated glial cells (astrocytes and microglia) in the brain, which release cytokines and chemokines that are toxic to neurons. Finally, protein misfolding and aggregation of specific proteins into toxic products is a common feature of neurodegenerative diseases. Depending on the type of protein involved and the pathology in question, its aggregation promotes different consequences. For example, in Alzheimer's disease, amyloid beta peptide (Aβ), originating from the fragmentation of amyloid precursor protein (APP), accumulates in the brain in the form of senile plaques. In Parkinson's disease, α-synuclein (α-syn) is often found accumulated and aggregated and has several harmful effects. GR: Glutathione reductase; GSH: Reduced glutathione; GSSG: Glutathione disulfide.

Mitochondria are essential organelles for eukaryotic life, producing most of the energy or adenosine triphosphate (ATP) required by the cell, being responsible for cellular respiration and oxidative phosphorylation, and also being involved in maintaining calcium levels at physiological concentrations in the cytosol and intervening in the apoptotic cell death mechanism. The process of oxidative phosphorylation occurs via electron transport chain, consisting of four complexes that transfer electrons from NADH (nicotinamide adenine dinucleotide) and FADH2 (flavin adenine dinucleotide) to molecular oxygen. The energy released by the oxidation of these substrates is used to generate a proton gradient in the mitochondrial membrane that will be used in complex V for the synthesis of ATP. Changes in the correct functioning or structures of this process originates a decrease in ATP production, to the accumulation of ROS, and to the release of apoptosis-inducing factors, leading to cell death [38]. This organelle is the main generator of ROS, but also its main target. The process of oxidative phosphorylation involves the interaction between unpaired electrons with molecular oxygen (O_2), leading to the generation of superoxide anion ($O2^{\bullet-}$). This radical is further converted in H_2O_2 by SOD. In the presence of Ferrous iron (Fe^{2+}), H_2O_2 can be converted into the highly reactive hydroxyl radical though the Fenton reaction, leading to oxidative damage [39–41].

Mitochondria undergo constant morphological changes by the process of continuous cycles of fusion and fission. The balance between these two processes determines the function of this organelle, controls its bioenergetic function and mitochondrial turnover, and protects mitochondrial DNA [42,43]. Besides, as mentioned, mitochondria play a pivotal role in maintaining the normal Ca^{2+} homeostasis. This cation is transported across the inner mitochondrial membrane via the electrogenic mitochondrial calcium transporter [44]. Changes in the mitochondrial influx/efflux of Ca^{2+} leads to a deregulation of mitochondrial Ca^{2+} homeostasis and, consequently, in mitochondrial Ca^{2+} overload. This Ca^{2+} overload induces oxidative stress and the opening of permeability transition pore, which can be an initial trigger for apoptotic and necrotic cell death. Besides that, it can also stimulate the activity of nitric oxide synthetase to generate NO•, which results in inhibition of via electron transport chain and leads to subsequent ROS production [45].

The connection of Parkinson's disease, mitochondrial dysfunction, and oxidative stress has been proven in many studies. For example, in 2016 a study concluded that Parkinson's disease is associated with increased levels of oxidative biomarkers, such as lipid peroxides and malondialdehyde and SOD activity, and inversely correlated with the levels of antioxidant defenses, such as the total radical trapping antioxidant parameter, SH-groups, and catalase activity, promoting oxidative stress and cell damage [46]. In the case of amyotrophic lateral sclerosis, a relationship was found between disease progression and glutathione peroxidase 4 (GPX4) levels, an enzyme belonging to the antioxidant system, which is responsible for preventing the formation of lipid peroxides. A group observed that in a mouse model of ferroptosis with GPX4 neuronal inducible knockout, the ablation of GPX4 in neurons resulted in a rapid paralysis and severe muscle atrophy, which are features of amyotrophic lateral sclerosis [47].

For Alzheimer's disease, Zweig and colleagues analyzed the protective effects of *Centella asiatica* (a natural compound with antioxidant properties) in five FAD mice. The group concluded that *Centella asiatica* improved spatial and contextual memory, with concomitant increased antioxidant gene expression and a decrease in the Aβ plaque burden relative to control animals, demonstrating the importance of antioxidant compounds in the treatment of Alzheimer's disease [48]. In addition, autopsy studies of multiple sclerosis patients revealed that active lesions of the white matter and cerebral cortex, demyelination, and neurodegeneration were associated with the presence of oxidized lipids in myelin membranes and apoptotic oligodendrocytes [49]. Overall, oxidative stress and mitochondrial dysfunction have been extensively reported as major contributors to the neuronal loss observed in several neurodegenerative diseases [50–59].

2.1.2. Neuroinflammation

Neuroinflammation is the complex innate immune response of neural tissue to foreign bodies of the body. This process plays a role in neural tissue fix and resolution. However, in neurological diseases, neuroinflammation becomes persistent and detrimental to neuronal cells [60].

The inflammatory process in the central nervous system (CNS) results primarily from the presence of chronically activated glial cells (astrocytes and microglia) in the brain. Glial cells are the most abundant and widely distributed cells in the CNS, which interact with neurons and immune cells, as well as with blood vessels. Microglia are immune cells of the brain, being the neural tissue's defense system. Their main functions in the CNS include removal of accumulated or deteriorated neuronal and tissue elements, interacting with neurons, regulating synaptic processes, and maintaining brain homeostasis. Upon stimulation or alterations at the brain level, microglia are morphologically altered, and inflammatory molecules, cytokines, and chemokines are released, which leads to neuroinflammation [61].

Astrocytes play a direct and important role in mediating neuronal survival and function in neurodegenerative diseases. The function of astrocytes (neuroprotective or neurodegenerative functions) depends on the microenvironment that astrocytes and neurons share. Astrocytes release neurotrophic factors such as nerve growth factor (NGF), glial cell line-derived neurotrophic factor (GDNF), mesencephalic astrocyte-derived neurotrophic factor (MANF), neurotrophin-3, and basic fibroblast growth factor (bFGF), and metabolic substrates, such as lactate and glutathione, to counteract neuronal death. Additionally, they provide protection by siphoning off the excess of excitotoxic agents, such as glutamate, potassium, and calcium [62,63]. Nonetheless, when astrocytes undergo a state of gliosis in response to neuronal injury, they release cytokines and chemokines that are toxic to neurons, further contributing, together with microglia, to neuronal damage [63].

Neuroinflammation is present in many neurodegenerative diseases. In Alzheimer's disease, increased levels of tumor necrosis factor (TNF)-α and lower levels TNF-β were detected in the cerebrospinal fluid (CSF) of mild cognitive impairment patients when compared with the controls [64]. Regarding Parkinson's disease, *postmortem* analyses indicated that the levels of cytokines are significantly elevated in the *substantia nigra* of patients [65,66]. In amyotrophic lateral sclerosis patients, an increase in active microglia and astrocytes was observed [67,68]. Lastly, in the cuprizone-induce demyelination experimental autoimmune encephalomyelitis (EAE) model, activated microglia were found in lesions of the CNS and were associated with CNS inflammation in multiple sclerosis [69]. Overall, several studies reported the presence and contribution of neuroinflammation to the progression of distinct neurodegenerative diseases [70–78].

2.1.3. Protein Misfolding

Protein misfolding and aggregation of specific proteins into toxic products is a common feature of neurodegenerative diseases. Under physiological conditions, cells are normally exposed to misfolded proteins (due to alterations in biogenesis, diseases-causing mutations, or endogenous inducers), but have the capability to counteract this effect by degrading or refolding misfolded proteins though the activity of chaperone proteins. However, under pathological stress, the protein misfolding promotes synaptic dysfunction and neuronal cell death. The mechanisms by which they exert their toxicity are not clearly defined, but it appears to act primarily by toxic gain-of-function and dominant-negative effects.

Depending on the type of protein involved and the pathology in question, its aggregation promotes different consequences. For example, in Alzheimer's disease, Aβ peptide originating from the fragmentation of amyloid precursor proteins (APP) accumulates in the brain in the form of senile plaques [79]. As a consequence, the Aβ overproduction induces its aggregation into oligomers, forming amyloid plaques that are visible in pathologic samples [80]. These plaques are toxic and can induce inflammation, hyperphosphorylation of the tau protein, excitotoxicity, and oxidative stress, and in the presence of iron, can also promote ROS generation [80].

In Parkinson's disease, α-synuclein is often found accumulated and aggregated and has several harmful effects. The phosphorylation and fibrilization of α-synuclein leads to Lewy bodies formation, which is mainly responsible for the death of dopaminergic neurons [81]. Additionally, α-synuclein can induce the loss of presynaptic proteins, the decrease of neurotransmitter release, the enlargement of synaptic vesicles, the inhibition of synaptic vesicle recycling, and also perturbations in calcium homeostasis [82]. Besides, it inhibits mitochondrial complex I, inducing the selective oxidation of ATP synthase and causing mitochondrial lipid peroxidation, leading to generation of ROS and cell death [83].

Several misfolded proteins are also associated with amyotrophic lateral sclerosis, such as SOD1, TDP-43, ubiquilin-2, and p62, which are produced through the unconventional repeat associated non-ATG translation of the repeat expansion in C9ORF72, which can promote the inhibition of essential cellular functions, leading to neuronal loss [84]. Mutations in SOD1 gene account for 20% of amyotrophic lateral sclerosis cases, and promote activation of caspases, cytoskeletal abnormalities, and mitochondrial dysfunction [85]. Although involving distinct proteins, protein misfolding was extensively reported as a pathophysiological mechanism present in distinct neurodegenerative diseases [86–91].

2.1.4. Iron Overload and Ferroptosis

Iron is a metal widely distributed in biological systems and its high availability and chemical properties (capability to form complexes with organic ligands and favorable redox potential to switch between its ferrous and ferric states) makes it a key component in energy-generating processes. This metal plays a remarkably important role in cellular processes (such as neurotransmission, DNA synthesis, oxygen transport), apart from catalyzing many chemical reactions. Regulating iron levels by controlling its absorption, use, storage, and excretion is extremely important, as low or high levels of this metal can have harmful effects on the human body [92,93].

Iron has essential functions in the brain and, therefore, needs to cross the BBB to reach this organ. The most elucidating hypothesis of the passage of iron through the luminal membrane of the capillary endothelium is through the transferrin/transferrin receptor (Tf/TfR) pathway. This process starts with the binding of iron-Tf to the extracellular portion of TfR, followed by the endocytosis of the complex of iron-Tf-TfR, formation of endosome, and acidification of the microenvironment within endosome. Next occurs the dissociation of iron from Tf and the reduction of ferric iron (Fe^{3+}) to Fe^{2+} by the ferrireductase six-transmembrane epithelial antigen of prostate 3 (STEAP3). Lastly, the translocation of Fe^{2+} across the endosomal membrane occurs, in a process mediated by the divalent metal transporter 1 (DMT1), forming the labile iron pool (LIP) that is located in cytoplasm. The excess intracellular iron is then stored in the form of ferritin and, when this metal is needed, it can be exported across the membrane via ferroportin (FPN) [94,95].

The regulation of iron levels is systemically controlled by hepcidin (which regulates its intestinal absorption), and cellularly by iron regulatory proteins (IRPs). These proteins bind to iron responsive elements (IREs) implicated in iron metabolism. When there is a decrease in iron levels, IRPs bind to the IRE located in the $5'$ untranslated regions of the mRNA of iron-responsive proteins (such as FPN and ferritin), inhibiting the translation of these proteins, leading to a reduction in iron export and free iron storage. In contrast, IRPs bind to IRE in the $3'$ untranslated regions of TfR1 and DMT1 mRNA, promoting the translation of TfR1 and DMT1, and consequently increasing the iron uptake [96]. A dysregulation of iron metabolism can lead to an imbalance in the normal iron redox status and levels of Fe^{2+}, which can participate in the Fenton reaction, leading to a cycle between the two redox states and prompting the generation of •OH [92].

Several studies have demonstrated the involvement of iron (in excess) in the progression of neurodegenerative diseases. For example, Bao et al. observed a decrease in FPN expression in both brains of mouse model and Alzheimer's disease patients, with concomitant iron deposition [97]. In Parkinson's disease, Sofic et al. found that the levels of total iron and ferric iron were increased (176% and 225%, respectively) in the *substantia nigra pars compacta* of Parkinson's disease patients, relative to age-matched controls [98]. Jeong et al. evaluated the accumulation of iron in SOD1G37R transgenic mice (representative of amyotrophic lateral sclerosis), and observed iron accumulation in the spinal cord of mice at 12 months of age. In addition, through a colorimetric ferrozine assay for the determination of the total iron amount, a 56% increase in iron levels was observed in SOD1G37R mice when compared to age-matched wild-type control animals [99]. Finally, using a cuprizone mouse model of multiple sclerosis, reduced immunofluorescence labelling for ferritin and reduced mRNA expression of ferritin heavy chain was reported in the animal's *corpus callosumn* [100].

Recently, a new type of programmed cell death has been identified called ferroptosis. According to the Nomenclature Committee on Cell Death (NCCD), ferroptosis is "a form of regulated cell death initiated by oxidative perturbations of the intracellular microenvironment that is under constitutive control by GPX4 and which can be inhibited by iron chelators and lipophilic antioxidants" [101]. Iron and lipid peroxides are the main participants, but in a ferroptotic process, the depletion of glutathione, decrease in GPX4 activity, NADPH oxidation, and inhibition of System Xc- (an amino acid antiporter that exchanges extracellular L-cystine and intracellular L-glutamate across the plasma membrane, impacting the synthesis of glutathione) also occurs. Through System Xc- inhibition, the entry of cystine into cells is interrupted, decreasing its conversion to cysteine, which participates in the synthesis of glutathione, therefore, reducing the synthesis of this important antioxidant [102]. This type of cell death has been increasingly associated with neurodegeneration. A study performed by Ashraf et al. analyzed the occurrence of iron dyshomeostasis, augmented lipid peroxidation, and impaired System Xc- in Alzheimer's disease patients. It was observed that the expression of iron-storage proteins was increased in Alzheimer's disease patients when compared with the medial temporal cortex of cognitively normal samples, and the levels of 4-hydroxy-2-nonenal [4-HNE, a lipid peroxidation product) were also significantly increased. Nonetheless, the expression of DMT1 and FPN were decreased in Alzheimer's disease patients, and an impairment of System Xc- was also observed [103]. In another study performed in zebrafish and in SH-SY5Y cells, 6-hydroxydopamine (6-OHDA, neurotoxin used to mimic PD) significantly reduced the levels of glutathione and increased the levels of iron and malondialdehyde (MDA, a lipid peroxidation marker), which indicates that this compound can induce ferroptosis in both models of Parkinson's disease [104].

In order to understand the involvement of ferroptosis in amyotrophic lateral sclerosis, namely lipid peroxidation, a group measured 4-HNE levels in amyotrophic lateral sclerosis patients and observed an increased level of this lipid peroxidation product in the serum and cerebrospinal fluid of sporadic amyotrophic lateral sclerosis patients when compared with controls. In addition, the group observed that the levels of 4-HNE were elevated in advanced stages of the disease when compared with earlier or moderate disease stages, which means that the 4-HNE levels were positively correlated with the disease stage [105]. In the case of multiple sclerosis, dimethyl fumarate (an approved therapeutic for this disease) was reported to modulate ferroptosis [46]. For example, the administration of dimethyl fumarate (100 mg/kg/day, for 28 days) promoted a reduction in iron and MDA levels in the hippocampus of a rat model of chronic cerebral hypoperfusion, as well as increased glutathione and SOD levels. Besides, the decreased expression of System Xc-, GPX4, and FTH1 transporter observed in the hippocampus of the chronic cerebral hypoperfusion rat model was recovered following dimethyl fumarate treatment [46].

Alterations in iron homeostasis promote the pathophysiological effects observed in several neurodegenerative diseases [106–108]. Furthermore, the occurrence of ferroptosis as a type of recent cell death has been receiving increased attention given its apparent occurrence in neurodegenerative diseases and the positive effect of inhibitors of this process in the disease progression [109–116]. Targeting ferroptosis can thus be proposed as a potential new therapeutic target to stop/delay neurodegenerative disease progression.

3. Marine Derived Biomolecules with Antioxidant Properties

The origin of the inflammatory events that trigger several diseases, such as cancer, cardiovascular diseases, diabetes, and neurodegenerative diseases, is related to oxidative stress resulting from the high production of ROS and RNS, which are not counterbalanced by the body's antioxidant defenses [117–119]. Thus, the understanding of oxidative stress mechanisms, as well as the discovery of new compounds with antioxidant properties, have been the focus of various investigations that have already demonstrated the existence of a strong relationship between the use of antioxidant compounds and the reduction of the risk of developing these diseases [117,120].

In recent years, the biotechnological industry has been searching for antioxidant compounds from natural sources to replace artificial antioxidants, such as butylated hydroxyanisole (BHA) and butylated hydroxytoluene (BHT), whose safety profiles are increasingly controversial as they have been associated with liver damage and carcinogenesis. In this context, natural antioxidant molecules extracted from marine bio-waste, in particular carotenoids, bioactive peptides, and polysaccharides, constitute promising alternatives to the synthetic antioxidants [5,117,118]. Table 1 presents examples of antioxidant biomolecules from marine organisms, and their properties and potential therapeutic applications.

Table 1. Examples of antioxidant biomolecules from marine organisms.

Biomolecule	Natural Source	Therapeutic Properties and Potential	References
Astaxanthin	Shrimp/crab shells *Haematococcus pluvialis*	Antioxidant and anti-inflammatory properties. Prevention and treatment of cardiovascular and neurodegenerative diseases.	[117,121–125]
Fucoxanthin	Brown algae *Laminaria japonica*	Antioxidant and anti-inflammatory properties. Prevention and treatment of neurodegenerative diseases.	[7,121,126]
β-carotene	Turban shell Microalga *Dunaliella salina*	Antioxidant properties. Prevention of liver fibrosis, acute and chronic coronary syndrome, and neurodegenerative diseases. Protection against UV radiation.	[117,127–130]
Collagen	Cod skin	Antioxidant properties. Anti-aging.	[2,131,132]
Gelatin	Tuna (*Thunnus* spp.) Flying squid (*Ommastrephes batramii*)	Antioxidant and anti-proliferative properties. Prevention of cancer.	[131]
Chitin	Crustaceans Cuttlefish Squid pen	Antioxidant, anticancer, antimicrobial, and anticoagulant properties. Immune system boosting. Wound healing.	[133–136]

3.1. Carotenoids

Carotenoids share a C40 isoprene structure, called a terpenoid, and are divided into carotenes, which consist only of hydrocarbons, and xanthophylls, which are oxygenated products of carotenes [4,7,117]. These lipophilic compounds of different colors (e.g., yellow, orange, and red) have been widely used in the pharmaceutical and biotech industries, mainly due to their antioxidant properties [7,121]. For instance, astaxanthin is a red xanthophyll predominantly isolated from the microalga *Haematococcus pluvialis*, which accumulates very high levels of this compound under stress conditions, such as high salinity, high temperature, and nitrogen deficiency. However, astaxanthin can also be extracted from marine bio-waste, including shrimps and crab shells, where it is responsible for their orange pigmentation [137,138]. Chemically, astaxanthin is a high lipophilic molecule with the IUPAC name 3,3'-dihydroxy-β-β-carotene-4,4'-dione, whose structure contains two rings with a hydroxyl group and a carbonyl group separated by an unsaturated chain of carbon–carbon double bonds. This specific configuration, namely polyene chain, confers to astaxanthin a powerful antioxidant activity in scavenging free radicals, being 40 and 100 times more effective as antioxidant than β-carotene and vitamin E, respectively [137,139–142]. For this reason, the use of astaxanthin has been highlighted in several investigations due to its valuable impact on human health, namely in the prevention of cancer and in reducing the risk of developing cardiovascular and neurodegenerative diseases [117,141,143].

β-carotene is the main carotenoid produced by the halotolerant microalgae *Dunaliella salina*, although it can also be found in turban shells [117,130]. This compound is recognized for its antioxidant activity, in particular, its great ability to eliminate ROS due to its structure with conjugated double bonds that allow accepting electrons of reactive species, transforming them into neutral species [117,144]. Several investigations have shown that, in addition to its antioxidant properties and potential in the prevention of neurodegenerative diseases, β-carotene has other benefits for human health, such as the prevention of liver fibrosis, acute and chronic coronary syndrome, and the protection of the skin against UV radiation [117,127,144].

3.2. Bioactive Peptides

Bioactive peptides are small proteins with various physiological functions, in particular antioxidant activity. Generally, these peptides contain 2 to 20 amino acid residues and have the ability to scavenge ROS, chelate metal ions, and inhibit lipid peroxidation [2,5,131].

In recent years, there has been much research focused on the use of bioactive peptides, obtained from the enzymatic hydrolysis of marine bio-waste, in the promotion of human health as well as the prevention of chronic diseases. In particular, collagen, a protein found in the structure of fish skin, bones, and scales, and its partially hydrolyzed form, gelatin, are rich in hydrophobic amino acids, which appear to have a high free radical scavenging capacity. Peptides derived from the gelatin of the skin of marine animals, such as flying squid (*Ommastrephes batramii*) and tuna (*Thunnus* spp.), have demonstrated high antioxidant activity, similar to that of the potent natural antioxidant α-tocopherol [2,131]. Collagen has gained great interest in the cosmetic industry, in anti-ageing creams, and in nutritional supplements for bone and cartilage regeneration, vascular and cardiac reconstruction, and skin substitutes [132].

3.3. Polysaccharides

Several studies have reported that polysaccharides derived from marine organism's exhibit antioxidant activity, suggesting that these compounds could be used to mitigate diseases mediated by oxidative stress, such as liver damage, diabetes, obesity, colitis, some types of cancer, and neurodegenerative diseases [118].

Among the different polysaccharides that can be extracted from marine organisms, chitin is the most exploited as it can be easily obtained from the exoskeletons of marine arthropods, such as crustaceans, cuttlefish, and squid. Through chemical or enzymatic processes of chitin, it is possible to obtain its derivative chitosan, which is of interest to the pharmaceutical industry due to its anticancer, antimicrobial, anticoagulant, immunological, and antioxidant properties that enable it to act in the prevention of various diseases, including neurodegenerative ones [133,145].

4. Intranasal Lipid Nanoparticles Containing Marine Bioactive Compounds for the Management of Neurodegenerative Diseases

Marine organisms are considered a large reservoir of bioactive compounds with high therapeutic value, and several studies have demonstrated the efficacy of marine biomolecules with antioxidant properties in the prevention and treatment of different diseases. Some of these biomolecules have been described as having neuroprotective effects, and their use has been suggested for the prevention and treatment of neurodegenerative diseases [121,146,147]. Among these compounds, carotenoids, such as astaxanthin, fucoxanthin, and β-carotene, have gained particular interest due to their high antioxidant activity, which can prevent/delay the onset of oxidative stress-related diseases, such as neurodegenerative diseases [122,148].

Astaxanthin has a protective effect on neuronal cells, being able to prevent and modulate the severity of neuronal death following oxidative stress-induced injury related to a high level of ROS [121–123,149]. Furthermore, results from recent studies support the beneficial effect of astaxanthin on the activation of antioxidant mechanisms, increasing the levels or stimulating the activity of endogenous enzymes, such as SOD and CAT [122,124,150]. Recently, astaxanthin is receiving attention for its effect on the prevention or co-treatment of Alzheimer's and Parkinson's diseases. The administration of astaxanthin as an adjunctive therapy for Alzheimer's dieses has demonstrated that the compound is able to attenuate microglial activation and simultaneously decrease the release of pro-inflammatory cytokines and reduce ROS levels. Similarly, the administration of astaxanthin as an adjuvant therapy for Parkinson's disease suggested that the biological activity of this compound could neutralize the pathophysiological characteristics of the disease, revealing a promising therapeutic potential in preventing or delaying the onset of symptoms in patients with Parkinson's disease [121,122,151].

Fucoxanthin and β-carotene have also been shown to have a protective effect on cells against oxidative stress due to their antioxidant activity that attenuates pro-inflammatory secretion by microglial cells and activates endogenous antioxidant enzyme mechanisms capable of inhibiting free radical-induced DNA oxidation [7,121,127–129].

Human studies on the beneficial effects of carotenoids in the treatment and prevention of neurodegenerative diseases showed that the use of an antioxidant supplement containing astaxanthin and β-carotene reduced ROS production and Aβ accumulation in Alzheimer's disease patients, showing the potential of these compounds in the prevention and treatment of the disease [129,152–154].

In addition to carotenoids, chitosan extracted from marine bio-waste, whose hydrolysis results in the formation of chito-oligosaccharides (COS), has shown good neuroprotective properties, with anti-neuroinflammatory and anti-apoptosis effects, suggesting the potential of COS as protective agents against neurodegeneration [134–136,155].

4.1. Intranasal Administration

Despite the progress that has been made in investigations of the pathogenic mechanisms underlying neurodegenerative diseases, the development of effective molecules and/or delivery systems that stop or slow their progression remains limited. One of the main drawbacks associated with current treatments is the occurrence of adverse effects since high doses usually have to be administered for the molecules to reach the brain in therapeutically effective concentrations [156–158].

According to the Food and Drug Administration (FDA), more than 90% of new drugs used to treat CNS diseases have not been approved due to the difficulty of molecules to cross the BBB and reach the brain, especially hydrophilic, ionized, or high molecular weight ones [14,157,159–162].

For this reason, several studies have investigated alternative and effective strategies to improve drug transport to the CNS by avoiding passage through the BBB, such as using the intranasal route that allows direct passage from the nasal cavity to the brain [14,156,163,164]. In addition to this important benefit, this route has demonstrated other advantages, including easy and non-invasive administration, avoidance of gastrointestinal and hepatic metabolism, high drug bioavailability, large surface area available for drug absorption, and rapid onset of action. However, several factors may limit the use of this route, such as short residence time in the nasal cavity, the small volume available for administration, and enzymatic degradation [14,156,165–167]. The main advantages and limitations of the intranasal route are summarized in Table 2.

Table 2. Main advantages and limitations of the intranasal route.

Advantages	Limitations
• Non-invasive and easy self-administration; • Possibility of transporting drugs directly to the CNS, avoiding the need to cross the BBB; • Prevention of hepatic first-pass metabolism of drugs; • Avoidance of degradation of drugs in the gastrointestinal tract; • Fast drug absorption; • High bioavailability of the drugs, providing the administration of low doses.	• Small volume administration (<200 μL); • Rapid elimination of drugs due to the mucociliary clearance mechanism; • Enzymatic degradation of drugs by P-glycoprotein, carboxypeptidases or endopeptidases; • Low permeability for drugs with high molecular weight (>1 kDa); • Interindividual variability.

BBB: blood–brain barrier; CNS: central nervous system.

4.1.1. Nose-to-Brain Transport

The mechanism of direct transport of compounds from the nose to the brain has been extensively studied, although there is no consensus about the exact path taken by the molecules upon intranasal administration (Figure 2). Several investigations have reported that, after entering the nasal cavity (in the vestibule region), the molecules undergo the mucociliary clearance mechanism. Subsequently, the molecules that are not eliminated in this process move to the posterior part of the cavity, where they contact the respiratory and olfactory regions. From here, they can be transported directly to the brain. Alternatively, molecules can be absorbed through the nasal mucosa into the bloodstream, having to cross the BBB to reach the brain [13–16,168].

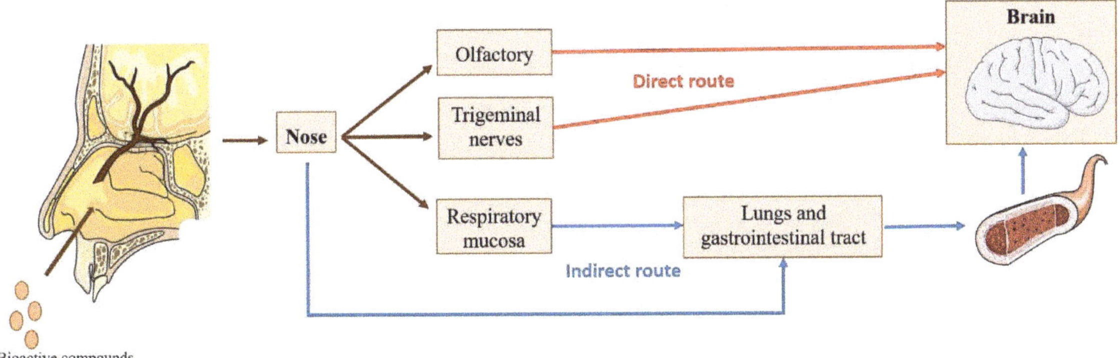

Figure 2. Possible transport routes of bioactive compounds or drugs to the brain after intranasal administration. Direct route: passage through the olfactory or trigeminal nerves, avoiding crossing the blood–brain barrier (BBB). Indirect route: absorption through the respiratory mucosa into the systemic circulation and across the BBB (adapted from Nguyen et al. [15,169]).

The contribution of the indirect route to the transport of bioactive compounds or drugs to the brain is poor, since most molecules show difficulty in bypassing the BBB, especially hydrophilic and high molecular weight ones [16,157]. Thus, the direct route constitutes the main transport pathway to the brain. In particular, transport through the olfactory region, where the molecules pass through the olfactory nerves, has been described as the most relevant. The passage of the compounds through this pathway can be divided into two types of transport [13–16,170,171]: (i) intraneuronal, where olfactory neurons internalize the molecules by endocytosis or pinocytosis, releasing them by exocytosis and distributing them to the different brain regions; (ii) extraneuronal transport, where the molecules can cross the olfactory mucosa through the supporting cells (transcellular transport) or along the supporting cells (paracellular transport).

The passage of compounds through the trigeminal nerves (intracellularly or extracellularly) also constitutes a direct transport route to the brain, since this nerve has three different branches (mandibular, ophthalmic, and maxillary) that connect the nasal cavity to the CNS. However, this route is less significant for the transport of compounds to the brain [13,16,172].

4.1.2. Factors Affecting Intranasal Absorption

Following intranasal administration, to ensure that direct transport of the compounds from the nose to the brain occurs, several factors must be considered, including the physicochemical properties of the molecules, the physiological and anatomical characteristics of the nasal cavity, and the particularities of the formulation [14].

Regarding the physicochemical properties of the molecules, factors such as molecular weight, lipophilic/hydrophilic characteristics, degree of ionization, and ability to solubilize in or penetrate mucus are important to determining the effectiveness of the nose-to-brain transport. In particular, molecules with a molecular weight greater than 1 kDa have difficulty in passing through the tight junctions between nasal cells, as opposed to molecules with a molecular weight of less than 300 Da, which pass easily through the nasal mucosa and are rapidly absorbed. The lipophilic/hydrophilic characteristics of the molecules, in particular those with a molecular weight between 300 Da and 1 kDa, determines the transport pathway these molecules follow, with lipophilic molecules passing through lipid-layered cells (transcellular pathway), and hydrophilic molecules passing cells through tight junctions (paracellular pathway) [13,16,171,173,174].

The physiological mechanism of mucociliary clearance of the nasal cavity is also one of the factors responsible for the inefficient transport of compounds to the brain since it can compromise the absorption of molecules in the nasal cavity [16,158,170]. Herein, the physicochemical properties of the molecules are quite decisive, since lipophilic molecules are less soluble in mucus, demonstrating a greater capacity for absorption in the nasal mucosa [166]. In addition, enzymes in the nasal cavity (carboxypeptidases and endopeptidases) promote the degradation of molecules, in particular peptides and proteins [16,174], while the expression of the efflux protein P-glycoprotein on the surface of ciliated nasal epithelium cells restricts absorption of the compounds [16,175]. Thus, when developing intranasal formulations, absorption promoters, enzyme inhibitors, and mucoadhesive agents can be used to improve the absorption of the compounds and increase their residence time in the nasal mucosa. Another approach that can be used is to encapsulate the compounds in lipid nanoparticles, which improves their absorption and protects them from enzymatic degradation [13,14,176]. Furthermore, intranasal formulations must have adequate viscosity and pH compatible with the nasal mucosa [6.4–6.8], avoiding irritation and discomfort after administration. They should also be isotonic so as not to interfere with normal cilia movement [16,177], composed of biocompatible and odorless excipients, and the administered volume should not exceed 200 µL [14,178].

Of note, intranasal formulations should be included in specific devices that direct them to the olfactory region of the nasal cavity, avoiding the losses that can occur after administration [14,168,179]. Nasal pharmaceutical dosage forms are generally presented in the form of drops and sprays. Drops, although simpler, show limitations in quantifying the amount of compound present in each drop, meaning that an excess can be easily administered. Thus, nasal sprays are preferable to drops because they are safer and easier to administer. However, the droplet diameter of the sprays should be greater than or equal to 10 μm to avoid deposition in the lower respiratory tract (i.e., in the lungs and bronchia) [16,180].

4.2. Using Lipid Nanoparticles for Nose-to-Brain Transport of Marine Bioactive Compounds

Several bioactive compounds and drugs proposed for the treatment of neurodegenerative diseases have limitations resulting from physicochemical instability and/or low bioavailability related to brain targeting difficulties [6,7,181]. To overcome these limitations, the use of lipid nanoparticles, namely SLN and NLC, have shown great efficiency in encapsulating and protecting these molecules, showing promising results in the treatment of these diseases. There have been several reviews published that provide detailed knowledge of the different characteristics and uses of lipid nanoparticle formulations. Interested readers are advised to read these works. Briefly, SLN contains a solid lipid matrix formed by a lipid, while NLC contain a solid lipid matrix formed by a solid and a liquid lipid, which allows to incorporate a larger amount of molecules and provides greater stability during storage when compared to SLN [13,14,17,170,182–188].

Although SLN and NLC share some advantages with other nanosystems, they have been showing better outcomes that are attributed to their particular characteristics. For example, they show superior biocompatibility than polymeric nanoparticles and inorganic nanoparticles; and they are more effective for brain targeting due to their lipidic nature that facilitates passage through the BBB. In addition, it has been reported that polymeric nanoparticles have less ability than SLN and NLC to prolong drug release, as the burst effect has been more frequently observed for the former. When compared to liposomes, the manufacture of SLN and NLC is cheaper as they use less expensive lipids. The latter also show greater long-term stability [12–17,185,189–192].

Several advantages have been described for the intranasal use of lipid nanoparticles, such as [16,158,166]: improved permeation through nasal mucosa; increased adhesion to the olfactory epithelium, avoiding mucocilliary clearance; protection of the encapsulated molecules from enzymatic degradation and P-glycoprotein efflux; ability to target the CNS, which increases the amount of compound reaching the brain, reducing the dose and frequency of administration. However, it is important that lipid nanoparticles have sizes below 200 nm and are composed of GRAS (generally recognized as safe) excipients in non-toxic concentrations so as not to damage the nasal mucosa [16,193]. The lipids and emulsifier(s) used must allow the formation of SLN or NLC with appropriate size, polydispersity index (PDI), and surface charge; high encapsulation ability and sustained release profile of encapsulated compounds, which is essential to the success of treatments [191]. Furthermore, after developing nasal lipid nanoparticles formulations, it is essential to assess their biocompatibility, first, in vitro, and then in vivo, to predict their clinical performance [14,194,195].

Several studies on the intranasal administration of natural bioactive compounds, obtained from different sources and encapsulated or on the surface of SLN and NLC, have demonstrated relevant outcomes in the treatment of neurodegenerative diseases. Specifically, for compounds obtained from marine bio-waste, only three studies were found (astaxanthin-loaded SLN, and SLN and NLC coated with chitosan), which shows the potential of this field. Table 3 summarizes the most relevant outcomes of these studies.

Table 3. Examples of the most relevant results from studies with natural bioactive compounds, encapsulated or on the surface of intranasal lipid nanoparticles (SLN or NLC), for the treatment of neurodegenerative diseases.

Type of Lipid Nanoparticle	Natural Bioactive Compound	Relevant Outcomes	Reference
SLN	Astaxanthin	• In vitro studies demonstrated the antioxidant potential of astaxanthin-loaded SLN against H_2O_2 induced toxicity. • In vivo biodistribution studies demonstrated a higher accumulation of astaxanthin-loaded SLN in the brain after intranasal administration ($1.70 \pm 0.13\%$ injected dose/gram organ), when compared to the intravenous route ($0.844 \pm 0.12\%$ injected dose/gram organ).	[141]
SLN	Dopamine combined with antioxidant grape seed-derived polyphenol compounds (GSE)	• In vitro studies demonstrated that the dopamine/GSE-loaded SLN formulations did not exert toxicity on olfactory ensheathing cells (OECs) and on neuroblastoma cells (SH-SY5Y). • Co-administration of dopamine/GSE-SLN and the oxidative stress-inducing neurotoxin 6-hydroxydopamine (6-OHDA) (100 μM) clearly demonstrated that formulation of dopamine/GSE-SLN determined an increase in cell viability, compared to cells treated with 6-OHDA alone.	[196]
SLN coated with chitosan	Ferulic acid	• In vivo, the ferulic acid intake via the intranasal route was found to be much more beneficial in upregulating the biochemical parameters, in relation to the oral treatment. • Intranasal ferulic acid/chitosan-loaded SLN showed superior concentration of ferulic acid in the rat's brain, when compared to the uncoated ferulic acid-loaded SLN.	[197]
SLN in situ gel	Paeonol	• In vitro studies with paenol-loaded SLN and an in situ gel with paenol-loaded SLN showed a low level of toxicity in RPMI 2650 cells. • In vivo biodistribution studies showed an effective accumulation of the in situ gel in the brain, after intranasal administration.	[198]
SLN	Geraniol combined with ursodeoxycholic acid (GER/UDCA)	• In vivo studies demonstrated a selective uptake of GER/UDCA to the cerebrospinal fluid, after nasal administration of GER/UDCA-loaded SLN.	[199]
SLN and NLC	Curcumin	• In vitro studies with curcumin-loaded SLN and NLC showed no toxicity in mouse fetal fibroblast cells for concentrations up to 10 μg/mL. • In vivo studies showed that curcumin-loaded NLC were able to promote the brain uptake of curcumin more than 4-fold, compared to curcumin-loaded SLN.	[200]
NLC	Nicergoline	• In vivo, bioavailability and brain distribution studies of nicergoline-loaded NLC showed a 4.57-fold increase of the compound in the brain, compared to nicergoline solution. • Results of in vivo studies indicated efficient direct nose-to-brain transport, with brain-targeting efficiency (BTE) and direct transport percentage (DTP) of 187.3% and 56.6%, respectively.	[201]
NLC coated with chitosan	Berberine	• In vivo studies showed that animals treated with intranasal berberine/chitosan-loaded NLC had substantially higher levels of the compound in the brain, compared to animals treated with intranasal berberine solution.	[202]

Although NLC have been preferred over SLN due to their apparent superiority for encapsulating compounds, the number of studies with these two types of nanoparticles is similar (Table 3). For instance, Bhatt et al. encapsulated astaxanthin in SLN for intranasal administration to improve brain targeting of the compound for the treatment of neurodegenerative disorders. The optimized astaxanthin-loaded SLN had a particle size of 213.23 nm and a PDI of 0.367. In vivo biodistribution studies, where the astaxanthin-loaded SLN were administered by the intravenous and intranasal routes, indicated that 1 h after administration, a higher concentration of astaxanthin was achieved in the brain with the intranasal formulation (1.70 ± 0.1312% injected dose/gram organ), compared to the intravenous (0.844 ± 0.12 injected dose/gram organ). These results demonstrated that intranasal administration of astaxanthin-loaded SLN improved the brain uptake of astaxanthin compared to intravenous administration, suggesting that direct nose-to-brain transport occurs. Furthermore, in vitro studies in pheochromocytoma-12 cell line (PC12) demonstrated the antioxidant potential of astaxanthin-loaded SLN against H_2O_2 induced toxicity. In conclusion, the results of these investigations support the use of astaxanthin-loaded SLN for brain targeting, which allows protection against various neurodegenerative diseases [141]. In another study, Sun et al. developed an in situ gel with paeonol-loaded SLN for direct nose-to-brain transport. Paenol is a phenolic compound with therapeutic potential in different neurodegenerative diseases. The nanoparticles developed had a particle size of 166.79 ± 2.92 nm and a PDI of 0.241 ± 0.030. In vitro studies showed that in situ gel with PAE-loaded SLN exerted low toxicity in RPMI 2650 cells. In vivo biodistribution studies showed that the effective accumulation of the in situ gel in the brain area after intranasal administration proved that it could effectively transport the paenol-loaded SLN to the brain, suggesting its potential use in the treatment of neurodegenerative diseases [198].

Regarding Parkinson's disease, Trapani et al. studied the effects of co-administration of dopamine combined with antioxidant grape seed-derived polyphenol compounds (GSE) encapsulated in SLN for intranasal administration as a novel approach in the treatment of this disease. The developed dopamine/GSE-loaded SLN had a particle size of 184 ± 34 nm and a PDI of 0.32 ± 0.07, and showed no toxicity in olfactory ensheathing cells (OECs) and neuroblastoma (SH-SY5Y) cells. Furthermore, in vitro evaluation of the effects on cell viability of incubating dopamine/GSE-loaded SLN and the oxidative stress-inducing neurotoxin 6-hydroxydopamine (6-OHDA) (100 μM) clearly demonstrated that DA/GSE-loaded SLN increased cell viability compared to cells treated with 6-OHDA alone. Therefore, it was concluded that dopamine/GSE-loaded SLN are promising for direct nose-to-brain transport of the tested compounds in the treatment of Parkinson's disease [196]. In another study, Junior et al. combined the anti-inflammatory properties of geraniol (GER), a natural compound known to promote the survival of dopaminergic neurons, with the mitochondrial rescue effects of ursodeoxycholic acid (UDCA) to improve the treatment of Parkinson's patients. The nanoparticles developed GER/UDCA-loaded SLN had a particle size of 121 ± 8.4 nm and a PDI of 0.164 ± 0.03. In vivo studies with intranasally administered of these nanoparticles demonstrated selective uptake of GER/UDCA into the cerebrospinal fluid, suggesting that direct nose-to-brain transport of the compounds occurs. Furthermore, histopathological evaluation demonstrated that, in contrast to pure GER, nasal administration of GER/UDCA-loaded SLN did not damage the structure of the nasal mucosa. In conclusion, these studies indicate that co-encapsulation of GER/UDCA in SLN may constitute an effective non-invasive approach to direct the compounds to the brain in the treatment of Parkinson's disease [199].

Concerning Alzheimer's disease, Saini et al. developed ferulic acid-loaded SLN coated with chitosan to improve the efficacy of this natural compound in the management of Alzheimer's disease. The optimized ferulic acid/chitosan-loaded SLN had a particle size of 184.9 nm. In vivo pharmacodynamic studies showed a marked improvement in cognition after administration of ferulic acid/chitosan-loaded SLN compared to uncoated ferulic acid-loaded SLN and pure ferulic acid solution. In addition, administration of ferulic acid intranasally was found to be more beneficial in upregulating biochemical parameters over the oral route and resulted in higher brain concentrations of the compound compared to uncoated ferulic acid-loaded SLN. Thus, surface coating the SLN with chitosan originated remarkably higher brain levels of ferulic acid, probably owing to a prolonged retention time of the formulation in the nasal cavity, which is due to the SLN positive charge provided by the chitosan coating [197].

Malvajerd et al. encapsulated curcumin in SLN and NLC to increase the concentration of compound in the brain due to its great therapeutic potential to manage CNS diseases. The developed curcumin-loaded SLN and NLC had particle size and PDI of 204.76 ± 0.36 nm and 0.194 ± 0.04 for curcumin-loaded SLN, and 117.36 ± 1.36 nm and 0.188 ± 0.020 for curcumin-loaded NLC, respectively. The in vitro toxicity of the formulations on rat fetal fibroblast cells was evaluated, and high cell viability was observed for concentrations up to 10 µg/mL. Furthermore, in vivo studies showed that curcumin-loaded NLC were able to increase brain uptake of the compound more than 4-fold compared to curcumin-loaded SLN. In view of these results, it was concluded that the use of curcumin-loaded NLC in the treatment of CNS diseases is promising [200]. In another study, Abourehab et al. optimized nicergoline-loaded sesame oil-based NLC for intranasal administration to achieve synergistic and enhanced neuroprotective properties, since nicergoline is described to be used in the treatment of dementia and other cerebrovascular diseases and sesame oil slows and reverses the cognitive symptoms of neurodegenerative diseases. The nicergoline-loaded NLC had a particle size of 111.18 ± 6.33 nm and a PDI of 0.251 ± 0.04. In vivo bioavailability and brain distribution studies showed a 4.57-fold increase of the compound in the brain compared to a nicergoline-free solution, after intranasal administration of the formulation to rats. The results of the in vivo experiments also showed effective brain targeting efficiency (BTE) and direct transport percentage (DTP) of 187.3% and 56.6%, respectively, indicating the efficacy of the nicergoline-loaded NLC for direct nose-to-brain transport [201].

Recently, El-Enin et al. optimized berberine-loaded NLC coated with chitosan for brain targeting via the intranasal route, as recent investigations have shown this natural compound to be effective against Alzheimer's disease, among other neurodegenerative diseases. The developed berberin/chitosan-loaded NLC had a particle size of 180.9 ± 4.3 nm. In vivo brain accumulation experiments showed that animals treated intranasally with berberin/chitosan-loaded NLC had substantially higher levels of the compound in the brain compared to those that were administered intranasally with a berberine solution. According to these results, the researchers concluded that berberin/chitosan-loaded NLC might be a successful approach to potentiate the effect of intranasal berberin in the treatment of CNS diseases, such as Alzheimer's [202].

5. Conclusions

The use of marine bio-waste with antioxidant properties promotes greater sustainability and awareness of the importance of recovery and valorization of waste resulting from the processing of marine organisms and, in particular, the concept of circular economy.

Intranasal administration of lipid nanoparticles, namely SLN and NLC, containing natural bioactive compounds obtained from different sources has potential in the prevention and treatment of neurodegenerative diseases, as these compounds can be transported directly from the nose to the brain, without crossing the BBB. In particular, for bioactive compounds obtained from marine bio-waste, few studies have been reported, showing the open potential of this research area. More in-depth knowledge about the potential neuroprotective effects of bioactive compounds from marine bio-waste is needed to enable their future clinical use.

Clinical studies are needed to evaluate the efficacy of using bioactive compounds loaded in SLN or NLC for intranasal administration. Although preclinical studies in animals have already shown evidence of the occurrence of a direct transport of molecules from the nose to the brain, the exact mechanism of this transport is not fully understood and its efficacy in humans remains undefined. Further knowledge should be gained about the effects of these nanoparticles within the body, including the degradation/elimination of excipients, release of molecules, and interactions with organs and tissues. It is also important to highlight the fact that anatomical and physiological differences between animals and humans can provide incomplete information that may lead to the failure of clinical trials.

Noteworthy, although not excluding the need to perform in vivo studies, investigations conducted in 3D models of the human nasal cavity may provide a deeper understanding of the factors that interfere with intranasal administration, such as, for example, the type and angle of the administration device, and the inclusion of mucoadhesive excipients in the formulations.

Despite the lacks identified, in the near future, the use of SLN and NLC via the nose-to-brain route could play a pivotal role in improving treatments of neurodegenerative diseases.

Author Contributions: Conceptualization, A.C.S. and J.T.; investigation, J.T. and I.C.; writing—original draft preparation, J.T., I.C. and A.C.S.; writing—review and editing, A.C.S., A.F.P., R.S. and J.M.S.L. All authors have read and agreed to the published version of the manuscript.

Funding: This work was supported by the Applied Molecular Biosciences Unit—UCIBIO, which is financed by national funds from Fundação para a Ciência e a Tecnologia—FCT (UIDP/04378/2020 and UIDB/04378/2020).

Institutional Review Board Statement: Not applicable.

Informed Consent Statement: Not applicable.

Data Availability Statement: Not applicable.

Conflicts of Interest: The authors declare no conflict of interest.

References

1. Maschmeyer, T.; Luque, R.; Selva, M. Upgrading of marine (fish and crustaceans) biowaste for high added-value molecules and bio(nano)-materials. *Chem. Soc. Rev.* **2020**, *49*, 4527–4563. [CrossRef]
2. Harnedy, P.A.; FitzGerald, R.J. Bioactive peptides from marine processing waste and shellfish: A review. *J. Funct. Foods* **2012**, *4*, 6–24. [CrossRef]
3. Ben-Othman, S.; Joudu, I.; Bhat, R. Bioactives From Agri-Food Wastes: Present Insights and Future Challenges. *Molecules* **2020**, *25*, 510. [CrossRef] [PubMed]
4. Shavandi, A.; Hou, Y.; Carne, A.; McConnell, M.; Bekhit, A.E.A. Marine Waste Utilization as a Source of Functional and Health Compounds. *Adv. Food Nutr. Res.* **2019**, *87*, 187–254. [PubMed]
5. Jo, C.; Khan, F.F.; Khan, M.I.; Iqbal, J. Marine bioactive peptides: Types, structures, and physiological functions. *Food Rev. Int.* **2016**, *33*, 44–61. [CrossRef]
6. Rehman, A.Q.T.; Jafari, S.M.; Assadpour, E.Q.S.; Aadil, R.M.; Iqbal, M.W.; Rashed, M.M.A.; Sajid, B.; Mushtaq, W.A. Carotenoid-loaded nanocarriers: A comprehensive review. *Adv. Colloid. Interface Sci.* **2020**, *275*, 102048. [CrossRef]
7. Genç, Y.; Bardakci, H.; Yücel, Ç.; Karatoprak, G.Ş.; Küpeli Akkol, E.; Hakan Barak, T.; Sobarzo-Sánchez, E. Oxidative Stress and Marine Carotenoids: Application by Using Nanoformulations. *Mar. Drugs* **2020**, *18*, 423. [CrossRef]
8. Nagappan, H.; Pee, P.P.; Kee, S.H.Y.; Ow, J.T.; Yan, S.W.; Chew, L.Y.; Kong, K.W. Malaysian brown seaweeds Sargassum siliquosum and Sargassum polycystum: Low density lipoprotein (LDL) oxidation, angiotensin converting enzyme (ACE), α-amylase, and α-glucosidase inhibition activities. *Food Res. Int.* **2017**, *99 Pt 2*, 950–958. [CrossRef]
9. *The State of the World Fisheries and Aquaculture, Meeting the Sustainable Development Goals*; Food and Agriculture Organization of the United Nations: Rome, Italy, 2018; ISBN 978-92-5-130562-1.
10. Yan, N.; Chen, X. Sustainability: Don't waste seafood waste. *Nature* **2015**, *524*, 155–157. [CrossRef]
11. Kabir, T.; Uddin, S.; Jeandet, P.; Emran, T.; Mitra, S.; Albadrani, G.; Sayed, A.; Abdel-Daim, M.; Simal-Gandara, J. Anti-Alzheimer's Molecules Derived from Marine Life: Understanding Molecular Mechanisms and Therapeutic Potential. *Mar. Drugs* **2021**, *19*, 251. [CrossRef]
12. Lamptey, R.N.L.; Chaulagain, B.; Trivedi, R.; Gothwal, A.; Layek, B.; Singh, J. A Review of the Common Neurodegenerative Disorders: Current Therapeutic Approaches and the Potential Role of Nanotherapeutics. *Int. J. Mol. Sci.* **2022**, *23*, 1851. [CrossRef] [PubMed]
13. Correia, A.C.; Monteiro, A.R.; Silva, R.; Moreira, J.N.; Sousa Lobo, J.M.; Silva, A.C. Lipid nanoparticles strategies to modify pharmacokinetics of central nervous system targeting drugs: Crossing or circumventing the blood-brain barrier (BBB) to manage neurological disorders. *Adv. Drug Deliv. Rev.* **2022**, *189*, 114485. [CrossRef] [PubMed]

14. Costa, C.P.; Moreira, J.N.; Sousa Lobo, J.M.; Silva, A.C. Intranasal delivery of nanostructured lipid carriers, solid lipid nanoparticles and nanoemulsions: A current overview of in vivo studies. *Acta Pharm. Sin. B* **2021**, *11*, 925–940. [CrossRef] [PubMed]

15. Cunha, S.; Forbes, B.; Sousa Lobo, J.M.; Silva, A.C. Improving Drug Delivery for Alzheimer's Disease through Nose-to-Brain Delivery Using Nanoemulsions, Nanostructured Lipid Carriers (NLC) and in situ Hydrogels. *Int. J. Nanomed.* **2021**, *16*, 4373–4390. [CrossRef] [PubMed]

16. Costa, C.; Moreira, J.N.; Amaral, M.H.; Sousa Lobo, J.M.; Silva, A.C. Nose-to-brain delivery of lipid-based nanosystems for epileptic seizures and anxiety crisis. *J. Control. Release Off. J. Control. Release Soc.* **2019**, *295*, 187–200. [CrossRef] [PubMed]

17. Costa, C.P.; Barreiro, S.; Moreira, J.N.; Silva, R.; Almeida, H.; Sousa Lobo, J.M.; Silva, A.C. In Vitro Studies on Nasal Formulations of Nanostructured Lipid Carriers (NLC) and Solid Lipid Nanoparticles (SLN). *Pharmaceuticals* **2021**, *14*, 711. [CrossRef] [PubMed]

18. Kovacs, G.G. Molecular pathology of neurodegenerative diseases: Principles and practice. *J. Clin. Pathol.* **2019**, *72*, 725–735. [CrossRef]

19. Kovacs, G.G. Concepts and classification of neurodegenerative diseases. *Handb. Clin. Neurol.* **2017**, *145*, 301–307.

20. Erkkinen, M.G.; Kim, M.-O.; Geschwind, M.D. Clinical Neurology and Epidemiology of the Major Neurodegenerative Diseases. *Cold Spring Harb. Perspect. Biol.* **2018**, *10*, a033118. [CrossRef]

21. Hou, Y.; Dan, X.; Babbar, M.; Wei, Y.; Hasselbalch, S.G.; Croteau, D.L.; Bohr, V.A. Ageing as a risk factor for neurodegenerative disease. *Nat. Rev. Neurol.* **2019**, *15*, 565–581. [CrossRef]

22. 2021 Alzheimer's disease facts and figures. *Alzheimers Dement.* **2021**, *17*, 327–406. [CrossRef]

23. Möller, H.J.; Graeber, M.B. The case described by Alois Alzheimer in 1911. Historical and conceptual perspectives based on the clinical record and neurohistological sections. *Eur. Arch. Psychiatry Clin. Neurosci.* **1998**, *248*, 111–122. [PubMed]

24. Lane, D.J.R.; Ayton, S.; Bush, A.I. Iron and Alzheimer's Disease: An Update on Emerging Mechanisms. *J. Alzheimers Dis.* **2018**, *64*, S379–S395. [CrossRef]

25. Lyketsos, C.G.; Carrillo, M.C.; Ryan, J.M.; Khachaturian, A.S.; Trzepacz, P.; Amatniek, J.; Cedarbaum, J.; Brashear, R.; Miller, D.S. Neuropsychiatric symptoms in Alzheimer's disease. *Alzheimer's Dement. J. Alzheimer's Assoc.* **2011**, *7*, 532–539. [CrossRef] [PubMed]

26. Jagadeesan, A.J.; Murugesan, R.; Vimala Devi, S.; Meera, M.; Madhumala, G.; Vishwanathan Padmaja, M.; Ramesh, A.; Banerjee, A.; Sushmitha, S.; Khokhlov, A.; et al. Current trends in etiology, prognosis and therapeutic aspects of Parkinson's disease: A review. *Acta Biomed.* **2017**, *88*, 249–262. [PubMed]

27. Schapira, A.H.; Jenner, P. Etiology and pathogenesis of Parkinson's disease. *Mov. Disord.* **2011**, *26*, 1049–1055. [CrossRef] [PubMed]

28. Beitz, J.M. Parkinson's disease: A review. *Front. Biosci.* **2014**, *6*, 65–74. [CrossRef]

29. Leray, E.; Moreau, T.; Fromont, A.; Edan, G. Epidemiology of multiple sclerosis. *Rev. Neurol.* **2016**, *172*, 3–13. [CrossRef]

30. Yeung, M.S.Y.; Djelloul, M.; Steiner, E.; Bernard, S.; Salehpour, M.; Possnert, G.; Brundin, L.; Frisén, J. Dynamics of oligodendrocyte generation in multiple sclerosis. *Nature* **2019**, *566*, 538–542. [CrossRef]

31. Zwibel, H.L. Contribution of impaired mobility and general symptoms to the burden of multiple sclerosis. *Adv. Ther.* **2009**, *26*, 1043–1057. [CrossRef]

32. Moreau, C.; Danel, V.; Devedjian, J.C.; Grolez, G.; Timmerman, K.; Laloux, C.; Petrault, M.; Gouel, F.; Jonneaux, A.; Dutheil, M.; et al. Could Conservative Iron Chelation Lead to Neuroprotection in Amyotrophic Lateral Sclerosis? *Antioxid. Redox Signal.* **2018**, *29*, 742–748. [CrossRef]

33. Masrori, P.; Van Damme, P. Amyotrophic lateral sclerosis: A clinical review. *Eur. J. Neurol.* **2020**, *27*, 1918–1929. [CrossRef] [PubMed]

34. Talbott, E.O.; Malek, A.M.; Lacomis, D. The epidemiology of amyotrophic lateral sclerosis. *Handb. Clin. Neurol.* **2016**, *138*, 225–238. [PubMed]

35. Saberi, S.; Stauffer, J.E.; Schulte, D.J.; Ravits, J. Neuropathology of Amyotrophic Lateral Sclerosis and Its Variants. *Neurol. Clin.* **2015**, *33*, 855–876. [CrossRef]

36. Schieber, M.; Chandel, N.S. ROS function in redox signaling and oxidative stress. *Curr. Biol.* **2014**, *24*, R453–R462. [CrossRef] [PubMed]

37. Rao, A.V.; Balachandran, B. Role of oxidative stress and antioxidants in neurodegenerative diseases. *Nutr. Neurosci.* **2002**, *5*, 291–309. [CrossRef]

38. Morán, M.; Moreno-Lastres, D.; Marín-Buera, L.; Arenas, J.; Martín, M.A.; Ugalde, C. Mitochondrial respiratory chain dysfunction: Implications in neurodegeneration. *Free Radic. Biol. Med.* **2012**, *53*, 595–609. [CrossRef]

39. Andreyev, A.Y.; Kushnareva, Y.E.; Starkov, A.A. Mitochondrial metabolism of reactive oxygen species. *Biochemistry* **2005**, *70*, 200–214. [CrossRef]

40. Cadenas, E.; Davies, K.J. Mitochondrial free radical generation, oxidative stress, and aging. *Free Radic. Biol. Med.* **2000**, *29*, 222–230. [CrossRef]

41. Gutteridge, J.M. Superoxide-dependent formation of hydroxyl radicals from ferric-complexes and hydrogen peroxide: An evaluation of fourteen iron chelators. *Free Radic. Res. Commun.* **1990**, *9*, 119–125. [CrossRef]

42. Popov, L.-D. Mitochondrial biogenesis: An update. *J. Cell Mol. Med.* **2020**, *24*, 4892–4899. [CrossRef] [PubMed]

43. Breuer, M.; Koopman, W.; Koene, S.; Nooteboom, M.; Rodenburg, R.; Willems, P.H.; Smeitink, J. The role of mitochondrial OXPHOS dysfunction in the development of neurologic diseases. *Neurobiol. Dis.* **2013**, *51*, 27–34. [CrossRef] [PubMed]

44. Gunter, T.E.; Pfeiffer, D.R. Mechanisms by which mitochondria transport calcium. *Am. J. Physiol.* **1990**, *258 Pt 1*, C755–C786. [CrossRef] [PubMed]

45. Bernardi, P.; Di Lisa, F.; Fogolari, F.; Lippe, G. From ATP to PTP and Back: A Dual Function for the Mitochondrial ATP Synthase. *Circ. Res.* **2015**, *116*, 1850–1862. [CrossRef]

46. Yan, N.; Xu, Z.; Qu, C.; Zhang, J. Dimethyl fumarate improves cognitive deficits in chronic cerebral hypoperfusion rats by alleviating inflammation, oxidative stress, and ferroptosis via NRF2/ARE/NF-κB signal pathway. *Int. Immunopharmacol.* **2021**, *98*, 107844. [CrossRef]

47. Chen, L.; Hambright, W.S.; Na, R.; Ran, Q. Ablation of the Ferroptosis Inhibitor Glutathione Peroxidase 4 in Neurons Results in Rapid Motor Neuron Degeneration and Paralysis. *J. Biol. Chem.* **2015**, *290*, 28097–28106. [CrossRef]

48. Zweig, J.A.; Brandes, M.S.; Brumbach, B.H.; Caruso, M.; Wright, K.M.; Quinn, J.F.; Soumyanath, A.; Gray, N.E. Prolonged Treatment with Centella asiatica Improves Memory, Reduces Amyloid-β Pathology, and Activates NRF2-Regulated Antioxidant Response Pathway in 5xFAD Mice. *J. Alzheimers Dis.* **2021**, *81*, 1453–1468. [CrossRef]

49. Haider, L.; Fischer, M.T.; Frischer, J.M.; Bauer, J.; Höftberger, R.; Botond, G.; Esterbauer, H.; Binder, C.J.; Witztum, J.L.; Lassmann, H. Oxidative damage in multiple sclerosis lesions. *Brain* **2011**, *134 Pt 7*, 1914–1924. [CrossRef]

50. Puspita, L.; Chung, S.Y.; Shim, J. Oxidative stress and cellular pathologies in Parkinson's disease. *Mol. Brain* **2017**, *10*, 53. [CrossRef]

51. Pegoretti, V.; Swanson, K.A.; Bethea, J.R.; Probert, L.; Eisel, U.L.M.; Fischer, R. Inflammation and Oxidative Stress in Multiple Sclerosis: Consequences for Therapy Development. *Oxidative Med. Cell. Longev.* **2020**, *2020*, 7191080. [CrossRef]

52. Barber, S.C.; Shaw, P.J. Oxidative stress in ALS: Key role in motor neuron injury and therapeutic target. *Free Radic. Biol. Med.* **2010**, *48*, 629–641. [CrossRef]

53. Ohl, K.; Tenbrock, K.; Kipp, M. Oxidative stress in multiple sclerosis: Central and peripheral mode of action. *Exp. Neurol.* **2016**, *277*, 58–67. [CrossRef] [PubMed]

54. Cunha-Oliveira, T.; Montezinho, L.; Mendes, C.; Firuzi, O.; Saso, L.; Oliveira, P.J.; Silva, F.S.G. Oxidative Stress in Amyotrophic Lateral Sclerosis: Pathophysiology and Opportunities for Pharmacological Intervention. *Oxidative Med. Cell. Longev.* **2020**, *2020*, 5021694. [CrossRef] [PubMed]

55. Cunha-Oliveira, T.; Franco Silva, D.; Segura, L.; Baldeiras, I.; Marques, R.; Rosenstock, T.; Oliveira, P.J.; Silva, F.S. Oxidative stress profiles of lymphoblasts from Amyotrophic Lateral Sclerosis patients with or without known SOD1 mutations. *bioRxiv*. 2022. Available online: http://biorxiv.org/content/early/2022/03/04/2022.03.03.482309.abstract (accessed on 1 January 2023). [CrossRef]

56. Dias, V.; Junn, E.; Mouradian, M.M. The role of oxidative stress in Parkinson's disease. *J. Park. Dis.* **2013**, *3*, 461–491. [CrossRef] [PubMed]

57. Kim, G.H.; Kim, J.E.; Rhie, S.J.; Yoon, S. The Role of Oxidative Stress in Neurodegenerative Diseases. *Exp. Neurobiol.* **2015**, *24*, 325–340. [CrossRef]

58. Huang, W.-J.; Zhang, X.; Chen, W.-W. Role of oxidative stress in Alzheimer's disease. *Biomed Rep.* **2016**, *4*, 519–522. [CrossRef] [PubMed]

59. Cassidy, L.; Fernandez, F.; Johnson, J.B.; Naiker, M.; Owoola, A.G.; Broszczak, D.A. Oxidative stress in alzheimer's disease: A review on emergent natural polyphenolic therapeutics. *Complement. Ther. Med.* **2020**, *49*, 102294. Available online: https://www.sciencedirect.com/science/article/pii/S0965229919315237 (accessed on 1 January 2023). [CrossRef]

60. Yang, Q.-Q.; Zhou, J.-W. Neuroinflammation in the central nervous system: Symphony of glial cells. *Glia* **2019**, *67*, 1017–1035. [CrossRef]

61. Badanjak, K.; Fixemer, S.; Smajić, S.; Skupin, A.; Grünewald, A. The Contribution of Microglia to Neuroinflammation in Parkinson's Disease. *Int. J. Mol. Sci.* **2021**, *22*, 4676. [CrossRef]

62. Phatnani, H.; Maniatis, T. Astrocytes in neurodegenerative disease. *Cold Spring Harb. Perspect. Biol.* **2015**, *7*, a020628. [CrossRef] [PubMed]

63. Acioglu, C.; Li, L.; Elkabes, S. Contribution of astrocytes to neuropathology of neurodegenerative diseases. *Brain Res.* **2021**, *1758*, 147291. Available online: https://www.sciencedirect.com/science/article/pii/S0006899321000160 (accessed on 1 January 2023). [CrossRef]

64. Tarkowski, E.; Andreasen, N.; Tarkowski, A.; Blennow, K. Intrathecal inflammation precedes development of Alzheimer's disease. *J. Neurol. Neurosurg. Psychiatry* **2003**, *74*, 1200–1205. [CrossRef] [PubMed]

65. Brodacki, B.; Staszewski, J.; Toczyłowska, B.; Kozłowska, E.; Drela, N.; Chalimoniuk, M.; Stępien, A. Serum interleukin (IL-2, IL-10, IL-6, IL-4), TNFalpha, and INFgamma concentrations are elevated in patients with atypical and idiopathic parkinsonism. *Neurosci. Lett.* **2008**, *441*, 158–162. [CrossRef]

66. Pieper, H.C.; Evert, B.O.; Kaut, O.; Riederer, P.F.; Waha, A.; Wüllner, U. Different methylation of the TNF-alpha promoter in cortex and substantia nigra: Implications for selective neuronal vulnerability. *Neurobiol. Dis.* **2008**, *32*, 521–527. [CrossRef]

67. Turner, M.R.; Cagnin, A.; Turkheimer, F.E.; Miller, C.C.J.; Shaw, C.E.; Brooks, D.J.; Leigh, P.N.; Banati, R.B. Evidence of widespread cerebral microglial activation in amyotrophic lateral sclerosis: An [11C](R)-PK11195 positron emission tomography study. *Neurobiol. Dis.* **2004**, *15*, 601–609. [CrossRef] [PubMed]

68. Johansson, A.; Engler, H.; Blomquist, G.; Scott, B.; Wall, A.; Aquilonius, S.-M.; Långström, B.; Askmark, H. Evidence for astrocytosis in ALS demonstrated by [11C](L)-deprenyl-D2 PET. *J. Neurol. Sci.* **2007**, *255*, 17–22. [CrossRef] [PubMed]

69. Luo, C.; Jian, C.; Liao, Y.; Huang, Q.; Wu, Y.; Liu, X.; Zou, D.; Wu, Y. The role of microglia in multiple sclerosis. *Neuropsychiatr. Dis. Treat.* **2017**, *13*, 1661–1667. [CrossRef]
70. Leng, F.; Edison, P. Neuroinflammation and microglial activation in Alzheimer disease: Where do we go from here? *Nat. Rev. Neurol.* **2021**, *17*, 157–172. [CrossRef]
71. Cao, M.C.; Cawston, E.E.; Chen, G.; Brooks, C.; Douwes, J.; McLean, D.; Graham, E.S.; Dragunow, M.; Scotter, E.L. Serum biomarkers of neuroinflammation and blood-brain barrier leakage in amyotrophic lateral sclerosis. *BMC Neurol.* **2022**, *22*, 216. [CrossRef]
72. Grotemeyer, A.; McFleder, R.L.; Wu, J.; Wischhusen, J.; Ip, C.W. Neuroinflammation in Parkinson's Disease—Putative Pathomechanisms and Targets for Disease-Modification. *Front. Immunol.* **2022**, *13*, 2301. [CrossRef]
73. Liu, E.; Karpf, L.; Bohl, D. Neuroinflammation in Amyotrophic Lateral Sclerosis and Frontotemporal Dementia and the Interest of Induced Pluripotent Stem Cells to Study Immune Cells Interactions With Neurons. *Front. Mol. Neurosci.* **2021**, *14*, 310. [CrossRef] [PubMed]
74. Bjelobaba, I.; Savic, D.; Lavrnja, I. Multiple Sclerosis and Neuroinflammation: The Overview of Current and Prospective Therapies. *Curr. Pharm. Des.* **2017**, *23*, 693–730. [CrossRef] [PubMed]
75. Liu, J.; Wang, F. Role of Neuroinflammation in Amyotrophic Lateral Sclerosis: Cellular Mechanisms and Therapeutic Implications. *Front. Immunol.* **2017**, *8*, 1005. [CrossRef] [PubMed]
76. Araújo, B.; Caridade-Silva, R.; Soares-Guedes, C.; Martins-Macedo, J.; Gomes, E.D.; Monteiro, S.; Teixeira, F.G. Neuroinflammation and Parkinson's Disease-From Neurodegeneration to Therapeutic Opportunities. *Cells* **2022**, *11*, 2908. [CrossRef]
77. Wang, Q.; Liu, Y.; Zhou, J. Neuroinflammation in Parkinson's disease and its potential as therapeutic target. *Transl. Neurodegener.* **2015**, *4*, 19. [CrossRef] [PubMed]
78. Heneka, M.T.; Carson, M.J.; El Khoury, J.; Landreth, G.E.; Brosseron, F.; Feinstein, D.L.; Jacobs, A.; Wyss-Coray, T.; Vitorica, J.; Ransohoff, R.; et al. Neuroinflammation in Alzheimer's disease. *Lancet Neurol.* **2015**, *14*, 388–405. [CrossRef]
79. Soria Lopez, J.A.; González, H.M.; Léger, G.C. Alzheimer's disease. *Handb. Clin. Neurol.* **2019**, *167*, 231–255.
80. Harris, M.E.; Hensley, K.; Butterfield, D.A.; Leedle, R.A.; Carney, J.M. Direct evidence of oxidative injury produced by the Alzheimer's beta-amyloid peptide (1-40) in cultured hippocampal neurons. *Exp. Neurol.* **1995**, *131*, 193–202. [CrossRef]
81. Khan, A.U.; Akram, M.; Daniyal, M.; Zainab, R. Awareness and current knowledge of Parkinson's disease: A neurodegenerative disorder. *Int. J. Neurosci.* **2019**, *129*, 55–93. [CrossRef]
82. Stefanis, L. α-Synuclein in Parkinson's disease. *Cold Spring Harb. Perspect. Med.* **2012**, *2*, a009399. [CrossRef]
83. Ludtmann, M.H.R.; Angelova, P.R.; Horrocks, M.H.; Choi, M.L.; Rodrigues, M.; Baev, A.Y.; Berezhnov, A.V.; Yao, Z.; Little, D.; Banushi, B.; et al. α-synuclein oligomers interact with ATP synthase and open the permeability transition pore in Parkinson's disease. *Nat. Commun.* **2018**, *9*, 2293. [CrossRef] [PubMed]
84. Parakh, S.; Atkin, J.D. Protein folding alterations in amyotrophic lateral sclerosis. *Brain Res.* **2016**, *1648 Pt B*, 633–649. [CrossRef]
85. Liu, J.; Lillo, C.; Jonsson, P.; Velde, C.V.; Ward, C.M.; Miller, T.M.; Subramaniam, J.R.; Rothstein, J.D.; Marklund, S.; Andersen, P.M.; et al. Toxicity of familial ALS-linked SOD1 mutants from selective recruitment to spinal mitochondria. *Neuron* **2004**, *43*, 5–17. [CrossRef]
86. Paré, B.; Lehmann, M.; Beaudin, M.; Nordström, U.; Saikali, S.; Julien, J.-P.; Gilthorpe, J.D.; Marklund, S.L.; Cashman, N.R.; Andersen, P.M.; et al. Misfolded SOD1 pathology in sporadic Amyotrophic Lateral Sclerosis. *Sci. Rep.* **2018**, *8*, 14223. [CrossRef] [PubMed]
87. Srinivasan, E.; Chandrasekhar, G.; Anbarasu, K.; Vickram, A.S.; Karunakaran, R.; Rajasekaran, R.; Srikumar, P.S. Alpha-Synuclein Aggregation in Parkinson's Disease. *Front. Med.* **2021**, *8*, 736978. Available online: https://www.frontiersin.org/articles/10.3389/fmed.2021.736978 (accessed on 1 January 2023). [CrossRef]
88. Sun, X.; Chen, W.-D.; Wang, Y.-D. β-Amyloid: The Key Peptide in the Pathogenesis of Alzheimer's Disease. *Front. Pharmacol.* **2015**, *6*, 221. Available online: https://www.frontiersin.org/articles/10.3389/fphar.2015.00221 (accessed on 1 January 2023). [CrossRef] [PubMed]
89. Gitler, A.D.; Bevis, B.J.; Shorter, J.; Strathearn, K.E.; Hamamichi, S.; Su, L.J.; Caldwell, K.A.; Caldwell, G.A.; Rochet, J.-C.; McCaffery, J.M.; et al. The Parkinson's disease protein a-synuclein disrupts cellular Rab homeostasis. *Proc. Natl. Acad. Sci. USA* **2008**, *105*, 145–150. Available online: https://www.pnas.org/doi/abs/10.1073/pnas.0710685105 (accessed on 1 January 2023). [CrossRef]
90. Chisholm, C.G.; Yerbury, J.J.; McAlary, L. Protein Aggregation in Amyotrophic Lateral Sclerosis. In *Spectrums of Amyotrophic Lateral Sclerosis*; John Wiley & Sons, Ltd.: Hoboken, NJ, USA, 2021; pp. 105–121. Available online: https://onlinelibrary.wiley.com/doi/abs/10.1002/9781119745532.ch6 (accessed on 1 January 2023).
91. Murphy, M.P.; LeVine, H., 3rd. Alzheimer's disease and the amyloid-beta peptide. *J. Alzheimers Dis.* **2010**, *19*, 311–323. [CrossRef] [PubMed]
92. Uranga, R.M.; Salvador, G.A. Unraveling the Burden of Iron in Neurodegeneration: Intersections with Amyloid Beta Peptide Pathology. *Oxidative Med. Cell. Longev.* **2018**, *2018*, 2850341. [CrossRef] [PubMed]
93. Lieu, P.T.; Heiskala, M.; Peterson, P.A.; Yang, Y. The roles of iron in health and disease. *Mol. Asp. Med.* **2001**, *22*, 1–87. [CrossRef]
94. Ndayisaba, A.; Kaindlstorfer, C.; Wenning, G.K. Iron in Neurodegeneration—Cause or Consequence? *Front. Neurosci.* **2019**, *13*, 180. [CrossRef] [PubMed]

95. Ke, Y.; Qian, Z.M. Brain iron metabolism: Neurobiology and neurochemistry. *Prog. Neurobiol.* **2007**, *83*, 149–173. [CrossRef] [PubMed]

96. Muckenthaler, M.U.; Galy, B.; Hentze, M.W. Systemic iron homeostasis and the iron-responsive element/iron-regulatory protein (IRE/IRP) regulatory network. *Annu. Rev. Nutr.* **2008**, *28*, 197–213. [CrossRef] [PubMed]

97. Bao, W.-D.; Pang, P.; Zhou, X.-T.; Hu, F.; Xiong, W.; Chen, K.; Wang, J.; Wang, F.; Xie, D.; Hu, Y.-Z.; et al. Loss of ferroportin induces memory impairment by promoting ferroptosis in Alzheimer's disease. *Cell Death Differ.* **2021**, *28*, 1548–1562. [CrossRef]

98. Sofic, E.; Riederer, P.; Heinsen, H.; Beckmann, H.; Reynolds, G.P.; Hebenstreit, G.; Youdim, M.B.H. Increased iron (III) and total iron content in post mortem substantia nigra of parkinsonian brain. *J. Neural. Transm.* **1988**, *74*, 199–205. [CrossRef]

99. Jeong, S.Y.; Rathore, K.I.; Schulz, K.; Ponka, P.; Arosio, P.; David, S. Dysregulation of iron homeostasis in the CNS contributes to disease progression in a mouse model of amyotrophic lateral sclerosis. *J. Neurosci.* **2009**, *29*, 610–619. [CrossRef]

100. Jhelum, P.; Santos-Nogueira, E.; Teo, W.; Haumont, A.; Lenoël, I.; Stys, P.K.; David, S. Ferroptosis Mediates Cuprizone-Induced Loss of Oligodendrocytes and Demyelination. *J. Neurosci.* **2020**, *40*, 9327–9341. [CrossRef]

101. Galluzzi, L.; Vitale, I.; Aaronson, S.A.; Abrams, J.M.; Adam, D.; Agostinis, P.; Alnemri, E.S.; Altucci, L.; Amelio, I.; Andrews, D.W.; et al. Molecular mechanisms of cell death: Recommendations of the Nomenclature Committee on Cell Death 2018. *Cell Death Differ.* **2018**, *25*, 486–541. [CrossRef]

102. Han, C.; Liu, Y.; Dai, R.; Ismail, N.; Su, W.; Li, B. Ferroptosis and Its Potential Role in Human Diseases. *Front. Pharmacol.* **2020**, *11*, 239. Available online: https://www.frontiersin.org/article/10.3389/fphar.2020.00239/full (accessed on 1 January 2023). [CrossRef]

103. Ashraf, A.; Jeandriens, J.; Parkes, H.G.; So, P.-W. Iron dyshomeostasis, lipid peroxidation and perturbed expression of cystine/glutamate antiporter in Alzheimer's disease: Evidence of ferroptosis. *Redox Biol.* **2020**, *32*, 101494. [CrossRef]

104. Sun, Y.; He, L.; Wang, T.; Hua, W.; Qin, H.; Wang, J.; Wang, L.; Gu, W.; Li, T.; Li, N.; et al. Activation of p62-Keap1-Nrf2 Pathway Protects 6-Hydroxydopamine-Induced Ferroptosis in Dopaminergic Cells. *Mol. Neurobiol.* **2020**, *57*, 4628–4641. [CrossRef] [PubMed]

105. Simpson, E.P.; Henry, Y.K.; Henkel, J.S.; Smith, R.G.; Appel, S.H. Increased lipid peroxidation in sera of ALS patients: A potential biomarker of disease burden. *Neurology* **2004**, *62*, 1758–1765. [CrossRef] [PubMed]

106. Liu, J.-L.; Fan, Y.-G.; Yang, Z.-S.; Wang, Z.-Y.; Guo, C. Iron and Alzheimer's Disease: From Pathogenesis to Therapeutic Implications. *Front. Neurosci.* **2018**, *12*, 632. [CrossRef] [PubMed]

107. Yu, J.; Wang, N.; Qi, F.; Wang, X.; Zhu, Q.; Lu, Y.; Zhang, H.; Che, F.; Li, W. Serum ferritin is a candidate biomarker of disease aggravation in amyotrophic lateral sclerosis. *Biomed Rep.* **2018**, *9*, 333–338. [CrossRef]

108. Ma, L.; Azad, M.G.; Dharmasivam, M.; Richardson, V.; Quinn, R.J.; Feng, Y.; Pountney, D.L.; Tonissen, K.F.; Mellick, G.D.; Yanatori, I.; et al. Parkinson's disease: Alterations in iron and redox biology as a key to unlock therapeutic strategies. *Redox Biol.* **2021**, *41*, 101896. Available online: https://www.sciencedirect.com/science/article/pii/S2213231721000446 (accessed on 1 January 2023). [CrossRef] [PubMed]

109. Thapa, K.; Khan, H.; Kanojia, N.; Singh, T.G.; Kaur, A.; Kaur, G. Therapeutic Insights on Ferroptosis in Parkinson's disease. *Eur. J. Pharmacol.* **2022**, *930*, 175133. Available online: https://www.sciencedirect.com/science/article/pii/S0014299922003946 (accessed on 1 January 2023). [CrossRef]

110. Jakaria, M.; Belaidi, A.A.; Bush, A.I.; Ayton, S. Ferroptosis as a mechanism of neurodegeneration in Alzheimer's disease. *J. Neurochem.* **2021**, *159*, 804–825. Available online: https://onlinelibrary.wiley.com/doi/abs/10.1111/jnc.15519 (accessed on 1 January 2023). [CrossRef]

111. Majerníková, N.; den Dunnen, W.F.A.; Dolga, A.M. The Potential of Ferroptosis-Targeting Therapies for Alzheimer's Disease: From Mechanism to Transcriptomic Analysis. *Front. Aging Neurosci.* **2021**, *13*, 745046. Available online: https://www.frontiersin.org/articles/10.3389/fnagi.2021.745046 (accessed on 1 January 2023). [CrossRef]

112. White, A.R. Ferroptosis drives immune-mediated neurodegeneration in multiple sclerosis. *Cell Mol. Immunol.* **2023**, *20*, 112–113. [CrossRef]

113. Wang, T.; Tomas, D.; Perera, N.D.; Cuic, B.; Luikinga, S.; Viden, A.; Barton, S.K.; McLean, C.A.; Samson, A.L.; Southon, A.; et al. Ferroptosis mediates selective motor neuron death in amyotrophic lateral sclerosis. *Cell Death Differ.* **2022**, *29*, 1187–1198. [CrossRef]

114. Matsuo, T.; Adachi-Tominari, K.; Sano, O.; Kamei, T.; Nogami, M.; Ogi, K.; Okano, H.; Yano, M. Involvement of ferroptosis in human motor neuron cell death. *Biochem. Biophys. Res. Commun.* **2021**, *566*, 24–29. Available online: https://www.sciencedirect.com/science/article/pii/S0006291X2100886X (accessed on 1 January 2023). [CrossRef] [PubMed]

115. Zhang, G.; Zhang, Y.; Shen, Y.; Wang, Y.; Zhao, M.; Sun, L. The Potential Role of Ferroptosis in Alzheimer's Disease. *J. Alzheimers Dis.* **2021**, *80*, 907–925. [CrossRef] [PubMed]

116. Mahoney-Sánchez, L.; Bouchaoui, H.; Ayton, S.; Devos, D.; Duce, J.A.; Devedjian, J.-C. Ferroptosis and its potential role in the physiopathology of Parkinson's Disease. *Prog. Neurobiol.* **2021**, *196*, 101890. [CrossRef] [PubMed]

117. Hamidi, M.; Kozani, P.S.; Kozani, P.S.; Pierre, G.; Michaud, P.; Delattre, C. Marine Bacteria versus Microalgae: Who Is the Best for Biotechnological Production of Bioactive Compounds with Antioxidant Properties and Other Biological Applications? *Mar. Drugs* **2019**, *18*, 28. [CrossRef] [PubMed]

118. Zhong, Q.; Wei, B.; Wang, S.; Ke, S.; Chen, J.; Zhang, H.; Wang, H. The Antioxidant Activity of Polysaccharides Derived from Marine Organisms: An Overview. *Mar. Drugs* **2019**, *17*, 674. [CrossRef]

119. Singh, A.; Kukreti, R.; Saso, L.; Kukreti, S. Oxidative Stress: A Key Modulator in Neurodegenerative Diseases. *Molecules* **2019**, *24*, 1583. [CrossRef]
120. Romano, G.; Costantini, M.; Sansone, C.; Lauritano, C.; Ruocco, N.; Ianora, A. Marine microorganisms as a promising and sustainable source of bioactive molecules. *Mar. Environ. Res.* **2017**, *128*, 58–69. [CrossRef]
121. Catanesi, M.; Caioni, G.; Castelli, V.; Benedetti, E.; d'Angelo, M.; Cimini, A. Benefits under the Sea: The Role of Marine Compounds in Neurodegenerative Disorders. *Mar. Drugs* **2021**, *19*, 24. [CrossRef]
122. Galasso, C.; Orefice, I.; Pellone, P.; Cirino, P.; Miele, R.; Ianora, A.; Brunet, C.; Sansone, C. On the Neuroprotective Role of Astaxanthin: New Perspectives? *Mar. Drugs* **2018**, *16*, 247. [CrossRef]
123. Sztretye, M.; Dienes, B.; Gönczi, M.; Czirják, T.; Csernoch, L.; Dux, L.; Szentesi, P.; Keller-Pintér, A. Astaxanthin: A Potential Mitochondrial-Targeted Antioxidant Treatment in Diseases and with Aging. *Oxidative Med. Cell. Longev.* **2019**, *2019*, 3849692. [CrossRef]
124. Barros, M.P.; Poppe, S.C.; Bondan, E.F. Neuroprotective properties of the marine carotenoid astaxanthin and omega-3 fatty acids, and perspectives for the natural combination of both in krill oil. *Nutrients* **2014**, *6*, 1293–1317. [CrossRef] [PubMed]
125. Hu, J.; Lu, W.; Lv, M.; Wang, Y.; Ding, R.; Wang, L. Extraction and purification of astaxanthin from shrimp shells and the effects of different treatments on its content. *Rev. Bras. Farmacogn.* **2019**, *29*, 24–29. [CrossRef]
126. Meresse, S.; Fodil, M.; Fleury, F.; Chenais, B. Fucoxanthin, a Marine-Derived Carotenoid from Brown Seaweeds and Microalgae: A Promising Bioactive Compound for Cancer Therapy. *Int. J. Mol. Sci.* **2020**, *21*, 9273. [CrossRef] [PubMed]
127. Mullan, K.; Williams, M.A.; Cardwell, C.R.; McGuinness, B.; Passmore, P.; Silvestri, G.; Woodside, J.V.; McKay, G.J. Serum concentrations of vitamin E and carotenoids are altered in Alzheimer's disease: A case-control study. *Alzheimers Dement.* **2017**, *3*, 432–439. [CrossRef]
128. Hughes, K.C.; Gao, X.; Kim, I.Y.; Rimm, E.B.; Wang, M.; Weisskopf, M.G.; Schwarzschild, M.A.; Ascherio, A. Intake of antioxidant vitamins and risk of Parkinson's disease. *Mov. Disord.* **2016**, *31*, 1909–1914. [CrossRef]
129. Cho, K.S.; Shin, M.; Kim, S.; Lee, S.B. Recent Advances in Studies on the Therapeutic Potential of Dietary Carotenoids in Neurodegenerative Diseases. *Oxidative Med. Cell. Longev.* **2018**, *2018*, 4120458. [CrossRef]
130. Maoka, T. Carotenoids in marine animals. *Mar. Drugs* **2011**, *9*, 278–293. [CrossRef]
131. Suarez-Jimenez, G.M.; Burgos-Hernandez, A.; Ezquerra-Brauer, J.M. Bioactive peptides and depsipeptides with anticancer potential: Sources from marine animals. *Mar. Drugs* **2012**, *10*, 963–986. [CrossRef]
132. Avila Rodríguez, M.I.; Rodríguez Barroso, L.G.; Sánchez, M.L. Collagen: A review on its sources and potential cosmetic applications. *J. Cosmet. Dermatol.* **2018**, *17*, 20–26. [CrossRef]
133. Muthu, M.; Gopal, J.; Chun, S.; Devadoss, A.J.P.; Hasan, N.; Sivanesan, I. Crustacean Waste-Derived Chitosan: Antioxidant Properties and Future Perspective. *Antioxidants* **2021**, *10*, 228. [CrossRef]
134. Zhang, J.; Xia, W.; Liu, P.; Cheng, Q.; Tahi, T.; Gu, W.; Li, B. Chitosan modification and pharmaceutical/biomedical applications. *Mar. Drugs* **2010**, *8*, 1962–1987. [CrossRef] [PubMed]
135. Hao, C.; Wang, W.; Wang, S.; Zhang, L.; Guo, Y. An Overview of the Protective Effects of Chitosan and Acetylated Chitosan Oligosaccharides against Neuronal Disorders. *Mar. Drugs* **2017**, *15*, 89. [CrossRef] [PubMed]
136. Shahidi, F.; Abuzaytoun, R. Chitin, chitosan, and co-products: Chemistry, production, applications, and health effects. *Adv. Food Nutr. Res.* **2005**, *49*, 93–135. [PubMed]
137. Rodriguez-Ruiz, V.; Salatti-Dorado, J.; Barzegari, A.; Nicolas-Boluda, A.; Houaoui, A.; Caballo, C.; Caballero-Casero, N.; Sicilia, D.; Venegas, J.B.; Pauthe, E.; et al. Astaxanthin-Loaded Nanostructured Lipid Carriers for Preservation of Antioxidant Activity. *Molecules* **2018**, *23*, 2601. [CrossRef] [PubMed]
138. Li, M.; Zahi, M.R.; Yuan, Q.; Tian, F.; Liang, H. Preparation and stability of astaxanthin solid lipid nanoparticles based on stearic acid. *Eur. J. Lipid Sci. Technol.* **2015**, *118*, 592–602. [CrossRef]
139. Santonocito, D.; Raciti, G.; Campisi, A.; Sposito, G.; Panico, A.; Siciliano, E.; Sarpietro, M.; Damiani, E.; Puglia, C. Astaxanthin-Loaded Stealth Lipid Nanoparticles (AST-SSLN) as Potential Carriers for the Treatment of Alzheimer's Disease: Formulation Development and Optimization. *Nanomaterials* **2021**, *11*, 391. [CrossRef]
140. Kogure, K. Novel Antioxidative Activity of Astaxanthin and Its Synergistic effect with vitamin E. *J. Nutr. Sci. Vitaminol.* **2019**, *65*, S109–S112. [CrossRef]
141. Chandra Bhatt, P.; Srivastava, P.; Pandey, P.; Khan, W.; Panda, B.P. Nose to brain delivery of astaxanthin-loaded solid lipid nanoparticles: Fabrication, radio labeling, optimization and biological studies. *RSC Adv.* **2016**, *6*, 10001–10010. [CrossRef]
142. Kim, S.H.; Kim, H. Inhibitory Effect of Astaxanthin on Oxidative Stress-Induced Mitochondrial Dysfunction-A Mini-Review. *Nutrients* **2018**, *10*, 1137. [CrossRef]
143. Geng, Q.; Zhao, Y.; Wang, L.; Xu, L.; Chen, X.; Han, J. Development and Evaluation of Astaxanthin as Nanostructure Lipid Carriers in Topical Delivery. *AAPS PharmSciTech* **2020**, *21*, 318. [CrossRef]
144. Milani, A.; Basirnejad, M.; Shahbazi, S.; Bolhassani, A. Carotenoids: Biochemistry, pharmacology and treatment. *Br. J. Pharmacol.* **2017**, *174*, 1290–1324. [CrossRef] [PubMed]
145. Xu, C.; Nasrollahzadeh, M.; Selva, M.; Issaabadi, Z.; Luque, R. Waste-to-wealth: Biowaste valorization into valuable bio(nano)materials. *Chem. Soc. Rev.* **2019**, *48*, 4791–4822. [CrossRef] [PubMed]
146. Fakhri, S.; Aneva, I.Y.; Farzaei, M.H.; Sobarzo-Sanchez, E. The Neuroprotective Effects of Astaxanthin: Therapeutic Targets and Clinical Perspective. *Molecules* **2019**, *24*, 2640. [CrossRef] [PubMed]

147. Ye, Q.; Hai, K.; Liu, W.; Wang, Y.; Zhou, X.; Ye, Z.; Liu, X. Investigation of the protective effect of heparin pre-treatment on cerebral ischaemia in gerbils. *Pharm. Biol.* **2019**, *57*, 519–528. [CrossRef] [PubMed]
148. Berthon, J.Y.; Nachat-Kappes, R.; Bey, M.; Cadoret, J.P.; Renimel, I.; Filaire, E. Marine algae as attractive source to skin care. *Free Radic. Res.* **2017**, *51*, 555–567. [CrossRef]
149. Xue, Y.; Qu, Z.; Fu, J.; Zhen, J.; Wang, W.; Cai, Y.; Wang, W. The protective effect of astaxanthin on learning and memory deficits and oxidative stress in a mouse model of repeated cerebral ischemia/reperfusion. *Brain Res. Bull.* **2017**, *131*, 221–228. [CrossRef]
150. Haider, S.; Saleem, S.; Perveen, T.; Tabassum, S.; Batool, Z.; Sadir, S.; Liaquat, L.; Madiha, S. Age-related learning and memory deficits in rats: Role of altered brain neurotransmitters, acetylcholinesterase activity and changes in antioxidant defense system. *Age* **2014**, *36*, 9653. [CrossRef] [PubMed]
151. Liu, X.; Shibata, T.; Hisaka, S.; Osawa, T. Astaxanthin inhibits reactive oxygen species-mediated cellular toxicity in dopaminergic SH-SY5Y cells via mitochondria-targeted protective mechanism. *Brain Res.* **2009**, *1254*, 18–27. [CrossRef]
152. Kiko, T.; Nakagawa, K.; Satoh, A.; Tsuduki, T.; Furukawa, K.; Arai, H.; Miyazawa, T. Amyloid β levels in human red blood cells. *PLoS ONE* **2012**, *7*, e49620. [CrossRef]
153. de Oliveira, B.F.; Veloso, C.A.; Nogueira-Machado, J.A.; de Moraes, E.N.; dos Santos, R.R.; Cintra, M.T.G.; Chaves, M.M. Ascorbic acid, alpha-tocopherol, and beta-carotene reduce oxidative stress and proinflammatory cytokines in mononuclear cells of Alzheimer's disease patients. *Nutr. Neurosci.* **2012**, *15*, 244–251. [CrossRef]
154. Mohammadzadeh Honarvar, N.; Saedisomeolia, A.; Abdolahi, M.; Shayeganrad, A.; Taheri Sangsari, G.; Hassanzadeh Rad, B.; Muench, G. Molecular Anti-inflammatory Mechanisms of Retinoids and Carotenoids in Alzheimer's Disease: A Review of Current Evidence. *J. Mol. Neurosci.* **2017**, *61*, 289–304. [CrossRef]
155. Nidheesh, T.; Salim, C.; Rajini, P.S.; Suresh, P.V. Antioxidant and neuroprotective potential of chitooligomers in Caenorhabditis elegans exposed to Monocrotophos. *Carbohydr. Polym.* **2016**, *135*, 138–144. [CrossRef] [PubMed]
156. Singh, K.; Ahmad, Z.; Shakya, P.; Kumar, A.; Arif, M. Nano formulation: A novel approach for nose to brain drug delivery. *J. Chem. Pharm. Res.* **2016**, *8*, 208–215.
157. Bourganis, V.; Kammona, O.; Alexopoulos, A.; Kiparissides, C. Recent advances in carrier mediated nose-to-brain delivery of pharmaceutics. *Eur. J. Pharm. Biopharm.* **2018**, *128*, 337–362. [CrossRef]
158. Khan, A.R.; Liu, M.; Khan, M.W.; Zhai, G. Progress in brain targeting drug delivery system by nasal route. *J. Control. Release* **2017**, *268*, 364–389. [CrossRef] [PubMed]
159. Shadab; Bhattmisra, S.K.; Zeeshan, F.; Shahzad, N.; Mujtaba, A.; Meka, V.S.; Radhakrishnan, A.; Kesharwani, P.; Baboota, S.; Ali, J. Nano-carrier enabled drug delivery systems for nose to brain targeting for the treatment of neurodegenerative disorders. *J. Drug Deliv. Sci. Technol.* **2018**, *43*, 295–310.
160. Fernandes, F.; Dias-Teixeira, M.; Delerue-Matos, C.; Grosso, C. Critical Review of Lipid-Based Nanoparticles as Carriers of Neuroprotective Drugs and Extracts. *Nanomaterials* **2021**, *11*, 563. [CrossRef] [PubMed]
161. Singh, V.; Lalotra, A.S.; Agrawal, S.; Mishrai, G. Nose-to-Brain drug delivery via nanocarriers for the management of neurodegenerative disorders: Recent advances and future. *Biol. Sci.* **2021**, *1*, 19–34. [CrossRef]
162. Beloqui, A.; Solinis, M.A.; Rodriguez-Gascon, A.; Almeida, A.J.; Preat, V. Nanostructured lipid carriers: Promising drug delivery systems for future clinics. *Nanomedicine* **2016**, *12*, 143–161. [CrossRef]
163. Devkar, T.B.; Tekade, A.R.; Khandelwal, K.R. Surface engineered nanostructured lipid carriers for efficient nose to brain delivery of ondansetron HCl using Delonix regia gum as a natural mucoadhesive polymer. *Colloids Surf. B Biointerfaces* **2014**, *122*, 143–150. [CrossRef]
164. Rajput, A.P.; Butani, S.B. Resveratrol anchored nanostructured lipid carrier loaded in situ gel via nasal route: Formulation, optimization and in vivo characterization. *J. Drug Deliv. Sci. Technol.* **2019**, *51*, 214–223. [CrossRef]
165. Khosa, A.; Reddi, S.; Saha, R.N. Nanostructured lipid carriers for site-specific drug delivery. *Biomed Pharmacother.* **2018**, *103*, 598–613. [CrossRef]
166. Cunha, S.; Amaral, M.H.; Lobo, J.M.S.; Silva, A.C. Lipid Nanoparticles for Nasal/Intranasal Drug Delivery. *Crit. Rev. Ther. Drug Carr. Syst.* **2017**, *34*, 257–282. [CrossRef] [PubMed]
167. Erdo, F.; Bors, L.A.; Farkas, D.; Bajza, A.; Gizurarson, S. Evaluation of intranasal delivery route of drug administration for brain targeting. *Brain Res. Bull.* **2018**, *143*, 155–170. [CrossRef] [PubMed]
168. Agrawal, M.; Saraf, S.; Saraf, S.; Antimisiaris, S.G.; Chougule, M.B.; Shoyele, S.A.; Alexander, A. Nose-to-brain drug delivery: An update on clinical challenges and progress towards approval of anti-Alzheimer drugs. *J. Control. Release* **2018**, *281*, 139–177. [CrossRef]
169. Nguyen, T.-T.-L.; Maeng, H.-J. Pharmacokinetics and Pharmacodynamics of Intranasal Solid Lipid Nanoparticles and Nanostructured Lipid Carriers for Nose-to-Brain Delivery. *Pharmaceutics* **2022**, *14*, 572. [CrossRef] [PubMed]
170. Cunha, S.; Almeida, H.; Amaral, M.H.; Lobo, J.M.S.; Silva, A.C. Intranasal lipid nanoparticles for the treatment of neurodegenerative diseases. *Curr. Pharm. Des.* **2018**, *23*, 6553–6562. [CrossRef] [PubMed]
171. Illum, L. Nasal drug delivery—Possibilities, problems and solutions. *J. Control. Release* **2003**, *87*, 187–198. [CrossRef]
172. Feng, Y.; He, H.; Li, F.; Lu, Y.; Qi, J.; Wu, W. An update on the role of nanovehicles in nose-to-brain drug delivery. *Drug Discov. Today* **2018**, *23*, 1079–1088. [CrossRef]
173. Costantino, H.R.; Illum, L.; Brandt, G.; Johnson, P.H.; Quay, S.C. Intranasal delivery: Physicochemical and therapeutic aspects. *Int. J. Pharm.* **2007**, *337*, 1–24. [CrossRef]

174. Grassin-Delyle, S.; Buenestado, A.; Naline, E.; Faisy, C.; Blouquit-Laye, S.; Couderc, L.-J.; Le Guen, M.; Fischler, M.; Devillier, P. Intranasal drug delivery: An efficient and non-invasive route for systemic administration: Focus on opioids. *Pharmacol. Ther.* **2012**, *134*, 366–379. [CrossRef] [PubMed]

175. Rassu, G.; Soddu, E.; Cossu, M.; Brundu, A.; Cerri, G.; Marchetti, N.; Ferraro, L.; Regan, R.F.; Giunchedi, P.; Gavini, E.; et al. Solid microparticles based on chitosan or methyl-β-cyclodextrin: A first formulative approach to increase the nose-to-brain transport of deferoxamine mesylate. *J. Control. Release* **2015**, *201*, 68–77. [CrossRef] [PubMed]

176. Pires, P.C.; Santos, A.O. Nanosystems in nose-to-brain drug delivery: A review of non-clinical brain targeting studies. *J. Control. Release* **2018**, *270*, 89–100. [CrossRef] [PubMed]

177. Kumar, A.; Pandey, A.N.; Jain, S.K. Nasal-nanotechnology: Revolution for efficient therapeutics delivery. *Drug Deliv.* **2016**, *23*, 681–693. [CrossRef] [PubMed]

178. Alavian, F.; Shams, N. Oral and Intra-nasal Administration of Nanoparticles in the Cerebral Ischemia Treatment in Animal Experiments: Considering its Advantages and Disadvantages. *Curr. Clin. Pharmacol.* **2020**, *15*, 20–29.

179. Wang, Z.; Xiong, G.; Tsang, W.C.; Schatzlein, A.G.; Uchegbu, I.F. Nose-to-Brain Delivery. *J. Pharmacol. Exp. Ther.* **2019**, *370*, 593–601. [CrossRef] [PubMed]

180. Kälviäinen, R. Intranasal therapies for acute seizures. *Epilepsy Behav.* **2015**, *49*, 303–306. [CrossRef] [PubMed]

181. Rostamabadi, H.; Falsafi, S.R.; Jafari, S.M. Nanoencapsulation of carotenoids within lipid-based nanocarriers. *J. Control. Release* **2019**, *298*, 38–67. [CrossRef] [PubMed]

182. Borges, A.; Freitas, V.; Mateus, N.; Fernandes, I.; Oliveira, J. Solid Lipid Nanoparticles as Carriers of Natural Phenolic Compounds. *Antioxidants* **2020**, *9*, 998. [CrossRef]

183. Ghasemiyeh, P.; Samani, S. Solid Lipid nanoparticles and nanostructure lipid carriers as novel drug delivery systems: Applications, advantages and disadvantages. *Res. Pharm. Sci.* **2018**, *13*, 288.

184. Scioli Montoto, S.; Muraca, G.; Ruiz, M.E. Solid Lipid Nanoparticles for Drug Delivery: Pharmacological and Biopharmaceutical Aspects. *Front. Mol. Biosci.* **2020**, *7*, 587997. [CrossRef] [PubMed]

185. Müller, R.H.; Mäder, K.; Gohla, S. Solid lipid nanoparticles (SLN) for controlled drug delivery—A review of the state of the art. *Eur. J. Pharm. Biopharm.* **2000**, *50*, 161–177. [CrossRef]

186. Garces, A.; Amaral, M.H.; Sousa Lobo, J.M.; Silva, A.C. Formulations based on solid lipid nanoparticles (SLN) and nanostructured lipid carriers (NLC) for cutaneous use: A review. *Eur. J. Pharm. Sci.* **2018**, *112*, 159–167. [CrossRef]

187. Rainer, M.; Shegokar, R.; Keck, C. 20 Years of Lipid Nanoparticles (SLN & NLC): Present State of Development & Industrial Applications. *Curr. Drug Discov. Technol.* **2011**, *8*, 207–227.

188. Muller, R.H.; Petersen, R.D.; Hommoss, A.; Pardeike, J. Nanostructured lipid carriers (NLC) in cosmetic dermal products. *Adv. Drug Deliv. Rev.* **2007**, *59*, 522–530. [CrossRef] [PubMed]

189. Gastaldi, L.; Battaglia, L.; Peira, E.; Chirio, D.; Muntoni, E.; Solazzi, I.; Gallarate, M.; Dosio, F. Solid lipid nanoparticles as vehicles of drugs to the brain: Current state of the art. *Eur. J. Pharm. Biopharm.* **2014**, *87*, 433–444. [CrossRef]

190. Kaur, I.P.; Bhandari, R.; Bhandari, S.; Kakkar, V. Potential of solid lipid nanoparticles in brain targeting. *J. Control. Release* **2008**, *127*, 97–109. [CrossRef]

191. Tapeinos, C.; Battaglini, M.; Ciofani, G. Advances in the design of solid lipid nanoparticles and nanostructured lipid carriers for targeting brain diseases. *J. Control. Release* **2017**, *264*, 306–332. [CrossRef]

192. Wong, H.L.; Wu, X.Y.; Bendayan, R. Nanotechnological advances for the delivery of CNS therapeutics. *Adv. Drug Deliv. Rev.* **2012**, *64*, 686–700. [CrossRef]

193. Silva, A.C.; Amaral, M.H.; Lobo, J.M.; Lopes, C.M. Lipid nanoparticles for the delivery of biopharmaceuticals. *Curr. Pharm. Biotechnol.* **2015**, *16*, 291–302. [CrossRef]

194. Labouta, H.I.; Sarsons, C.; Kennard, J.; Gomez-Garcia, M.J.; Villar, K.; Lee, H.; Cramb, D.T.; Rinker, K.D. Understanding and improving assays for cytotoxicity of nanoparticles: What really matters? *RSC Adv.* **2018**, *8*, 23027–23039. [CrossRef]

195. Silva, A.H.; Filippin-Monteiro, F.B.; Mattei, B.; Zanetti-Ramos, B.G.; Creczynski-Pasa, T.B. In vitro biocompatibility of solid lipid nanoparticles. *Sci. Total Environ.* **2012**, *432*, 382–388. [CrossRef] [PubMed]

196. Trapani, A.; Guerra, L.; Corbo, F.; Castellani, S.; Sanna, E.; Capobianco, L.; Monteduro, A.; Manno, D.; Mandracchia, D.; Di Gioia, S.; et al. Cyto/Biocompatibility of Dopamine Combined with the Antioxidant Grape Seed-Derived Polyphenol Compounds in Solid Lipid Nanoparticles. *Molecules* **2021**, *26*, 916. [CrossRef] [PubMed]

197. Saini, S.; Sharma, T.; Jain, A.; Kaur, H.; Katare, O.P.; Singh, B. Systematically designed chitosan-coated solid lipid nanoparticles of ferulic acid for effective management of Alzheimer's disease: A preclinical evidence. *Colloids Surf. B Biointerfaces* **2021**, *205*, 111838. [CrossRef] [PubMed]

198. Sun, Y.; Li, L.; Xie, H.; Wang, Y.; Gao, S.; Zhang, L.; Bo, F.; Yang, S.; Feng, A. Primary Studies on Construction and Evaluation of Ion-Sensitive in situ Gel Loaded with Paeonol-Solid Lipid Nanoparticles for Intranasal Drug Delivery. *Int. J. Nanomed.* **2020**, *15*, 3137–3160. [CrossRef] [PubMed]

199. de Oliveira Junior, E.R.; Truzzi, E.; Ferraro, L.; Fogagnolo, M.; Pavan, B.; Beggiato, S.; Rustichelli, C.; Maretti, E.; Lima, E.M.; Leo, E.; et al. Nasal administration of nanoencapsulated geraniol/ursodeoxycholic acid conjugate: Towards a new approach for the management of Parkinson's disease. *J. Control. Release* **2020**, *321*, 540–552. [CrossRef]

200. Sadegh Malvajerd, S.; Azadi, A.; Izadi, Z.; Kurd, M.; Dara, T.; Dibaei, M.; Zadeh, M.S.; Javar, H.A.; Hamidi, M. Brain Delivery of Curcumin Using Solid Lipid Nanoparticles and Nanostructured Lipid Carriers: Preparation, Optimization, and Pharmacokinetic Evaluation. *ACS Chem. Neurosci.* **2019**, *10*, 728–739. [CrossRef]
201. Abourehab, M.A.S.; Khames, A.; Genedy, S.; Mostafa, S.; Khaleel, M.A.; Omar, M.M.; El Sisi, A.M. Sesame Oil-Based Nanostructured Lipid Carriers of Nicergoline, Intranasal Delivery System for Brain Targeting of Synergistic Cerebrovascular Protection. *Pharmaceutics* **2021**, *13*, 581. [CrossRef]
202. Abo El-Enin, H.A.; Elkomy, M.H.; Naguib, I.A.; Ahmed, M.F.; Alsaidan, O.A.; Alsalahat, I.; Ghoneim, M.M.; Eid, H.M. Lipid Nanocarriers Overlaid with Chitosan for Brain Delivery of Berberine via the Nasal Route. *Pharmaceuticals* **2022**, *15*, 281. [CrossRef]

MDPI

St. Alban-Anlage 66

4052 Basel

Switzerland

www.mdpi.com

Pharmaceuticals Editorial Office

E-mail: pharmaceuticals@mdpi.com

www.mdpi.com/journal/pharmaceuticals

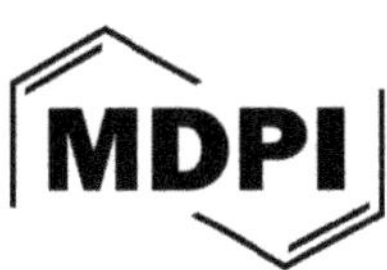